Imaging in
Photodynamic Therapy

Series in Cellular and Clinical Imaging

Series Editor
Ammasi Periasamy

PUBLISHED

Coherent Raman Scattering Microscopy
edited by Ji-Xin Cheng and Xiaoliang Sunney Xie

Imaging in Cellular and Tissue Engineering
edited by Hanry Yu and Nur Aida Abdul Rahim

Second Harmonic Generation Imaging
edited by Francesco S. Pavone and Paul J. Campagnola

The Fluorescent Protein Revolution
edited by Richard N. Day and Michael W. Davidson

Natural Biomarkers for Cellular Metabolism:
Biology, Techniques, and Applications
edited by Vladimir V. Gukasyan and Ahmed A. Heikal

Optical Probes in Biology
edited by Jin Zhang, Sohum Mehta, and Carsten Schultz

Super-Resolution Imaging in Biomedicine
edited by Alberto Diaspro and Marc A. M. J. van Zandvoort

Imaging in Photodynamic Therapy
edited by Michael R. Hamblin and Yingying Huang

SERIES IN CELLULAR AND CLINICAL IMAGING

Ammasi Periasamy, series editor

Imaging in Photodynamic Therapy

Edited by

Michael R. Hamblin, PhD
Yingying Huang, MD

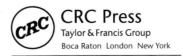

CRC Press
Taylor & Francis Group
Boca Raton London New York

CRC Press is an imprint of the
Taylor & Francis Group, an **informa** business

CRC Press
Taylor & Francis Group
6000 Broken Sound Parkway NW, Suite 300
Boca Raton, FL 33487-2742

First issued in paperback 2020

© 2017 by Taylor & Francis Group, LLC
CRC Press is an imprint of Taylor & Francis Group, an Informa business

No claim to original U.S. Government works

ISBN-13: 978-1-4987-4145-3 (hbk)
ISBN-13: 978-0-367-78235-1 (pbk)

Library of Congress Cataloging-in-Publication Data

Names: Hamblin, Michael R., editor. | Huang, Ying-Ying, editor.
Title: Imaging in photodynamic therapy / [edited by] Michael R. Hamblin,
Ying-Ying Huang.
Description: Boca Raton: Taylor & Francis, 2017. | Includes bibliographical
references and index.
Identifiers: LCCN 2016032241 | ISBN 9781498741453 (hardback: alk. paper)
Subjects: | MESH: Photochemotherapy--methods | Photosensitizing
Agents--therapeutic use
Classification: LCC RC271.P43 | NLM WB 480 | DDC 615.8/31--dc23
LC record available at https://lccn.loc.gov/2016032241

**Visit the Taylor & Francis Web site at
http://www.taylorandfrancis.com**

**and the CRC Press Web site at
http://www.crcpress.com**

"To the love of my life, my beautiful wife Angela, to whom I have been devoted for thirty-four years".

Michael R Hamblin

Contents

Series preface

A picture is worth a thousand words.

This proverb says everything. Imaging began in 1021 with use of a pinhole lens in a camera in Iraq; later in 1550, the pinhole was replaced by a biconvex lens developed in Italy. This mechanical imaging technology migrated to chemical-based photography in 1826 with the first successful sunlight picture made in France. Today, digital technology counts the number of light photons falling directly on a chip to produce an image at the focal plane; this image may then be manipulated in countless ways using additional algorithms and software. The process of taking pictures ("imaging") now includes a multitude of options—it may be either invasive or noninvasive, and the target and details may include monitoring signals in two, three, or four dimensions.

Microscopes are an essential tool in imaging used to observe and describe protozoa, bacteria, spermatozoa, and any kind of cell, tissue, or whole organism. Pioneered by Antonie van Leeuwenhoek in the 1670s and later commercialized by Carl Zeiss in 1846 in Jena, Germany, microscopes have enabled scientists to better grasp the often misunderstood relationship between microscopic and macroscopic behavior, by allowing for the study of the development, organization, and function of unicellular and higher organisms, as well as structures and mechanisms at the microscopic level. Further more, the imaging function preserves temporal and spatial relationships that are frequently lost in traditional biochemical techniques and gives two- or three-dimensional resolution that other laboratory methods cannot. For example, the inherent specificity and sensitivity of fluorescence and the high-temporal, spatial, and three-dimensional resolution that is possible and the enhancement of contrast resulting from detection of an absolute rather than relative signal (i.e., unlabeled features do not emit) are the advantages of fluorescence techniques. Additionally, the plethora of well-described spectroscopic techniques providing different types of information and the commercial availability of fluorescent probes such as visible fluorescent proteins (many of which exhibit an environment- or analytic-sensitive response) increase the range of possible applications, such as the development of biosensors for basic and clinical research. Recent advancements in optics, light sources, digital imaging systems, data acquisition methods, and image enhancement, analysis, and display methods have further broadened the applications in which fluorescence microscopy can be applied successfully.

Another development has been the establishment of multiphoton microscopy as a three-dimensional imaging method of choice for studying biomedical specimens from single cells to whole animals with submicron resolution. Multiphoton microscopy methods utilize naturally available endogenous fluorophores—including NADH, TRP, and FAD—whose autofluorescent properties provide a label-free approach. Researchers may then image various functions and organelles at molecular levels using two-photon and fluorescence lifetime imaging microscopy to distinguish normal from cancerous conditions. Other widely used nonlabeled imaging methods are coherent anti-Stokes Raman scattering spectroscopy and stimulated Raman scattering microscopy, which allow imaging of molecular function using the molecular vibrations in cells, tissues, and whole organisms. These techniques have been widely used in gene therapy, single-molecule imaging, tissue engineering, and stem cell research. Another nonlabeled method is harmonic generation (SHG and THG), which is also widely used in clinical imaging, tissue engineering, and stem cell research. There are many more advanced technologies developed for cellular and clinical imaging including multiphoton tomography, thermal imaging in animals, and ion imaging (calcium, pH) in cells.

The goal of this series is to highlight these seminal advances and the wide range of approaches currently used in cellular and clinical imaging. Its purpose is to promote education and new research across a broad spectrum of disciplines. The series emphasizes practical aspects, with each volume focusing on a particular theme that may cross various imaging modalities. Each title covers basic to advanced imaging methods, as well as detailed discussions dealing with interpretations of these studies. The series also provides cohesive, complete state-of-the-art, cross-modality overviews of the most important and timely areas within cellular and clinical imaging.

Since my graduate student days, I have been involved and interested in multimodal imaging techniques applied to cellular and clinical imaging. I have pioneered and developed many imaging modalities throughout my research career. The series manager, Luna Han, recognized my genuine enthusiasm and interest to develop a new book series on cellular and clinical imaging. This project would not have been possible without the support of Luna. I am sure that all the volume editors, chapter authors, and myself have benefited greatly from her continuous input and guidance to make this series a success.

Equally important, I personally thank the volume editors and the chapter authors. It has been an incredible experience working with colleagues who demonstrate such a high level of interest in educational projects, even though they are all fully occupied with their own academic activities. Their work and intellectual contributions based on their deep knowledge of the subject matter will be appreciated by everyone who reads this book series.

Ammasi Periasamy, PhD
Series Editor
Professor and Center Director
W.M. Keck Center for Cellular Imaging
University of Virginia
Charlottesville, Virginia

Preface

In this book, we have aimed to cover the broad field of cellular, molecular, preclinical, and clinical imaging associated or combined with photodynamic therapy (PDT). PDT uses a nontoxic photosensitizer, which is a colored dye, together with harmless visible light of the correct wavelength to be absorbed by the dye. The excited state dye can then undergo different chemical reactions with ambient oxygen-producing reactive oxygen species that damage biomolecules, kill targeted cells, and destroy unwanted tissues. Clinically, PDT is used for cancer, infections, and diseases such as atherosclerosis or blindness characterized by unwanted tissues. Because photosensitizers are also fluorescent, various imaging systems such as confocal microscopy and small animal imaging systems have been widely used to follow and optimize treatment and to answer important mechanistic questions. In several cases (skin, bladder, and brain) imaging has made an important contribution to clinical outcomes. PDT has made an important contribution to the development of theranostics (agents that can both detect and treat diseases).

Many of the advances in imaging and PDT have been technology driven. Highly sophisticated confocal microscopes have become readily available in most departments. *In vivo* small animal imaging systems again have made large strides and now will often cover several modalities that can be chosen from fluorescence, bioluminescence, and photoacoustic imaging, CT, PET, high-resolution ultrasound, etc. Because of the expansion in available technologies, many investigators have been able to take advantage of the new capabilities to answer questions that have until now remained elusive. Moreover, the advent of the field of "seek and destroy" theranostics has also increased the demand for research studies that are combinations of imaging and therapeutics. Photosensitizers can act as fluorescent reporters for imaging of tissue localization, can mediate photogeneration of reactive oxygen species, and can even monitor effectiveness of treatment due to photobleaching. They can also be incorporated into an array of nanoparticles and nanocarriers to take advantage of the nanotechnology revolution. As PDT becomes more often used clinically and as the awareness of imaging grows, more and more clinical studies are including an imaging element to optimize the treatment. This book is designed to reflect these advances and to provide a resource for physicians and research scientists in the fields of cell biology, microscopy, PDT, cell signaling, nanotechnology, and drug discovery. It is also aimed at scientists in optics, molecular imaging, lasers, cancer diagnostics and treatment, and pharmaceuticals.

Acknowledgment

The editors acknowledge the valuable assistance of Xiaoshen Zhang from Tongji University, School of Medicine, Shanghai, China.

Editors

Michael R. Hamblin, PhD, is a principal investigator at the Wellman Center for Photomedicine at Massachusetts General Hospital, an associate professor of dermatology at Harvard Medical School, and a member of the affiliated faculty of the Harvard-MIT Division of Health Science and Technology. His research interests lie in the areas of photodynamic therapy (PDT) for infections, cancer, and stimulation of the immune system and in low-level light therapy or photobiomodulation for wound healing, traumatic brain injuries, neurodegenerative diseases, and psychiatric disorders. He directs a laboratory of around a dozen postdoctoral fellows, visiting scientists, and graduate students. His research program is supported by the NIH, CDMRP, USAFOSR, and CIMIT, among other funding agencies. He has published more than 340 peer-reviewed articles and more than 150 conference proceedings, book chapters, and international abstracts and holds 8 patents. He is an associate editor and editorial board member on numerous journals and serves on NIH study sections. For the past several years, Dr. Hamblin has chaired the annual conference at SPIE Photonics West titled "Mechanisms for low level light therapy" and has edited proceedings, volumes, and major textbooks on PDT and photomedicine. In 2011 Dr. Hamblin was honored by election as a fellow of SPIE.

Ying-Ying Huang, MD, is a scientist in Dr. Michael Hamblin's lab at the Wellman Center for Photomedicine at Massachusetts General Hospital and an instructor of dermatology at Harvard Medical School. She was trained as a dermatologist in China. Her research interests lie in the areas of photodynamic therapy for infections and cancer and in the mechanism of low-level light therapy for traumatic brain injuries. She has published almost 50 peer-reviewed articles and numerous conference proceedings and book chapters. She is the coeditor of the recent publication *Handbook of Photomedicine*.

Contributors

Heidi Abrahamse
Faculty of Health Sciences
Laser Research Centre
Laser Applications in Health
University of Johannesburg
Doornfontein, South Africa

Vefa Ahsen
Department of Chemistry
Gebze Technical University
Gebze-Kocaeli, Turkey

Ron R. Allison
Department of Radiation Oncology
Brody School of Medicine
East Carolina University
Greenville, North Carolina

Devrim Atilla
Department of Chemistry
Gebze Technical University
Gebze-Kocaeli, Turkey

Isabel O.L. Bacellar
Institute of Chemistry
University of São Paulo
São Paulo, Brazil

Maurício S. Baptista
Institute of Chemistry
University of São Paulo
São Paulo, Brazil

Hubert van den Bergh
Laboratory of Organometallic and Medicinal
    Chemistry
Swiss Federal Institute of Technology
    in Lausanne
Lausanne, Switzerland

Jonathan P. Celli
Department of Physics
University of Massachusetts
Boston, Massachusetts

Bin Chen
Department of Pharmaceutical Sciences
University of the Sciences
Philadelphia, Pennsylvania

Jincan Chen
State Key Laboratory of Structural Chemistry
and
Danish-Chinese Centre for Proteases and
    Cancer
Fujian Institute of Research on the Structure
    of Matter
Chinese Academy of Sciences
Fuzhou, Fujian, People's Republic of China

Zhuo Chen
State Key Laboratory of Structural Chemistry
and
Danish-Chinese Centre for Proteases and Cancer
Fujian Institute of Research on the Structure
    of Matter
Chinese Academy of Sciences
Fuzhou, Fujian, People's Republic of China

Anthony Davies
Institute of Health and Biomedical Innovation
Queensland University of Technology
Woolloongabba, Brisbane, Australia

Marica B. Ericson
Department of Chemistry and Molecular
    Biology
University of Gothenburg
Gothenburg, Sweden

Kinya Furukawa
Department of Thoracic Surgery
Tokyo Medical University Ibaraki Medical Center
Ibaraki, Japan

Ayşe Gül Gürek
Department of Chemistry
Gebze Technical University
Gebze-Kocaeli, Turkey

Steffen Hackbarth
Department of Physics
Humboldt-Universität zu Berlin
Berlin, Germany

Michael R. Hamblin
Department of Dermatology
Harvard Medical School
and
Wellman Center for Photomedicine
    Massachusetts General Hospital
Boston, Massachusetts

Ping Hu
State Key Laboratory of Structural Chemistry
and
Danish-Chinese Centre for Proteases and Cancer
Fujian Institute of Research on the Structure
    of Matter
Chinese Academy of Sciences
Fuzhou, Fujian, People's Republic of China

Mingdong Huang
College of Chemistry
Fuzhou University
Fuzhou, People's Republic of China

Hsin-I Hung
Department of Drug Discovery and
    Biomedical Sciences
Medical University of South Carolina
Charleston, South Carolina

Zafar Iqbal
Department of Chemistry
COMSATS Institute of Information
    Technology
Abbottabad, Khyber Pakhtunkhwa, Pakistan

and

State Key Laboratory of Structural Chemistry
and
Danish-Chinese Centre for Proteases and Cancer
Fujian Institute of Research on the Structure
    of Matter
Chinese Academy of Sciences
Fuzhou, Fujian, People's Republic of China

Longguang Jiang
College of Chemistry
Fuzhou University
Fuzhou, People's Republic of China

Patrice Jichlinski
Department of Urology
CHUV Hospital
Lausanne, Switzerland

Despoina Kantere
Department of Dermatology and Venereology
University of Gothenburg
Gothenburg, Sweden

Harubumi Kato
Department of Thoracic Surgery
Niizashiki Central General Hospital
Saitama, Japan

and

Department of Surgery
Tokyo Medical University
International University of Health and Welfare
Tokyo, Japan

Yasufumi Kato
Department of Thoracic Surgery
Tokyo Medical University Ibaraki Medical Center
Ibaraki, Japan

Anil Kishen
Faculty of Dentistry
University of Toronto
Toronto, Ontario, Canada

Norbert Lange
School of Pharmaceutical Sciences
University of Geneva
University of Lausanne
Geneva, Switzerland

John J. Lemasters
Department of Drug Discovery and
    Biomedical Sciences
Medical University of South Carolina
Charleston, South Carolina

and

Institute of Theoretical and Experimental
    Biophysics
Russian Academy of Science
Pushchino, Russia

Buhong Li
MOE Key Laboratory of OptoElectronic
    Science and Technology for Medicine
Fujian Provincial Key Laboratory for Photonics
    Technology
Fujian Normal University
Fuzhou, People's Republic of China

Rui Li
State Key Laboratory of Structural Chemistry
and
Danish-Chinese Centre for Proteases
and Cancer
Fujian Institute of Research on the Structure
of Matter
Chinese Academy of Sciences
Fuzhou, Fujian, People's Republic of China

Lisheng Lin
MOE Key Laboratory of OptoElectronic
Science and Technology for Medicine
Fujian Provincial Key Laboratory for Photonics
Technology
Fujian Normal University
Fuzhou, Fujian, People's Republic of China

Hui Liu
Department of Physics
University of Massachusetts
Boston, Massachusetts

Jonathan F. Lovell
Department of Biomedical Engineering
University at Buffalo
State University of New York
Buffalo, New York

Kuniharu Miyajima
Department of Thoracic Surgery
Niizashiki Central General Hospital
Saitama, Japan

Pawel Mroz
Department of Pathology
University of Michigan Medical School
University of Michigan Health System
Ann Arbor, Michigan

Anna-Liisa Nieminen
Department of Drug Discovery and
Biomedical Sciences
Medical University of South Carolina
Charleston, South Carolina

Keishi Ohtani
Department of Surgery
Tokyo Medical University
Tokyo, Japan

John Paoli
Department of Dermatology and Venereology
University of Gothenburg
Gothenburg, Sweden

Leonardo Barcelos de Paula
Department of Chemistry
Center of Nanotechnology and Tissue
Engineering
Photobiology and Photomedicine Research
Group
Faculty of Philosophy, Sciences and Letters of
Ribeirão Preto
University of São Paulo
São Paulo, Brazil

Christiane Pavani
Postgraduate Program in Applied Biophotonics
in Science and Health
July Ninth University
São Paulo, Brazil

Rozhin Penjweini
Department of Radiation Oncology
University of Pennsylvania
Philadelphia, Pennsylvania

Michael Pfitzner
Department of Physics
Humboldt-Universität zu Berlin
Berlin, Germany

Claude-André Porret
Laboratory of Organometallic and Medicinal
Chemistry
Swiss Federal Institute of Technology
in Lausanne
Lausanne, Switzerland

Fernando Lucas Primo
Department of Bioprocess and
Biotechnology
São Paulo State University
Araraquara, Brazil

Marcin Ptaszek
Department of Chemistry and Biochemistry
University of Maryland
Baltimore, Maryland

Beate Röder
Department of Physics
Humboldt-Universität zu Berlin
Berlin, Germany

Ričardas Rotomskis
Biomedical Physics Laboratory
National Cancer Institute
and
Biophotonics Laboratory
Vilnius University
Vilnius, Lithuania

Sarah-Louise Ryan
Institute of Health and Biomedical Innovation
Queensland University of Technology
Woolloongabba, Brisbane, Australia

Jan C. Schlothauer
Department of Physics
Humboldt-Universität zu Berlin
Berlin, Germany

Oliver Schnell
Deparment of Neurosurgery
Klinikum der Universität München
München, Germany

and

Medical Center
University of Freiburg
Freiburg, Germany

Mathias O. Senge
School of Chemistry
Trinity College Dublin
University of Dublin
Dublin, Ireland

Wentao Song
Department of Biomedical Engineering
University at Buffalo
State University of New York
Buffalo, New York

Herbert Stepp
LIFE Center
Laser-Forschungslabor
Klinikum der Universität München
München, Germany

Giedre Streckyte
Biophotonics Laboratory
Vilnius University
Vilnius, Lithuania

Antonio Claudio Tedesco
Department of Chemistry
Center of Nanotechnology and Tissue
    Engineering
Photobiology and Photomedicine Research
    Group
Faculty of Philosophy, Sciences and Letters of
    Ribeirão Preto
University of São Paulo
São Paulo, Brazil

Duygu Aydın Tekdaş
Department of Chemistry
Gebze Technical University
Gebze-Kocaeli, Turkey

Tayana M. Tsubone
Institute of Chemistry
University of São Paulo
São Paulo, Brazil

Jitsuo Usuda
Department of Thoracic Surgery
Nippon Medical School
Tokyo, Japan

Gisela M.F. Vaz
Institute of Molecular Medicine
Trinity College Dublin
St. James's Hospital
Dublin, Ireland

Georges Wagnières
Laboratory of Organometallic and Medicinal
    Chemistry
Swiss Federal Institute of Technology
    in Lausanne
Lausanne, Switzerland

Danni Wang
Department of Chemistry and Molecular
    Biology
University of Gothenburg
Gothenburg, Sweden

Ann-Marie Wennberg
Department of Dermatology and Venereology
University of Gothenburg
Gothenburg, Sweden

Brian C. Wilson
Department of Medical Biophysics
University Health Network
and
University of Toronto
Toronto, Ontario, Canada

Cai Yuan
College of Bioscience and Biotechnology
Fuzhou University
Fuzhou, People's Republic of China

Matthieu Zellweger
Laboratory of Organometallic and Medicinal
    Chemistry
Swiss Federal Institute of Technology
    in Lausanne
Lausanne, Switzerland

Ke Zheng
State Key Laboratory of Structural Chemistry
and
Danish-Chinese Centre for Proteases
    and Cancer
Fujian Institute of Research on the Structure
    of Matter
Chinese Academy of Sciences
Fuzhou, Fujian, People's Republic of China

Xiaolei Zhou
State Key Laboratory of Structural Chemistry
and
Danish-Chinese Centre for Proteases
    and Cancer
Fujian Institute of Research on the Structure
    of Matter
Chinese Academy of Sciences
Fuzhou, Fujian, People's Republic of China

Yang Zhou
College of Chemistry
Shandong Normal University
Jinan, Shandong, People's Republic of China

Timothy C. Zhu
Department of Radiation Oncology
University of Pennsylvania
Philadelphia, Pennsylvania

PART 1

INTRODUCTION

Looking out the optical window
Physical principles and instrumentation of imaging in photodynamic therapy

HUI LIU AND JONATHAN P. CELLI

1.1 INTRODUCTION

As a light-based treatment modality, photodynamic therapy (PDT) is inherently conducive to integration with optical imaging. The central principle of PDT is to leverage photochemistry that occurs following activation of a photosensitizing chemical [photosensitizer (PS)] using a light source of the appropriate wavelength and mode of delivery to achieve destruction of target tissues (Dougherty et al. 1998). Importantly, some degree of specificity is achieved as PSs have been almost universally observed to exhibit quasi-selective accumulation in neoplastic tissues, going back to the early observations of Policard, who studied accumulation of hematoporphyrin in rat sarcomas (Policard 1924). Since clinical PS should have little or no dark toxicity, an additional degree of selectivity is afforded by restriction of light to the target tissue. This basic photodynamic process, the fundamentals of which are discussed more extensively throughout this volume, has been developed and adapted for treatment of numerous cancer and noncancer pathologies at diverse anatomical sites using appropriate chemical modifications of the PS and innovative light delivery strategies. Importantly, the same photosensitizing agents employed in PDT for targeted tissue destruction also have a finite probability to undergo a radiative transition back to the ground state following light absorption. In other words, PS can act as both therapeutic agents and diagnostic fluorophores. Therefore, upon illumination, longer wavelength fluorescence emission is generated from the malignant tissues in which the PS accumulates, thus marking the tumor location and margins otherwise difficult to visualize. This process has been extensively leveraged to confirm PS uptake and localization and to guide surgical resection as discussed at length in the literature and reviewed elsewhere (Celli et al. 2010).

In this chapter, we review the basic physical principles underlying PDT-related optical imaging and underscore points where these basic principles have particularly important implications for PDT and imaging and/or its key enabling technologies. This discussion will include a brief review of the fundamental nature of light itself, how it interacts with matter as both a particle and a wave, and how these interactions manifest in the propagation of light through tissue to allow therapy and imaging. Also of central importance to PDT and its associated imaging applications is the probabilistic nature of quantum mechanics and the allowability of transitions between quantum states, which ultimately determine excited state lifetimes. Finally, technological developments in light sources and light detectors will be briefly discussed in the context of their role in enabling PDT and associated optical imaging applications.

1.2 PHYSICAL PRINCIPLES: LIGHT PROPAGATION AND INTERACTIONS WITH MATTER

1.2.1 LIGHT AS WAVE AND PARTICLE

When we talk about light in this chapter, we are referring to the narrow slice of the spectrum of electromagnetic (EM) radiation that is visible to the human eye (Figure 1.1a). EM radiation, which includes radio waves, microwaves, infrared, visible light, ultraviolet, and x-ray and gamma radiation, is produced when charged particles accelerate, generating electric (**E**) and magnetic fields (**B**) propagating through space in a manner that satisfies the set of equations set down by James Clerk Maxwell (1865). For this to be true, the electric and magnetic fields are necessarily sinusoidal in space and time, and mutually perpendicular to the direction of propagation (Figure 1.1b). The descriptive categories of EM waves stated earlier are defined purely on the basis of their frequency, ν, or wavelength, λ, where $\lambda\nu = c$. The frequency of a wave is its oscillation rate, typically reported in the SI units of Hertz (Hz), oscillations per second. The wavelength of an EM wave is its propagation distance in a vacuum during a full oscillation cycle (between two adjacent crests or troughs). In a vacuum, all EM radiation propagates at the speed of light, c, approximately 3.00×10^8 m/s, though its speed is different in other media (such as biological tissue). However, although the propagation speed of EM radiation is medium dependent, it maintains the same frequency or wavelength. For the

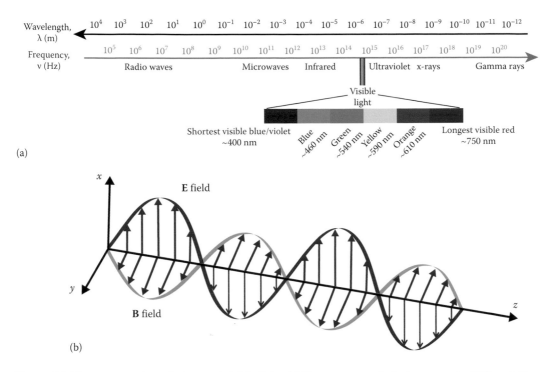

Figure 1.1 Electromagnetic radiation and visible light. (a) The spectrum of electromagnetic (EM) radiation. (b) The electrical field (red) and magnetic field (blue) are mutually perpendicular to the direction of propagation.

example of an EM wave propagating in the z-direction through a vacuum (empty space), this description can be written more succinctly as

$$E(z,t) = E_0 \cos\left(\frac{2\pi}{\lambda}(z - ct)\right)\hat{x}$$

$$B(z,t) = \frac{E_0}{c} \cos\left(\frac{2\pi}{\lambda}(z - ct)\right)\hat{y}$$

where $\hat{x}$ and $\hat{y}$ are the unit vectors in the x- and y-directions, respectively. The energy carried by EM radiation is reported by the Poynting vector, the vector cross-product of its electric and magnetic fields, with SI units of Watts per meter squared (W/m²). Notwithstanding this universality, however, the physical processes that are relevant to the interaction of EM radiation with matter are indeed highly dependent on wavelength. Hence, our review of the light–matter interaction in the following section will be limited to the discussion of processes that are energetically allowed and relevant for light of visible and near-infrared wavelengths used in PDT and optical imaging, approximately 400–750 nm (Figure 1.1a). For example, this chapter does not deal with effects such as Compton scattering or other important processes more relevant to the interaction of ionizing EM radiation with matter. For a more complete discussion of the basic principles of electrodynamics, the curious reader is referred to any number of texts on this subject, such as the classic by J.D. Jackson (1999).

Yet simultaneously, light can be described as photons, particles that carry discrete packets of energy, $E = h\nu$, where $h = 6.626 \times 10^{-34}$ J·s, is Planck's constant (Einstein 1905). Photons are massless particles and have no electronic charge, but do carry momentum, $p = h/\lambda$, such that interactions with other particles are governed by the conservation of momentum. This well-known duality, in which light can be described as both a particle and as a wave, is left over from historic debates on the quantum nature of light and matter in the early twentieth century. Although the wave description is used to describe certain phenomena (coherence, interference, diffraction, etc.) and the particle description is needed for other processes (quantized transitions, photoelectric effect, etc.), both descriptions must always coexist. Indeed, even a single photon can be modeled by wave propagation and, conversely, massive particles such as electrons can also be described as waves, having a de Broglie wavelength, $\lambda = h/p$. Here too, in this chapter, we will go back and forth between both descriptions as we discuss the physics of PDT and optical imaging.

1.2.2 PHASE AND COHERENCE

Phase, φ, is a parameter in any periodical sinusoidal function that specifies where in its oscillation cycle it is at $t = 0$:

$$y(t) = \sin(\omega t + \varphi)$$

In general, EM waves are out of phase, with a difference in φ from 0 to 2π radians (0°–360°). Only when $\Delta\varphi = 0$ or 2π are the waves in phase. This becomes important when calculating the power (P) or intensity (I), which are proportional to the square of the amplitude of electric field: $P \propto E^2$ and $I \propto E^2$.

Since EM waves are typically not in phase, the resultant amplitude is typically not just the direct addition of each amplitude. Hence, the power at a given point in space where two sources of EM radiation combine cannot in general be thought of as a direct addition. A mathematical illustration of this important point is provided next and also illustrates the phenomenon of interference:

$$E_1(t) = E_0 \sin(\omega t), \quad E_2(t) = E_0 \sin(\omega t + 2\pi), \quad E_3(t) = E_0 \sin(\omega t + \pi),$$

$$E_{12}(t) = E_1 + E_2 = 2E_0 \sin(\omega t), \quad I_{12} \propto 4E_0^2$$

$$E_{13}(t) = E_1 + E_3 = 0, \quad I_{13} = 0$$

Interference is critical for all aspects of image formation in optical systems and can also be exploited in various innovative ways. For example, the interference patterns formed from rays of a monochromatic and coherent (Figure 1.2) light source that are back reflected from different depths in tissue can be used to obtain depth-resolved specimen structure. This principle is at the heart of optical coherence tomography, a powerful 3D imaging approach that may be implemented in conjunction with PDT (Korde et al. 2007, Jung et al. 2012, Themstrup et al. 2014).

When two EM waves have a constant phase difference and have the same frequency, they are called perfectly coherent. Common light sources, such as sunlight and lamps, do not produce coherent waves. In fact, there is no truly perfectly coherent source since there is no absolute single-frequency source that is infinitely small. That being said, lasers are very nearly perfectly coherent light sources, a powerful property that has enabled myriad different technologies and even new industries, since the invention of lasers. The different light sources, along with their properties, are discussed in Section 1.3. The characteristics of different light sources with relevance to their applications in PDT and optical imaging are further developed later in this chapter.

1.2.3 LIGHT PROPAGATION

When light traveling through any given medium encounters a change in medium, the direction and speed of propagation will generally change. Depending on the details of the media involved, this interaction may give rise to reflection, refraction, scattering, and absorption processes (Figure 1.3; Jackson 1999).

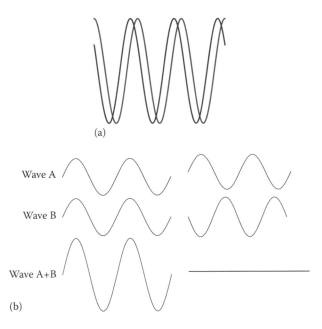

(a)

(b)

Figure 1.2 Phase and interference. (a) An example of phase difference between two waves. (b) Examples of constructive and destructive interference. When waves A and B, both of the same wavelength, are in phase, their amplitudes combine constructively. When waves A and B are out of phase, their amplitude cancels each other.

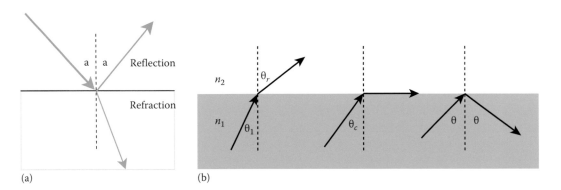

(a)   (b)

Figure 1.3 Reflection, refraction, and total internal reflection. (a) When light passes through an interface of two media with differing optical properties refraction and/or reflection may occur. (b) Total internal reflection occurs when the incident medium has lower refractive index than the propagating medium and the incident angle is bigger than the critical angle that is determined by the refractive index of the two media.

1.2.3.1 REFLECTION

Two types of reflection, specular and diffuse reflection, may occur depending on the nature of the receiving medium's surface. Specular reflection is the familiar reflection that typically occurs when light encounters the smooth surface of metal and dielectric materials. It is governed by the law of reflection, which stipulates that (1) the incident ray, the reflected ray, and the normal to the reflection surface at the point of the incidence lie in the same plane; (2) the incident and reflected rays are at equal angles to the normal; and (3) the reflected ray and the incident ray are on the opposite sides of the normal.

When the reflecting material is either nonsmooth or nonmetallic, the macroscopic reflection resulting from the superposition of many microreflections at the length scale of the roughness of the material sends light in multiple directions. Diffuse reflection is the reason for the general visibility of objects. For example, the moon is visible due to its diffuse reflection of the sunlight that falls upon it. A mixture of specular and diffuse reflection is exhibited by many common materials and is essential to any imaging modality that is based on reflectance. In general, materials that enable reflection consist of structures with dimensions much larger than the incident wavelength.

1.2.3.2 REFRACTION

Usually when reflection occurs at an interface between two media, some portion of the light will continue to propagate into the receiving medium. Refraction describes the behavior of light that is not reflected back to the incident medium (medium 1), but continues propagating in the transmission medium (medium 2) in a different direction (Figure 1.3a). Due to the medium change, the speed of the wave will change depending on the refractive indices (n) of the two media, according to Snell's law:

$$\frac{\sin(\theta_1)}{\sin(\theta_2)} = \frac{\upsilon_1}{\upsilon_2} = \frac{n_2}{n_1}$$

where n, the refractive index, is defined as $n = c/\upsilon$, where c is the speed of light.

However, when the second medium has smaller refractive index than the first one, and when the angle of the incident beam is larger than some critical value, all the incident light is reflected back to the first medium. This is called *total internal reflection* (Figure 1.3b), with critical angle defined as

$$\theta_c = \arcsin\left(\frac{n_2}{n_1}\right)$$

Total internal reflection is the essential principle in the design of waveguides, such as optical fibers (Figure 1.4), a revolutionary technology that has been used in therapeutic light delivery and medical imaging (Epstein 1982), as well as myriad other telecommunications application (Toge and Ito 2013). While light is propagating in a flexible fiber with higher index than the surrounding medium, as long the fiber is not bent so far that rays encountering the interface will exceed θ_c, then propagation will continue with near total efficiency until the end of the fiber. The design of fibers does not require selection of materials with large difference in refractive index. For a typical single-mode fiber used for telecommunications, the cladding is made of pure silica, with an index of 1.444 (at $\lambda = 1500$ nm), and its core is doped silica with an index around 1.4475. The refractive index of air is close to 1. It goes without saying that optical fibers have had huge consequences for PDT light delivery and endoscopic imaging (discussed further later), shedding light on internal spaces that would otherwise be inaccessible due to light attenuation by tissue (also discussed later).

Refraction also plays a fundamental role in determining how the light collection of optical systems, and as we will see, the ability of imaging systems to spatially resolve objects. The numerical aperture (NA) is the

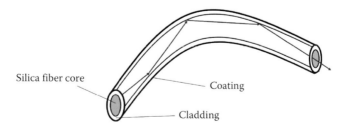

Figure 1.4 Fiber optics. Optical fibers, made of core, cladding and coating, are a key enabling technology for imaging and PDT. The slight refractive index difference between core and cladding guides the light to propagate inside the fiber via total internal reflection, provided that the fiber is not bent too sharply, causing light to be incident on the boundary interface at an angle exceeding the critical angle.

product of the refractive index of the medium and the sine of the angle that a marginal ray (a ray that exits the lens system at its outer edge) makes with the optical axis.

$$NA = n \sin \theta$$

In other words, the NA describes the maximum acceptance angle of a lens system (such as objective) or waveguide (such as fibers). NA is an important parameter of microscopes since it is related to the light-gathering ability of the objectives and resolution of the system.

1.2.3.3 DIFFRACTION

As with any propagating wave, EM waves will bend around small obstacles and spread out as they propagate through small openings. This process, called diffraction, becomes significant when waves encounter a slit or opening that is comparable in size to the wavelength. When diffraction of EM radiation occurs, the waves that recombine at later points will produce characteristic interference patterns (Figure 1.5), and it is the observation of such interference patterns that originally motivated the wave description of light.

For our purposes, it is important that the discussion of diffraction leads directly into the very important and practical consideration of resolution. In any imaging system, there is a fundamental physical limit that determines the closest distance between two objects that can be resolved. If light is incident on multiple point objects, it can generate one diffraction pattern for each object. When the objects are close, their diffraction patterns overlap. When they move closer still, the excessive overlap can prevent the two points from being resolved in the image. Or more precisely, using the criterion established by Lord Rayleigh, the cutoff for two objects being resolved is that the central bright spot of one point object must overlap with the first dark ring of the other object. If the two objects are closer than this, their diffraction patterns are no longer distinguishable and they cannot be resolved. Mathematically, this minimum distance, d, is

$$d = \frac{0.61\lambda}{NA}$$

Since a high-quality objective may have an NA of 1.4 (but not much higher than this), a good rule of thumb is that the highest resolution achievable with an optical microscope is about half the wavelength of the light used to illuminate the specimen. Of course with other technologies higher resolutions can be achieved. For example, electron microscopy uses accelerated electrons which may have wavelengths orders of magnitude smaller than that of visible light. Additionally, super-resolution optical techniques have been developed that can surpass the diffraction-limited resolution (Huang 2010, Huang et al. 2010, Schermelleh et al. 2010).

By analyzing the diffraction pattern, the geometry of the object can be revealed. At the same time, the geometry of the obstacle can be designed to generate the desired diffraction pattern. A diffraction grating, an object of great practical utility in optical systems, has periodic structures that can separate the different wavelength at high resolution.

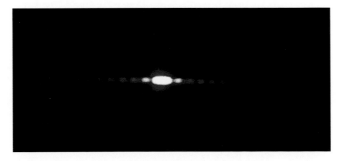

Figure 1.5 Diffraction. A photograph of the diffraction pattern resulting from a Helium Neon laser illuminating a 500 nm single slit.

1.2.4 LIGHT–MATTER INTERACTIONS AND THE OPTICAL WINDOW

In most practical scenarios, as light is moving through a medium, the dissipation of energy that occurs as light is scattered, absorbed, and reemitted cannot be ignored. This is particularly important for light propagating through tissues consisting of water, proteins, cells, and subcellular organelles, all of which present structures of heterogeneous size, structure, and optical properties. While the consideration of reflection, refraction, and diffraction relies on the wave property of light, here we will also use the particle description as we discuss scattering and absorption processes. The consequences of light interaction with tissue are obviously critical for both PDT and imaging. Calibrating the light dose for PDT in which light must propagate through a significant thickness of tissue before hitting the target cells (which is usually the case) must be informed by some understanding of how much light is absorbed before it gets there. Similarly, in any biomedical optical imaging scenario, propagation of light through a particular tissue plays a huge role in determining image depth, contrast, and quality.

1.2.4.1 SCATTERING

In thinking about light scattering, it is useful to recognize that photons must obey the law of conservation of momentum, just like with billiard balls or any other collision between particles. A particle cannot gain momentum without another object losing momentum. At the same time, the wavelike behavior we just described also comes into play, and as we will see the length scales of scattering structures relative to the wavelength of light play an important role.

When light is incident on a particle, the perpendicular electric field component may induce separation, or polarization, of the positive and negative charge in that object. Since the electric field is oscillatory (Figure 1.1), this gives rise to an oscillating dipole. The sinusoidally accelerating and decelerating charge distribution in turn gives rise to EM radiation (which results from accelerating electric charges) of the same frequency and wavelength. The amplitude of the electric field however is proportional to the frequency of the incident radiation squared. As noted earlier, intensity depends on the square of the electric field, so in this scenario the wavelength dependence of the intensity of scattered light is

$$I_{scattered} \propto \lambda^{-4}$$

This relationship, called Rayleigh scattering (named for Lord Rayleigh), is the description best suited to EM radiation scattered from particles that are small relative to the wavelength of the radiation. A full derivation of dipole scattering is a straightforward mathematical exercise for which the reader is again referred to Jackson (1999). The dependence on frequency to the fourth power is noteworthy. For example, blue-violet light with a wavelength of 400 nm is scattered with seven times the intensity of red light with a wavelength of 650 nm. The most ubiquitous example of Rayleigh scattering is what we see when we look up on a sunny day as the highly scattered blue light is scattered throughout the sky, while sun itself appears yellow. Rayleigh scattering certainly plays some role in light scattering from structures within biological tissues as well, but because it is combined with so many other processes the net wavelength dependence of light scattered in tissue will be different from λ^{-4}.

When the size of the scattering particles is comparable to the wavelength, the scattering can become quite complex, such that closed form analytical solutions cannot easily be written down. This scenario is described by Mie scattering and is generally solved numerically (Bassan et al. 2010, Hergert and Wriedt 2012). When the particle size is much bigger (>10 times) than the wavelength of the light, the scattering behavior can be explained by geometric optics. It is important to note again here that we are restricting ourselves to scattering processes relevant to visible light. For higher-energy EM radiation, such as x-rays used in radiation therapy, other physical processes become important, but fall outside the scope of this text.

1.2.4.2 ABSORPTION

EM radiation can also be absorbed by matter. Photon absorption occurs on the order 10^{-15} s, an extremely rapid process relative to the time scale of events subsequent to the molecular vibrational transition, intersystem crossing, and radiative emission time scales. How EM energy is absorbed and how the absorbing molecules subsequently dissipate their increased energy are again highly dependent on the wavelengths involved. Quantum mechanics tells us that atoms and molecules have well-defined energy states that only allow for absorption and emission of energy in discrete packets that correspond to specific changes in the physical state of the system. For our purposes, we are most concerned with quantized energy gaps that correspond to different allowed electron orbitals, and the quantized gaps between specific, discretely spaced vibrational frequencies, like tuning forks of different sizes. The former are relatively larger energy gaps that match up with photon energies of visible light. The allowed vibrational energy levels of atoms and molecules are more closely spaced, corresponding to the energies of infrared photon. Again, there are many other states with associated quantized transitions corresponding to, for example, changes in electron spin states, nuclear spin. These other transitions play critical roles in other medical imaging technologies (e.g., magnetic resonance imaging), but here we focus on absorption mediated by electronic and vibrational transitions relevant to optical and near-infrared frequencies used for PDT. After light is absorbed, the newly energetically excited molecule will ultimately find a path to drop back down to its lowest available energy state, as discussed further in the next section.

The absorption of visible light also affects the perceived colors of objects. For example, red ink looks black when in a bottle. Its red color is only perceived when it is placed on a scattering material, like paper. This is because the light path through the paper fibers (and through the very thin layer of ink) is only a fraction of a millimeter long; while light from the ink bottle has crossed several centimeters of ink and has been heavily absorbed, even in its red wavelengths.

In biological tissues, the combined effects of absorption processes by prevalent structures and chemical species give rise to surprisingly well-defined wavelength boundaries, between which light propagates with relatively low absorption. This wavelength window in tissue is called the *optical window* (Figure 1.6a) and is a critical consideration for PDT and all its imaging applications. Biological molecules like heme, flavins, and melanin strongly absorb visible light through electronic transitions. Absorption via transitions in vibrational energy levels of water molecules is the strongest absorption contributor in the infrared. Overall, the absorption in tissue increases toward shorter wavelengths due to protein, DNA, and other molecules, and toward longer wavelengths due to water absorption. In the 400–600 nm range, absorption by hemoglobin is very significant and residual hemoglobin staining of vessel walls can be a strong influence and can be seen in some of

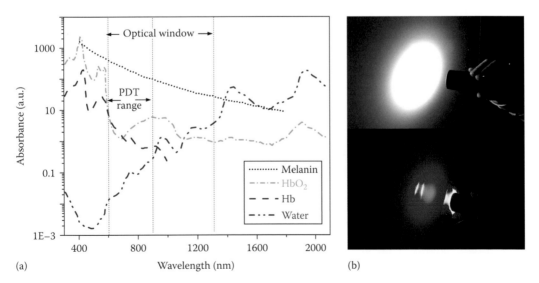

Figure 1.6 The optical window. (a) In the visible and near-infrared range, melanin, oxy, and de-oxy hemoglobin (HbO$_2$ and Hb) and water are four important absorptive molecules in tissue, which contribute to light attenuation. The region between approximately 600 and 1300 nm is known as the optical window, where absorption by these species is relatively small. The 600–900 nm window is the range of wavelengths typically useful for PDT. (Spectral data is compiled from published sources: Beard, 2011; Hamblin et al., 2006; Kim et al., 2011.) (b) A simple visual demonstration of the optical window in which white light from a flashlight is either incident directly on a screen (upper panel) or after having passed through a hand placed over the flashlight. Red light is absorbed least by skin tissue among the visible wavelengths generated by the flash light.

the spectra in this region. In the region between 600 and 1300 nm, tissue absorption is lowest. Superimposed on top of these absorption processes, scattering also takes place, and as we know from the discussion given earlier, shorter wavelengths will be far more strongly scattered than longer wavelengths.

A familiar visual representation of the optical window is given in Figure 1.6b, showing the spot from a flashlight, which emits white light, incident on a white screen. In the lower panel, the author's hand is placed over the front of the flashlight and the light incident on the screen after passing through tissue is predominantly red. This simple demonstration reflects the fact that the vast majority of lower wavelength light (400–600 nm) emitted by the flashlight is absorbed or scattered by tissue.

In Figure 1.6a, it is also noted that only a subset of the optical transmission window is energetically useful for PDT. This is because, at least for the standard assumption of an oxygen-dependent PDT process, the excited triplet state of the PS must have at least 22.4 kcal/mol required to excite ground state oxygen to its excited singlet state via collisional quenching (Turro et al. 2010). If this energy requirement of the photosensitizing molecule is to be met, then of course the incident photon must carry enough energy to excite the PS to its initial singlet excited state in the first place, which will be higher in energy than the triplet state from whence oxygen interaction will occur. Applying $E = h\nu$, this effectively stipulates an upper wavelength boundary of around 900 nm. This consideration is discussed more later as we consider photophysical processes following the absorption of light.

The difference in light transmission through tissue for wavelengths within the optical window versus those outside the window is so large that clinical PDT is virtually always performed using red or near-infrared excitation of photosensitizing molecules with accordingly strong absorption in this window. In fact, the porphyrin molecules used as PDT photosensitizers typically absorb blue light (around 400 nm) far more strongly than red light. For example, benzoporphyrin derivative monoacid ring-A (verteporfin) has excellent absorption around 690 nm, but in any given solvent the extinction coefficient for blue (Soret) absorption band is 2–2.5 times higher (Aveline et al. 1994). At first glance, it may appear that it is more efficient to excite this molecule with blue light. However, looking closely at the difference in absorption (vertical axis of Figure 1.6a) for these wavelengths, we see that even accounting for just one of these chemical species the absorption by tissue is easily 100 times greater for the blue excitation band, far dwarfing any benefit of the higher probability of PS excitation at these wavelengths. Although the blue light could perhaps generate more efficient PS activation in the top layer of cells, any therapeutic effect of PDT would be limited to only this very shallow depth of penetration. One might then ask why PS imaging applications almost always use blue light, but for this consideration we defer to the discussion of fluorescence and how it is applied in PS imaging.

1.2.4.3 ATTENUATION MODELS AND TISSUE OPTICS

It is often more useful not to identify each specific mechanism of light scattering and absorption in tissue, but rather to establish some scaling relationships that report how much light is attenuated overall as a function of wavelength and depth in tissue. When one considers the inherent heterogeneity and multitude of possible light interactions with all the structures and chemical species within tissue, it quickly becomes clear that writing down any kind of deterministic relationship is difficult, and even making many assumptions and simplifications, tissue optics still presents a challenging mathematical problem. A well-established approach is to model light transport as a diffusion process, in which photons are so highly scattered their motion can be modeled as a random walk using the mathematical approach developed by Einstein to describe Brownian motion of small particles (e.g., pollen grains) in a thermal bath. This approach works well for light, provided that the path length through tissue is large enough to allow sufficient scattering to occur for diffusion to become a good description. For visible wavelengths propagating in tissue, this length works out to be on the order of 1–2 mm (Jacques and Pogue 2008), making diffusive transport a good model in general for light transport through tissue at PDT wavelengths (Sandell and Zhu 2011).

At the simplest level, Beer's law provides a general relation between the attenuation of light and the optical properties of a material. T is the transmission of the light; μ_1, μ_2, etc., each represent a contribution from some physical process to a total attenuation per unit length:

$$T = \frac{P_{out}}{P_{in}} = e^{-(\mu_1 z + \mu_2 z + \mu_3 z + \cdots)}$$

In tissue optics, the total attenuation is described by the wavelength-dependent absorption coefficient, μ_a, and scattering coefficient, μ_s, which are the probability of absorption and scattering, respectively, per unit length at a given wavelength. As it turns out, for typical PDT wavelengths in the optical window, the scattering is usually much larger than the absorption (Wilson 2002), though we nevertheless need to account for both types of processes. Since scattering is also influenced by an optical anisotropy factor g, with value between −1 and 1, this property is expressed more compactly in the form of a reduced scattering coefficient, $\mu_s' = \mu_s(1-g)$. In the diffusive scattering regime, we can further combine the contributions from scattering and absorption into a single effective attenuation coefficient, $\mu_{eff} = \sqrt{3\mu_a \mu_s'}$ (Wilson and Patterson 1986). Putting these metrics together, with an additional depth-dependent backscattering factor $k_a(z)$, and adopting traditional PDT dosimetry notation, we can write down simple relationships to describe light transport as a function of tissue depth, depending on the geometry of illumination. For example, in the case of a uniform surface illumination of a tissue surface with irradiance E, the fluence rate, Φ, as a function of depth (z) becomes

$$\Phi = k_a(z) E e^{-\mu_{eff} z}$$

It is noteworthy that this relationship, unlike Beer's law, is not a simple monotonic decay, but due to the backscatter factor there is a fluence rate peak just below the tissue surface due to backward propagating photons combining with the forward illumination incident upon that depth of tissue. This is particularly important in a closed cavity environment, such as the oral cavity or bladder, where the effective fluence rate can be large relative to the delivered irradiance. In a bladder or esophagus treatment, this increase could be as high as five to seven times. Because this backscatter factor may be significantly different on different patients, adjustment of dosage of light delivery needs to be considered to prevent the increase of normal tissue damage (Star et al. 1987). For a useful summary of typical values of μ_s' and μ_a at PDT-relevant wavelengths in various tissues, the reader is referred to the review by Sandell and Zhu (2011).

1.3 PHYSICAL PROCESSES FOLLOWING LIGHT ABSORPTION: IMAGING AND THERAPEUTIC APPLICATIONS

In the discussion of light absorption given earlier, we briefly mentioned the importance of energy dissipation mechanisms following light absorption, by which an excited state molecule drops back down to its ground (lowest energy) state. Energy dissipation pathways include radiative decay via fluorescence emission, converting energy directly to heat, colliding and transferring energy to another molecule (which then will undergo a quantized excitation), or by transitioning to a new excited state with different spin structure, which will itself then dissipate energy by one of these possible mechanisms. As an excited state molecule is a quantum system, these processes should be thought of in terms of probabilities. For a given photon excitation, the energy dissipation route is not predetermined, though the symmetry of the molecule and the microenvironment (solvent) in which it is located will have a huge effect on the relative probabilities of different processes. To describe this, we use the term "quantum yield," the number of instances of a particular event, divided by the number of photons absorbed. So, for example, the quantum yield for fluorescence for a particular molecule is the ratio of photons emitted to photons absorbed. We will discuss later what properties of the absorbing species make it a good PS and imaging agent, and how dynamic changes in excited states can produce both fluorescence and induce cell death via the PDT process by transferring energy to other substrates such as oxygen to form potent reactive species.

1.3.1 RADIATIONLESS DISSIPATION ➜ HEAT

The absorbed energy of the incident photon can be transferred directly into heat without any intermediate radiative process. A molecule with sufficient density of vibrational states can undergo the process of internal conversion, transferring electronic excitation to the vibrational modes of the system and transferring the energy as heat to the local solvent bath (Bixon and Jortner 1968). An important example of this process is the internal conversion of the melanin molecule following ultraviolet excitation, a key physiological protection mechanism for photodamage (Wolbarsht et al. 1981). Generation of heat following laser irradiation can also be leveraged to great advantage in photothermal and photoacoustic imaging (Grauby et al. 1999, Xu and Wang 2006, Gobin et al. 2007, Huang et al. 2016). Therapeutically, heat generation can be exploited for laser surgery, where tissue is ablated by a high-intensity laser source (Trokel et al. 1983).

1.3.2 FLUORESCENCE

Fluorescence is a three-stage process that can occur with some probability depending on the chemical structure and symmetry of the electronically excited molecule. Generally, polyaromatic hydrocarbons or heterocycles dissipate a significant amount of energy via fluorescence and therefore make good fluorophores. As noted earlier, almost all known PDT PSs also act as fluorophores. Fluorescence is a rapid process where light is emitted within a fraction of a second after excitation. Figure 1.7a illustrates this process in which the players involved are the incident excitation photon $h\nu_{ex}$, the longer wavelength emitted photon, $h\nu_{em}$, electronic ground state S_0, the first excited electronic state S_1 (the next highest allowed energy state), and state S_1', a vibrational excited state that is higher in energy than S_1. The excitation and emission process follows three steps as follows.

Step 1: An orbital electron at ground state S_0 receives a photon carrying sufficient energy for excitation to state S_1':

$$S_0 + h\nu_{ex} \rightarrow S_1'$$

Step 2: The exited state is unstable, which usually lasts for a few nanoseconds. Afterward, the excited electron will dissipate excess vibrational energy to its surroundings and fall to a more stable transient state S_1, the lowest accessible vibrational state within that electronic excitation. This process is called relaxation oscillation:

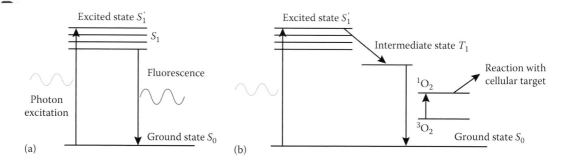

Figure 1.7 Fluorescence, intersystem crossing, and PDT. (a) In the fluorescence process, an electron absorbs the incident photon and jumps to excited state S_1' before rapidly transitioning to the lowest vibrational state S_1 through relaxation oscillation. Radiative decay to the ground state occurs, releasing a photon with less energy (longer wavelength) than the incident photon. (b) Alternatively, some excited electrons will undergo intersystem crossing, in which electron spin states change to a triplet configuration, T_1. This state is forbidden to undergo radiative decay back to the ground state and therefore has a long lifetime on the order of microseconds. Interaction via collisions with nearby ground state (triplet) oxygen molecules, $^3O_2$ simultaneously provides an energy dissipation mechanism for the excited triplet state photosensitizer while exciting $^3O_2$ to its excited singlet state, $^1O_2$. The highly reactive $^1O_2$ will then be rapidly quenched by nearby biological targets, leading to destruction of proteins and membranes.

$$S_1' \rightarrow \text{Dissipated energy} + S_1$$

Step 3: Finally, S_1 will return to its ground state via emission a lower energy photon $h\nu_{em}$. This process is fluorescence emission:

$$S_1 \rightarrow h\nu_{em} + S_0$$

The typical implementation of fluorescence imaging requires a set of filters, such that incident light is filtered to match the known excitation wavelength of the fluorescent molecule being imaged then reflected onto the sample by means of a dichroic mirror. Then, the longer wavelength light emitted from the sample passes (undeflected) through the dichroic mirror and onto an emission filter before it is incident on the camera or detector. Although there are many variations on this basic approach, some form of these basic components are used both for laboratory-based microscopy and in vivo fluorescence imaging applications (Klaunberg and Klaunberg 2004). Using this approach, extremely high contrast images can be generated, where regions of a tissue that are positively stained for a fluorophore (or express fluorescent protein) appear as bright objects against a nearly black background. Of course, endogenous molecules in tissue may be intrinsically fluorescent, at excitation and emission wavelengths that overlap with the target fluorophore, so care is needed in quantitative interpretation of fluorescence signals (more on this later). Nevertheless, this approach is clearly of enormous practical benefit and widely versatile in its applications in biomedical imaging. Fluorescent labels can be traditional fluorophores (e.g., AlexaFluor dyes), genetically encoded proteins (e.g., green fluorescent protein (GFP)), or quantum dots. Panels of fluorescent labels can be attached to target proteins or subcellular structures for multiplexed imaging, provided that each fluorescent dye is sufficiently spectrally distinct.

Coming back to an important point introduced earlier, PDT PSs can also be imaged in this manner. Since these compounds exhibit some degree of quasi-selective localization in neoplastic tissues, PDT PSs inherently behave as tumor-targeted fluorescence contrast agents. Indeed, there are an enormous number of studies, of which only a representative handful are cited here, that have demonstrated highly significant gains in sensitivity and specificity using PS fluorescence, rather than white light, to identify malignant tissues (Gregorie et al. 1968, Hemming et al. 1993, Megerian et al. 1993, Kriegmair 1996, Andrejevic-Blant et al. 1997, Allison et al. 1998, Chang et al. 1998, Koenig et al. 1999, Stummer et al. 2000, Zaak 2001, Yang et al. 2003, Bogaards et al. 2004, Loning et al. 2004, Olivo and Wilson 2004, Bogaards et al. 2005, Kostron et al. 2006). Most such examples of PS-enabled tumor imaging have used 5-aminolevulinic acid (ALA)-induced protoporphyrin IX as the photosensitizing strategy (Kennedy et al. 1990, Kennedy and Pottier 1992), though several examples also exist with exogenous PSs. This approach has become highly significant in enabling fluorescence-guided resection, with particularly noteworthy clinical results for bladder cancers (Kriegmair 2002) and malignant glioma (Stummer et al. 2006).

It is worth noting that in all the examples cited earlier blue light is used for PS excitation, even though these compounds all have the desirable feature of also being activated by red light. Regardless of which quantized transition corresponds to the initial photon absorption, the loner wavelength fluorescence emission is always initiated following relaxation oscillation to the lower vibration level, resulting in the same emission spectrum. In fact, this is the reason that blue light must be used for activation. Even though there is an available red wavelength excitation peak, it is not practical, even with the best optical filters, to spectrally separate the excitation light from the emission light. By using blue light for excitation, it leverages the extremely strong efficient absorption from the Soret band, with excellent separation (Stokes shift), though the tissue penetration is so limited that the approach dose gathers light only from the tissue surface. In many of the clinical studies, the emission light is actually unfiltered, so that the fluorescence images also show the blue excitation and malignant regions appear as a mix of backscattered blue light and red fluorescence emission.

Using PSs as fluorescence contrast agents also presents some challenges as these molecules tend to have an inherently low quantum yield for fluorescence. Indeed, this fact is by design as the molecules that have high quantum yield for fluorescence must in turn have a lower yield for intersystem crossing to the excited triplet state, which, as discussed in the following section, is the crucial process for PDT. And for the same reason, these molecules are less photostable, and the reactive species generated subsequent to light activation (which make them potent PDT agents) also leads more quickly to inactivation (photobleaching) of the PS itself.

1.3.3 INTERSYSTEM CROSSING → PHOTODYNAMIC THERAPY

Figure 1.7b shows the most important competing process following absorption of light for photosensitizing molecules. Following its initial activation to the excited singlet state, it is possible for a rearrangement of electron spins to occur such that the spin states' lowest unoccupied and highest occupied molecular orbitals flip to a parallel triplet configuration, denoted by the excited state T_1 (Turro et al. 2010). This process is called intersystem crossing, and an effective PS will generally have a high quantum yield for this event. It is significant that the transition from T_1 to S_0 is spin-forbidden, thereby making T_1 a long-lived intermediate quantum state. It is also significant that the ground state electronic configuration of the diatomic oxygen molecules is a triplet, $^3O_2$, enhancing the likelihood of energy transfer from the T_1 PS. Collisions resulting in energy transfer from T_1 to $^3O_2$ simultaneously provide a mechanism for dissipation so the PS can return to $S0$, while exciting oxygen to its excited singlet state, $^1O_2$. For this process to proceed, T_1 must have sufficient energy to transfer the required 22.4 kcal/mol for the transition from $^3O_2$ to $^1O_2$. Singlet oxygen, once created, reacts almost immediately with nearby cellular targets. It may also react with PS itself, which leads to its irreversible destruction (photobleaching), reduce the concentration of the PS, and decrease the effectiveness of PDT (Zhu and Finlay 2006). The majority of singlet oxygen reactions are irreversible, which results in a net consumption of oxygen during PDT. Although this explanation does not account for all competing photochemical and photophysical processes, the generation of singlet oxygen is widely believed to be the most important process mediating cytotoxic response by current clinically approved PSs. PDT can also generate a cytotoxic response by non-oxygen-dependent processes, or type I photochemistry. Here, we have focused on the more common oxygen-dependent type II process. The curious reader seeking to obtain a deeper understanding of the selection rules that determine the allowability of transitions that play such an important role in the PDT is encouraged to refer to the excellent text on photochemistry by Turro, Ramamurthy and Scaiano (2010).

1.3.4 NONLINEAR OPTICAL PROCESSES

When the incident light intensity is high enough that the electric field component of the EM radiation is comparable with interatomic electric fields, nonlinear optical processes may occur (Boyd and ebrary Inc. 2003). Usually, a pulsed laser with high power delivered in a short interval (less than 100 fs) is needed to generate such high peak power. An important nonlinear optical process is multiphoton absorption, where the electron absorbs more than one photon simultaneously such that they provide sufficient total energy for a quantized transition by the sum of more than one photon energy quanta. This nonlinear excitation event has extremely low probability requiring two or more phase-matched excitation photons with the appropriate energy to arrive at nearly the same point in space and time. The cross section for the two photon absorption process is expressed in units of Goeppert-Mayer (GM), where $1\ GM = 10^{-50}\ cm^4 \cdot s \cdot photon^{-1}$, named after Maria Goeppert-Mayer who predicted this nonlinear excitation process in her PhD thesis, decades before pulsed femtosecond near infrared laser sources were available (Göppert-Mayer 1931).

The two-photon excitation process can also lead to fluorescence emission as illustrated in Figure 1.8. Two-photon fluorescence microscopes based on these principles were first developed in the lab of Watt Webb at Cornell University in 1990 (Denk et al. 1990). As a biomedical imaging tool, this has huge implications. This approach provides a practical benefit similar to confocal microscopy, in that the excitation volume is so inherently small that scanning in a plane provides a depth-resolved optical section. The longer wavelengths used for two photon excitation also provide deeper penetration to allow deeper tissue imaging (Zipfel et al. 2003). Two photon microscopes are now commercially available from major microscope manufacturers and enable myriad applications in biological imaging (So et al. 2000, Rubart 2004, Helmchen and Denk 2005). The development of more affordable and reliable femtosecond NIR laser sources (Backus et al. 1998, Fermann et al. 2003, Wise 2013, Sugioka and Cheng 2014), including fiber lasers (Chong et al. 2012,

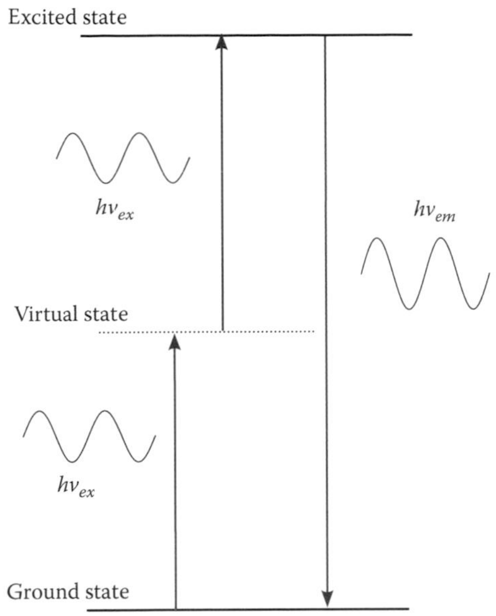

Figure 1.8 Two-photon excitation and fluorescence. When the incident photon flux is high enough, nonlinear optical processes may occur. This process can also generate fluorescence emission as shown here.

Horton et al. 2013, Xu and Wise 2013), has the potential to make this field even more approachable and will likely broaden its application space.

Two-photon absorption for PDT has also been evaluated (Drobizhev et al. 2006, Karotki et al. 2006, Horton et al. 2013). There are a couple of notable potential advantages of two-photon PDT. As with imaging, the use of near-infrared light for PS activation provides deeper tissue penetration. Secondly, the possibility for precision damage control exists since the two-photon absorption only happens within a tiny excitation volume. This has been aptly demonstrated by Collins et al. (2008), who used modified porphyrins with higher two-photon cross-sectional absorption to achieve selective closure of blood vessels in a mouse model. The small excitation volume cuts both ways of course, and for more typical applications where PDT treatment of a larger tissue volume is required, the traditional single-photon excitation process remains more practical. Going forward, the development of affordable and reliable fs NIR laser sources, such as fiber lasers (Chong et al. 2006), could make this strategy more approachable by researchers and clinicians in the future.

1.4 INSTRUMENTATION AND TECHNOLOGIES FOR IMAGING AND PDT

Here, we discuss some of the key instrumentation for imaging and PDT, including common illumination sources, detectors, and cameras, and some relevant examples of approaches enabled by these technologies.

1.4.1 LIGHT SOURCES

Lamps, lasers, and LED light sources have all been used extensively in imaging and PDT with some tradeoffs in cost, spectral properties, versatility, and coherence.

1.4.1.1 LASERS

The word "laser" is an acronym for "light amplification by stimulated emission of radiation" (Siegman 1986). As discussed earlier, lasers provide extraordinary coherence, both spatially and temporally. They are also nearly monochromatic (though even laser sources do have some finite spectral width). Two key components of a laser to achieve these properties are its gain medium and pump. The gain medium must have energy state structures that allows the possibility of having more electrons in the higher energy state than the lower energy state through pumping, in a process called population inversion. When this happens, stimulated emission can win over incoherent spontaneous emission (as occurs in other processes given earlier) to generate amplified and coherent emission.

Lasers are typically classified by the material used as the gain medium: semiconductor lasers, solid state lasers, gas lasers, fiber lasers, etc. These different types of lasers have different emission wavelength range and power range. For example, the red or green laser pointer is a semiconductor laser that can generate as low as a few milliwatts. The CO_2 lasers used in industrial cutting can achieve 3000 W, with peak emission in the infrared at 10.6 µm.

Laser can also be classified according to whether light is emitted continuously [continuous wave (CW)] or whether light output is packed into high intensity pulses, as short as a few femotoseconds (10^{-15} s). CW lasers have traditionally been employed for PDT and are used in most laser-based devices from CD players to laser scanning confocal microscopes. When integrated over time, the total power of a pulsed laser may not be as high as that of a powerful CW laser, but the short pulse duration can provide the high peak intensity to enable non-linear optical processes mentioned earlier. As such, pulsed lasers are a crucial enabling technology for nonlinear optics and multiphoton imaging.

The high spatial coherence of laser sources also affords some additional practical benefits for a very long distance while keeping concentration of its power in almost the same beam size. Lasers can be focused to a very tiny spot to get very high irradiance at low total power. Also, the very tiny spot can enable more than 90% high coupling to a single optical fiber used in light delivery for medical practice such as endoscopy. The monochromaticity property of laser light gives the maximum efficiency of photoactivation. However, different PSs may need different wavelength to activate them, which would require a separate diode laser system for each of them.

In biological microscopy, laser sources have also had a significant impact in enabling scanning confocal fluorescence microscopy (Robert 1996, Cox 2002). In contrast to the whole field illumination in traditional wide-field microscopes, a confocal microscope uses point illumination and a pinhole in an optically conjugate plane in front of the detector to eliminate light from above or below the focal plane, providing a thin "optical section" of a specimen. In this approach, a laser of appropriate wavelength for excitation of a target fluorophore is scanned by means of rapidly rotating deflecting mirrors to reconstruct successive XY image planes in series. The fluorescence emission from each point in each sample plane is detected after passing through the pinhole to construct the image pixel by pixel. By scanning over successive focal depths, this approach provides stacks of confocal image planes that can be reconstructed into 3D images. The implementation of this approach requires careful consideration of tradeoffs in laser power, scan speed (how long the laser spot resides at one point), and detector gain (which also amplifies background noise). In particular for imaging PS s, which as noted earlier are prone to rapid photobleaching and generally have low quantum yield for fluorescence, care must be taken to choose settings that maximize weak fluorescent signal and minimize noise, while avoiding photobleaching. It is also important to note that confocal microscopy is still constrained by the same tissue optics considerations discussed earlier, and just because fluorescence emission from out of the focal plane is rejected, it does not mean that light from deeper in tissue can be accessed. So, sections closer to the collection optics or objective will have a better signal to noise ratio than optical sections that arise at significant sample depth.

It cannot be overstated the extent to which laser light sources have revolutionized almost all aspects of optical imaging and photomedicine. Virtually all interferometry-based and nonlinear optical imaging processes were enabled by this breakthrough. Yet, having said that, the key features of lasers, their high coherence and extremely narrow (monochromatic) spectral width, are not actually requirements for PDT. So, while a great many PDT and PDT imaging applications rely on laser sources as an available light source to provide the desired irradiance at the target wavelength for a specific PS, it is important to recognize that incoherent lamps and LED sources may be just as applicable and win out in other areas such as cost and robustness as discussed later.

1.4.1.2 LIGHT-EMITTING DIODES

A light-emitting diode (LED) is a two-lead semiconductor light source that emits light when a voltage is applied. Compared with traditional incandescent lighting, LED lighting can be more efficient, durable, and compact. The color of LEDs depends on the semiconductor band gap structure. Different energy band gaps will result in different LED colors, so there is no "white" LED, although white light is produced by mixing multiple colors or using a phosphor material to produce longer wavelength emission. To date, LED colors are available across the visible, ultraviolet, and infrared wavelengths, with very high brightness. LED emission is narrow in its spectral width compared with lamps but has a much wider bandwidth than lasers, which makes it a useful candidate for fluorescence imaging and well suited to providing an efficient spectral overlap with a PS absorption peak.

The power output of LEDs range from a couple of milliWatts to several Watts. With the increase of LED power, due to its efficiency of generation, high-power LEDs require external heat sinks for heat dissipation. Otherwise, the temperature of the diode itself can increase, causing short lifetimes of operation. Depending on the material used, LEDs can have other useful features. For example, organic LEDs (OLEDs) made from organic material in a crystal phase or in polymers can be very flexible and even printable at low cost with a big viewing angle, an exciting development for potentially flexible and conformable PDT light sources. Despite its high total power, the power densities of LEDs are still low compared with lasers and lamp. Nevertheless, in some applications of fluorescence imaging LEDs can be used to replace lasers or lamps as the light source. In recent years, there have been many applications with LEDs in microscope systems (Burroughes et al. 1990, Moser et al. 2006, Robertson et al. 2009) and also LEDs as PDT light sources (Schmidt et al. 1999, Tsai et al. 2004, Bogaards et al. 2005, Mallidi et al. 2015).

There are some interesting tradeoffs that warrant consideration in contrasting LED and laser sources for PDT treatment and imaging. Compared with diode lasers, the cost per Watt from an LED is relatively low. LEDs are generally more robust and, unlike laser diodes, do not need high precision control systems to minimize fluctuation of the power and temperature. Because of their low cost, it is easy to integrate a few LEDs at different wavelength in the same driving system, which is useful when multifunctional light sources are needed to provide different wavelengths for different PSs. Similar to laser diodes, fluctuations in electric current could easily cause damage to the LED. LEDs are also easy to configure into various geometry tailored for applications, potentially user-configurable geometry to match to the treatment area. However, due to the poor efficiency of electrical to light conversion, the excessive heat generated from LED operation must be removed to prevent heat damage to the tissue, especially when operating at high power. This consideration is potentially problematic for the idea of using an LED inside the body for PDT or imaging inside an enclosed cavity. To overcome this, fiber-coupled LED devices can separate the heat-emitting light source from the light delivery in the tissue. However, another consideration is that the efficiency of LED to fiber coupling is not as high as in the case of laser to fiber coupling. So, when it comes to choosing between LED and laser sources for PDT, it will depend on the specific application in terms of treatment area, cost, electrical requirements, and power needed. The development of novel LED sources is still undergoing, such as OLEDs (Burroughes et al. 1990), and chemiluminescence-based sources, for example, in the form of "light patches" (Zelickson et al. 2005).

1.4.1.3 LAMPS

While clearly the oldest of light sources discussed here, incandescent lamps remain useful as bright light sources offering the versatility of a continuous emission spectrum that can then be selectively filtered to provide excitation for a wide range of target wavelengths from a single source. The white light lamp sources typically found in microscopes are usually either tungsten–halogen, gas discharge arc lamps, or metal halide lamps. Tungsten–halogen lamps provide 100W level output power with very small temporal and spatial fluctuation from the central ultraviolet (above 400 nm) through the visible and into the infrared wavelength regions. These sources are most useful for simple transmitted light imaging in microscopes. In fluorescence imaging, mercury and xenon arc lamps have historically been the most widely used sources, with high output and very closely approaching the ideal model for a point source of light. The lifetime of these lamps is about

200 hours. First commercialized in 1930, the mercury arc lamp is still considered to be one of the best illumination sources, especially for fluorescence microscopy. One-third of its spectral output lies in the visible region, and the rest of the spectrum confined to the ultraviolet and infrared region. It has a few prominent emission lines across the whole spectrum, where some specialized fluorophores have been developed to have maximum absorption. One of the drawbacks of the mercury lamp is its significant temporal and spatial instability. Xenon arc lamps have better stability than mercury arc lamps. The xenon lamp generates a continuous and uniform output across the entire visible spectral region. Therefore, the xenon arc lamp is a better candidate for stringent applications requiring the simultaneous excitation of multiple fluorophores over a wide wavelength range in quantitative fluorescence microscopy. More recently, metal halide lamps have increasingly replaced traditional arc lamps. They have much longer life spans compared with arc lamps (2000 hours versus 200 hours). The spectral features of metal halide lamps are similar to mercury lamps but with higher radiance level, making them an alternative source for exciting fluorophores that were designed for mercury arc lamps. They can be efficiently coupled into optical fiber bundles or liquid light guides of 5–10 mm diameter. However, these sources have not yet been integrated with single-fiber coupling for endoscopic use.

1.4.2 ENDOSCOPES

Optical imaging is clearly a powerful technique for treatment guidance and diagnosis. It offers excellent spatial resolution relative to other clinical imaging modalities, providing detailed structural information down to the cellular and subcellular level, and does so without the use of ionizing radiation, which itself can be carcinogenic. However, in most cases, it is limited to tissues that are readily accessible using visible wavelengths. Compact light sources, combined with mirrors, provide some degree of access to areas that are partially enclosed, as in the case of dental examination. However, a transformative development for clinical optical imaging has been the development of endoscopes, using flexible imaging fibers (see earlier text) that can be inserted directly inside the body to reach spaces otherwise inaccessible to light. The basic design concept consists of a flexible bundle of optical fibers coupled to a light source and a camera (Epstein 1980). This basic design is often combined with additional flexible tools that enable endoscopic-guided biopsies and laparoscopic surgery. This approach is in wide clinical use for accessing the gastrointestinal tract and transurethral imaging of the bladder. For PDT, this allows for the possibility of "seek and destroy" treatments in these lumenal cavities, where PS fluorescence can be imaged endoscopically, then targeted for therapeutic light delivery using another fiber to deliver higher irradiance red light for PS activation alongside the endoscope. PDT endoscopic imaging applications have been extensively developed, mostly with ALA-induced PpIX, in the context of transurethral guided bladder cancer resection (Riedl et al. 2001, Kriegmair 2002), fluorescence bronchoscopy (Weigel et al. 2000, Zargi et al. 2000, Zellweger et al. 2001) and for imaging Barrett's esophagus (Endlicher et al. 2001, Stepinac et al. 2003). This approach has also been demonstrated in the clinic for imaging ovarian cancer micrometastses that escaped detection by traditional white light endoscopy (Loning et al. 2004).

1.4.3 PHOTODETECTORS AND CAMERAS

Here, we discuss three particularly important types of photodetectors, the photodiode, thermal power meter, and photomultiplier tube (PMT). Each one converts light into an electrical signal in some physical manner. PMTs are vacuum phototubes that are extremely sensitive detectors of light in the ultraviolet, visible, and near-infrared regions. PMTs are a truly miraculous invention at the heart of such diverse systems as confocal microscopes and detectors of cosmic rays. PMTs are fundamentally enabled by the photoelectric effect (Einstein 1905), in which a single-photon incident upon the photocathode can eject a photoelectron that is in turn amplified as it travels through a series of dynode stages inside the tube. PMTs use high voltage (on the order of several hundred to a thousand volts) to accelerate the electron and multiply the current produced by incident light by as much as 100 million times, which is critical for applications where the signal light is very low, such as in some fluorescence microscopy. PMTs are highly sensitive and somewhat fragile. While high voltage is applied, the photocathode needs to be shielded from ambient light that could cause overexcitation and lead to destruction of the detector.

Photodiodes also use the photoelectric effect to convert light into current. Only when a photon carries enough energy into the semiconductor sensor material will it cause emission of a photoelectron. The semiconductor materials used in a photodiode determine the bandwidth of EM waves that can be measured. For example, silicon photodetectors measure wavelength range from 190 to 1100 nm while indium gallium arsenide detectors measure from 800 to 2600 nm.

Thermal power meters use thermal sensors that convert heat into voltage. The light hit on the sensor is absorbed and efficiently converted to heat (see processes following light absorption given earlier), which is proportional to the voltage it creates. Although thermal power meters have lower power resolution and longer response time compared with photodiode, they generally have a wider wavelength and power range that are needed for many applications. For example, a typical thermal power meter can measure from 190 nm to 20 μm. In addition, they are useful for applications with ultrashort pulses where high peak power would saturate a photodiode sensor.

1.4.3.1 CAMERAS

The development of image sensors based on charge-coupled devices (CCDs; Boyle and Smith 1970) has truly revolutionized optical imaging, both in the laboratory and clinical settings. The CCD image sensor can be thought of as a grid of tiny capacitors, each storing an electric charge that is proportional to the intensity of light incident at that pixel element. When appropriate optics are used to project an image onto the sensor plane, a digital image is formed. The number of pixels on the sensor determines the resolution, which also refers to the sharpness and clarity of an image. The sensitivity of cameras is determined by both the minimum number of photons needed for detection by the optical sensor and the number of photons needed to change from one digital brightness level to the next. The number of brightness levels, n, that can be recorded is described as the bit depth, d, of the camera, where $n = 2^d$. So, with a 12-bit camera, there are 2^{12} or 4096 possible brightness levels. Another important parameter of cameras is the speed, which is also the shutter speed determined by the length of time (called exposure time) required to obtain an image, typically from 0.001 to 1 second. By convention, cameras that acquire more than 250 fps are dubbed high-speed cameras. Because the number of photons reaching the image sensors is proportional to the exposure time, a bright light source is needed for high-speed camera for the sensor to receive enough photons within a short exposure time.

1.4.4 IMAGE PROCESSING

Finally, we note that an imaging study is not truly complete upon image acquisition, but virtually always requires the additional step of some quantitative image processing. The full depth of information that can be obtained from quantitative analysis of PDT image data is enormous and has yet to be fully realized. Indeed, the term "bioimage informatics" has been used in reference to the pursuit of advanced image processing strategies to unlock rich content encoded in biological image data sets (Eliceiri et al. 2012, Myers 2012), and this concept is directly applicable to imaging in PDT. Regardless of whether a digital image is constructed by a point scanning detector system, or from a CCD or CMOS sensor array, images are fundamentally matrices, $I(x, y)$, in which each pixel (each xy position) has a numerical value associated with it. The range of possible values is determined by the bit depth of the camera. At the most basic level, pixel values in fluorescence image data scale with the brightness of the fluorophore. So, typically a bright spot with high pixel values corresponds to a locally high concentration or (higher degree of activity) of a fluorophore. Even a simple analysis of changes in fluorescence intensity, obtained via measuring average pixel values over regions of interest in an image, can be extremely useful. For example, we noted earlier that PS fluorescence decreases following therapeutic light activation due to photobleaching. Hence, it is often useful to analyze fluorescence images of a target tissue that has PS accumulated in it, both before and after therapeutic light activation of the PS, to quantify the fractional photobleaching as a measure of the PDT dose deposited (Mang et al. 1987, Iinuma et al. 1999, Bonnett 2001, Finlay et al. 2004, Pogue et al. 2008).

In the laboratory setting, beyond just looking at fluorescence signals from the PS itself, this type of intensity-based analysis is widely used to analyze PDT (or any) treatment response. For example, a well-established way to quantify PDT treatment response in cell cultures is to quantify signal from fluorescent reporters of cell viability and cell death (Anbil et al. 2013, Celli et al. 2014). Another very basic image processing task is segmentation by which a cutoff in the distribution of pixel intensity values is identified that separates relatively bright foreground pixels from relatively dark background pixels. Segmentation itself can be performed using a variety of algorithms such as Otsu's method, which identifies this cutoff value by iterating over candidate values to identify a point with minimum intraclass variance between foreground and background. Automated segmentation can of course be combined with patterns of fluorescence intensity fluctuations in selected subregions and structures and images to inform specific spatial patterns of PS uptake, localization, and photobleaching (Glidden et al. 2012), which can be of course co-registered with fluorescent labels of particular biomarkers and virtually anything else that can be fluorescently tagged in an image.

Increasingly, image acquisition systems now often provide spectral information at each pixel, providing additional opportunities and challenges for image processing. Rather than the traditional practice described earlier, of using an emission filter in front of the camera or detector, optical systems are increasingly using multispectral detectors that use a prism to spread the full spectral profile of fluorescence emission over a detector array, wherein each element records the light intensity of a narrow spectral width at one particular spatial position. There are several variations on this basic approach, all generally known as hyperspectral imaging (Zimmermann et al. 2003, Mansfield et al. 2005, Chang et al. 2008). Hyperspectral image data can be processed by linear spectral unmixing to separate the full spectral signature of each contributing chemical species contributing to the total fluorescence signal at each spatial position in an image (Zimmermann et al. 2003, Mansfield et al. 2005). In one example, multispectral images of articular cartilage results were analyzed to reveal changes in collagen content of the tissue (Kaufman et al. 1987). Having full spectral data at each pixel is extremely powerful, particularly for imaging PDT PSs with low quantum yield, since endogenous tissue autofluorescence often makes a significant contribution to the overall fluorescence signal collected (Hewett et al. 2001).

1.5 CONCLUSION, PERSPECTIVES, AND EMERGING DIRECTIONS

It is clear that fundamental principles of physics are deeply involved in almost all aspects of PDT imaging applications, from the classical electrodynamics descriptions of light itself, light propagation, and its interaction with matter, to quantum mechanics ideas that govern PDT photophysics. The technology of PDT imaging applications has also been driven by physics and engineering innovations such as the development of lasers, LEDs, fiber optics, digital cameras, and PMTs, which are so fundamental as to be taken for granted. Nevertheless, a conscious awareness of the underlying principles is invaluable to understanding device operation and to get the best results, and this remains true even for the most well-designed turnkey, user-friendly imaging systems.

There is no doubt that cameras, detectors, and optoelectronics will continue to become smaller, faster, lighter, and more sensitive. It is entirely possible that the next technological breakthrough will come from a completely unexpected development, possibly even in a different field. One potentially exciting area, coming out of the increasingly widespread use of low-cost embedded microcontrollers in electronic devices, is the potential for "smarter" interfaced PDT/imaging devices. For example, it is well known that PDT efficacy is determined by complex tradeoffs in the rate of PS activation relative to reoxygenation and other physiological processes. Yet, treatment protocols are still largely static, designed to deliver a fixed fluence rate, in a fixed amount of time, based on previous experience that is almost certainly not patient specific. This suggests the need for better-integrated multifunctional fluorescence imaging and treatment devices could that utilize dynamic feedback from multimodal image data (e.g., photobleaching, derived measurements of hemoglobin oxygenation, etc.) to modulate light delivery in real time.

Moreover, exciting possibilities for the broader application of PDT may come not only from cutting-edge breakthroughs in optics that improve speed, sensitivity, and resolution, but from the adaptation of PDT and imaging devices into lower-cost, easier-to-use formats. In recent years, smart phones, which are widely available throughout the world, have become increasingly leveraged as low-cost, compact, portable platforms with built-in computing power and increasingly high-quality cameras that can be implemented in impressively sophisticated fluorescence imaging applications (Shen et al. 2012, Wei et al. 2013). As such, it is not surprising that smart phone–based fluorescence imaging has also been adopted in the context of PDT (Hempstead et al. 2015, Kulyk et al. 2015), with the potential for broad impact in resource-limited settings where there is limited medical infrastructure and reliable electricity may not be available. Combining this idea with the discussion of LED light sources for PDT and better-integrated PDT/imaging systems with low-cost embedded control suggests the potential for enabling image-guided PDT in global health settings.

REFERENCES

Allison, R. R., T. S. Mang, and B. D. Wilson. 1998. Photodynamic therapy for the treatment of nonmelanomatous cutaneous malignancies. *Semin Cutan Med Surg* **17**(298332271):153–163.

Anbil, S., I. Rizvi, J. P. Celli, N. Alagic, B. W. Pogue, and T. Hasan. 2013. Impact of treatment response metrics on photodynamic therapy planning and outcomes in a three-dimensional model of ovarian cancer. *J Biomed Opt* **18**(9):098004. doi: 10.1117/1.JBO.18.9.098004.

Andrejevic-Blant, S., C. Hadjur, J. P. Ballini, G. Wagnieres, C. Fontolliet, H. van den Bergh, and P. Monnier. 1997. Photodynamic therapy of early squamous cell carcinoma with tetra(m-hydroxyphenyl)chlorin: Optimal drug-light interval. *Br J Cancer* **76**(8):1021–1028.

Aveline, B., T. Hasan, and R. W. Redmond. 1994. Photophysical and photosensitizing properties of benzoporphyrin derivative monoacid ring A (BPD-MA). *Photochem Photobiol* **59**(3):328–335.

Backus, S., C. G. Durfee III, M. M. Murnane, and H. C. Kapteyn. 1998. High power ultrafast lasers. *Rev Sci Instrum* **69**(3):1207–1223.

Bassan, P., A. Kohler, H. Martens, J. Lee, E. Jackson, N. Lockyer, P. Dumas, M. Brown, N. Clarke, and P. Gardner. 2010. RMieS-EMSC correction for infrared spectra of biological cells: Extension using full Mie theory and GPU computing. *J Biophotonics* **3**(8–9):609–620. doi: 10.1002/jbio.201000036.

Beard, P. 2011. Biomedical photoacoustic imaging. *Interface Focus* **1**(4):602–631. doi: 10.1098/rsfs.2011.0028.

Bixon, M. and J. Jortner. 1968. Intramolecular radiationless transitions. *J Chem Phys* **48**(2):715–726.

Bogaards, A., A. Varma, S. P. Collens, A. H. Lin, A. Giles, V. X. D. Yang, J. M. Bilbao, L. D. Lilge, P. J. Muller, and B. C. Wilson. 2004. Increased brain tumor resection using fluorescence image guidance in a pre-clinical model. *Lasers Surg Med* **35**(3):181–190. doi: 10.1002/lsm.20088.

Bogaards, A., A. Varma, K. Zhang, D. Zach, S. K. Bisland, E. H. Moriyama, L. Lilge, P. J. Muller, and B. C. Wilson. 2005. Fluorescence image-guided brain tumour resection with adjuvant metronomic photodynamic therapy: Pre-clinical model and technology development. *Photochem Photobiol Sci* **4**(5):438–442. doi: 10.1039/b414829k.

Bonnett, R. and M. Gabriel. 2001. Photobleaching of sensitisers used in photodynamic therapy. *Tetrahedron* **57**(591):9513–9547.

Boyd, R. W. and ebrary Inc. 2003. *Nonlinear Optics*. San Diego, CA: Academic Press. http://site.ebrary.com/lib/rockefeller/Doc?id=10185952.

Boyle, W. S. and G. E. Smith. 1970. Charge coupled semiconductor devices. *Bell Syst Tech J* **49**(4):587–593.

Burroughes, J. H., D. D. C. Bradley, A. R. Brown, R. N. Marks, K. MacKay, R. H. Friend, P. L. Burns, and A. B. Holmes. 1990. Light-emitting diodes based on conjugated polymers. *Nature* **347**(6293):539–541.

Celli, J. P., I. Rizvi, A. R. Blanden, I. Massodi, M. D. Glidden, B. W. Pogue, and T. Hasan. 2014. An imaging-based platform for high-content, quantitative evaluation of therapeutic response in 3D tumour models. *Sci Rep* **4**: 3751. doi: 10.1038/srep03751. http://www.nature.com/srep/2014/140117/srep03751/abs/srep03751.html#supplementary-information.

Celli, J. P., B. Q. Spring, I. Rizvi, C. L. Evans, K. S. Samkoe, S. Verma, B. W. Pogue, and T. Hasan. 2010. Imaging and photodynamic therapy: Mechanisms, monitoring, and optimization. *Chem Rev* **110**(5):2795–2838. doi: 10.1021/cr900300p.

Chang, C. J., Y. L. Lai, and C. J. Wong. 1998. Photodynamic therapy for facial squamous cell carcinoma in cats using Photofrin. *Chang Keng I Hsueh* **21**(198270182):13–19.

Chang, S. K., I. Rizvi, N. Solban, and T. Hasan. 2008. In vivo optical molecular imaging of vascular endothelial growth factor for monitoring cancer treatment. *Clin Cancer Res* **14**(13):4146–4153. doi: 10.1158/1078-0432.ccr-07-4536.

Chong, A., J. Buckley, W. Renninger, and F. Wise. 2006. All-normal-dispersion femtosecond fiber laser. *Opt Express* **14**(21):10095–10100.

Chong, A., H. Liu, B. Nie, B. G. Bale, S. Wabnitz, W. H. Renninger, M. Dantus, and F. W. Wise. 2012. Pulse generation without gain-bandwidth limitation in a laser with self-similar evolution. *Opt Express* **20**(13):14213–14220. doi: 10.1364/OE.20.014213.

Collins, H. A., M. Khurana, E. H. Moriyama, A. Mariampillai, E. Dahlstedt, M. Balaz, M. K. Kuimova et al. 2008. Blood-vessel closure using photosensitizers engineered for two-photon excitation. *Nat Photon* **2**(7): 420–424. doi: http://www.nature.com/nphoton/journal/v2/n7/suppinfo/nphoton.2008.100_S1.html.

Cox, G. 2002. Biological confocal microscopy. *Mater Today* **5**(3):34–41. doi: http://dx.doi.org/10.1016/S1369-7021(02)05329-4.

Denk, W., J. H. Strickler, and W. W. Webb. 1990. Two-photon laser scanning fluorescence microscopy. *Science* **248**(4951):73–76.

Dougherty, T. J., C. J. Gomer, B. W. Henderson, G. Jori, D. Kessel, M. Korbelik, J. Moan, and Q. Peng. 1998. Photodynamic therapy: Review. *J Natl Cancer Inst* **90**(12):889–905.

Drobizhev, M., F. Meng, A. Rebane, Y. Stepanenko, E. Nickel, and C. W. Spangler. 2006. Strong two-photon absorption in new asymmetrically substituted porphyrins: Interference between charge-transfer and intermediate-resonance pathways. *J Phys Chem B* **110**(20):9802–9814. doi: 10.1021/jp0551770.

Einstein, A. 1905. Über einen die Erzeugung und Verwandlung des Lichtes betreffenden heuristischen Gesichtspunkt. *Ann Phys* **17**(6):132–148. doi: 10.1002/andp.19053220607.

Eliceiri, K. W., M. R. Berthold, I. G. Goldberg, L. Ibanez, B. S. Manjunath, M. E. Martone, R. F. Murphy et al. 2012. Biological imaging software tools. *Nat Methods* **9**(7):697–710. doi: 10.1038/nmeth.2084.

Endlicher, E., R. Knuechel, T. Hauser, R.-M. Szeimies, J. Schölmerich, and H. Messmann. 2001. Endoscopic fluorescence detection of low and high grade dysplasia in Barrett's oesophagus using systemic or local 5-aminolaevulinic acid sensitisation. *Gut* **48**(3):314–319.

Epstein, M. 1980. Endoscopy: Developments in optical instrumentation. *Science* **210**(4467):280–285.

Epstein, M. 1982. Fiber optics in medicine. *Crit Rev Biomed Eng* **7**(2):79–120.

Fermann, M. E., A. Galvanauskas, and G. Sucha. 2003. *Ultrafast Lasers: Technology and Applications*. Taylor & Francis, CRC Press, New York.

Finlay, J. C., S. Mitra, M. S. Patterson, and T. H. Foster. 2004. Photobleaching kinetics of Photofrin in vivo and in multicell tumour spheroids indicate two simultaneous bleaching mechanisms. *Phys Med Biol* **49**(21):4837–4860.

Glidden, M. D., J. P. Celli, I. Massodi, I. Rizvi, B. W. Pogue, and T. Hasan. 2012. Image-based quantification of benzoporphyrin derivative uptake, localization, and photobleaching in 3D tumor models, for optimization of PDT parameters. *Theranostics* **2**(9):827–839. doi: 10.7150/thno.4334.

Gobin, A. M., M. H. Lee, N. J. Halas, W. D. James, R. A. Drezek, and J. L. West. 2007. Near-infrared resonant nanoshells for combined optical imaging and photothermal cancer therapy. *Nano Lett* **7**(7):1929–1934. doi: 10.1021/nl070610y.

Göppert-Mayer, M. 1931. Über Elementarakte mit zwei Quantensprüngen. *Ann Phys* **401**(3):273–294. doi: 10.1002/andp.19314010303.

Grauby, S., B. C. Forget, S. Holé, and D. Fournier. 1999. High resolution photothermal imaging of high frequency phenomena using a visible charge coupled device camera associated with a multichannel lock-in scheme. *Rev Sci Instrum* **70**(9):3603–3608. doi: http://dx.doi.org/10.1063/1.1149966.

Gregorie, H. B., Jr., E. O. Horger, J. L. Ward, J. F. Green, T. Richards, H. C. Robertson, Jr., and T. B. Stevenson. 1968. Hematoporphyrin-derivative fluorescence in malignant neoplasms. *Ann Surg* **167**(6):820–828.

Hamblin, M. R., R. W. Waynant, T. N. Demidova, and J. Anders. 2006. Mechanisms of low level light therapy. *Proc SPIE* **6140**:614001. doi: 10.1117/12.646294.

Helmchen, F. and W. Denk. 2005. Deep tissue two-photon microscopy. *Nat Methods* **2**(12):932–940.

Hemming, A. W., N. L. Davis, B. Dubois, N. F. Quenville, and R. J. Finley. 1993. Photodynamic therapy of squamous cell carcinoma. An evaluation of a new photosensitizing agent, benzoporphyrin derivative and new photoimmunoconjugate. *Surg Oncol* **2**(3):187–196.

Hempstead, J., D. P. Jones, A. Ziouche, G. M. Cramer, I. Rizvi, S. Arnason, T. Hasan, and J. P. Celli. 2015. Low-cost photodynamic therapy devices for global health settings: Characterization of battery-powered LED performance and smartphone imaging in 3D tumor models. *Sci Rep* **5**:10093. doi: 10.1038/srep10093. http://www.nature.com/srep/2015/150512/srep10093/abs/srep10093.html#supplementary-information.

Hergert, W. and T. Wriedt. 2012. *The Mie Theory: Basics and Applications*. Berlin, Germany: Springer.

Hewett, J., V. Nadeau, J. Ferguson, H. Moseley, S. Ibbotson, J. W. Allen, W. Sibbett, and M. Padgett. 2001. The application of a compact multispectral imaging system with integrated excitation source to in vivo monitoring of fluorescence during topical photodynamic therapy of superficial skin cancers. *Photochem Photobiol* **73**(3):278–282. doi: 10.1562/0031-8655(2001)073<0278:TAOACM>2.0.CO;2.

Horton, N. G., K. Wang, D. Kobat, C. G. Clark, F. W. Wise, C. B. Schaffer, and C. Xu. 2013. Three-photon microscopy of subcortical structures within an intact mouse brain. *Nat Photonics* **7**(3):205–209.

Huang, B. 2010. Super-resolution optical microscopy: Multiple choices. *Curr Opin Chem Biol* **14**(1):10–14. doi: 10.1016/j.cbpa.2009.10.013.

Huang, B., H. Babcock, and X. Zhuang. 2010. Breaking the diffraction barrier: Super-resolution imaging of cells. *Cell* **143**(7):1047–1058. doi: 10.1016/j.cell.2010.12.002.

Huang, X., I. H. El-Sayed, W. Qian, and M. A. El-Sayed. 2016. Cancer cell imaging and photothermal therapy in the near-infrared region by using gold nanorods. *J Am Chem Soc* **128**(6):2115–2120. doi: 10.1021/ja057254a.

Iinuma, S., K. T. Schomacker, G. Wagnieres, M. Rajadhyaksha, M. Bamberg, T. Momma, and T. Hasan. 1999. In vivo fluence rate and fractionation effects on tumor response and photobleaching in photodynamic therapy with two photosensitizers in an orthotopic rat tumor model. *Cancer Res* **59**:6164–6170.

Jackson, J. D. 1999. *Classical Electrodynamics*, 3rd edn. New York: Wiley.

Jacques, S. L. and B. W. Pogue. 2008. Tutorial on diffuse light transport. *J Biomed Opt* **13**(4):041302. doi: 10.1117/1.2967535.

Jung, Y., A. J. Nichols, O. J. Klein, E. Roussakis, and C. L. Evans. 2012. Label-free, longitudinal visualization of PDT response in vitro with optical coherence tomography. *Isr J Chem* **52**(8–9):728–744. doi: 10.1002/ijch.201200009.

Karotki, A., M. Khurana, J. R. Lepock, and B. C. Wilson. 2006. Simultaneous two-photon excitation of Photofrin in relation to photodynamic therapy. *Photochem Photobiol* **82**(2):443–452. doi: 10.1562/2005-08-24-RA-657.

Kaufman, J. L., K. Stark, and R. E. Brolin. 1987. Disseminated atheroembolism from extensive degenerative atherosclerosis of the aorta. *Surgery* **102**(1):63–70.

Kennedy, J. C. and R. H. Pottier. 1992. Endogenous protoporphyrin IX, a clinically useful photosensitizer for photodynamic therapy. *J Photochem Photobiol B* **14**:275–292.

Kennedy, J. C., R. H. Pottier, and D. C. Pross. 1990. Photodynamic therapy with endogenous protoporphyrin IX: Basic principles and present clinical experience. *J Photochem Photobiol B* **6**:143–148.

Kim, H. W., D. G. Moon, H. M. Kim, J. H. Hwang, S. C. Kim, S. G. Nam, and J. T. Park. 2011. Effect of shifting from combination therapy to monotherapy of α-blockers or 5α-reductase inhibitors on prostate volume and symptoms in patients with benign prostatic hyperplasia. *Korean J Urol* **52**(10):681–686. doi: 10.4111/kju.2011.52.10.681.

Klaunberg, M. H. and B. A. Klaunberg 2004. Biomedical applications of fluorescence imaging in vivo. *Comp Med* **54**(6):635–644.

Koenig, F., F. J. McGovern, R. Larne, H. Enquist, K. T. Schomacker, and T. F. Deutsch. 1999. Diagnosis of bladder carcinoma using protoporphyrin IX fluorescence induced by 5-aminolaevulinic acid. *BJU Int* **83**(1):129–135.

Korde, V. R., G. T. Bonnema, W. Xu, C. Krishnamurthy, J. Ranger-Moore, K. Saboda, L. D. Slayton et al. 2007. Using optical coherence tomography to evaluate skin sun damage and precancer. *Lasers Surg Med* **39**(9):687–695. doi: 10.1002/lsm.20573.

Kostron, H., T. Fiegele, and E. Akatuna. 2006. Combination of FOSCAN mediated fluorescence guided resection and photodynamic treatment as new therapeutic concept for malignant brain tumors. *Med Laser Appl* **21**:285–290. doi: 10.1016/j.mla.2006.08.001.

Kriegmair, M. 1996. Detection of early bladder cancer by 5-aminolevulinic acid induced porphyrin fluorescence. *J Urol* **155**:105–109.

Kriegmair, M. 2002. Transurethral resection for bladder cancer using 5-aminolevulinic acid induced fluorescence endoscopy versus white light endoscopy. *J Urol* **168**:475–478.

Kulyk, O., S. H. Ibbotson, H. Moseley, R. M. Valentine, and I. D. W. Samuel. 2015. Development of a hand-held fluorescence imaging device to investigate the characteristics of protoporphyrin IX fluorescence in healthy and diseased skin. *Photodiagnosis Photodyn Ther* **12**(4):630–639.

Loning, M., H. Diddens, W. Kupker, K. Diedrich, and G. Huttmann. 2004. Laparoscopic fluorescence detection of ovarian carcinoma metastases using 5-aminolevulinic acid-induced protoporphyrin IX. *Cancer* **100**(8):1650–1656. doi: 10.1002/cncr.20155.

Mallidi, S., Z. Mai, I. Rizvi, J. Hempstead, S. Arnason, J. Celli, and T. Hasan. 2015. In vivo evaluation of battery-operated light-emitting diode-based photodynamic therapy efficacy using tumor volume and biomarker expression as endpoints. *J Biomed Opt* **20**(4):048003.

Mang, T. S., T. J. Dougherty, W. R. Potter, D. G. Boyle, S. Somer, and J. Moan. 1987. Photobleaching of porphyrins used in photodynamic therapy and implications for therapy. *Photochem Photobiol* **45**(4):501–506.

Mansfield, J. R., K. W. Gossage, C. C. Hoyt, and R. M. Levenson. 2005. Autofluorescence removal, multiplexing, and automated analysis methods for in-vivo fluorescence imaging. *J Biomed Opt* **10**:041207.

Maxwell, J. C. 1865. A dynamical theory of the electromagnetic field. *Philos Trans R Soc Lond* **155**:459–512. doi: 10.1098/rstl.1865.0008.

Megerian, C. A., S. I. Zaidi, R. C. Sprecher, S. Setrakian, D. W. Stepnick, N. L. Oleinick, and H. Mukhtar. 1993. Photodynamic therapy of human squamous cell carcinoma in vitro and in xenografts in nude mice. *Laryngoscope* **103** (9):967–975.

Moser, C., T. Mayr, and I. Klimant. 2006. Filter cubes with built-in ultrabright light-emitting diodes as exchangeable excitation light sources in fluorescence microscopy. *J Microsc* **222**(Pt 2):135–140. doi: 10.1111/j.1365-2818.2006.01581.x.

Myers, G. 2012. Why bioimage informatics matters. *Nat Methods* **9**(7):659–660. doi: 10.1038/nmeth.2024.

Olivo, M. and B. C. Wilson. 2004. Mapping ALA-induced PPIX fluorescence in normal brain and brain tumour using confocal fluorescence microscopy. *Int J Oncol* **25**(1):37–45.

Pogue, B. W., C. Sheng, J. Benevides, D. Forcione, B. Puricelli, N. Nishioka, and T. Hasan. 2008. Protoporphyrin IX fluorescence photobleaching increases with the use of fractionated irradiation in the esophagus. *J Biomed Opt* **13**(3):10. doi: 034009.10.1117/1.2937476.

Policard, A. 1924. Etudes sur les aspects offerts par des tumeurs experimentales examinees a la lumiere de Wood. *C R Soc Biol* **91**:1423–1428.

Riedl, C. R., D. Daniltchenko, F. Koenig, R. Simak, S. A. Loening, and H. Pflueger. 2001. Fluorescence endoscopy with 5-aminolevulinic acid reduces early recurrence rate in superficial bladder cancer. *J Urol* **165**(4):1121–1123.

Robert, H. W. 1996. Confocal optical microscopy. *Rep Prog Phys* **59**(3):427.

Robertson, J. B., Y. Zhang, and C. H. Johnson. 2009. Light-emitting diode flashlights as effective and inexpensive light sources for fluorescence microscopy. *J Microsc* **236**(1):1–4. doi: 10.1111/j.1365-2818.2009.03208.x.

Rubart, M. 2004. Two-photon microscopy of cells and tissue. *Circ Res* **95** (12):1154–1166. doi: 10.1161/01. RES.0000150593.30324.42.

Samkoe, K. S., A. A. Clancy, A. Karotki, B. C. Wilson, and D. T. Cramb. 2007. Complete blood vessel occlusion in the chick chorioallantoic membrane using two-photon excitation photodynamic therapy: Implications for treatment of wet age-related macular degeneration. *J Biomed Opt* **12**(3):034025. doi: 10.1117/1.2750663.

Sandell, J. L. and T. C. Zhu. 2011. A review of in-vivo optical properties of human tissues and its impact on PDT. *J Biophotonics* **4**(11–12):773–787.

Schermelleh, L., R. Heintzmann, and H. Leonhardt. 2010. A guide to super-resolution fluorescence microscopy. *J Cell Biol* **190**(2):165–175. doi: 10.1083/jcb.201002018.

Schmidt, M. H., K. W. Reichert, 2nd, K. Ozker, G. A. Meyer, D. L. Donohoe, D. M. Bajic, N. T. Whelan, and H. T. Whelan. 1999. Preclinical evaluation of benzoporphyrin derivative combined with a light-emitting diode array for photodynamic therapy of brain tumors. *Pediatr Neurosurg* **30**(5):225–231.

Shen, L., J. A. Hagen, and I. Papautsky. 2012. Point-of-care colorimetric detection with a smartphone. *Lab Chip* **12**(21):4240–4243.

Siegman, A. E. 1986. *Lasers*. Mill Valley, CA: University Science Books.

So, P. T. C., C. Y. Dong, B. R. Masters, and K. M. Berland. 2000. Two-photon excitation fluorescence microscopy. *Annu Rev Biomed Eng* **2**(1):399–429.

Star, W. M., H. P. Marijnissen, H. Jansen, M. Keijzer, and M. J. van Gemert. 1987. Light dosimetry for photodynamic therapy by whole bladder wall irradiation. *Photochem Photobiol* **46**(5):619–624.

Stepinac, T., C. Felley, P. Jornod, N. Lange, T. Gabrecht, C. Fontolliet, P. Grosjean et al. 2003. Endoscopic fluorescence detection of intraepithelial neoplasia in Barrett's esophagus after oral administration of aminolevulinic acid. *Endoscopy* **35**(8):663–668.

Stummer, W., A. Novotny, H. Stepp, C. Goetz, K. Bise, and H. J. Reulen. 2000. Fluorescence-guided resection of glioblastoma multiforme by using 5-aminolevulinic acid-induced porphyrins: A prospective study in 52 consecutive patients. *J Neurosurg* **93**(6):1003–1013.

Stummer, W., U. Pichlmeier, T. Meinel, O. D. Wiestler, F. Zanella, and H.-J. Reulen. 2006. Fluorescence-guided surgery with 5-aminolevulinic acid for resection of malignant glioma: A randomised controlled multicentre phase III trial. *Lancet Oncol* **7**(5):392–401.

Sugioka, K. and Y. Cheng. 2014. Ultrafast lasers—Reliable tools for advanced materials processing. *Light: Sci Appl* **3**(149). doi: 10.1038/lsa.2014.30.

Themstrup, L., C. A. Banzhaf, M. Mogensen, and G. B. Jemec. 2014. Optical coherence tomography imaging of non-melanoma skin cancer undergoing photodynamic therapy reveals subclinical residual lesions. *Photodiagnosis Photodyn Ther* **11**(1):7–12. doi: 10.1016/j.pdpdt.2013.11.003.

Toge, K. and F. Ito. 2013. Recent research and development of optical fiber monitoring in communication systems. *Photonic Sens* **3**(4):304–313. doi: 10.1007/s13320-013-0127-2.

Trokel, S. L., R. Srinivasan, and B. Braren. 1983. Excimer laser surgery of the cornea. *Am J Ophthalmol* **96**(6):710–715.

Tsai, J. C., C. P. Chiang, H. M. Chen, S. B. Huang, C. W. Wang, M. I. Lee, Y. C. Hsu, C. T. Chen, and T. Tsai. 2004. Photodynamic Therapy of oral dysplasia with topical 5-aminolevulinic acid and light-emitting diode array. *Lasers Surg Med* **34**(1):18–24. doi: 10.1002/lsm.10250.

Turro, N. J., V. Ramamurthy, and J. C. Scaiano. 2010. *Modern Molecular Photochemistry of Organic Molecules*. Sausalito, CA: University Science Books.

Wei, Q., H. Qi, W. Luo, D. Tseng, S. J. Ki, Z. Wan, Z. Gorocs et al. 2013. Fluorescent imaging of single nanoparticles and viruses on a smart phone. *ACS Nano* **7**(10):9147–9155. doi: 10.1021/nn4037706.

Weigel, T. L., S. Yousem, S. Dacic, P. J. Kosco, J. Siegfried, and J. D. Luketich. 2000. Fluorescence bronchoscopic surveillance after curative surgical resection for non-small-cell lung cancer. *Ann Surg Oncol* **7**(3):176–180.

Wilson, B. C. 2002. Photodynamic therapy for cancer: Principles. *Can J Gastroenterol* **16** (6):393–396.

Wilson, B. C. and M. S. Patterson. 1986. The physics of photodynamic therapy. *Phys Med Biol* **31**(4):327–360.

Wise, F. 2013. Lasers for nonlinear microscopy. *Cold Spring Harb Protoc* **2013**(3):205–209.

Wolbarsht, M. L., A. W. Walsh, and G. George. 1981. Melanin, a unique biological absorber. *Appl Optics* **20**(13):2184–2186. doi: 10.1364/AO.20.002184.

Xu, C. and F. W. Wise. 2013. Recent advances in fiber lasers for nonlinear microscopy. *Nat Photonics* **7**:205–209.

Xu, M. and L. V. Wang. 2006. Photoacoustic imaging in biomedicine. *Rev Sci Instrum* **77**(4):041101. doi: http://dx.doi.org/10.1063/1.2195024.

Yang, V. X., P. J. Muller, P. Herman, B. C. Wilson, V. X. D. Yang, P. J. Muller, P. Herman, and B. C. Wilson. 2003. A multispectral fluorescence imaging system: Design and initial clinical tests in intra-operative Photofrin-photodynamic therapy of brain tumors. *Lasers Surg Med* **32**(3):224–232.

Zaak, D. 2001. Endoscopic detection of transitional cell carcinoma with 5-aminolevulinic acid: Results of 1012 fluorescence endoscopies. *Urology* **57**:690–694.

Zargi, M., I. Fajdiga, and L. Smid. 2000. Autofluorescence imaging in the diagnosis of laryngeal cancer. *Eur Arch Otorhinolaryngol* **257**(1):17–23.

Zelickson, B., J. Counters, C. Coles, and M. Selim. 2005. Light patch: Preliminary report of a novel form of blue light delivery for the treatment of actinic keratosis. *Dermatol Surg* **31**(3):375–378.

Zellweger, M., D. Goujon, R. Conde, M. Forrer, H. van den Bergh, and G. Wagnieres. 2001. Absolute autofluorescence spectra of human healthy, metaplastic, and early cancerous bronchial tissue in vivo. *Appl Optics* **40**(22):3784–3791.

Zhu, T. C. and J. C. Finlay. 2006. Prostate PDT dosimetry. *Photodiagnosis Photodyn Ther* **3**(4):234–246. doi: 10.1016/j.pdpdt.2006.08.002.

Zimmermann, T., J. Rietdorf, and R. Pepperkok. 2003. Spectral imaging and its applications in live cell microscopy. *FEBS Lett* **546**(1):87–92.

Zipfel, W. R., R. M. Williams, and W. W. Webb. 2003. Nonlinear magic: Multiphoton microscopy in the biosciences. *Nat Biotechnol* **21**(11):1369–1377. doi: 10.1038/nbt899.

Photochemistry and photophysics of PDT and photosensitizers

MARCIN PTASZEK

2.1 INTRODUCTION

Photodynamic therapy (PDT) relies on the generation of highly cytotoxic species upon illumination of a specific molecular agent known as a photosensitizer.[1,2] In most cases, the photosensitizer itself does not react with biomolecules, but upon illumination reacts with molecular oxygen to generate actual toxic agents, namely, reactive oxygen species (ROS), which includes singlet oxygen $^1O_2$, superoxide radical $O_2^{-\bullet}$, hydroxyl radical $HO^\bullet$, and hydrogen peroxide H_2O_2.[3] The high yield of production of these species upon illumination with light is the key prerequisite for the efficacy of PDT. Selection of the molecular platform with a set of optimized optical and photochemical properties is usually the first step in the development of a useful photosensitizer. This step requires knowledge of both photochemical and chemical processes occurring when a photosensitizer interacts with oxygen, as well as properties of the photosensitizer, particularly in its excited state. This chapter provides a concise overview of key photochemical processes involved in the generation of ROS and a survey of photosensitizers commonly used in PDT, together with the discussion of their properties, relevant to ROS generation.

2.2 BASIC PHOTOCHEMISTRY OF PDT

2.2.1 ABSORPTION OF LIGHT AND PROPERTIES OF EXCITED STATE

The absorption of light to achieve an excited state of the photosensitizer is the first step in the generation of ROS in PDT. The processes of light absorption and energy levels in the excited state can be conveniently described using a Jablonski diagram (Figure 2.1).[4] An organic molecule (which constitutes the vast majority of photosensitizers tested in PDT) in the ground state (the energetically lowest state) possesses an even number of electrons with paired spins (singlet ground state S_0). Absorption of a photon leads to the rearrangement of an electronic configuration in the molecule and formation of a higher-energy excited state, still with all electrons spins paired (the singlet excited states S_1, S_2, etc.). The wavelength of absorption depends on the energy gap between S_1 (or S_2, etc.), and S_0 (ΔE) by the following relation:

$$\lambda_{abs} = \frac{hc}{\Delta E} \tag{2.1}$$

where

λ_{abs} is the wavelength of absorption
h is Planck's constant
c is speed of light

Another important parameter is the probability that a photon with energy matching ΔE will be absorbed by the molecule of interest. From a practical point of view, this probability is described by the molar absorption coefficient ε (also termed the extinction coefficient), which links the absorbance to the concentration of absorbing molecules in Beer's law[4]:

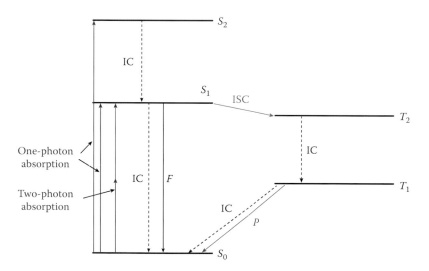

Figure 2.1 Simplified Jablonski diagram.

$$A = \log\left(\frac{I_0}{I}\right) = \varepsilon c l \tag{2.2}$$

where

ε is the molar absorption coefficient $[M^{-1} \cdot cm^{-1}]$

I is the intensity of light after passing through the sample solution

I_0 is the intensity of incident light

c is the concentration of absorbing molecules $[M]$

l is the distance light travels through the sample solution $[cm]$

Both the wavelength of absorption, which is determined by ΔE, and the molar absorption coefficient are important parameters characterizing a photosensitizer. The wavelength of absorption tells us what range of light needs to be used for illumination of the photosensitizer to achieve its excited state. This is particularly critical when the photosensitizer needs to be used for actual medical applications. Human tissue is a highly complex structure, into which light has limited penetration. Generally, two processes can occur that both severely attenuate light intensity in tissue: absorption and scattering.[2,5] Absorption is caused by the certain chemical species present in tissue and cells: hemoglobin, proteins and their cofactors, nucleotides, etc. Most of the cellular components, such as amino acids, flavins, and nucleotides, absorb in the short wavelength spectral window, for example, <500 nm, while hemoglobin absorbs up to 650 nm.[2] The other phenomenon that reduces light intensity in deep tissue is scattering. The degree of light scattering in a given medium, according to the Rayleigh Law, is proportional to $1/\lambda^w$, where w depends on the type of medium; therefore, scattering is more pronounced for light at shorter wavelengths.[2,4] Both absorption and scattering result in light having very limited tissue penetration and both factors (absorption and scattering) are less pronounced for light at longer wavelengths (>650 nm). On the other hand, light with λ > 900 nm is absorbed by water in the body, which may generate excessive and dangerous heating.[2] It is generally recommended, to use deep red and near-infrared (NIR) light with λ range 650–900 nm (sometimes called the first biological window or NIR-I),[5-7] and 1000–1400 nm (second biological window or NIR-II[5]) could be used for the deepest tissue penetration. The large majority of ROS photosensitizers absorb in NIR-I.

Considering that a high absorption coefficient facilitates efficient photosensitizer excitation, ε should be as high as possible (often a value ε > 100,000 $M^{-1} \cdot cm^{-1}$ is cited as most desirable).[8] For many singlet-oxygen photosensitizers, ε falls between 40,000 and 100,000 $M^{-1} \cdot cm^{-1}$ (see Table 2.1 for examples).

In addition to the above-discussed one-photon absorption, where photosensitizers absorb one photon with energy matching $\Delta E = E(S_n) - E(S_0)$, it is possible under certain conditions and for certain molecules to simultaneously absorb two photons of the same energy, equal to the $1/2\Delta E$ each. The probability of two-photon absorption is proportional to the square of the light intensity at the given wavelength and is often quantitatively expressed by two-photon absorption cross-sectional δ (unit 1 Göppert–Meyer, 1 GM = 10^{-50} $cm^4 \cdot s \cdot photons^{-1} \cdot molecule^{-1}$).[9] Some carefully designed, efficient two-photon absorbers possess δ > 10,000 GM at the wavelength of maximum of two-photon absorbance,[9] while typical photosensitizers used in PDT exhibit δ < 100 GM (e.g., for tetraphenyl-porphyrin (TPP) (**1**, Table 2.1) δ = 24 GM at 760 nm).[10]

Two-photon absorption allows utilization of light with twice the wavelength relative to one-photon excitation. Therefore, this technique enables excitation in the NIR-I range for many photosensitizers, which lack strong one-photon absorbance in that range. Secondly, two-photon excitation allows using a very focused laser beam for illumination, providing a high spatial resolution of excitation since the photosensitizer can be selectively excited in a small volume of tissue.[9]

Even a brief discussion of the relationship between the structure and absorption properties of molecules (absorption wavelength, molar absorption coefficient, and two-photon absorption cross section) is far beyond the scope of this chapter. Organic molecules with high molar absorption coefficients in NIR-I usually possess a large, often polycyclic conjugated system of double bonds. For efficient two-photon excitation, even a larger conjugated system, with the proper symmetry and careful choice of electron-withdrawing and electron-donating substituents, is required.[9]

Table 2.1 Photochemical properties of representative ROS photosensitizers

Compound	Compound	Properties
1	Protoporphyrin-IX dimethyl ester	λ_{max} = 631 nm[30] ε_{max} = 5000 M$^{-1}\cdot$cm^{-1} [30] Φ_{ISC} = 0.68 (0.73 in the presence of air) τ_T = 320 μs Φ_Δ = 0.57 (0.62 in oxygen saturated)[31] All data in benzene.
2	Tetraphenylporphyrin (TPP)	λ_{max} = 648 nm[12] ε_{max} = 4000 M$^{-1}\cdot$cm^{-1} [12] Φ_f = 0.11[12] τ_S = 9.3 ns[12] Φ_{ISC} = 0.69 (air-free benzene), 0.71 (air-equilibrated benzene)[31] τ_T = 115 μs[12] τ_T = 200 μs[31] Φ_Δ = 0.68 (air-saturated benzene)[31] All data in toluene, unless noted otherwise.
3	Tetrakis(*m*-hydroxyphenyl)porphyrin	λ_{max} = 644 nm ε_{max} = 3400 M$^{-1}\cdot$cm^{-1} Φ_f = 0.12 Φ_{ISC} = 0.69 τ_T = 120 μs E_T = 137 kJ/mol Φ_Δ = 0.46 (0.59 in oxygen saturated) All data in MeOH[32].
4	Tetrakis(*m*-hydroxyphenyl)chlorin (FOSCAN)	λ_{max} = 650 nm ε_{max} = 29,600 M$^{-1}\cdot$cm^{-1} Φ_f = 0.089 Φ_{ISC} = 0.89 τ_T = 50 μs E_T = 140.5 kJ/mol Φ_Δ = 0.43 (0.59 in oxygen saturated) All data in MeOH[32].

(Continued)

Table 2.1 (*Continued*) Photochemical properties of representative ROS photosensitizers

Compound	Compound	Properties
5	 Tetrakis(*m*-hydroxyphenyl)bacteriochlorin	λ_{max} = 735 nm ε_{max} = 91,000 M$^{-1}\cdot$cm^{-1} Φ_f = 0.11 Φ_{ISC} = 0.83 τ_T = 53 µs E_T = 119 kJ/mol Φ_Δ = 0.43 (0.62 in oxygen saturated) All data in MeOH[32].
6	 Purlytin	λ_{max} = 656 nm ε_{max} = 42,800 M$^{-1}\cdot$cm^{-1} Φ_f = 0.024 τ_S = 1.0 ns Φ_{ISC} = 0.86 (DMSO) τ_T = 34 µs (DMSO) Φ_Δ = 0.71 (MeCN) All data in MeOH, except noted otherwise.[33]
7	 TOOKAD	λ_{max} = 760 nm (water/liposome) ε_{max} = 100,000 M$^{-1}\cdot$cm^{-1} τ_S = 0.091 ns Φ_{ISC} > 0.98 τ_T = 5 µs Φ_Δ = 1 All data in acetone, except noted otherwise.[24]
8	 Dicyanobacteriochlorin	λ_{max} = 748 nm Φ_f = 0.14 τ_S = 4.1 ns Φ_{ISC} = 0.43 τ_T = 84 µs (THF) E_T = 1.11 eV All data in toluene, except noted otherwise.[17]
9	 Zinc complex of dicyanobacteriochlorin	λ_{max} = 761 nm Φ_f = 0.15 τ_S = 3.9 ns Φ_{ISC} = 0.63 τ_T = 121 µs (THF) E_T = 1.09 eV All data in toluene, except noted otherwise.[17]

(*Continued*)

Table 2.1 (*Continued*) Photochemical properties of representative ROS photosensitizers

Compound	Compound	Properties
10	Palladium complex of dicyanobacteriochlorin	λ_{max} = 753 nm Φ_f < 0.007 τ_S = 0.023 ns Φ_{ISC} = 0.99 τ_T = 7 µs (THF) E_T = 1.11 eV All data in toluene, except noted otherwise.[17]
11	Strongly conjugated porphyrin dyad	λ_{max} = 669 and 728 nm ε_{max} = 58,900 $M^{-1} \cdot cm^{-1}$ and 79,400 $M^{-1} \cdot cm^{-1}$ Φ_{ISC} = 0.74 τ_T = 400 µs E_T = 1.30 eV (average from three methods) Φ_Δ = 0.70 (phosphorescence), 0.80 (DPBF) All data in toluene.[34]
12	Zinc complex of phthalocyanine	λ_{max} = 669 nm ε_{max} = 270,000 $M^{-1} \cdot cm^{-1}$ Φ_f = 0.32 τ_S = 4.73 ns Φ_{ISC} = 0.50 τ_T = 250 µs Φ_Δ = 0.40 All data in DMSO.[35]
13	Silicon complex of naphthocyanine	λ_{max} = 776 nm ε_{max} = 650,000 $M^{-1} \cdot cm^{-1}$ τ_S = 2.83 ns Φ_{ISC} = 0.39 τ_T = 331 µs Φ_Δ = 0.35 (air saturated) All data in benzene.[36]

(Continued)

Table 2.1 (*Continued*) Photochemical properties of representative ROS photosensitizers

Compound	Compound	Properties
14	\n\nLutetium complex of texaphyrin	λ_{max} = 733 nm\n$\varepsilon_{max}$ = 22,730 $M^{-1} \cdot cm^{-1}$\n$\Phi_f$ = 0.01\n$\tau_S$ = 0.380 ns\n$\Phi_{ISC}$ = 0.40\n$\tau_T$ = 17 μs\n$E_T$ = 1.30 eV\n$\Phi_\Delta$ = 0.11 (oxygen-saturated H_2O)\nAll data in H_2O, pH = 7.[26]
15	\n\nTetraphenylporphycene	λ_{max} = 659 nm\n$\varepsilon_{max}$ = 50,100 $M^{-1} \cdot cm^{-1}$\n$\Phi_{ISC}$ = 0.33\n$\Phi_\Delta$ = 0.23\nAll data in toluene.[10]
16	\n\nIodinated BODIPY	λ_{max} = 534 nm\n$\varepsilon_{max}$ = 110,000 $M^{-1} \cdot cm^{-1}$\n$\Phi_f$ = 0.02\n$\Phi_\Delta$ = comparable to Rose Bengal\nAll data in MeOH.[37]
17	\n\nBODIPY with styryl substituents	λ_{max} = 648 nm\n$\varepsilon_{max}$ = 45,000 $M^{-1} \cdot cm^{-1}$\n$\Phi_f$ = 0.095\n$\Phi_\Delta$ = 0.10 (in PBS)\nAll data in acetonitrile, except\n noted otherwise.[38]
18	\n\naza-BODIPY	λ_{max} = 660 nm\n$\varepsilon_{max}$ = 83,000\n$\Phi_{ISC}$ = 0.68\n$\tau_T$ = 1.9 μs\n$\Phi_\Delta$ = 0.34 (oxygen-saturated\n solution)\nAll data in DMSO.[27]

(*Continued*)

Table 2.1 (*Continued*) Photochemical properties of representative ROS photosensitizers

Compound	Compound	Properties
19	BODIPY with fused thiophene ring	λ_{max} = 694 nm ε_{max} = 230,000 $M^{-1} \cdot cm^{-1}$ Φ_f = 0.04 Φ_Δ = 0.63 All data in CH_2Cl_2.[39]
20	BODIPY dyad	λ_{max} = 506 nm ε_{max} = 136,000 Φ_f = 0.022 τ_T = 115.6 μs Φ_Δ = 0.64 All data in CH_2Cl_2.[40]
21	Iodinated squaraine	λ_{max} = 610 nm (20% vol./vol. MeOH/H_2O) ε_{max} = 47,000 $M^{-1} \cdot cm^{-1}$ (20% vol./vol. MeOH/H_2O) Φ_f = 0.002 (2% vol./vol. MeOH/H_2O) Φ_{ISC} = 0.5 τ_T = 36 μs Φ_Δ = 0.47 All data in MeOH, unless noted otherwise).[41]
22	Thiosquaraine	λ_{max} = 687 nm ε_{max} = 157,000 $M^{-1} \cdot cm^{-1}$ Φ_f < 0.001 Φ_{ISC} = 0.97 τ_T = 245 μs Φ_Δ = 1.0 All data in toluene.[42]

Absorption of a photon with suitable energy results in a molecule in the excited state (S_1, S_2, etc., depending on the energy of absorbed photon). A molecule in any singlet excited state higher than S_1 very quickly (within picoseconds, 10^{-12} s) loses the energy nonradiatively (i.e., without emission of photons in a process called internal conversion [IC]) and relaxes to the first singlet excited state S_1.[4] The S_1 relaxes then to the ground S_0 state, usually within hundreds of picoseconds to tens of nanoseconds either nonradiatively by IC, or emitting a photon, through the process called fluorescence. The third possible process for the deactivation of S_1 is nonradiative flipping of the spin of the electron by the process called intersystem crossing (ISC), and formation of the so-called triplet state T, which posses two electrons of unpaired spin. Depending on the specific molecule, and energies of the given states, either the first triplet excited state T_1 or higher triplet excited states T_2, T_3, etc., can be formed. The important observation is that, according to Hund's rule, T_1 is always lower in energy than S_1, and similarly T_2 is lower in energy than S_2, etc.[11] In analogy to the singlet states, the higher excited triplet states (T_2, T_3, etc.) quickly relax to T_1 via IC, and T_1 relaxes to the ground state either nonradiatively through IC, or emitting a photon in the process called phosphorescence P. Both processes, $S_1 \rightarrow T_1$ and $T_1 \rightarrow S_1$, are so-called forbidden processes, which means that their occurrence is not allowed by the quantum mechanical rules.[4,11] The process of spin–orbit coupling, that is, mixing of the orbital wave function and spin wave function, allows ISC ($S_1 \rightarrow T_1$, $T_1 \rightarrow S_0$, etc.) to occur under certain circumstances (see later text); however, these processes are usually less probable than processes that do not change the spin. Therefore, deactivation of T_1 typically occurs within a longer timescale (usually tens to hundreds of microseconds).[4,11]

Quantitatively, the processes of deactivation of excited states can be described using rate constants for each deactivation process: k_{ic}, k_f, k_{ISC}, and k_p.[4] The rate of deactivation of S_1 is given by

$$r(S_1) = (k_{ic} + k_f + k_{ISC})[S_1] \tag{2.3}$$

Conversely, the rate of deactivation of the triplet state is given by

$$r(T_1) = (k_{ic} + k_p)[T_1] \tag{2.4}$$

where
  $r(S_1)$ and $r(T_1)$ are the rates of decay [$mol \cdot dm^{-3} \cdot s^{-1}$] for S_1 and T_1, respectively
  $[S_1]$ and $[T_1]$ are concentrations of the molecule in the first excited singlet and triplet states, respectively, at a given time point

Both expressions are valid assuming the absence of deactivation processes other than these discussed earlier.

The values $\tau_S = 1/(k_{ic} + k_f + k_{ISC})$ and $\tau_T = 1/(k_{ic} + k_p)$ are called singlet excited state lifetime and triplet excited state lifetime, respectively. The physical interpretation of the excited state lifetime is the time after excitation with an infinitely short pulse of light, at which the concentration of molecules in the excited state is equal to e^{-1} (37%) of the initial concentration.[4]

The quantum yield for a given process is defined as a ratio of the rate constant for that process over the sum of rate constants for each process contributing to deactivation of the given excited state. For example, the quantum yield of fluorescence is defined as

$$\Phi_f = \frac{k_f}{(k_{ic} + k_f + k_{ISC})} \tag{2.5}$$

while quantum yield of the triplet state formation (ISC) is defined as

$$\Phi_{ISC} = \frac{k_{ISC}}{(k_{ic} + k_f + k_{ISC})}. \tag{2.6}$$

The definition of Φ_f given earlier is equivalent with "operational" definition of fluorescence quantum yield as a ratio of photon emitted in fluorescence to the number of the photons absorbed.[4]

The rate constants, lifetimes, and quantum yields for given processes and states can be determined by spectroscopic measurements and are important parameters in evaluation of the effectiveness of an individual photosensitizer. For typical organic molecules, the values for k_f and k_{ic} are in the range of 10^8–10^9 s^{-1}, τ_S in the range of 500 ps to 10 ns, and τ_T in the range of 1–1000 µs.[4,11] Values of quantum yields Φ_f and Φ_{ISC} vary broadly from 0 to 1. The presence of other deactivation processes (such as the interaction of the excited state with oxygen) can dramatically reduce lifetimes of the excited states and decrease quantum yields of fluorescence and ISC. For example, for TPP **2** τ_T in deoxygenated toluene is 115 µs while in air-equilibrated toluene drops more than 400 times to 0.279 µs.[12]

2.2.2 GENERATION OF THE SINGLET OXYGEN

Singlet oxygen $^1O_2$ is a highly reactive state of oxygen, and it is assumed to be one of the major ROS responsible for the efficiency of PDT.[1,3,13] Oxygen in its ground state, $^3O_2$, has two unpaired electrons, and therefore, it is in the triplet state (contrary to the majority of organic molecules, for which the ground state is the singlet state).[3,11,13] The lowest excited state of oxygen is $^1O_2$, the formation of which requires flipping of the spin of an electron. The generation of $^1O_2$ by an excited photosensitizer is often referred to as the type II mechanism.[3,13]

The formation of $^1O_2$ requires physical collision of ground state triplet oxygen with an excited state of the photosensitizer; energy from the photosensitizer is transferred to oxygen, accompanied by flipping the spins of electrons in both oxygen and photosensitizer.[11] The photosensitizer excited state decays to a state with lower energy and different spin. The most common process in PDT is the collision of the photosensitizer in T_1 with triplet oxygen, which produces singlet oxygen and photosensitizer in the ground singlet state (Equation 2.7).[11,13] This process is allowed since the sums of the spins in the photosensitizer and oxygen before and after process are the same.[11]

$$T_1\left(-\,-\right)+\,^3O_2\left(\downarrow\downarrow\right)\rightarrow S_0\left(-\downarrow\right)+\,^1O_2\left(\downarrow-\right) \tag{2.7}$$

There are several important requirements that need to be met for efficient photosensitization of $^1O_2$. The difference in energy between $^3O_2$ and $^1O_2$ is 94 kJ/mol = 0.974 eV[8,11]; therefore, the energy of the T_1 must be at least this level. For irreversible formation of the singlet oxygen, the photosensitizer T_1 energy should be around 15 kJ/mol above the energy of $^1O_2$, which gives the minimal energy for T_1 $E(T_1) = 109$ kJ/mol = 1.13 eV.[8] The majority of organic molecules absorbing in NIR-I fulfills this requirement.

Considering the formation of $^1O_2$ requires physical collision of $^3O_2$ with the photoexcited photosensitizer, it can be described as a dynamic quenching of the excited state photosensitizer by oxygen.[11] The efficiency of this process can be measured, for example, by determining the reduction of the lifetime of the T_1 photosensitizer in the presence of oxygen, as described by the Stern–Volmer law[4,11]:

$$\frac{\tau_0}{\tau}=1+k_q\tau_0[^3O_2] \tag{2.8}$$

where

τ_0 is the lifetime of the triplet state in the absence of oxygen
τ is the lifetime of the triplet state in the presence of oxygen
k_q is the quenching constant
$[^3O_2]$ is the concentration of the ground state oxygen

Generally, a more pronounced reduction of the triplet excited state lifetime (higher value on the left side) indicates more efficient production of $^1O_2$. The value of k_q in cells for typical organic photosensitizers is estimated as $0.8–5.0 \cdot 10^8$ $mol \cdot dm^{-3} \cdot s^{-1}$.[14] The concentration of $^3O_2$ in the tissue strongly depends on the distance from blood vessels, and it is estimated as 6.75–19.8 µM.[15] Therefore, a long lifetime for T_1 is essential for efficient singlet-oxygen photosensitization. It is generally recommended that the lifetime of the excited state (determined in homogenous solution) in the absence of oxygen should be >100 µs,[8] which is in most cases fulfilled by the T_1 of typical organic photosensitizers. This is also the reason why the triplet excited state of a photosensitizer is much better suited for $^1O_2$ photosensitization than the S_1, for which the lifetime rarely exceeds 10 ns. It is worth noting, however, that there are examples of efficient $^1O_2$ photosensitizers, for which the lifetime of T_1 falls in the range of 1–5 µs (see Table 2.1 for examples).

2.2.3 Photosensitized generation of oxygen radicals

Although $^1O_2$ is generally considered as the main cytotoxic agent generated and operating in PDT, it has become apparent that generation of oxygen radicals is equally, and in the case of some photosensitizers, more important than generation of $^1O_2$. Generation of oxygen radicals by a photosensitizer is often referred to as the type I mechanism[3,13] and involves formation of superoxide radical ($O_2^{\bullet-}$), hydroxyl radical ($HO^\bullet$), and hydrogen peroxide (H_2O_2).[3] The process of oxygen radicals formation has been studied in detail for some photosensitizers (e.g., bacteriochlorins, see later text). It is generally accepted that generation of oxygen radicals is initiated by electron transfer from excited photosensitizers to molecular oxygen, which results in formation of $O_2^{\bullet-}$ and cation radical of photosensitizers ($P^{+\bullet}$, oxidation of photosensitizer).[3,16–18]

$$P^* + {}^3O_2 \rightarrow P^{+\bullet} + O_2^{\bullet-} \tag{2.9}$$

Electron transfer is accompanied by degradation of photosensitizers as the resulting $P^{+\bullet}$ is unstable and highly reactive. However, in the presence of secondary electron donors, such as amino acid side chains in proteins, the transient $P^{+\bullet}$ is reduced back to the neutral form of P.

$$P^{+\bullet} + D \rightarrow P + D^{+\bullet} \tag{2.10}$$

For example, it has been shown that illumination of an aqueous solution of bacteriochlorin derivative (WT11) results in generation of superoxide radicals (with no detectable $^1O_2$) and fast degradation of photosensitizers.[18] However, irradiation of aqueous solution of the noncovalent complex of the same bacteriochlorin with bovine serum albumin (BSA) results in equally efficient formation of oxygen radicals and significantly slower degradation of photosensitizers. It has been postulated that redox-active amino acid side chains from BSA serve as an electron donor, which reduces $P^{+\bullet}$.[18]

The exact mechanism of electron transfer from a photosensitizer to oxygen was studied in detail for selected photosensitizers, for example, bacteriochlorins.[16] It is proposed that the first step is formation of a complex (exciplex) between a photoexcited photosensitizer and ground state oxygen, followed by charge transfer (CT) in the resulting exciplex.[16] The occurrence of CT from a photosensitizer to oxygen requires that the free energy for CT complex formation is negative. ΔG can be calculated from the following Rehm–Weller equation[19]:

$$\Delta G = E_{ox} - E_{red} - E_{00} + e^2/\varepsilon R_{DA} \tag{2.11}$$

where

E_{ox} is the oxidation potential of the photosensitizer
E_{red} is the reduction potential of oxygen
E_{00} is the energy of the excited state of the photosensitizer
e is the charge of electron
ε is the dielectric constant of medium
R is the distance between the photosensitizer and oxygen

Therefore, the CT process is facilitated by a low ionization potential (i.e., low oxidation potential E_{ox}) of the photosensitizer and a highly polar medium (e.g., water, high ε). For example, it has been shown that for porphyrin generation of $^1O_2$ is the main pathway of ROS production, whereas for bacteriochlorins, a significant contribution of superoxide generation is observed. This observation can be rationalized by the markedly higher oxidation potential of porphyrins compared to the structurally analogous bacteriochlorins, and therefore, formation of the CT state in the case of porphyrins is energetically unfavorable.[16]

There has been an alternative mechanism proposed for the generation of $O_2^{-\bullet}$ by photosensitizers.[17] It has been proposed that a photosensitizer in T_1 reacts first with an electron donor, to undergo reduction, rather than oxidation. This produces a radical anion, which subsequently reacts with $^3O_2$ to produce $O_2^{-\bullet}$ (Equations 2.12 and 2.13).

$$P^* + D \rightarrow P^{-\bullet} + D^{+\bullet} \tag{2.12}$$

$$P^{-\bullet} + {}^3O_2 \rightarrow P + O_2^{-\bullet} \tag{2.13}$$

Ascorbate has been proposed to act as an electron donor, capable of reducing the excited photosensitizer. For this mechanism, the electron affinity (i.e., reduction potential) of the photosensitizer in its excited state is important as a less-negative reduction potential facilitates reduction of the photosensitizer.

The photogenerated superoxide $O_2^{-\bullet}$ is a highly reactive species and reacts readily with biomolecules.[3] Alternatively, it can disproportionate to produce hydroxyl radical $HO^{\bullet}$ and hydrogen peroxide H_2O_2.[3]

$$2O_2^{-\bullet} + 2H^+ \rightarrow H_2O_2 + O_2 \tag{2.14}$$

Electron transfer from a photosensitizer to oxygen requires a collisional, diffusion-controlled interaction between the photoexcited photosensitizer and oxygen, and similarly to $^1O_2$ generation this is facilitated by a long-lived excited state of the former. Thus, formation of superoxide radical is much more probable in the case of T_1 of photosensitizers.

In the view of these, efficient production of the triplet state photosensitizer upon excitation (high value of Φ_{ISC}) is a prerequisite for efficient photosensitization of $^1O_2$ and oxygen radicals. As it was mentioned, the transition $S_1 \rightarrow T_1$ is a forbidden process, and for most of the organic compounds $\Phi_{ISC} \sim 0$. The design of a photosensitizer that produces a long-lived triplet state with a high quantum yield upon excitation is one of the challenging tasks in the development of efficient photosensitizers. Recall that ISC is possible due to spin–orbit coupling, that is, mixing of the orbital and spin wave functions.[11] Spin–orbit coupling for many simple organic compounds is negligible; however, it can be greatly enhanced by introducing a heavy element, most commonly Br, I, Zn, Pd, Pt, In, etc., see later for examples. This is because spin–orbit coupling is proportional to Z^4, where Z is the atomic number (so-called heavy atom effect).[11] This approach allows for a significant increase of Φ_{ISC} for many organic compounds; however, the heavy atom effect also increases the rate of $T_1 \rightarrow S_0$ IC and therefore decreases in the T_1 lifetime (see examples given later). There are several classes of organic compounds with high Φ_{ISC} without the presence of heavy elements (e.g., oligopyrrolic macrocycles, see later text).

2.2.4 SINGLET-OXYGEN QUANTUM YIELD

Singlet-oxygen quantum yield Φ_Δ is defined as the number of molecules of $^1O_2$ per number of photons absorbed by a photosensitizer.[11] Sometimes, also the efficiency of singlet-oxygen generation $S = \Phi_\Delta / \Phi_{ISC}$ is defined, which describes how efficiently the triplet state of a photosensitizer produces $^1O_2$.[11] Φ_Δ is often used for the initial evaluation of the efficiency of photosensitizers; however, some care needs to be taken in the interpretation and comparison of the results of Φ_Δ measurements. First, measured Φ_Δ depends on the properties of the solvent (or other medium in which the sample is measured), such as polarity, viscosity, and oxygen concentration. Therefore, it is reasonable to compare values obtained under identical conditions (solvent, temperature) and oxygen concentration (e.g., in solvent that is air- or oxygen-saturated). Moreover, there are different methods used for the determination of Φ_Δ, which do not always provide the same results. The most direct method of those prevalent in the literature relies on the quantification of the $^1O_2$ luminescence at 1270 nm, and comparison with a reference of known Φ_Δ.[20] This method allows for selective quantification of photosensitized $^1O_2$. While this method allows for accurate determination of the amount of $^1O_2$ produced by a photosensitizer, it does not provide any information about oxygen radicals production; therefore, it does not necessarily accurately reflect the photosensitizer efficiency.[18] The other methods for the determination of Φ_Δ utilizes a chemical trap, which reacts with $^1O_2$.[21] The amount of $^1O_2$ can be quantified by monitoring the amount of products formed or the fraction of consumed trap.[21] The most popular trap is 2,5-diphenylisobenzofuran (DPBF), which reacts with $^1O_2$ to give 1,2-benzoylbenzene.[21] DPBF absorbs strongly at 414 nm, and fluoresces at 450 nm, whereas the resulting product is not fluorescent and does not absorb in the same spectral window. Therefore, monitoring the rate of disappearance of either absorption or emission of DPBF and comparing this rate with the rate for the reference photosensitizer allows for the determination of Φ_Δ. However, there is a report that DPBF also reacts with superoxide radical, and the resulting "Φ_Δ" may potentially consist of contributions from both $^1O_2$ and $O_2{}^{\bullet-}$.[21,22] There are several fluorescent probes, which allow selective detection of $^1O_2$ or reactive oxygen radicals.[23] In principle, this enables selective quantification of both species.[23] Alternatively, oxygen radicals can be trapped with certain radical spin traps, and resulting radicals can be detected using electron paramagnetic resonance (EPR).[24]

2.3 PHOTOCHEMISTRY OF COMMON ROS PHOTOSENSITIZERS

The ROS photosensitizers for PDT can be categorized in four generations: (1) photosensitizers capable of producing ROS upon illumination, (2) photosensitizers with spectral and photochemical properties optimized for application in the deep tissue, (3) photosensitizers with an additional targeting unit that enhances their selective accumulation in the target tissue or tumor, and (4) photosensitizers for which photosensitization of ROS is selectively activated only in the target cancer cells.[13,25] All four generations of photosensitizers have been investigated, while those that have been clinically tested or approved for clinical use belong to the first and second generations of photosensitizers.[25]

The properties of "ideal" photosensitizers for use in PDT have been listed by several authors.[8,25] In the view of these consideration, the photochemical properties of photosensitizers that allow for efficient generation of ROS in the tissue or cells include (1) strong absorption band in NIR-I spectral window (650–900 nm), with $\varepsilon > 100,000$ $M^{-1} \cdot cm^{-1}$, (2) high yield of ISC ($\Phi_{ISC} > 0.70$), and (3) long-lived triplet state (with $\tau_T > 100$ μs). It is also desirable that a photosensitizer is fluorescent, so it can be conveniently tracked and localized using fluorescence imaging.[8] Note that fluorescence is competitive with ISC; therefore, highly fluorescent molecules usually posses only moderate-to-low Φ_{ISC}. Ideally, a photosensitizer should also be photostable; for example, it should not undergo photoinduced degradation called photobleaching. Obviously, these are basic spectral and photochemical properties of photosensitizers; there are several other important requirements to be fulfilled, such as chemical purity, proper lipophilicity/hydrophilicity balance, ease of synthesize, lack of nonsystemic toxicity, etc. which will not be discussed here.

There are many examples of efficient photosensitizers for which spectral properties are significantly "below" those listed earlier. For example, a lutetium complex of texaphyrin possesses very moderate Φ_Δ (0.11).[26] Many photosensitizers with high Φ_{ISC} possess short τ_T (<10 μs; e.g., see 7,[24] 10,[17] 18[27]). One of the challenges in proper assessment of photochemical properties of ROS photosensitizers for PDT is that the crucial properties are often optimized based on their performance in vitro, in homogenous solutions and often in organic solvents. The same properties can be significantly altered at the site of their operation, in cells or in tissue, where the local physicochemical microenvironment, such as polarity, viscosity, redox microenvironment, and interaction with certain ions or (bio)molecules, can significantly affect the properties of photosensitizers. For example, the Pd(II) complex of bacteriochlorin 7 exhibits Φ_Δ in acetone of 1.0, while in aqueous micelles it drops to 0.5.[24]

There are a large number of compounds that have been tested as potential photosensitizers for PDT or for which high Φ_Δ or just the ability to generate ROS has been reported. Here, the most important or most promising photosensitizers are described, together with their photochemical characteristics. For a comprehensive review of singlet-oxygen photosensitizers and their properties, see Reference 28.

2.3.1 TETRAPYRROLIC MACROCYCLES AND RELATED COMPOUNDS

Tetrapyrrolic macrocycles are by far the most intensively exploited photosensitizers in PDT.[6,7] Most of the photosensitizers approved for clinical use or clinically tested belong to this class of compounds.[6] The majority of research on mechanistic aspects of PDT has been done using tetrapyrrolic macrocycles.[5,6,8] Photochemistry of these macrocycles has also been very broadly studied.[29] This class of compounds includes (1) tetrapyrrolic, porphyrinic macrocycles (porphyrins, chlorins, bacteriochlorins); (2) phthalocyanines; and (3) expanded and modified porphyrins. The photochemical properties of representative macrocycles, including those that have undergone clinical trials, and model compounds used in research, are presented in Table 2.1.

The "parent" family of tetrapyrrolic macrocycles includes porphyrins (e.g., **1**, **2**, **3**, **11**), chlorins (e.g., **4**, **6**), and bacteriochlorins (e.g., **5**, **7–10**). The porphyrin backbone is a fully unsaturated macrocycle, where 4 five-membered pyrrole rings are connected with four methine carbons (called *meso* carbons). The partially saturated congener of porphyrin, with one partially saturated pyrrole ring is called a chlorin, while the congener with two partially saturated pyrrole rings on opposite sides is called a bacteriochlorin.[29] The latter, partially saturated tetrapyrrolic macrocycles, are called in general hydroporphyrins. Porphyrins and hydroporphyrins are all aromatic by virtue of a conjugated 18π-electron system. Porphyrins and hydroporphyrins posses multiple absorption bands; B_x and B_y bands located in UV/blue spectral window (330–370 nm for bacteriochlorins, 400–420 nm for chlorins and porphyrins), Q_x band (500–520 nm), and Q_y band (650 nm, chlorins and porphyrins, >700 nm, bacteriochlorins).[29] The presence of long-wavelength Q_y bands located in the therapeutic optical windows makes these macrocycles suitable for applications in deep tissue; however, the molar absorption coefficient for that band varies significantly between the classes of tetrapyrrolic macrocycles: 4000 $M^{-1} \cdot cm^{-1}$ for simple porphyrins, 40,000–60,000 for chlorins, and 100,000 for bacteriochlorins.[6,29] Each macrocycle can coordinate a central metal cation through four nitrogen–metal coordination bonds.[29] Tetrapyrrolic macrocycles exhibit inherently high quantum yields of ISC, without the presence of a heavy element, with typical values of $\Phi_{ISC} > 0.5$ (see data in Table 2.1). The lifetime of the triplet state varies significantly: for metal-free porphyrins, they are typically >100 µs; however, for metal complexes they can drop as short as 1 µs. The coordination of heavy non-open-shell metal cations greatly increases the Φ_Δ value, up to unity; however, it is accompanied by large reduction of T_1 lifetime. The different metal atoms that greatly enhance ISC include Pd(II), Pt(III), and Sn(IV).[29]

Coordination to most of the transition metal cations (e.g., Fe(II), Fe(III), Ni(II), Cu(II), Co(III), etc.) results in fast and efficient quenching of the excited state and negligible ISC.[29]

Porphyrin derivatives have been very intensively investigated as singlet-oxygen photosensitizers, and they constitute the first clinically approved therapeutic photosensitizer—Photofrin, which is mixture of oligomers of hematoporphyrin.[6,7] The major limitation of porphyrins as a photosensitizer in PDT is their low extinction coefficient in the therapeutic window. Therefore, chlorins and bacteriochlorins have recently received much more attention. Chlorin derivatives include [tetra(*m*-hydroxy)phenylchlorin],[32] and purlytin (tin complex of a chlorin called etiopurpurin),[33] while bacteriochlorin derivatives include Tookad (palladium complex of bacteriochlorophyll).[24] Bacteriochlorins seem to possess the most promising sets of optical properties to be applied as photosensitizers for PDT, including strong absorption in near-IR spectral window and high Φ_{ISC} (typically >0.50, which can reach near unity for metal complexes). It is worth noting that Pd bacteriochlorin **10** exhibits the highest PDT efficiency in intracellular studies compared to analogous Zn complex **9** and metal-free bacteriochlorin **8**, despite having a significantly shorter τ_T (7 µs for **10** compared to 84 µs and 121 µs for **8** and **9**).[17] Apparently even such a short triplet lifetime is sufficient for generation of ROS. Bacteriochlorins are also very efficient in generation of oxygen radicals due to their low oxidation potential (via oxidative mechanism, Equation 2.10).[16] The recent results suggest that bacteriochlorins may also photosensitize oxygen radicals via the reductive mechanism (Equations 2.12 and 2.13).[17] If that is the case, the reduction potential of bacteriochlorins also needs to be properly adjusted. Both oxidation and reduction potential, as well as wavelength of absorption and emission, as well as Φ_{ISC} can be broadly tuned either by structural modification of the macrocycle (placing electron-withdrawing, electron-donating, or conjugated substituents) or by metal coordination.[16]

The chief drawback in the applications of bacteriochlorins (from the photochemical point of view) is their low photostability, specifically those derivatives that produce ROS via electron transfer.[17]

Several classes of porphyrin derivatives have been synthesized and examined in order to improve their photochemical properties and develop better photosensitizers.[6,29] One of the notable approaches includes strongly conjugated porphyrin oligomers, that is, arrays of two or more porphyrins that are connected by a linker that provides strong electronic conjugation between macrocycles (exemplified by structure **11**).[34] It has been found that in strongly conjugated porphyrin arrays absorption in the NIR-I was significantly increased compared to the parent monomers.[34] Interestingly, increasing the number of conjugated porphyrins in arrays has led to a marked decrease of ISC, and consequently singlet-oxygen yield.[34] The strongly conjugated porphyrin dimers possess much larger two-photon absorption cross section than porphyrin monomers and therefore are better suited for two-photon PDT.[34]

2.3.1.1 PHTHALOCYANINES

Phthalocyanines are macrocyclic compounds composed of four isoindole moieties linked by nitrogen atoms. Phthalocyanines possess a strong absorption band around 670 nm (with $\varepsilon > 100,000 \text{ M}^{-1} \cdot \text{cm}^{-1}$, e.g., **12**[35]), which can be further shifted toward longer wavelength (760 nm), and intensified ($\varepsilon > 600,000 \text{ M}^{-1} \cdot \text{cm}^{-1}$) by expanding the aromatic system (e.g., naphthocyanines, **13**[36]). Phthalocyanines possess moderate-to-high Φ_{ISC}, which, similarly to porphyrins, can be significantly enhanced by coordination to heavy metals (e.g., see Reference 29). The chief obstacle in broader applications of phthalocyanines is their large aromatic, hydrophobic system, which causes difficulties in their solubilization in organic, and especially aqueous media. One of the solutions to this lack of solubility is the complexation with hexacoordinating metals (e.g., Si, analogously to that in **13**), to which axial water-solubilizing substituents can be attached. Such substituents, localized above and below the macrocyclic plane, prevent facial aggregation of macrocycles and increase solubility.[43]

2.3.1.2 EXPANDED AND MODIFIED PORPHYRINS

There are a huge number of pyrrolic macrocycles described in the literature with modified structures, for example, with different numbers of pyrrolic units, different connection between them, and/or different heterocyclic or carbocyclic units incorporated into the macrocycle.[44] One of the chief motivations for the development of such a rich palette of compounds was an interest in whether the optical properties of parent porphyrins could be further modified or expanded for a variety of applications. Many expanded porphyrins have been tested as ROS-generating photosensitizers, and some of them have been proven to be efficient ROS sensitizers. Two examples from representative classes of such macrocycles are given in Table 2.1. Texaphyrins (e.g., **14**) are expanded porphyrins, where one pyrrole moiety has been replaced by *o*-phenylenediamine.[26] Texaphyrins, and their metal complexes, similarly to porphyrins, show a high Φ_{ISC} with an absence of heavy elements and, contrary to porphyrins, show a relatively high absorption in NIR-I. Lutetium complex of texaphyrins (Lutex) is currently under phase II clinical trials.[26]

Porphycenes (e.g., **15**) are porphyrin isomers, with a different arrangement of the *meso* carbons, they exhibit moderate Φ_{ISC}, which can be greatly enhanced by palladium complexation, and relatively high absorbance in NIR-I.[10] Porphycene exhibits a high two-photon cross section compared to porphyrins. The determined value of δ for **10** is 2280 GM (at 770 nm), while δ for TPP is 24 GM (at 760 nm).[10]

2.3.2 BODIPY AND RELATED COMPOUNDS

BODIPYs are boron complexes of dipyrrin, that is, compounds where two pyrrolic units are linked by an sp^2 methane carbon. BODIPY dyes have been used for a long time as fluorescent probes and imaging agents due to their strong fluorescence in the visible spectral window (>500 nm).[45] BODIPY derivatives without heavy elements show a negligible Φ_{ISC}, and therefore very low Φ_Δ. Both Φ_{ISC} and Φ_Δ can be significantly increased by substitution of iodine or bromine at the pyrrolic rings (e.g., **16**).[37] Furthermore, simple BODIPY derivatives absorb at rather short wavelengths (500 nm), which is not suitable for in vivo applications. The wavelength of absorption can be shifted toward longer wavelengths in order to obtain derivatives absorbing in NIR-I by structural modifications. Such modifications may include, for example, placing conjugated substituents (e.g., styrene, **17**),[38,46] replacing the bridging carbon atom by nitrogen (so-called aza-BODIPY, e.g., **18**),[27] or fusing an additional heterocyclic ring on the pyrrole moieties (e.g., **19**, in the latter case the sulfur atoms in thiophene moieties likely increase spin–orbit coupling and facilitate ISC).[39] In all examples listed here, a heavy element was necessary to impart a high Φ_Δ. Recently, an interesting approach to increase both Φ_{ISC} and Φ_Δ without the use of a heavy element has been proposed.[40] It has been shown that BODIPY dimers (e.g., **20**) possess a high long-living T_1 ($\tau_T = 115$ μs) and high $\Phi_\Delta = 0.64$.

Little is known about the photosensitization of other ROS by BODIPY derivatives. In many works, it is assumed that $^1O_2$ is produced, without consideration of other ROS.[45] However, it has been shown that HO· is produced, in addition to $^1O_2$, by derivative **17**.[38] BODIPY derivatives are currently being very intensively investigated as singlet ROS photosensitizers. The chief advantage of BODIPY relative to other photosensitizers seems to be their apparent easier and less labor-intensive synthetic chemistry, and availability of a large number of synthetic methods for their modification. Therefore, synthesis of their diverse derivatives with desirable optical and chemical properties seems to be often more straightforward than in the case of tetrapyrrolic macrocycles.

2.3.3 SQUARAINES

Squaraines are another class of organic molecules, which have been recently examined as ROS photosensitizers with potential applications in PDT. Squaraines exhibit a strong absorbance in NIR-I, which can be broadly tuned (600–800 nm) by structural modification.[47] Similar to BODIPY derivatives, simple squaraine does not exhibit appreciable Φ_{ISC}, making substitution with a heavy element necessary (e.g., **21**,[41] **22**[42]). One such highly efficient modification was the replacement of oxygen atoms with sulfur in the central squaric acid moiety, which provides derivatives with nearly unity Φ_{ISC} and Φ_Δ (e.g., **22**).[42] One of the chief problems with the use of squaraines in PDT seems to be their relatively low chemical stability, specifically high reactivity of squaraines toward biologically relevant nucleophiles (e.g., thiols).[48] An elegant solution was proposed to overcome this problem, which involves protection of the squaraine core by a mechanical entrapping inside the larger macrocycle, to form an interlocked compound, known as rotaxane.[48] It has been shown that rotaxane containing sulfur squaraine, analogous to **22**, degrades four times slower in nucleophilic solvents than non-threaded squaraine.[43]

2.4 CONCLUSION

The intensive research over the last half century has led to fairly good understanding of the processes underlying ROS, particularly $^1O_2$ photosensitization, and establishing the design principles for highly efficient photosensitizers. Now, the major challenge seems to be to fully understand the properties of ROS photosensitizers in the cellular environment, and optimizing their photochemical properties to achieve optimal performance in vivo. The recent results have also underpinned the importance of type I photochemistry (generation of oxygen radicals) in PDT. The detailed understanding of these processes and optimization of oxygen radical photosensitizers' properties is expected to be the area of vigorous research.

ACKNOWLEDGMENTS

The author thanks Adam Meares for thorough proofreading of the manuscript. UMBC and NSF (Grant No. CHE-1301109) are acknowledged for supporting the author's work on ROS photosensitizers.

REFERENCES

1. Dougherty, T. J., Gomer, C. J., Henderson, B. W., Jori, G., Kessel, D., Korbelik, M., Moan, J., and Peng, Q. 1998. Photodynamic therapy. *J. Natl. Cancer Inst.* **90**, 889–905.

2. Wilson, B. C. and Patterson, M. S. 2008. The physics, biophysics and technology of photodynamic therapy. *Phys. Med. Biol.* **53**, R61–R109.

3. (a) Foote, C. S. 1968. Mechanism of photosensitized oxidation. *Science* **162**, 963–970. (b) Ochsner, M. 1997. Photophysical and photobiological processes in the photodynamic therapy of tumor. *J. Photochem. Photobiol.* **39**, 1–18.

4. Valeour B. and Berberan-Santos, M. N. 2012. *Molecular Fluorescence Principles and Applications.* Wiley-VCH, Weinheim, Germany.

5. Welsher, K., Sherlock, S. P., and Dai, H. 2011. Deep-tissue anatomical imaging of mice using carbon nanotube fluorophores in the second near-infrared window. *Proc. Natl. Acad. Sci. USA* **108**, 8943–8948.

6. Ethirajan, M., Chen, Y., Joshi, P., and Pandey, R. K. 2011. The role of porphyrin chemistry in tumor imaging and photodynamic therapy. *Chem. Soc. Rev.* **40**, 340–362.

7. Sternberg, E. D., Dolphin, D., and Brückner, C. 1998. Porphyrin-based photosensitizers for use in photodynamic therapy. *Tetrahedron* **54**, 4151–4202.

8. Arnaut, L. G. and Formosinho, S. J. 2013. From elementary reaction to chemical relevance in the photodynamic therapy of cancer. *Pure Appl. Chem.* **85**, 1389–1403.

9. Pawlicki, M., Collins, H. A., Denning, R. G., and Anderson, H. L. 2009. Two-photon absorption and the design of two-photon dyes. *Angew. Chem. Int. Ed.* **48**, 3244–3266.

10. Ambjerg, J., Jiménez-Banzo, A., Paterson, M. J., Nonell, S., Borrell, J. I., Christiansen, O., and Ogilby, P. R. 2007. Two-photon absorption in tetraphenylporphycenes: Are porphycenes better candidates than porphyrins for providing optimal optical properties for two-photon photodynamic therapy? *J. Am. Chem. Soc.* **129**, 5188–5199.

11. Turro, N. J., Ramamurthy, V., and Scaiano, J. C. 2010. *Modern Molecular Photochemistry of Organic Molecules.* University Science Books, Sausalito, CA.

12. Ventura, B., Flamingi, L., Marconi, G., Lodato, F., and Officer, D. L. 2008. Extending the porphyrin core: synthesis and photophysical characterization of porphyrins with π-conjugated ß-substituents. *New J. Chem.* **32**, 166–178.

13. DeRosa, M. and Crutchley, R. J. 2002. Photosensitized singlet oxygen and its applications. *Coord. Chem. Rev.* **233–234**, 351–371.

14. Firey, P. A., Jones, T. W., Jori, G., and Rodgers, M. A. J. 1988. Photoexcitation of zinc phthalocyanine in mouse myeloma cells: The observation of triplet states but not of singlet oxygen. *Photochem. Photobiol.* **48**, 357–360.

15. Helmlinger, G., Yusn, F., Delian, M., and Jain, R. K. 1997. Interstitial pH and pO$_2$ gradients in solid tumors *in vivo*. High-resolution meassurements reveal a lack of correlation. *Nat. Med.* **3**, 177–182.

16. Silva, E. F. F., Serpa, C., Dabrowski, J. M., Monteiro, C. J. P., Formosinho, S. J., Stochel, G., Urbanska, K., Simões, S., Pereira, M. M., and Arnaut, L. 2010. Mechanism of singlet-oxygen and superoxide-ion generation by porphyrin and bacteriochlorin and their implication in photodynamic therapy. *Chem. Eur. J.* **16**, 9273–9286.

17. Yang, E., Diers, J. R., Huang, Y.-Y., Hamblin, M. R., Lindsey, J. S., Bocian, D. F., and Holten, D. 2013. Molecular electronic tuning of photosensitizers to enhance photodynamic therapy: Synthetic dicyanobacteriochlorins as a case study. *Photochem. Photobiol.* **89**, 605–618.

18. Ashur, I., Goldschmidt, R., Pinkas, I., Salomon, Y., Szewczyk, G., Sarna, T., and Scherz, A. 2009. Photocatalytic generation of oxygen radicals by the water-soluble bacteriochlorophyll derivative WST11, noncovalently bound to serum albumin. *J. Phys. Chem. A* **113**, 8027–8037.

19. Weller, A. 1982. Photoinduced electron transfer in solution: Exciplex and ion-pair formation free enthalpies and their solvent dependence. *Z. Phys. Chem.* **133**, 93–98.

20. Nonell, S. and Braslavsky, S. E. 2000. Time-resolved singlet oxygen detection. *Methods Enzymol.* **319**, 37–49.
21. Gomes, A., Fernandes, E., and Lima, J. F. C. 2005. Fluorescence probes used for detection of reactive oxygen species. *J. Biochem. Biophys. Methods* **65**, 45–80.
22. Ohyashiki, T., Nunomura, M., and Katoh, T. 1999. Detection of superoxide anion radicals in phospholipid liposomal membranes by fluorescence quenching method using 1,3-diphenylisobenzofuran. *Biochim. Biophys. Acta* **1421**, 131–139.
23. Chen, X., Tian, X., Shin, I., and Yoon, J. 2011. Fluorescent and luminescent probes for detection of reactive oxygen and nitrogen species. *Chem. Soc. Rev.* **40**, 4783–4804.
24. Vakrat-Haglili, Y., Weiner, L., Brumfeld, V., Brandis, A., Salomon, Y., McIlroy, B., Wilson, B. C. et al. 2005. The microenvironment effect on the generation of reactive oxygen species by Pd-bacteriopheophorbide. *J. Am. Chem. Soc.* **127**, 6487–6497.
25. Lovell, J. F., Liu, T. W. B., Chen, J., and Zheng, G. 2010. Activatable photosensitizers for imaging and therapy. *Chem. Rev.* **110**, 2839–2857.
26. Sessler, J. L., Dow, W. C., O'Connor, D., Harriman, A., Hemmi, G., Mody, T. D., Miller, R. A. et al. 1997. Biomedical applications of lanthanide(III) texaphyrins. Lutetium(III) texaphyrins as potential photodynamic therapy photosensitizers. *J. Alloys Compd.* **249**, 146–152.
27. Adarsh, N., Shanmugasundaram, M., Avirah, R. R., and Ramaiah, D. 2012. Aza-BODIPY derivatives: Enhanced quantum yields of triplet excited states and the generation of singlet oxygen and their role as facile sustainable photooxygenation catalysts. *Chem. Eur. J.* **18**, 12655–12662.
28. Redmond, R. W. and Gamlin, J. N. 1999. A compilation of singlet oxygen yields from biologically relevant molecules. *Photochem. Photobiol.* **70**, 391–475.
29. Arnaut, L. G. 2011. Design of porphyrin-based photosensitizers for photodynamic therapy. *Adv. Inorg. Chem.* **63**, 167–233.
30. Dixon, J. M., Taniguchi, M., and Lindsey, J. S. 2005. PhotochemCAD 2: A refined program with accompanying spectral databases for photochemical calculations. *Photochem. Photobiol.* **81**, 212–2123. Data taken from Photochemcad: http://photochemcad.com.
31. Tanielian, C. and Wolff, C. 1995. Porphyrin-sensitized generation of singlet molecular oxygen: Comparison of steady-state and time-resolved methods. *J. Phys. Chem.* **99**, 9825–9830.
32. Bonnett, R., Charlsworth, P., Djelal, B. D., Foley, S., McGarvey, D. J., and Truscott T. G. 1999. Photophysical properties of 5,10,15,20-tetrakis(*m*-hydroxyphenyl)porphyrin (*m*-THPP), 5,10,15,20-tetrakis(*m*-hydroxyphenyl)chlorin (*m*-THPC) and 5,10,15,20-tetrakis(*m*-hydroxyphenyl)bacteriochlorin (*m*-THPBC): A comparative study. *J. Chem. Soc. Perkin Trans.* **2**, 325–328.
33. Pogue, B. W., Redmond, R. W., Trivedi, N., and Hasan, T. 1998. Photophysical properties of tin ethyl etiopurpurin I (SnET$_2$) and tin octaethylbenzochlorin (SnOEBC) in solution and bound to albumin. *Photochem. Photobiol.* **68**, 809–815.
34. Kuimova, M. K., Hoffmann, M., Winters, M. U., Eng, M., Balaz, M., Clark, I. P., Collins, H. A. et al. 2007. Determination of the triplet state energies of a series of conjugated porphyrin oligomers. *Photochem. Photobiol. Sci.* **6**, 675–682.
35. Zhang, X.-F. and Xu, H.-J. 1993. Influence of halogenation and aggregation on photosensitizing properties of zinc phthalocyanine (ZnPC). *J. Chem. Soc. Faraday Trans.* **89**, 3347–3351.
36. Firey, P. A. and Rodgers, M. A. J. 1987. Photoproperties of a silicon naphthalocyanine: A potential photosensitizer for photodynamic therapy. *Photochem. Photobiol.* **45**, 535–538.
37. Yogo, T., Urano, Y., Ishitsuka, Y., Maniwa, F., and Nagano, T. 1995. Highly efficient and photostable photosensitizer based on BODIPY chromophore. *J. Am. Chem. Soc.* **127**, 12162–12163.
38. Wang, J., Hou, Y., Lei, W., Zhou, Q., Li, C., Zhang, B., and Wang, X. 2012. DNA photocleavage by a cationic BODIPY dye through both singlet oxygen and hydroxyl radical: New insight into the photodynamic mechanism of BODIPYs. *Chemphyschem* **13**, 2739–2747.
39. Yang, Y., Guo, Q., Chen, H., Zhou, Z., Guo, Z., and Shen, Z. 2013. Thienopyrrole-expanded BODIPY as a potential NIR photosensitizer for photodynamic therapy. *Chem. Commun.* **49**, 3940–3942.

40. (a) Cakmak, Y., Kolemen, S., Duman, S., Dede, Y., Doden, Y., Kilic, B., Kostereli, Z. et al. 2011. Designing excited states: Theory-guided access to efficient photosensitizers for photodynamic action. *Angew. Chem. Int. Ed.* **50**, 11937–11941. (b) Wu, W., Cui, J., and Zhao, J. 2013. Hetero BODIPY-dimers as heavy atom-free triplet photosensitizers showing a long-lived triplet excited state for triplet-triplet anhilation upconversion. *Chem. Commun.* **49**, 9009–9011.

41. Ramaiah, D., Joy, A., Chandrasekhar, N., Eldho, N. V., Das, S., and George, M. V. 1997. Halogentaed squaraine dyes as potential photochemotherapeutic agents. Synthesis and study of photophysical properties and quantum efficiencies of singlet oxygen generation. *Photochem. Photobiol.* **65**, 783–790.

42. Webster, S., Peceli, D., Hu, H., Padilha, L. A., Przhonska, O. V., Masunov, A. E., Gerasov, A. O. et al. 2010. Near-unity quantum yields for intersystem crossing and singlet oxygen generation in polymethine-like molecules: Design and experimental realization. *J. Phys. Chem. Lett.* **1**, 2354–2360.

43. Devlin, R. F., Dandliker, W. B., and Arrhenius, P. O. G. 2000. Fluorescence immunoassays using fluorescent dyes free of aggregation and serum binding. U.S. Patent 6,060,598.

44. Sessler, J. L. and Seidel, D. 2003. Synthetic expanded porphyrin chemistry. *Angew. Chem. Int. Ed.* **42**, 5134–5175.

45. (a) Loudet, A. and Burgess K. 2007. BODIPY dyes and their derivatives: Synthesis and spectroscopic properties. *Chem. Rev.* **107**, 4891–4932. (b) Kamkaew, A., Lim, S. H., Lee, H. B., Kiew, L. V., Chung, L. Y., and Burgess, K. 2013. BODIPY dyes in photodynamic therapy. *Chem. Soc. Rev.* **42**, 77–88.

46. Atilgan, S., Ekmekci, Z., Dogan, A. L., Guc, D., and Akkaya, E. U. 2006. Water soluble distyryl-boradiazaindacenes as efficient photosensitizers for photodynamic therapy. *Chem. Commun.* 4398–4400.

47. Avirah, R. R., Jayaram, D. T., Adarsh, N., and Ramaiah, D. 2012. Squaraine dyes in PDT: From basic design to *in vivo* demonstration. *Org. Biomol. Chem.* **10**, 911–920.

48. Peck, E. M., Collins, C. G., and Smith, B. G. 2013. Thiosquaraine rotaxanes: Synthesis, dynamic structure, and oxygen photosensitization. *Org. Lett.* **15**, 2762–2765.

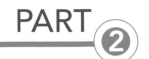
IN VITRO MICROSCOPY FOR PHOTOSENSITIZER LOCALIZATION IN CELLS

Phthalocyanines in photodynamic therapy

HEIDI ABRAHAMSE

3.1 INTRODUCTION

In photodynamic therapy (PDT), photosensitizers (PSs) allow the transfer and translation of light energy into a type II chemical reaction. Rapid cyto and vascular toxicity due to the reactive end products of this pathway is the result of photochemical reactions. PDT requires a sensitizing agent, light energy, and oxygen, which, when successfully combined, create a photodynamic reaction (Alison et al., 2004a). Metallophthalocyanines (PC) have drawn considerable attention in recent years for their potential use as second-generation PSs for PDT of neoplastic diseases. The major advantage of PCs currently is their strong absorption of red light at approximately 675 nm (extinction coefficient 2.5×10^5 mol^{-1} dm^3 cm^{-1}), which allows light penetration into tissues to almost twice the depth. In addition, PCs have low absorption of light in other parts of the solar spectrum, thus lowering the risk of skin photoreaction that often occurs in patients after PDT. Water-soluble sulfonated derivatives were used for demonstrating PC photoefficacy in the destruction of in vivo tumors. Numerous lipophilic PC derivatives have proven to be effective PDT agents in vivo, although the success of these agents relies upon their incorporation into carrier vehicles or their formulation in specific reagents, such as liposomes and oil emulsions that circumvent the problem of aggregation in biological fluids (Zaidi et al., 1993).

Aluminum phthalocyanine (AlPc) is chemically stable and is relatively easy to synthesize while yielding a single isomeric product that is highly effective in photoinactivating cultured cells (Chan et al., 1997).

3.2 PHTHALOCYANINES USED IN PHOTODYNAMIC THERAPY

Treatment of cancerous tumors involves aggressive, invasive methods such as surgery, chemotherapy, and radiotherapy. The development of PDT as an alternative treatment that is able to selectively destroy cancerous tumor cells, together with the superior photophysical attributes of PCs, allows for powerful cancer treatment (Ben-Hur and Chan, 2003). PCs strongly absorb light in the near-infrared (NIR) region where it has low toxicity, but potent skin photosensitizing. It has high selectivity to tumor cells where it produces singlet-oxygen species upon irradiation. In addition, PDT is a noninvasive, oxygen-dependent process that uses a specific wavelength of light allowing the PSs to generate cytotoxic oxygen species (e.g., $^1O_2$, O_2^-, $O_2^{\bullet}$, and $OH^{\bullet}$). These cytotoxic oxygen species are produced by type I or type II processes (Figure 3.1), mediated by the excited triplet state of the PS.

It is difficult to establish which reaction mechanism is involved in PDT as contributions from both type I and II processes are likely. Electron/hydrogen transfer from the PS to generate ions or radicals, which react rapidly, usually with oxygen, to form highly reactive oxygen species (ROS) is termed type I mechanism. Following excitation of the PS to the triplet state, the direct interaction of the PS with ground state molecular oxygen results in the formation of reactive singlet oxygen (type II mechanism). The PS then returns to its singlet ground state (S0). Studies suggest that singlet-oxygen formation is the more dominant process in PDT (MacDonald and Dougherty, 2001). Lipophilic as well as water-soluble PCs have been used in PDT studies, and those that have already been accepted for use in clinical trials include Photosens® (a mixture of sulfonated AlPc (AlPcSmix)), AlPcS2, and liposomal formulations of phthalocyanine 4 (Pc-4) and ZnPc [36] (Figure 3.2; Nyokong and Antunes, 2013).

PCs are tetrapyrrolic macrocycles that have nitrogen atoms linking the individual pyrrole units instead of methine bridges. The macrocycle is extended by benzene rings, which strengthens the absorption at longer wavelengths. PCs have been used as dyes and coloring agents as well as photoconducting agents in photocopying machines. They have been extensively studied as PDT agents because of their favorable photophysical properties and because their properties (such as solubility) can be altered through the addition of substituents to the periphery of the macrocycle. Ciba–Geigy Ltd. (Basel, Switzerland), in partnership with QLT PhotoTherapeutics, has developed a liposomal preparation of zinc PC (CGP55847) used for squamous cell carcinoma clinical trials in Switzerland (Ochsner, 1996). The oncological center of the Russian Academy of Medical Sciences (Moscow, Russia) and the surgical clinic of the Moscow Medical Academy (Moscow, Russia) have carried out trials using a mixture of sulfonated aluminum PC derivatives (Photosense) against malignancies such as skin, breast, lung, and gastrointestinal cancer (Sobolev and Stranadko, 1997). The addition of sulfonate groups to the PC increases the solubility of these compounds, removing the need for liposomal delivery vehicles. In addition,

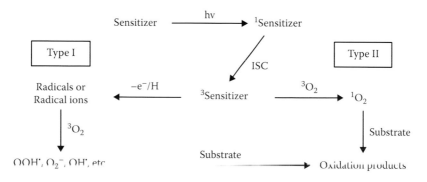

Figure 3.1 Photosensitization and reactive oxygen species generation during PDT.

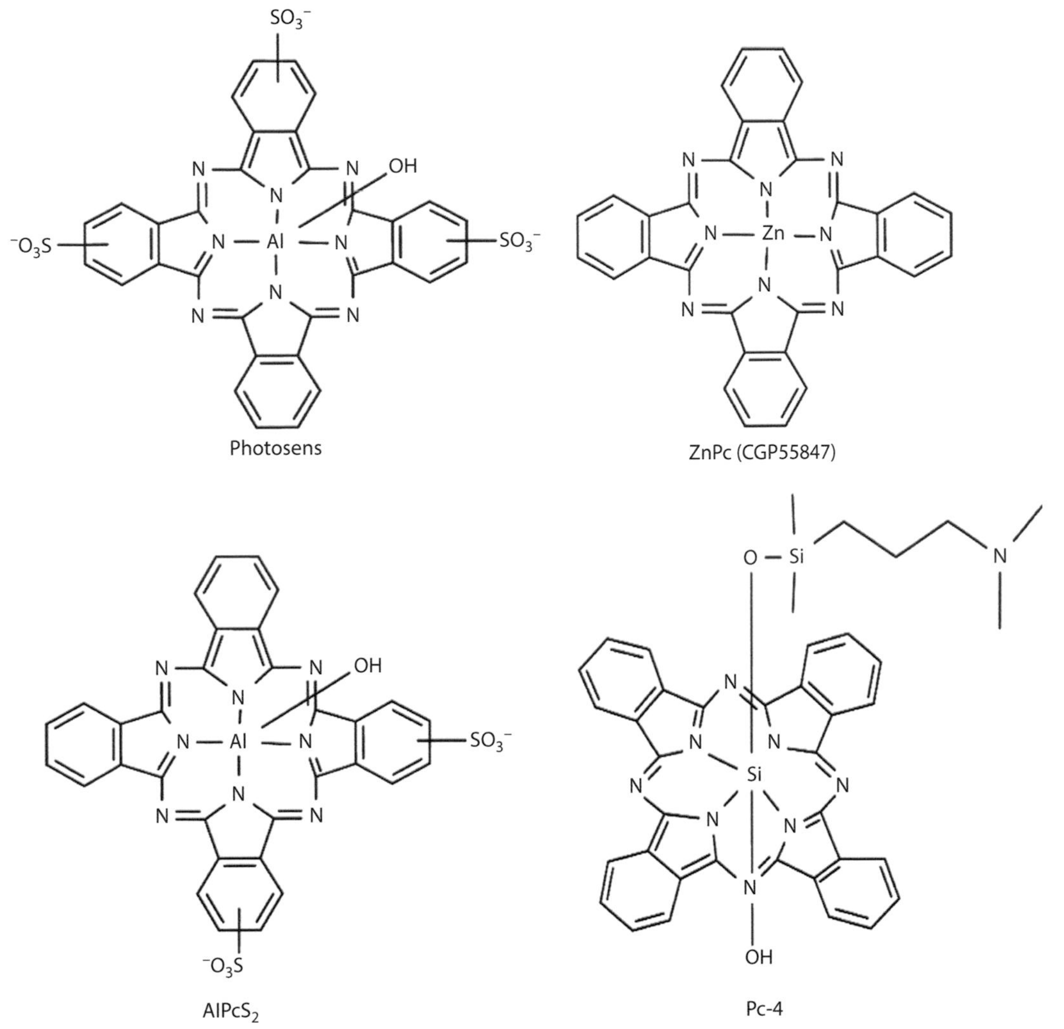

Figure 3.2 PCs currently used and tried in clinical trials.

a silicon-based PC (PC4) has been studied for the sterilization of blood components by V.I. Technologies (Vitex, Melville, NY, USA), who are based at the New York Blood Center. The addition of a second benzene ring to the periphery of the PC produces naphthalocyanines 57, which absorb at a higher wavelength than PCs (770 nm vs. 680 nm), increasing the therapeutic penetration depth (Sharman et al., 1999).

3.3 CLINICALLY APPROVED PSs

PSs should be nontoxic, should not generate toxic or mutagenic catabolites, exhibit low-to-no dark toxicity, be chemically pure and photostable, absorb maximally in the therapeutic window (650–850 nm), have a high triplet-state quantum yield, have a high ROS production efficiency, and accumulate selectively in the tumor tissue (Allison et al., 2004). The four most frequently utilized clinical PSs include (1) hematoporphyrin derivative (HpD); (2) a semi-purified form of HpD known as porfimer sodium; (3) 5-aminolevulinic acid (5-ALA), which is a precursor of the mitochondrially produced PS protoporphyrin IX (PpIX); and (4) m-tetrahydroxyphenyl-chlorin (mTHPC), albeit these PSs are associated with a considerable level of phototoxicity that is caused by long clearance times after systemic administration and extensive PS retention in the skin (Table 3.1).

Table 3.1 Pharmacokinetic, pharmacodynamic, and toxicity parameters of clinically applied and experimental photosensitizers

	Administration route	Tumor: healthy tissue ratio	Mutagenicity	Elimination (half-life)	Photosensitivity	LD$_{50}$ dark toxicity (µM)[a]
HpD	IV[a]	NA[a]	Yes	12–22 d	1–12 wk	367–1136[a]
Porfimer sodium	IV	1.7–2:1	Yes	12 d	4–12 wk	5.3
5-ALA	Oral/IV	2:1	Yes	5-ALA 0.75 h PpIX:8 h	1–2 d	9041
	Topical	1.7–30:1				
mTHPC	IV	2–3:1	No	45 h	2–6 wk	8.46–26.4
ZnPC	IV	6.3:1 [3.7–9:1]	No	NA	NA	>5
ZnPCS$_4$	IV	NA	No	NA	NA	>31.6
AlPC	IV	NA	No	NA	NA	>10
AlPCS$_4$	IV	10:1	No	NA	NA	>500

Source: Weijer, R. et al., J. Photochem. Photobiol. C: Photochem. Rev., 23, 103, 2015.

Abbreviations: LD$_{50}$, lethal 50% dose; Est., estimated; IV, intravenous; NA, not assessed; d, day; wk, week; NCA, not commercially available; h, hour; ZnPC, zinc phthalocyanine; ZnPCS$_4$, tetrasulfonated zinc phthalocyanine; AlPC, chloro aluminum phthalocyanine; AlPCS4, tetrasulfonated chloro aluminum phthalocyanine.

[a] LD$_{50}$ dark toxicity for HpD was calculated based on a molecular weight of 598.7 g/mol.

Another limitation of the clinically approved PSs is the relatively low main absorption peak in the red spectrum (Q-band) as demonstrated in Figure 3.3a. The position of the Q-band maximum influences the clinical efficiency since short-wavelength red light has a lower optical penetration depth into tissue than longer-wavelength red light because of the competitive absorption by melanin and hemoglobin (Figure 3.3b; Weijer et al., 2015).

The use of 690 nm light significantly reduces absorption by blood, which theoretically yields a 1.67-fold increase in optical penetration depth while sunlight is more intense at the shorter red wavelengths and therefore accounts for more ROS generation by PSs with more blue-positioned Q-band maxima compared to red-positioned Q-band maxima at equal concentrations. The need for more ideal characteristics in PSs has triggered the development of improved spectral and photochemical properties and more sophisticated PDT modalities (Weijer et al., 2015).

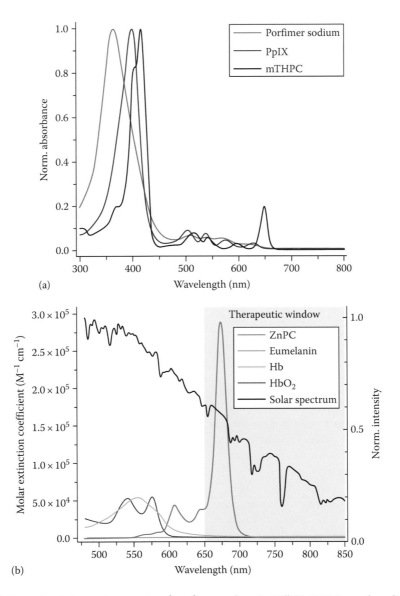

Figure 3.3 (a) Normalized absorption spectra of porfimer sodium (in MilliQ), PpIX (in methanol), and mTHPC (in ethanol:MilliQ (49:51, v/v)). (b) Molar extinction coefficient of eumelanin [383], hemoglobin (Hb), oxyhemoglobin (HbO$_2$) [384], and zinc phthalocyanine (ZnPC, in pyridine). The solar spectrum (black trace) was recorded from direct sunlight in the 250–1050 nm range, and the spectrum was normalized to the maximum intensity (secondary y-axis). The pink area represents the therapeutic window for clinical PDT (650–850 nm).

3.4 MECHANISMS OF PHOTODYNAMIC-THERAPY-MEDIATED CELL DEATH

PDT-induced mechanisms of cell death are in part dependent on the type of PS used and the intracellular localization of the PSs. Type II photochemical reaction–derived $^1O_2$ is the most predominant type of ROS that is produced upon PDT (Sharman et al., 2000; Weishaupt et al., 1976). Cytosolic $^1O_2$ diffusion is restricted to very short distances (220 nm) and is only capable of oxidizing biomolecules in close proximity to its production site. ROS normally have a short diffusion distance and are not generated close to nuclear material, hence do not result in sublethal oxidation of DNA and consequent malignant cell transformation in noncancerous cells. In addition, the short lifetimes of most ROS preclude cell damage to peritumoral healthy tissue and often target more than one subcellular location that will result in concomitant activation of different cell death pathways limiting the efficacy of simultaneously activated cell survival pathways and stress responses after PDT. Intracellular PS localization, cell type, intracellular PS concentration, light dose, local oxygen tension, and residual energy status govern the eventual mode of cell death and autophagy (Huang et al., 2008). PCs are initially confined to the plasma membrane, whereas at longer incubation times (>1–2 h) they become more prominently localized in distinct perinuclear areas. The effect of PS localization on PDT efficacy was evaluated in a so-called chase experiment. Human epidermoid carcinoma (A431) cells were incubated with ZnPC encapsulating cationic liposomes (ZnPC-ETLs) for 10 min, after which the liposome-containing medium was replaced with fresh culture medium. After specific time intervals, the cells were treated with PDT and examined for cell viability and the data revealed that a greater killing capacity was achieved when these cells were irradiated at early time points after incubation (<4 h) compared to later time points (>4 h). Confocal microscopy experiments were performed to examine the intracellular localization of ZnPC as a function of time revealing that ZnPC is highly associated with mitochondria after 30 min and to a lesser extent after 4 h. At the 4 h time point, ZnPC exhibited a more diffuse localization, which was even more pronounced after 24 h (Figure 3.4; Weijer, 2015; Gross et al., 2013).

This is in line with the previously alluded to spatiotemporal dynamics of PSs following uptake, attesting to the importance of a well-defined PDT protocol and the fact that systematic modulation of this protocol can culminate in the activation of distinct cell death pathways (Weijer et al., 2015).

3.5 CELL DEATH PATHWAYS AND PHTHALOCYANINE

Cell death is a biological process referring to the inability of a cell to preserve indispensable life functions required for both development and homeostasis. It removes damaged cells and superfluous cells that cause harm and need to be destroyed for the advantage of the whole organism (Engelberg-Kulka et al., 2006). Depending on cellular aspects such as morphology, enzymatic activity, functional and immunological responses, the mode of cell death is determined and designated as either a programmed or nonprogrammed mode (Kroemer et al., 2009).

3.5.1 APOPTOSIS

Apoptosis is characterized by nuclear and membrane degradation and is triggered by precise signals that lead to the activation of cascade pathways to finally deliver a suicidal response. It is an induced and regulated process that activates a family of proteins (known as caspase) and precise cellular events, which degrade nucleic and polypeptide materials. Caspases are cysteine aspartyl proteases and can further stimulate effectors agents to digest cellular contents. The apoptotic response is enhanced upon the binding of BH3-only members of B-cell lymphoma 2 (Bcl-2) family to inhibit the action of prosurvival proteins. Affected cells round up and cease communication with adjacent cells; their plasma membranes bleb and phosphatidylserines translocate in the outer layers (Table 3.1).

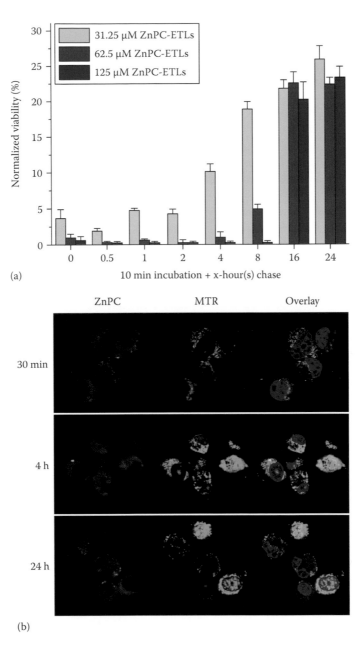

Figure 3.4 (a) Effect of intracellular ZnPC dispersion time on PDT-induced cell death and spatiotemporal dynamics of intracellular ZnPC distribution. A431 cells were incubated with ZnPC-encapsulating cationic liposomes (ZnPC–ETLs) composed of DPPC:DC-chol:Cholesterol:DSPE-PEG (66:25:5:4, molar ratio). ZnPC was incorporated at a ZnPC:Lipid ratio of 0.003. Concentrations in the legend indicate final lipid concentrations. After 10 min, the medium was refreshed and cells were treated with PDT at the indicated time points (x-axis) and kept under standard culture conditions until the time of viability testing. (b) Intracellular ZnPC localization as a function of time. A431 cells were incubated with ZnPC-ETLs (ZnPC:Lipid ratio of 0.030) for 10 min, after which the intracellular localization was visualized by confocal microscopy at different time points. ZnPC (red) MitoTracker red (MTR, mitochondria, green), DAPI (nuclei, blue).

These mechanisms are accompanied by additional cellular changes, including cross-linkage and polymerization of proteins, chromatin condensation, nuclear fragmentation from ±300,000 to 185 nucleotides through internucleosomal degradation by cation-dependent endonuclease, and finally cellular fragmentation into apoptotic bodies and removal. The intrinsic pathway of apoptosis is characterized by increased permeability of the mitochondrial membranes and the release of apoptogenic substances such as cytochrome C while the activation of death receptors such as tumor necrosis factor receptor 1 or Fas/CD95 on the plasma membrane characterizes the extrinsic pathway (Erental et al., 2012; Kang et al., 2011; Kim et al., 2012). The presence of Beclin 1 prevents caspase-dependent cell death events and demonstrates antiapoptotic potential. Silicon PCs (PC-4) used in PDT cause damage to CD4+ CD7-malignant T-lymphocytes. It is efficient in inducing cytodamage by destroying BCL-2 proteins and promoting apoptosis while in breast cancer cells leads to apoptotic cell death with nuclear fragmentation and increased expression of the Bcl-2, DNA fragmentation factor alpha, and caspase 2 genes (Lam et al., 2010; Mfouo-Tynga et al., 2014). PSs that accumulate in mitochondria and damage BCL-2 protein like PC generally are inducers of apoptosis while the level of calcium ions (Ca^{2+}) and transfer from endoplasmic reticulum (ER) to mitochondria represent further criteria for cell death induction. The overload of Ca^{2+} in the mitochondria may lead to change in morphology and eventually in a Ca^{2+}-dependent non-nuclear apoptosis while the presence of increased levels of intracellular Ca^{2+} by PDT can induce cytodamage, which appears to be p53 dependent (Giorgi et al., 2015).

3.5.2 NECROSIS

Necrosis is an accidental and nonprogrammed cell death event. It is characterized by an absence of signals associated with programmed cell death and an inflammatory response. External stimuli such as infections, toxins, and trauma are required to initiate a necrotic cell death response. Signal transduction and catabolic activities govern the execution of the necrotic pathway through death domain and toll-like receptors. The activity of the receptor interacting protein (RIP1) controls the promotion of this cell death. RIP1 is a serine/threonine kinase required for the death receptor signaling and necroptosis, which is a necrotic-like and caspase-independent programmed cell death (Table 3.2; Cho et al., 2011; Lemasters, 2005). Seven types of necrotic cell death pathways have been recognized, but the sequential events remain unchanged as it includes membrane permeability, movement of calcium ions across the ER, cytoplasmic swelling (oncosis), calcium dependent calpain activation, lysosomal rupture, followed by degradation of cell component and induction of inflammatory response. Necrosis is comprised of precise sequential events and occurs in a controlled manner. The efficiency of the liposomal aluminum chloro-PC (AlClPC) was studied in both in vitro and in vivo Ehrlich tumor cells and oral cancer cells. AlClPC-mediated PDT led to 90% necrotic cell death and disruption of blood vessels (Longo et al., 2009, 2013). Another PC, zinc PC tetra-sulfonated, exhibited antineoplastic activity after PDT and an increase of necrotic-related cell death was seen. Subcellular localizations with cell membrane disintegration, local depletion of oxygen and nutrient, are prone to receive PCs that would stimulate cell death by necrosis (FláviaArrudaPortilho et al., 2013). The uptake, cytodamage, and subcellular localization are all functions of the distinctive chemical features of each PC. Neutral PCs showed more diffuse localization and were likely to primary localize in the Golgi apparatus in the perinuclear area. Though both cationic and anionic PCs prefer lysosomes as their initial sites of localization, the cationic, followed by the neutral PCs, appeared to be more effective than their anionic counters. Following irradiation, PCs undergo relocalization, which is charge dependent and demonstrated that the secondary localization site is more important in predicting the outcome of any PC-mediated PDT (Wood et al., 1997).

3.5.3 AUTOPHAGY

Autophagy is a prosurviving mechanism initiated by cells that have to face sublethal levels of damage by promoting the induction of the immunogenic cell death mechanism. It plays a critical role in photodynamic-related cell damage in apoptosis-resistant cells. When autophagy is inhibited, cancer cells show resistance and increased cell survival after PDT treatment (Michaud et al., 2011; Xue et al., 2010). Thirty autophagy-related genes (Atg) and two ubiquitin-dependent mechanisms have been identified, but Atg7 protein is involved,

Table 3.2 Distinctive characteristics of cell death pathways

Distinctive features	Cell death pathways		
	Apoptosis	Autophagy	Necrosis
Morphologies	Shrinkage; blebbing; chromatin condensation; DNA degradation; nuclear fragmentation, apoptotic bodies	Decreased cell size; double membrane vesicles; organelle degradation	Cell swelling; loss of membrane integrity; organelle swelling; NO DNA laddering
Regulators	Death receptors; Bcl-2 family; Beclin 1; caspases; IAPs; adaptor proteins; kinases; phosphatases; calcium ions, calpains; BCNI1	mTOR; PI3 kinase; ATG family; UPR stress sensors; Beclin 1; kinase (JNK); Bcl-2 family; IP3 receptor	Calcium ions; ion channels; metabolic failure; PARB, calcium regulated proteins; RIP kinase; death receptors; ceramides
Stimuli	ROS; DNA damage; death receptors ligands; developmental programs; organelle stress; anticancer drugs; ER calcium release	Nutrient starvation; protein aggregation; ER stress; calcium overload; developmental programs; hypoxia; ischemia; damaged organelles; proteasome impairment	Bacterial toxins; metabolic poisons; ischemia; stroke; calcium overload
Response	Programmed, physiological	Survival, accidental, physiological	Accidental, pathological

Abbreviations: ATG, autophagy; Bcl-2, B-cell lymphoma 2; IAPs, inhibitor of apoptosis proteins; IP3 receptor, inositol 1,4,5-trisphosphate (IP3) receptors ER, endoplasmic reticulum; mTOR, (mammalian) target of rapamycin; PAR, poly(ADP-ribose); NO, nitrite oxide; PARB, PAR-binding site; PI3 kinase, phosphatidylinositide 3-kinases; UPR, unfolded protein response; ROS, reactive oxygen species; RIP1: a specific kinase that is recruited to the death-inducing signaling complex.

Notes: Different cell death pathways can be classified according to morphological appearance (apoptotic, autophagic, necrotic), enzymological criteria or regulators (distinctive classes of proteases, such as caspases, calpains, and kinases), functional aspects (programmed or accidental, physiological, or pathological).

in both mechanisms and participate in other Atg activation, autophagosomal assemblage, and molecular degradation. It is a catabolic process involving ROS accumulation, membrane lipid oxidation on the membrane, and loss of plasma membrane integrity in the absence of caspase activity. Caspase inhibition induces catalase degradation and ROS accumulation that is dependent on the activity of catalase and is related to autophagy (Xie and Klionsky, 2007; Yu et al., 2006). Four consecutive steps make up the process of autophagy: appropriation, transportation to lysosomes, degradation, and reutilization of residues (Table 3.2). Lysosomes are the sites for cellular degradation that prompts cell death through the release of lysosomal hydrolases into the cytoplasm that prompts cell death. Autophagic proteins protect neighboring cells from detrimental effects of lysosomal degradation. Regulated autophagy controls the cell metabolism by degrading, recycling, and synthesizing cell components (Patel et al., 2012, Peracchio et al., 2012; Separovic et al., 2011). PDT is recognized to activate apoptosis but it can as well induce autophagy in several types of cells, where autophagic responses can be either survival or cell death mechanisms. Autophagy-triggered PDT can add resistance to the therapy by inhibiting cell death signals. However, apoptosis-deficient cells depend upon autophagic responses to induce cell death after PC-4 PDT. Both apoptosis and autophagy are required for enhanced cell death response, and when blocking autophagy, Michigan Cancer Foundation (MCF)-7 (human breast adenocarcinoma cancer) cells develop resistance to PC-mediated PDT, resulting in increased cell survival. PCs that localize in the ER and affect the target of rapamycin (mTOR) activation and beclin-1 protein are likely to lead to a comprehensively autophagic cell death response (Garg et al., 2015; Mroz et al., 2011; Xue et al., 2010). Photochemotherapy of cancer, also known as PDT, is a sequential photochemical and photo-biological process that aims to irreversible target and damage malignant tissues. It is an evolving and clinically approved approach that exerts selective cytotoxic activities to malignant cells. The mechanisms of cell death include direct tumoricidal effects, microvascular damage, and induction of a potent local inflammatory responses and depend mainly on the type and dose of PS used, the intensity of irradiation, and the level of oxygen (Figure 3.5; Brackett and Gollnick, 2011; Firdous et al., 2012).

In both clinical and experimental settings, most PSs do not localize in nuclei but rather in plasma membrane, lysosomes, mitochondria, ER, and Golgi apparatus after entering the cell through the plasma membrane. Subcellular localization depends on the physicochemical properties of PSs (Pereira et al., 2014). Photodynamic actions are associated with acute inflammatory responses, including increased levels of inflammatory cytokines and accumulation of leukocytes in targeted tumor areas while antitumor immunity has also been reported (Allen et al., 2001; Guillard et al., 1998). In most photodynamic responses, the inductor stimulus is $^1O_2$ that increases the formation of receptor interacting protein 3 (RIP-3) complex; however, this mechanism is not well understood (Coupienne et al., 2011). Due to poor relatively yield and limited efficiency in photodynamic applications, porphyrins were subjected to chemical modifications in order to improve their photochemical features and photodynamic therapeutic effectiveness. Phthalocyanines evolved from porphyrins, and although they share some of the features, PCs are better photodynamic agents with higher yields and improved spectroscopic properties that are within the therapeutic window. Phthalocyanine-mediated PDT has been shown to enhance autophagy, caspase-3 activation, and increased cell killing, and are mostly red light–absorbing compounds and are referred to as tetrabenzotetraazaporphyrins, macrocyclic structured compounds with isoindole and nitrogen atoms at their meso-positions. Metallized PCs have been identified as strong inducers of cytodamage

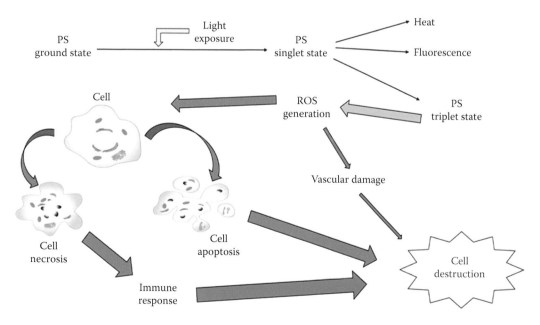

Figure 3.5 Photodynamic cancer therapy (PDT)–mediated cellular effects. Photosensitizer (PS) localizes in tumor cells and is converted from its ground to singlet state form through light activation. Singlet-state PS can lose energy in the form of heat or fluorescence but an ideal photodynamic PS undergoes intersystem crossing and transforms into triplet state form. Triplet-state PSs with a long lifespan mediate ROS generation within cells. ROS induce cytotoxic effects (predominantly apoptotic and necrotic type of responses at the exception of autophagy, which is more cytoprotecting than cytodamaging), causing cell damage and destruction (Mfouo-Tynga I. and Abrahamse H. (2015) Cell Death Pathways and Phthalocyanine as an Efficient Agent for Photodynamic Cancer Therapy. International Journal of Molecular Sciences. 16: 10228-10241; doi:10.3390/ijms160510228).

and preferentially accumulate in tumor cells where they stimulate photodamages in various tumor models. In vitro, they have been associated with induction apoptotic and necrotic pathways, while in vivo, PCs promote cell death through translocation of activated p38 to mitochondria, phosphorylation of BCL2 and/or BCL-X2, through facilitation of cytochrome C release from mitochondria, caspase-mediated PARP cleavage, and inhibition of the P13/Akt/mTOR pathway (Campidelli et al., 2008; Whitacre et al., 2000).

The phototherapeutic activity of metallized PCs has been studied in various cancer cell lines. A mixed sulfonated metallophthalocyanine with zinc as the central atom (ZnPcSmix) successfully entered cells and localized in vital organelles, including mitochondria, lysosomes, and Golgi apparatus inducing neoplastic damage in lung, colon, and breast cancer cells (Manoto et al., 2012; Mfouo-Tynga et al., 2012). Inlung cancer cells, a change in cell morphology, decrease in cell viability and proliferation, increase in cytotoxicity, and further cell damage were evident. Increased ROS production in both monolayer and multicellular tumor spheroid models of lung cancer were identified using this PC. In breast cancer, an abundance of apoptotic cells, degradation of nuclear material, and an increase in the level of expression of B-cell lymphoma-2, DNA fragmentation factor alpha, and caspase-2 genes concurred apoptosis as the induced mode of cell death (Manoto et al., 2011, 2013). Replacing the central metal ion with aluminum or germanium results in a dose-dependent increased cytotoxicity and effective targeting of the cancer cells especially for esophageal and breast cancer cells. Relative lower concentration of photoactivated AlPcSmix and GePcSmix showed greater apoptotic-inducing capabilities (Abrahamse et al., 2006). The effects of SnPcSmix and SiPcSmixas photochemotherapeutic agents were assessed in esophageal cancer and compared to GePcSmix. All three metallized PCs led to increased cellular damage when compared to an unmetallized mix PC and a binaphthalo PC. GePcSmix caused and induced an inflammatory response and high intracellular ATP, which could be an indication of a necroctic type of cell death (Seotsanyana-Mokhosi et al., 2006).

3.6 FUTURE DIRECTIVES FOR PHTHALOCYANINE PSs

3.6.1 Phthalocyanine-gold nanoparticle (AuNP) conjugates

Gold nanoparticles (NPs) have had a great impact on nanotechnology and are the subject of intense research. A physical characteristic of noble metal NPs is their ability to absorb visible light, as a consequence of the surface plasmon resonance (SPR) effect. For spherical AuNPs with diameters in the range of 2–100 nm, the SPR absorption band is found at 520 nm (Burda et al., 2005). AuNPs have been applied in imaging, sensing, medicine, photonics, and optics as well as plasmonic photothermal therapy (Gormley et al., 2012), where cancer cell death is induced by heat. This treatment relies on the fact that normal cells often remain undamaged by the use of high temperatures. The biocompatibility, coupled with the low toxicity and inert nature of AuNPs, makes them ideal for use as drug carriers in medicinal applications. Gold complexes have garnered interesting preclinical and clinical results in antiarthritic, anticancer, antimicrobial, antiparasitic, and anti-HIV studies (Shaw, 1999). NPs may be linked to recognition moieties, such as antibodies or oligonucleotides, in the detection of target biomolecules or to PC (Fonteh et al., 2010; Mthethwa et al., 2012). Strong interaction between sulfur and gold (Au) allows surface modification of AuNPs through self-assembly of thiol-substituted PSs on the AuNP surface. Since the AuNP surface is multivalent, it allows for covalent or noncovalent conjugation of the therapeutic drugs (Cho et al., 2008). Covalent conjugation of Pc-AuNP has an added stable PDT activity. Clinical trials have been carried out using polyethylene glycol–coated AuNPs as carriers for silicon PC 4 (Pc-4). The results showed that, once Pc-4 is injected in vivo, it takes a few days until a sufficient quantity of Pc-4 reaches the tumor site and the PEG-AuNP-Pc-4 conjugate significantly reduced the accumulation time to less than 2 h, while renal clearance of the NPs took place over 7 days (Baron et al., 2010; Cheng et al., 2008). Another study showed that labile amino adsorption on the AuNP surface allowed efficient drug release into the cancer cells that lead to an effective tumor killing when the delivery and PDT effect of covalently (via thiol groups) and noncovalently (via amide groups) attached Pc-4 to AuNPs were investigated in human cancer (HeLa) cells (Cheng et al., 2010).

3.6.2 PHTHALOCYANINE-SEMICONDUCTOR QUANTUM DOT CONJUGATES

Quantum dots (QDs) are defined as 0-D semiconductor materials with physical dimensions smaller than the exciton Bohr radius, usually less than 10 nm and quantized energy levels that lie between those of atomic and bulk materials (Bukowski, 2002; Juzenas et al., 2008). Their optical properties include a broad absorption spectrum, allowing for excitation over a broad range of wavelengths, and their size-tunable narrow emission spectra, which may span the ultraviolet to infrared region (Idowu et al., 2008; Seydel, 2003). QDs are well suited to fluorescence imaging applications because of their innate characteristics such as high-fluorescence quantum yields and low photobleaching rates. QD can be easily tuned and have potential applications in diverse fields such as high-density data storage, chemical sensing, optics, light-emitting diodes, and in bio-medicine as labels. QDs are seen as a new generation of PSs in PDT because they are capable of transferring energy to ground-state molecular oxygen to generate cytotoxic singlet oxygen and they may be used as imaging tools, thus enhancing the efficacy of PDT treatment (Nyokong and Antunes, 2013). Phthalocyanine molecules can form conjugates with QDs (Dayal, 2006). The enhanced PC triplet lifetimes in the presence of QDs allow the excited PC molecules to stay longer in the triplet state, allowing increased collisional and diffusional interactions between the PC molecules and ground-state molecular oxygen. This would result in a greater production of singlet oxygen, which is necessary for photosensitized reactions.

3.6.3 PHTHALOCYANINE-MAGNETIC IRON NANOPARTICLE CONJUGATES

Magnetic nanoparticles (MNPs) have been used in ultra-high-density magnetic storage media as versatile probes in biological, anticancer agents, and as magnetic resonance imaging (MRI) contrast agents (Chelebaeva et al., 2011; Gao et al., 2007). MNPs are good candidates for MRI as contrast agents and possess desirable attributes, including a narrow size distribution and tunable properties; high chemical stability; super paramagnetism; excellent mechanical, optical, and electrical properties; and ease of synthesis. MNPs can interact with induced electromagnetic fields of various frequencies and due to their small size are able to penetrate a wide range of materials, including bodily tissues, while their characteristics allow them to be tracked, manipulated, imaged, and remotely heated allowing numerous possibilities for cancer treatment (Ito et al., 2005). MNPs may also be used for tissue repair, immunoassays, detoxification of biological fluids, drug delivery, and cell separation and cellular (Gupta and Gupta, 2005). Superparamagnetic NPs have been used as MRI T2-shortening agents in clinical practice and have played an important role in the detection of small metastatic liver tumors and/or hepatocarcinomas (Karp et al., 2007). The conjugation of phthalocyanines to NPs such as QDs, gold, and magnetic NPs by an amide bond between NPs containing carboxy or amino functionalities and PC containing amino or carboxy functionalities, respectively, as well as their photochemical and photophysical behavior of the PCs indicates a significant improvement on current therapeutic possibilities. Investigations improving the water solubility of PCs, with appropriate functionalities for attachment to NPs, as well as advances in synthetic methods to produce less toxic QDs are required (Nyokong and Antunes, 2013).

3.7 CLINICAL PHOTODYNAMIC THERAPY

Clinicians have been practicing PDT despite the lack of complete knowledge and insight of the cell death mechanisms and effects. The basic concept of a sensitizer localizing in an anatomical area of interest followed by light activation to this anatomy is simple enough for clinicians to appreciate. Rapid cyto- and vasculotoxic reactions, together with visible tumor destruction amidst normal tissue remaining undamaged, have made this therapy appealing to both patient and clinician. The availability of mobile and reliable light sources, abundance of newly developed PSs, and a relatively side effect–free therapy has made PDT attractive as a therapeutic modality and it continues to grow. Significant improvements in PDT have been seen in a variety of cancers of the physiological system (Allison et al., 2004).

3.8 CONCLUSION

The need for new protocols for the treatment of cancer and other diseases is becoming acute. With the population aging and established therapies operating close to optimal levels, new therapies that can effectively treat cancer and other conditions while being cost effective are required. PDT offers the possibility of being an effective and specific method of destroying malignant, premalignant, and benign tissues while sparing surrounding normal healthy cells. Initial clinical studies have shown that PDT is effective against cancer, and a variety of other diseases and offers a promising treatment option for patients whose conditions have no established or effective cure or that has become refractory to existing therapies. As cancer encompasses a large family of diseases with widely different clinical patterns, it is very unlikely that a single PS will ever serve all the diseases in oncology. Metallized PCs are among the best currently used PSs in vitro, and their use in clinical settings should be encouraged for prospective means of managing cancer. It is also desirable to extend PDT into the treatment of other conditions and, hence, the need to develop new PSs with optimal properties for treating a given condition becomes obvious (Sharman et al., 1999).

REFERENCES

Abrahamse, H., Kresfelder, T., Horne, T., Cronje, M., Nyokong, T. (2006) Apoptotic inducing ability of a novel photosensitizing agent, Ge sulfophthalocyanine, on oesophageal and breast cancer cell lines. *Proceedings of SPIE Optical Methods for Tumor Treatment and Detection: Mechanisms and Techniques in Photodynamic Therapy XV*, San Jose, CA, Vol. 6139, pp. 17–29.

Abrahamse, H., Tynga, I. (2015) Cell death pathways and phthalocyanine as an efficient agent for photodynamic cancer therapy. *International Journal of Molecular Sciences* **16**: 10228–10241.

Agnello, M., Morici, G., Rinaldi, A.M. (2008) A method for measuring mitochondrial mass and activity. *Cytotechnology* **56**(3): 145–149.

Allen, C.M., Sharman, W.M., van Lier, J.E. (2001) Current status of phthalocyanines in the photodynamic therapy of cancer. *Journal of Porphyrines and Phthalocyanines* **5**: 161–169.

Allison, R.R., Downie, G.H., Cuenca, R., Hu, X., Childs, C.J.H., Sibata, C.H. (2004a) Photosensitizers in clinical PDT. *Photodiagnosis and Photodynamic Therapy* **1**: 27–42.

Allison, R.R., Mota, H.C., Sibata, C.H. (2004b) Clinical PD/PDT in North America: An historical review. *Photodiagnosis and Photodynamic Therapy* **1**: 263–277.

Baron, E.D., Malbasa, C.L., Santo-Domingo, D., Fu, P., Miller, J.D., Hanneman, K.K., Hsia, A.H., Oleinick, N.L., Colussi, V.C., Cooper, K.D. (2010) Silicon phthalocyanine (Pc 4) photodynamic therapy is a safe modality for cutaneous neoplasms: Results of a phase 1 clinical trial. *Lasers in Surgery and Medicine* **42**(10): 728–735.

Ben-Hur, E., Chan, W.S. (2003) Phthalocyanines in photobiology and their medical applications, in: K.M. Kadish, K.M. Smith, R. Guilard (Eds.), *Porphyrin Handbook, Phthalocyanine Properties and Materials*, Vol. 19, Chapter 117, Academic Press, New York.

Brackett, C., Gollnick, S. (2011) Photodynamic therapy enhancement of anti-tumour immunity. *Photochemistry and Photobiology* **83**(5): 1063–1068.

Bukowski, T.J. (2002) Drug delivery nanoparticles formulation and characterization. *Solid State Material Science* **27**(3–4): 119–142.

Burda, C., Chen, X., Narayanan, R., El-Sayed, M.A. (2005) Chemistry and properties of nanocrystals of different shapes. *Chemical Reviews* **105**: 1025.

Campidelli, S., Ballesteros, B., Filoramo, A., Diaz, D., de la Torre, G., Torres, T., Rahman, G.M.A. et al. (2008) Facile decoration of functionalized single-wall carbon nanotubes with phthalocyanines via "Click Chemistry". *Journal of the American Chemical Society* **130**: 11503–11509.

Chan, W.S., Brasseur, N., La Madeleine, C., Ouellet, R., van Lier, J.E. (1997) Efficacy and mechanism of aluminium phthalocyanine and its sulphonated derivatives mediated photodynamic therapy on murine tumours. *European Journal of Cancer* **33**(11): 1855–1859.

Chelebaeva, E., Larionova, J., Guari, Y., Ferreira, R.A.S., Carlos, L.D., Trifonov, A.A., Kalaivani, T. et al. (2011) Nanoscale coordination polymers exhibiting luminescence properties and NMR relaxivity. *Nanoscale* **3**(10): 1200–1203.

Cheng, Y., Samia, A.C., Li, J., Kenney, M.E., Resnick, A., Burda, C. (2010) Delivery and efficacy of a cancer drug as a function of the bond to the gold nanoparticle surface. *Langmuir* **26**(4): 2248–2255.

Cheng, Y., Samia, A.C., Meyers, J.D., Panagopoulos, I., Fei, B., Burda, C.J. (2008) Highly efficient drug delivery with gold nanoparticle vectors for in vivo photodynamic therapy of cancer. *American Journal of Chemical Society* **130**: 10643–10647.

Cho, K., Wang, X., Nie, S., Chen, Z.G., Shin, D.M. (2008) Therapeutic nanoparticles for drug delivery in cancer. *Clinical Cancer Research* **14**(5): 1310–1316.

Cho, Y., McQuade, T., Zhang, H., Zhang, J., Chan, F.K.M. (2011) RIP1-dependent and independent effects of necrostatin-1 in necrosis and T cell activation. *PLoS One* **6**(8): e23209.

Coupienne, I., Fettweis, G., Rubio, N., Agostinis, P., Piette, J. (2011) 5-ALA-PDT induces RIP3-dependent necrosis in glioblastoma. *Photochemistry Photobiology Sciences* **10**: 1868–1878.

Dayal, S., Krolicki, R., Lou, Y., Qiu, X., Berlin, J.C., Kenney, M.E., Burda, C. (2006) Femtosecond time-resolved energy transfer from CdSe nanoparticles to phthalocyanines. *Applied Physics B* **84**(1): 309–315.

Engelberg-Kulka, H., Amitai, S., Kolodkin-Gal, I., Hazan, R. (2006) Bacterial programmed cell death and multicellular behavior in bacteria. *PLoS Genetics* **2**(10): e135.

Erental, A., Sharon, I., Engelberg-Kulka, H. (2012) Two programmed cell death systems in *Escherichia coli*: An apoptotic-like death is inhibited by the mazEF-mediated death pathway. *PLoS Biology* **10**(3): e1001281.

Firdous, S., Nawaz, M., Ikram, M., Ahmed, M. (2012) In vitro study of cell death with 5-aminolevulinic acid based photodynamic therapy to improve the efficiency of cancer treatment. *Laser Physics* **22**(3): 626–633.

FláviaArrudaPortilho, F.A., Cavalcanti, C.E.O., Miranda-Vilela, A.L., Estevanato, L.L.C., Longo, J.P.F., Santos, M.F.M.A., Bocca, A.L. et al. (2013) Antitumor activity of photodynamic therapy performed with nanospheres containing zinc-phthalocyanine. *Journal of Nanobiotechnology* **11**: 41–65.

Fonteh, P.N., Keter, F.K., Meyer, D. (2010) HIV therapeutic possibilities of gold compounds. *Biometals D* **23**: 185–196.

Gao, J.H., Liang, G.L., Zhang, B. (2007) FePt@CoS2 yolk-shell nanocrystals as a potent agent to kill HeLa cells. *Journal of the American Chemical Society* **129**(5): 1428–1433.

Garg, A.D., Maes, H., Romanoa, E., Agostinis, P. (2015) Autophagy, a major adaptation pathway shaping cancer cell death and anticancer immunity responses following photodynamic therapy. *Photochemistry and Photobiology Science* **14**(8): 1410–1424.

Giorgi, C., Bonora, M., Missiroli, S., Poletti, F., Ramirez, F.G., Morciano, G., Morganti, C., Pandolfi, P.P., Mammano, F., Pinton, P. (2015) Intravital imaging reveals p53-dependent cancer cell death induced by phototherapy via calcium signaling. *Oncotargets* **6**(3): 1435–1445.

Gormley, A.J., Larson, N., Sadekar, S., Robinson, R., Ray, A., Ghandehari, H. (2012) Guided delivery of polymer therapeutics using plasmonic photothermal therapy. *NanoToday* **7**: 158.

Gross, N., Ranjbar, M., Evers, C., Hua, J., Martin, G., Schulze, B., Michaelis, U., Hansen, L.L. Agostini, H.T. (2013) Choroidal neovascularization reduced by targeted drug delivery with cationic liposome-encapsulated paclitaxel or targeted photodynamic therapy with verteporfin encapsulated in cationic liposomes. *Molecular Vision* **19**: 54–61.

Guillaud, G., Simon, J., Germain, J.P. (1998) Metallophthalocyanines: Gas sensors, resistors and field effect transistors. *Coordinated Chemical Reviews* **178–180**: 903–1846.

Gupta, A.K., Gupta, M. (2005) Synthesis and surface engineering of iron oxide nanoparticles for biomedical applications. *Biomaterials* **26**(18): 3995–4021.

Huang, Z., Xu, H.P., Meyers, A.D., Musani, A.I., Wang, L.W., Tagg, R., Barqawi, A.B., Chen, Y.K. (2008) Photodynamic therapy for treatment of solid tumors—Potential and technical challenges. *Technology of Cancer Research and Treatment* **7**: 309–320.

Idowu, M., Chen, J.-Y., Nyokong, T. (2008) Photoinduced energy transfer between water soluble CdTe quantum dots and aluminium tetrasulfonatedphthalocyanine. *New Journal of Chemistry* **32**: 290–296.

Ito, A., Shinkai, M., Honda, H., Kobayashi, T. (2005) Medical application of functional magnetic nanoparticles. *Journal of Bioscience and Bioengineering* **100**(1): 1–10.

Juzenas, P., Chen, W., Sun, Y.-P. Coelho, M.A.V.N., Generalova, R., Generalova, N., Christensen, I.L. (2008) Quantum dots and nanoparticles for photodynamic and radiation therapies of cancer. *Advances in Drug Delivery Reviews* **60**(15): 1600–1614.

Kang, R., Zeh, H.J., Lotze, M.T., Tang, D. (2011) The Beclin 1 network regulates autophagy and apoptosis. *Cell Death Differentiation* **18**: 571–580.

Karp, J.M., Peer, D., Hong, D., Farokhzad, S., Margalit, O., Langer, R.R. (2007) Nanocarriers as an emerging platform for cancer therapy. *National Nanotechnology* **2**(12): 751–760.

Kim, K.S., Cho, C.H., Park, E.K., Jung, M.H., Yoon, K.S., Park, H.K. (2012) AFM-detected apoptotic changes in morphology and biophysical property caused by paclitaxel in Ishikawa and HeLa cells. *PLoS One* **7**(1): e30066.

Kroemer, G., Galluzzi, L., Vandenabeele, P., Abrams, J., Alnemri, E.S., Baehrecke, E.H., Blagosklonny, M.V. et al. (2009) Classification of cell death. *Cell Death Differentiation* **16**(1): 3–11.

Lam, M., Lee, Y.J., Deng, M., Hsia, A.H., Morrissey, K.A., Yan, C., Azzizudin, K. et al. (2010) Photodynamic therapy with the silicon phthalocyanine Pc 4 induces apoptosis in mycosis fungoides and sezary syndrome. *Advances in Hematology* **2010**: 896161. doi:10.1155/2010/896161.

Lemasters, J.J. (2005) Dying a thousand deaths: Redundant pathways from different organelles to apoptosis and necrosis. *Gastroenterology* **129**(1): 351–360.

Longo, J.P.F., de Melo, L.N.D., Mijan, M.C., Valois, C.R.A., Joanitti, G.A., Simioni, A.R., Tedesco, A.C., de Azevedo, R.B. (2013) Photodynamic therapy mediated by liposomal chloroaluminum-phthalocyanine induces necrosis in oral cancer cells. *Journal of Biomaterials and Tissue Engineering* **3**(1): 148–156.

Longo, J.P.F., Lozzi, S.P., Simioni, A.R., Morais, P.C., Tedesco, A.C., Azevedo, R.B. (2009) Photodynamic therapy with aluminum-chloro-phthalocyanine induces necrosis and vascular damage in mice tongue tumors. *Journal of Photochemistry and Photobiology B* **94**(2): 143–146.

MacDonald, I.J., Dougherty, T.J. (2001) Advances in heterocyclic chemistry *Porphyrins Phthalocyanines* **5**: 105.

Manoto, S.L., Abrahamse, H. (2011) Effect of a newly synthesized Zn sulfophthalocyanine derivative on cell morphology, viability, proliferation, and cytotoxicity in a human lung cancer cell line (A549). *Lasers in Medical Science* **26**(4): 523–530.

Manoto, S.L., Houreld, N.N., Abrahamse, H. (2013) Phototoxic effect of photodynamic therapy on lung cancer cells grown as a monolayer and three dimensional multicellular spheroids. *Lasers in Surgery and Medicine* **45**(3): 186–194.

Manoto, S.L., Sekhejane, P.R., Houreld, N.N., Abrahamse, H. (2012) Localization and phototoxic effect of zinc sulfophthalocyanine photosensitizer in human colon (DLD-1) and lung (A549) carcinoma cells (in vitro). *Photodiagnosis and Photodynamic Therapy* **9**(1): 52–59.

Mfouo-Tynga, I., Abrahamse, H. (2015) Cell death pathways and phthalocyanine as an efficient agent for photodynamic cancer therapy. *International Journal of Molecular Sciences* **16**: 10228–10241. doi:10.3390/ijms16051022.

Mfouo-Tynga, I., Houreld, N.N., Abrahamse, H. (2012) The primary subcellular localization of zinc phthalocyanine and its cellular impact on viability, proliferation and structure of breast cancer cells (MCF-7). *Journal of Photochemistry and Photobiology B* **120**: 171–176.

Mfouo-Tynga, I., Houreld, N.N., Abrahamse, H. (2014) Induced cell death pathway post photodynamic therapy using a metallophthalocyanine photosensitizer in breast cancer cells. *Photomedicine and Laser Surgery* **32**(4): 205–211.

Michaud, M., Martins, I., Sukkurwala, A.Q., Adjemian, S., Ma, Y., Pellegatti, P., Shen, S. et al. (2011) Autophagy-dependent anticancer immune responses induced by chemotherapeutic agents in mice. *Science* **334**: 1573–1577.

Mroz, P., Yaroslavsky, A., Kharkwal, G.B., Hamblin, M.R. (2011) Cell death pathways in photodynamic therapy of cancer. *Cancers* **3**: 2516–2539.

Mthethwa, T.P., Arslanoglu, Y., Antunes, E., Nyokong, T. (2012) Photophysical behaviour of cationic 2-(dimethylamino) ethanethiotetrasubstitutedphthalocyanine complexes in the presence of gold nanoparticles. *Polyhedron* **38**: 169–177.

Nyokong, T., Antunes, E. (2013) Influence of nanoparticle materials on the photophysical behaviour of phthalocyanines. *Coordination Chemistry Reviews* **257**: 2401–2418.

Ochsner, M. (1996) Light scattering of human skin: A comparison between zinc(II)—Phthalocyanine and photofrin II. *Journal of Photochemistry and Photobiology B: Biology* **32**: 3–9.

Patel, A.S., Lin, L., Geyer, A., Haspel, J.A., An, C.H., Cao, J., Rosas, I.O., Morse, D. (2012) Autophagy in idiopathic pulmonary fibrosis. *PLoS One* 7(7): e41394.

Peracchio, C., Alabiso, O., Valente, G., Isidoro, C. (2012) Involvement of autophagy in ovarian cancer: A working hypothesis. *Journal of Ovarian Research* **5**: 22–32.

Pereira, P.M.R., Silva, S., Cavaleiro, J.A.S., Ribeiro, C.A.F., Tome, J.P.C., Fernandes, R. (2014) Galactodendritic phthalocyanine targets carbohydrate-binding proteins enhancing photodynamic therapy. *PLoS One* 9(4): e95529.

Seotsanyana-Mokhosi, I., Kresfelder, T., Abrahamse, H., Nyokong, T. (2006) The effect of Ge, Si and Sn phthalocyanine photosensitizers on cell proliferation and viability of human oesophageal carcinoma cells. *Journal of Photochemistry and Photobiology B* 83(1): 55–62.

Separovic, D., Joseph, N., Breen, P., Bielawski, J., Pierce, J.S., van Buren, E., Bhatti, G., Saad, Z.H., Bai, A., Bielawska, A. (2011) Combining anticancer agents photodynamic therapy and LCL85 leads to distinct changes in the sphingolipid profile, autophagy, caspase-3 activation in the absence of cell death, and long-term sensitization. *Biochemistry Biophysics Research Communications* **409**: 372–377.

Seydel, C. (2003) Quantum dots get wet. *Science* **300**(5616): 80–81.

Sharman, W.M., Allen, C.M., van Lier J.E. (1999) Photodynamic therapeutics: Basic principles and clinical applications. *Therapeutic Reviews* 4(11): 508–517.

Sharman, W.M., Allen, C.M., van Lier J.E. (2000) Role of activated oxygen species in photodynamic therapy. *Methods in Enzymology* **319**: 376–400.

Shaw, C.F. (1999) Gold-based therapeutic agents. *Chemical Reviews* **99**: 2589–2600.

Sobolev, A.S., Stranadko, E.F. (1997) Photodynamic therapy in Russia: Clinical and fundamental aspects. *International Photodynamics* 1(6): 2–3.

Weijer, R., Broekgaarden, M., Kos, M., Van Vught, R., Rauws, E.A.J., Breukink, E., Van Gulik, T.M., Storm, G., Heger, M. (2015) Enhancing photodynamic therapy of refractory solid cancers: Combining second-generation photosensitizers with multi-targeted liposomal delivery. *Journal of Photochemistry and Photobiology C: Photochemistry Reviews* 23(2015): 103–131.

Weishaupt, K.R., Gomer, C.J., Dougherty, T.J. (1976) Identification of singlet oxygen as cytotoxic agent in photo-inactivation of a murine tumor. *Cancer Research* **36**: 2326–2329.

Whitacre, C.M., Feyes, D.K., Satoh, T., Grossmann, J., Mulvihill, J.W., Mukhtar, H., Oleinick, N.L. (2000) Photodynamic therapy with the phthalocyanine photosensitizer Pc 4 of SW480 human colon cancer xenografts in athymic mice. *Clinical Cancer Research* 6(5): 2021–2027.

Wood, S.R., Holroyd, J.A., Brown, S.B. (1997) The subcellular localization of Zn (II) phthalocyanines and their redistribution on exposure to light. *Photochemistry and Photobiology* 65(3): 397–402.

Xie, Z., Klionsky, D.J. (2007) Autophagosome formation: Core machinery and adaptation. *Nature Cell Biology* **9**: 1102–1109.

Xue, L.Y., Chiu, S.M., Oleinick N.L. (2010) Atg7 deficiency increases resistance of MCF-7 human breast cancer cells to photodynamic therapy. *Autophagy* 6(2): 248–255.

Yu, L., Wan, F., Dutta, S., Welsh, S., Liu, Z., Freundt, E., Baehrecke, E.H., Lenardo, M. (2006) Autophagic programmed cell death by selective catalase degradation. *Proceedings of the Nathional Academy of Science USA* **103**(13): 4952–4957.

Zaidi, S.I.A., Oleinick, N.L., Zaim, M.T., Mukhtar, H. (1993) Apoptosis during photodynamic therapy-induced ablation of RIF 1 tumors in C3H mice: Electron microscopic, histopathologic and biochemical evidence. *Photochemistry Photobiology* **58**: 771–776.

Singlet oxygen luminescence imaging
A prospective tool in bioscience?

MICHAEL PFITZNER, JAN C. SCHLOTHAUER, LISHENG LIN,
BUHONG LI, AND BEATE RÖDER

4.1 INTRODUCTION

The concept of monitoring the distribution of photosensitizers (PSs) in biological systems is a well-known and common procedure in various medical and scientific applications. However, the registration of PS fluorescence is limited to obtain an impression of its localization. Evaluation of the PS fluorescence does not necessarily give information about $^1O_2$ generation efficiency.

It is well known that $^1O_2$ is the main mediator of the photodynamic therapy (PDT) effect.[1] For this, numerous efforts have been made to detect $^1O_2$ in vitro as well as in vivo. The detection methods of

$^1O_2$ range from indirect methods using monitor molecules, other indirect methods that do not require additional drugs, to direct $^1O_2$ detection via its weak near-infrared (NIR) phosphorescence at around 1270 nm.[2–9]

The registration of this NIR phosphorescence is believed to be a potent PDT dosimetry technique that may be used for improving the treatment efficiency. Furthermore, it can be used for quantitative investigations of the mechanism of $^1O_2$ generation and its interaction with the microenvironment of the PS.[10,11]

Elevating the ability of $^1O_2$ NIR detection to an imaging level will greatly improve knowledge about basic processes. The advantages, problems, and prospects of state-of-the art imaging methods will be discussed in this chapter.

4.1.1 SINGLET OXYGEN DETECTION METHODS

For imaging purposes, fluorescence microscopy is a useful approach since it is a well-established and widely used technique. The advantage of fluorescence microscopy using fluorescence markers is the high quantum yield ($>10^{-2}$) of such markers. Their fluorescence can easily be detected in contrast to the extremely weak (quantum yield $<10^{-5}$) NIR phosphorescence generated by $^1O_2$.

Fluorescence probes for indirect detection of $^1O_2$ such as singlet oxygen sensor green can be used in solution[12] and have been investigated for the use in leaves and mammalian cells.[4,13] Similar probes such as Aarhus sensor green overcome specific problems such as self-photosensitization.[14,15] However, the relative localization of the PS and the monitor molecule in the cell is of high importance to treat and understand the measurement results. For this reason, it is considered to be "difficult or impossible" to use such probes in complex systems as in vivo.[16] Another crucial factor one has to keep in mind when using monitor molecules is the reaction between $^1O_2$ and the monitor molecule [**This book - Chapter 15 by St. Hackbarth: "Photosensitizer activity imaging on the microscopic scale"**]. This reaction competes with the required reaction between $^1O_2$ and cell organelles and consequently the PDT effect.

Other common indirect detection methods do not allow spatial resolution, such as spin-trap markers detected with electron spin resonance,[17,18] or observation of the change of inherent parameters such as refractive index or the generation of acoustic waves.[19,20]

Singlet oxygen imaging is in principle also possible by using delayed fluorescence of the PS.[21,22] Approaches like the direct excitation of $^1O_2$ by a 1270 nm laser may be suitable to monitor the effect of localized $^1O_2$ generation.[23] Image generation might be feasible by combining it with a scanning approach.

Apart from the problem of colocalization of PS and monitor molecules, all indirect methods, at best, indicate the amount of $^1O_2$ generated. A major limitation of using indirect methods is the intrinsic inability to resolve the $^1O_2$ luminescence and PS triplet kinetics. In this chapter, we will focus on recent efforts and promising prospects of imaging techniques that rely on direct $^1O_2$ detection.

4.1.1.1 DIRECT SINGLET OXYGEN LUMINESCENCE DETECTION AND IMAGING

The possibility of direct $^1O_2$ measurements by its luminescence at 1270 nm was first demonstrated in 1976 using a cooled NIR photomultiplier. In this study, photodynamic reactions in air-saturated solutions of pigments were investigated.[24,25]

With the development of modern, high-sensitive NIR photomultiplier tubes (PMTs), NIR cameras, lasers with ns pulse duration and high repetition rates and different electronic systems for data acquisition, today there exists a technical basis that makes it reasonable to consider $^1O_2$ luminescence as a prospective tool in bioscience.

Two approaches for $^1O_2$ imaging exist. One method is based on the utilization of a NIR PMT in combination with a scanning device and fibers (Figure 4.1a) or conventional optics (Figure 4.1b). The second approach is based on the use of a NIR camera with a set of band-pass (BP) filters to discriminate the $^1O_2$ phosphorescence from background luminescence (Figure 4.1c). Reports of these approaches in literature are summarized in Table 4.1.

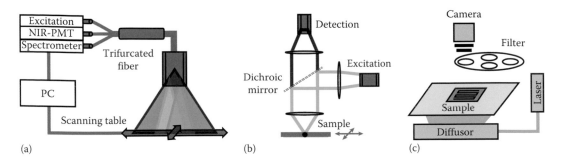

Figure 4.1 Illustration of scanning (a, b) and (c) steady-state wide-field imaging.

Table 4.1 Imaging systems for $^1O_2$ luminescence

NIR detector	Object	Scanning	Resolution (µm)	Integrated time (s)	Ref.
InGaAs linear array detector (Princeton Instrument)	Cells with D_2O	(Yes)	2.5	30	[26]
Camera (XEVA, Xenics)	Mouse skin	No	39.4	1	[5]
Camera (MOSIR 950, Intevac)	Tumor model	No	46.0	40–50	[6]
Camera (NIRvana:640, Princeton Instruments)	Cells with D_2O	No	1.4	5	[27]
Camera (XEVA, Xenics)	Dorsal skin window chamber	No	30	1	[28]
PMT (R5509, Hamamatsu)	Tumor model	Yes	1000	400	[29]
PMT (H10330-45, Hamamatsu)	Skin model	Yes	200	4000	[9]
PMT (R5509, Hamamatsu)	C_{60} powder	Yes	17.96	589.824	[30]

4.1.1.2 STEADY-STATE IMAGING

In 2002, Andersen et al. firstly obtained a $^1O_2$ luminescence image by developing a microscope with an InGaAs linear array.[26] Singlet oxygen images of single cells with 2.5 µm spatial resolution could be achieved by exchanging the intracellular H_2O with D_2O to enhance the lifetime of $^1O_2$ in the intracellular environment. For these $^1O_2$ images, data from each slice in the sample were recorded using an exposure time of 30 s. Major efforts on $^1O_2$ imaging on the microscopic scale have been made, for example, by the group of Ogilby.[31–33] Imaging on the microscopic scale will not be discussed in this chapter because medical relevance for PDT is currently not established. Its use for fundamental research, such as the investigation of cell signaling processes, is discussed in the literature.[34]

With regard to $^1O_2$ luminescence imaging, Hu et al. used a cooled NIR InGaAs camera combined with 1150 nm long-pass (LP) and 1270 nm BP optical filters.[5] The spatial resolution of the imaging system was around 50 µm, and the acquisition time for each image was about 1.0 s. However, a single LP filter with a 1270 nm BP filter is insufficient to differentiate $^1O_2$ luminescence from other long-wavelength background signals. This is especially true for in vivo measurements, where the $^1O_2$ luminescence is extremely weak relative to the tissue and PS luminescence background. In order to overcome this limitation, Lee et al. used a set of BP

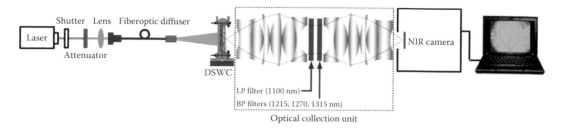

Figure 4.2 Schematic diagram of the $^1O_2$ luminescence imaging system. DSWC, dorsal skinfold window chamber; LP, long-pass; BP, band-pass; NIR, Near-infrared.

filters at 1220, 1270, and 1320 nm with 15 nm full width at half maximum (FWHM) bandwidth to discriminate the $^1O_2$ luminescence from other possible radiation sources.[6] The spatial resolution was estimated to be less than 100 μm. When measurements were made in a highly quenching fetal bovine serum environment, the images were obtained in 40–50 s at each optical filter position to improve signal-to-noise ratio (SNR).

Most recently, a novel configuration of the Xenics Model XEVA-1.7-320 NIR-sensitive InGaAs camera was developed to image the photodynamically generated $^1O_2$ luminescence using custom-designed NIR optics to collect the luminescence.[28] The system is illustrated in Figure 4.2. A semiconductor laser was coupled into a quartz fiberoptic diffuser for illumination, and the optimized collection optics provided accelerated image acquisition with acceptable SNR. The detection of $^1O_2$ luminescence in the acquired images was tested using the model photosensitizer rose bengal (RB) in aqueous solution. To demonstrate the system performance, luminescence images were recorded with each of three custom-made BP filters (25 nm FWHM) following an LP filter that reduces the background. The average of the 1215 and 1315 nm images was subtracted pixel by pixel from the image recorded at 1270 nm to obtain the $^1O_2$ luminescence image. Furthermore, attempts to correlate $^1O_2$ luminescence images, obtained with a camera, with the biological response during PDT were made.[35-37]

4.1.1.3 TIME-RESOLVED IMAGING

Analysis of the $^1O_2$ kinetics can give insights into the microenvironment of the PS and the amount of generated $^1O_2$. A strong interaction of $^1O_2$ with molecules located in the microenvironment of the PS results in a shorter $^1O_2$ lifetime, whereas oxygen depletion leads to longer PS triplet decay times. Under normal physiological conditions, the deactivation of the PS triplet state mainly occurs via energy transfer to O_2.

In 2005, Niedre et al. developed a scanning laser system to image $^1O_2$ luminescence in an intradermal tumor model in mice. In order to maintain adequate SNR, each image was acquired in four 100 s scans with 1.0 mm resolution.[29]

A major leap in methodology was reported in 2009 by Schlothauer et al. reporting high SNR measurements of cells (in vitro) and subsequent scanning of skin tissues (ex vivo). Schlothauer et al. reported a 2-D imaging system for scanning of $^1O_2$ luminescence kinetics in skin samples with spatial resolution of 0.2 mm using an integration time of 10.0 s per pixel. The collected data showed that the $^1O_2$ kinetics coincides with the microarchitecture of the epidermis, such as fissures and hair follicles.[9,38]

Most recently, the feasibility of $^1O_2$ luminescence lifetime imaging microscopy was studied on a modified fluorescence lifetime imaging microscope, and the $^1O_2$ luminescence intensity and lifetime image of a layer of loose C_{60} powder have been successfully obtained.[30]

4.2 DISCUSSION OF SINGLET OXYGEN LUMINESCENCE IMAGING IN SPECIFIC SYSTEMS

Here, several aspects of direct $^1O_2$ imaging of selected in vivo model systems will be presented, followed by a discussion of the benefits of the applied methods as well as current problems.

The evaluation of $^1O_2$ kinetics in complex systems is a very challenging task. Furthermore, a sound interpretation of the kinetics is a necessary basis for the interpretation of such data. Several fundamental aspects, including the effects by the measurement itself, have to be taken into account: Fundamentally, knowledge about the structure of the microenvironment is necessary to describe the $^1O_2$ kinetics in many different biological systems [**This book Chapter 15 by St. Hackbarth: "Photosensitizer activity imaging on the microscopic scale"**]. The luminescence signal may consist of light arising from different origins with different kinetics. Unwanted components have to be identified to discriminate the $^1O_2$ kinetics of interest. In addition, effects of the measurement, such as the duration or the light exposure during the measurement, affect the kinetics.

4.2.1 EVALUATION OF NIR LUMINESCENCE KINETICS IN MODEL SYSTEMS

To illustrate the fundamental problems associated with the $^1O_2$ detection in vivo, we give a short introduction of the evaluation of time-resolved $^1O_2$ luminescence kinetics for three model systems. The most basic system, which is well described in literature,[39] is that of a single PS in a homogeneous solution. The $^1O_2$ luminescence intensity $I(t)$ can be fitted with the biexponential model described by

$$I(t) = \frac{A}{1 - \frac{\tau_T}{\tau_\Delta}} \left(e^{-\frac{t}{\tau_\Delta}} - e^{-\frac{t}{\tau_T}} \right) + O, \tag{4.1}$$

including the PS triplet decay time τ_T, the $^1O_2$ decay time τ_Δ, an amplitude parameter A, and an offset O due to detector noise.

For chlorine e6 (Ce6) in water, a reduced χ^2 of 1.02 shows that the kinetics can be described with the biexponential $^1O_2$ model (Equation 4.1). The typical[38,40,41] $^1O_2$ decay time of (3.49 ± 0.04) µs for aqueous surroundings was observed and a PS triplet decay time of (1.99 ± 0.03) µs was obtained (compare Figure 4.3a).

Deviations from this signal form may have different reasons:

- Diffusion effects
- PS phosphorescence
- Endogenous NIR luminescence
- Superposition of $^1O_2$ signals from different environments

Diffusion effects influence kinetics if $^1O_2$ is generated inside a membrane and diffuses into the surroundings. A detailed explanation of this mechanism can be found in the respective chapter. [**This book Chapter 15 by St. Hackbarth: "Photosensitizer activity imaging on the microscopic scale"**].

Another mechanism preventing the usage of the biexponential model is the tail of the PS phosphorescence emission extending into the detection window around 1270 nm.[42–44] Depending on its intensity, it can be an almost undetectable disturbance of the signal. Depending on the PS and the environment, a strong additional exponential PS phosphorescence decay can occur, obscuring the typical signal form. Since the phosphorescence originates from triplet PS molecules, its decay time is the triplet decay time, and the following model has to be used to describe the luminescence signal:

$$I(t) = \frac{A}{1 - \frac{\tau_T}{\tau_\Delta}} \left(e^{-\frac{t}{\tau_\Delta}} - e^{-\frac{t}{\tau_T}} \right) + Be^{-\frac{t}{\tau_T}} + O \tag{4.2}$$

Such signals can be acquired, for example, from RB in water. The luminescence kinetics are shown in Figure 4.3b. The individual contributions of the PS and $^1O_2$ phosphorescence components are indicated.

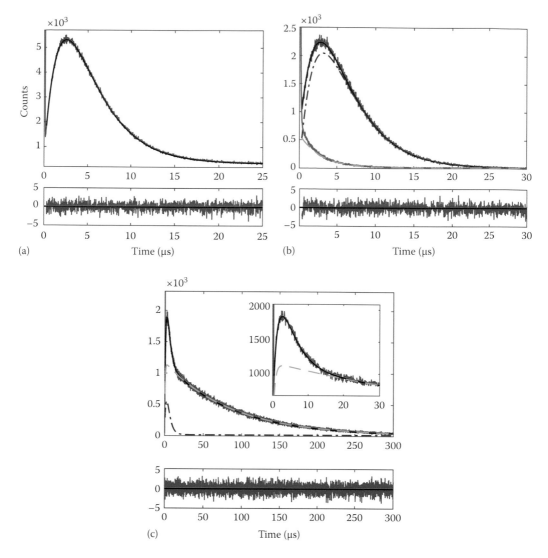

Figure 4.3 Luminescence signals of (a) Ce6 in PBS (τ_Δ = 3.49 μs and τ_T = 1.99 μs). (b) RB in water (τ_Δ = 3.5 μs and τ_T = 2.7 μs), and (c) layers of TMPyP in water and pheophorbide-a (Pheo) in ethanol.

As a first approximation for the description of the luminescence kinetics if an additional NIR luminescence from a source other than the PS triplet state occurs, the signal can be described by

$$I(t) = \frac{A}{1 - \dfrac{\tau_T}{\tau_\Delta}} \left(e^{-\frac{t}{\tau_\Delta}} - e^{-\frac{t}{\tau_T}} \right) + Be^{-\frac{t}{\tau_{NIR}}} + O \tag{4.3}$$

introducing the apparent decay time τ_{NIR} for the additional luminescence.

Additionally, a superposition of kinetics resulting from $^1O_2$ generated in different microenvironments can also be a cause for the deviation of the luminescence kinetics from the commonly used biexponential model.

To mimic a system in which we can detect $^1O_2$ generated in two distinct microenvironments, two PSs in different solvents were used as a model, specifically Pheo in DCM and TMPyP in water. Since neither the PS

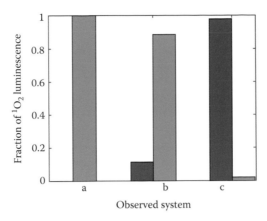

Figure 4.4 The contribution of integrated signals as they would contribute to the measured steady-state signal in these three systems is illustrated. Thereby in system "a" only $^1O_2$ luminescence, whereas in "b" $^1O_2$ luminescence as well as some additional phosphorescence are detected. In system "c," the shorter decaying $^1O_2$ luminescence of TMPyP in water is assumed to be the signal of interest. The ratios are valid only for the model systems to illustrate possible conditions in vivo.

is soluble in the other environment nor do the solvents intermix, we can prepare a two-layered arrangement with negligible interaction along the interface. If the detection volume covers partly the upper and partly the lower solvent, the described superposition of kinetics can be detected (compare Figure 4.3c). A fit to this kinetics with the appropriate double biexponential model (Equation 4.4) yields decay times of $\tau_{\Delta 1} = 3.6$ μs, $\tau_{T1} = 2.2$ μs, $\tau_{\Delta 2} = 84.7$ μs, and $\tau_{T2} = 0.5$ μs, which are in good agreement with the decay times obtained for the corresponding homogeneous solutions separately:

$$I(t) = \frac{A}{1 - \dfrac{\tau_{T1}}{\tau_{\Delta 1}}} \left(e^{-\frac{t}{\tau_{\Delta 1}}} - e^{-\frac{t}{\tau_{T1}}} \right) + \frac{B}{1 - \dfrac{\tau_{T2}}{\tau_{\Delta 2}}} \left(e^{-\frac{t}{\tau_{\Delta 2}}} - e^{-\frac{t}{\tau_{T2}}} \right) + O \tag{4.4}$$

The desired information is usually the amount of $^1O_2$ generated in a specific subsystem. As a result of the different possible kinetics, the total luminescence intensity such as that obtained by steady-state measurements does not reflect the amount of $^1O_2$ generated as illustrated in Figure 4.4. Only for the simple PS in solution without quenchers or PS phosphorescence the total luminescence signal is proportional to the amount of $^1O_2$. Time-resolved measurements as well as the knowledge about the system are necessary to calculate the $^1O_2$ quantity.

4.2.2 SKIN

PDT can be advantageously used in many different oncological and nononcological applications in dermatology.[45,46] Today, many conditions can be treated with high success rates and few side effects.[47] Due to the long-term experience from medical practice and a quite extensive use of PDT in dermatology, the investigation of $^1O_2$ generation in skin is consequentially a very important field of study.

Singlet oxygen luminescence detection in skin can be used to investigate a variety of questions. Upon the photophysical characterization of new PDT drugs, time-resolved detection is considered the most beneficial and informative tool.[48] It is relevant to tumor treatment by PDT for which $^1O_2$ luminescence is believed to be a prospective technique for optimizing protocols by direct dosimetry.[49] In addition, the possible reduction of photoprotection against PDT-drug-induced photosensitization of the skin[50] as well as the photoprotection of normal healthy skin by sunscreens[51,52] are questions that can be addressed by $^1O_2$ luminescence detection.

The most widely used model for in vivo human skin probably is the ex vivo pig ear. The ex vivo porcine ear is considered a model for healthy human skin with respect to several different parameters.[53–58] For some penetration experiments, for example, for follicular penetration, the ex vivo pig ear is even reported to be superior to, for example, ex vivo human skin.[59]

For experiments using photodynamic drugs, different procedures for incorporating the PS into the skin have been applied. The topical application of ALA-crème is a clinical procedure for photodynamic treatment of various skin diseases[60]; simulations of the response including $^1O_2$ have been reported.[61] Experiments using the medically approved PS Foscan® applied in a crème were reported for pig ear.[62] Also, experiments based on incubation of skin samples with a PS in solution were reported.[63]

A few single observations of $^1O_2$ luminescence kinetics from in vivo living skin have been reported in the literature. Rat skin was investigated after intravenous (IV) injection of AlS_4Pc,[64] human skin by UVA excitation of endogenous PS.[65] Ex vivo pig ear was investigated after incubation with an aqueous solution of TMPyP.[66] The time-resolved luminescence detection with a very high SNR has only been reported a few years ago,[67] which enabled skin $^1O_2$ luminescence detection under light doses relevant to PDT ex vivo pig ear upon topical application of Pheo.[3,9,68]

4.2.2.1 TIME-RESOLVED SINGLET OXYGEN LUMINESCENCE AND THE STRUCTURE OF SKIN

A comparative study of the time-resolved $^1O_2$ luminescence of two different PSs, topically applied to the pig ear skin, was conducted. Namely, the amphiphilic Pheo and the highly hydrophobic perfluoroalkylated zinc phthalocyanine ($F_{64}PcZn$) were used. Fluorescence microscopy (Figure 4.5) indicated the exclusive accumulation of Pheo in the stratum corneum, while $F_{64}PcZn$ accumulates also in deeper layers of the epidermis of the pig ear skin.

When the correlations between the differences in the accumulation pattern of the different PSs and the $^1O_2$ kinetics are examined, differences are apparent. The blue and red curves in Figure 4.6a and b show the kinetics for an initial measurement and a measurement after illumination. For Pheo, the triplet decay time of the first measurement is 0.3 ± 0.2 μs and increases after an illumination of the sample with 5.5. J/cm² to 0.9 ± 0.2 μs, while the $^1O_2$ decay time increases from 12.5 ± 0.5 μs to 16.7 ± 0.5 μs. $F_{64}PcZn$ exhibits a similar behavior with slightly different parameters: the decay times of the $F_{64}PcZn$ sample increase from $\tau_T = 0.4 \pm 0.2$ μs and $\tau_{O2} = 10.2 \pm 0.5$ μs to $\tau_T = 0.8 \pm 0.2$ μs and $\tau_{O2} = 15.0 \pm 0.5$ μs after delivery of 11 J/cm².

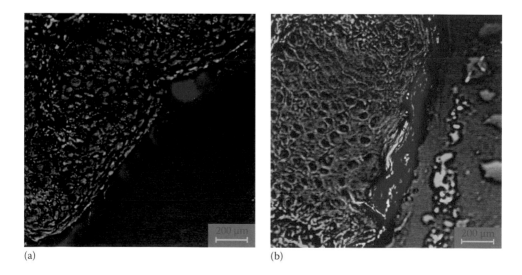

(a)   (b)

Figure 4.5 Fluorescence microscopy image of skin samples prepared with PS-crème. The fluorescence of the photosensitizers is shown in red, (a) Pheo and (b) $F_{64}PcZn$. Pheo shows fluorescence only in the stratum corneum while $F_{64}PcZn$ is also fluorescing in deeper layers of the epidermis. (Reprinted from Schlothauer, J.C. et al., *J. Biomed. Opt.*, 1711, 115005, 2012.)

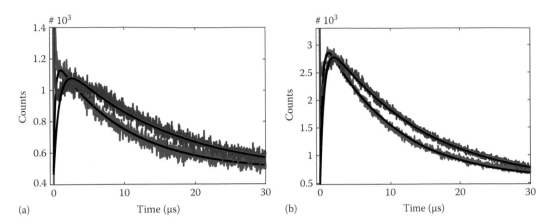

Figure 4.6 Luminescence decay of $^1O_2$ photosensitized generated by (a) Pheo and (b) $F_{64}PcZn$ in pig skin. Dark blue dots: initial measurement (1.1 J/cm²), light red squares: measurement after (a) 5.5 J/cm² resp. (b) 11 J/cm². Black lines are the fitting curves according to Equation 4.1. Fitted parameters (a) (1.1 J/cm²): $\tau_T = 0.3 \pm 0.2$ µs, $\tau_{O2} = 12.5 \pm 0.5$ µs, (5.5 J/cm²): $\tau_T = 0.9 \pm 0.2$ µs, $\tau_{O2} = 16.7 \pm 0.5$ µs, (b) (1.1 J/cm²): $\tau_T = 0.4 \pm 0.2$ µs, $\tau_{O2} = 10.2 \pm 0.5$ µs, (11 J/cm²): $\tau_T = 0.8 \pm 0.2$ µs, $\tau_{O2} = 15.0 \pm 0.5$ µs. (Reprinted from Schlothauer, J.C. et al., *J. Biomed. Opt.*, 1711, 115005, 2012.)

The systematic changes in the $^1O_2$ and PS triplet lifetimes as a function of the illumination light have been tracked up to a total dose of 20 J/cm², shown in Figure 4.7. For both PSs, it can be observed that the triplet decay times initially rise rapidly and then remain fairly constant after illumination with 5–10 J/cm². The variation of the PS triplet decay time can be attributed to a reduction of oxygen availability in the skin. Due to initial oxygen retention within the sample, a very short PS triplet decay time is observed at the beginning of the measurement followed by the consumption of oxygen within the skin by chemical reactions. Eventually, an equilibrium is reached when the rate of oxygen diffusion from the environment into the skin equals the rate of its local consumption. The increase of the $^1O_2$ decay time can be associated with a consumption of chemical quenchers.[38] As $^1O_2$ is generated, it reacts with chemical quenchers, such as endogenous antioxidants, proteins, unsaturated lipids, or other oxidative targets such as keratins,[69,70] occurring in the skin.

When the correlation between differences in the accumulation pattern of the different PSs and differences in the $^1O_2$ kinetics is examined, a significant difference between Pheo and $F_{64}PcZn$ is observed in the change of the $^1O_2$ decay time with illumination. While the Pheo sample shows an initially faster increase of the decay time, the $F_{64}PcZn$ sample shows a smoother increase with illumination.

The discrepancy could be attributed to the accumulation of the two PSs in different microenvironments. A preliminary investigation showed that intercellular lipids pose a likely accumulation site within the ultra-structure of the stratum corneum. Similar differences in the kinetics and the change of kinetics are also observed in films of extracted lipids from the stratum corneum with lower levels of tissue lipids. At this point, it must be assumed that the PSs, besides differences in their macroscopic localization, also have different microenvironments, which determine the kinetics.

In contrast to ex vivo pig ear skin, the PS triplet time in human in vivo skin changes less during illumination. Furthermore, the $^1O_2$ decay time of the in vivo sample is much lower than in the ex vivo skin. The $^1O_2$ decay time measured on the ex vivo pig ear also depends on the condition of the sample. Measurements performed on very fresh samples (at the day of slaughter) show lower decay times compared to samples measured one day later. It is reasonable to assume that the amount of $^1O_2$ scavengers would be higher in in vivo skin than in ex vivo skin, which is in agreement with the lower $^1O_2$ decay time observed in the human skin. Furthermore, the data indicate that quenchers in ex vivo pig ear skin are depleted during storage (Figure 4.8).

Despite the fact that a systematic evolution of the kinetics is observed, the order of magnitude of the parameters of signal rise and decay time matches previous reports in the literature. Decay times of 14 µs were

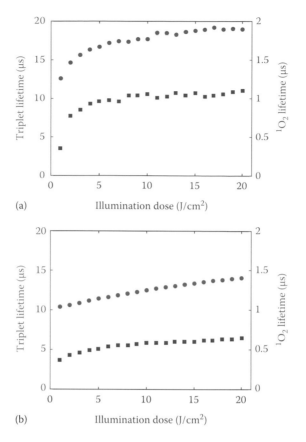

Figure 4.7 Variation of $^1O_2$ and Pheo triplet decay times in pig ear skin as a function of light doses (the scale is proportional to a time scale of 0–7 minutes). The photosensitizer is (a) Pheo and (b) F_{64}PcZn. Fitted parameters: (a) initial measurement (1.1 J/cm²): $\tau_T = 0.3 \pm 0.2$ µs, $\tau_{O2} = 12.5 \pm 0.5$ µs; final measurement (20 J/cm²): $\tau_T = 0.9 \pm 0.2$ µs, $\tau_{O2} = 19.2 \pm 0.5$ µs. (b) Initial measurement (1.1 J/cm²): $\tau_T = 0.4 \pm 0.2$ µs, $\tau_{O2} = 10.2 \pm 0.5$ µs; final measurement (20 J/cm²): $\tau T = 0.6 \pm 0.2$ µs, $\tau_{O2} = 16.1 \pm 0.5$ µs. (Reprinted from Schlothauer, J.C. et al., *J. Biomed. Opt.*, 1711, 115005, 2012.)

observed in different lipid compounds commonly found in skin.[16] These times are similar to reports by Baier et al.[65] and Nonell et al.[66] for $^1O_2$ kinetics obtained by direct excitation of pig ear samples and Jarvi et al. for experiments on rat skin.[49]

However, the statistics are not yet sufficient to draw general conclusions from the data. Nevertheless, the observed differences are in agreement with observations reported in literature. Baier et al.[65] reported a significant lower decay time of the 1270 nm luminescence signal in human skin in vivo compared to ex vivo pig ear skin upon excitation of endogenous PSs by UVA.

Even though information gained from this type of experiments is not imaging in the strict sense of the word, nevertheless it allows us to draw conclusions about the microenvironment. A more detailed discourse about the influence of the environment on the kinetics can be found in the corresponding chapter. [**This book Chapter 15 by St. Hackbarth: "Photosensitizer activity imaging on the microscopic scale"**].

4.2.2.2 TIME-RESOLVED SINGLET OXYGEN LUMINESCENCE AND THE MICROARCHITECTURE OF THE SKIN

Using a setup for macroscopic scanning, spatially resolved measurements of $^1O_2$ luminescence kinetics were acquired from a sample of pig ear skin, prepared with pheo-crème. A scanned area of about 4 mm by 4 mm is shown in Figure 4.9. The luminescence intensity distribution clearly shows several distinct maxima of the $^1O_2$

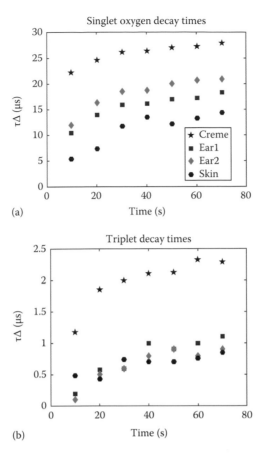

(a)

(b)

Figure 4.8 Variation of the fitted (a) $^1O_2$ decay times and (b) triplet decay times for crème, two samples of ex vivo pig ear skin and in vivo human skin, prepared with pheophorbide-a in crème, as a function of the measurement time (under constant illumination).

luminescence intensity. A correlation with a photo (Figure 4.9b) and of the scanned area (Figure 4.9c) suggests that the $^1O_2$ luminescence intensity maxima correlate with the macrostructure of the skin. Likely, the topography of the skin allows a higher accumulation of PS at certain locations. Structures like hair follicles and furrows seem to pose accumulation sites for the PS and show a higher luminescence intensity.

Even though it can be assumed that the follicular orifice acts as a location for the accumulation of the PS-crème, the luminescence kinetics allows disproving this assumption: The $^1O_2$ luminescence kinetics differs from the kinetics that would be expected for the PS in the crème. The luminescence kinetics in the skin sample shows a maximum of the $^1O_2$ decay time of 19 µs at the presumed location of follicles. Previously reported kinetics of $^1O_2$ luminescence in crème have yielded $^1O_2$ decay times of above 23 µs.[68] Taking into account the short diffusion range in the order of 100 nm, this leads to the conclusion that the $^1O_2$ is interacting with the skin. A significant accumulation of the PS-crème within the comparably large follicular orifice would show a much longer decay time—similar to crème. Cryo-biopsies of pig ear skin samples prepared with Pheo support this hypothesis: the samples show an accumulation of Pheo in the hair follicle as well as in the stratum corneum (Figure 4.10b).

Present results still do not allow us to clearly differentiate, whether the higher $^1O_2$ luminescence at the hair follicles is merely an effect of the much higher surface area due to the geometry of the hair follicle or the hair follicle provides a preferred accumulation site for Pheo.[71]

The discussed data as well as the available literature suggest very promising applications of the time-resolved $^1O_2$ imaging for PDT in dermatology. Nevertheless, the exact evaluation of the data and the conclusions to be drawn from it need further research.

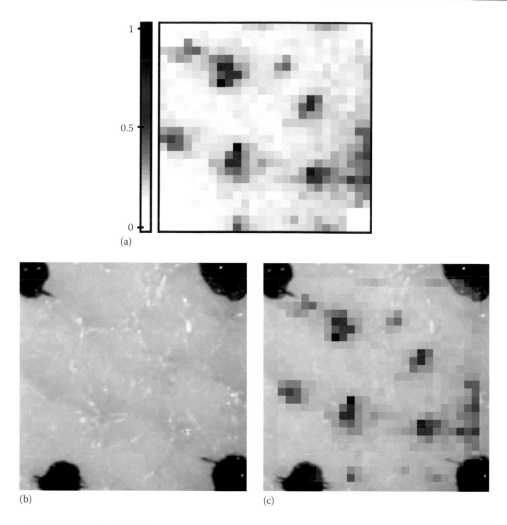

Figure 4.9 (a) Normalized $^1O_2$ luminescence intensity map. The size of the scanned area is approximately 4 × 4 mm². (b) Photo of the scanned area. The black dots on the photo are markings to correlate the scanning area with the location on the photo. (c) Overlay of (a) and (b). (Reprinted from Schlothauer, J.C. et al., *J. Biomed. Opt.*, 18(11), 115001, 2013.)

4.2.3 BLOOD VESSELS

Three interrelated mechanisms contribute to the antitumor effects of PDT: direct cytotoxic effects on tumor cells and damage to the tumor vasculature and induction of a robust inflammatory reaction that can lead to the development of systemic immunity.[72] Vascular-targeted photodynamic therapy (V-PDT) is based on site-directed delivery of a PS to tumor vasculature, which induces blood vessel closure upon light activation. V-PDT has been successfully used for the treatment of prostate cancer[73] and vascular-related diseases, including age-related macular degeneration,[74] port wine stains,[75] and bleeding gastrointestinal mucosal vascular lesions.[76] Blood vessels in the dorsal skin-fold window chamber model are widely utilized to conduct in vivo studies in order to elucidate the potential mechanisms of V-PDT treatment.

4.2.3.1 DORSAL SKINFOLD WINDOW CHAMBER MODEL

A number of both technical and conceptual reasons exist why measuring the volume-averaged $^1O_2$ concentration may fail in the complex and heterogeneous milieu of solid tumors. The well-controlled dorsal

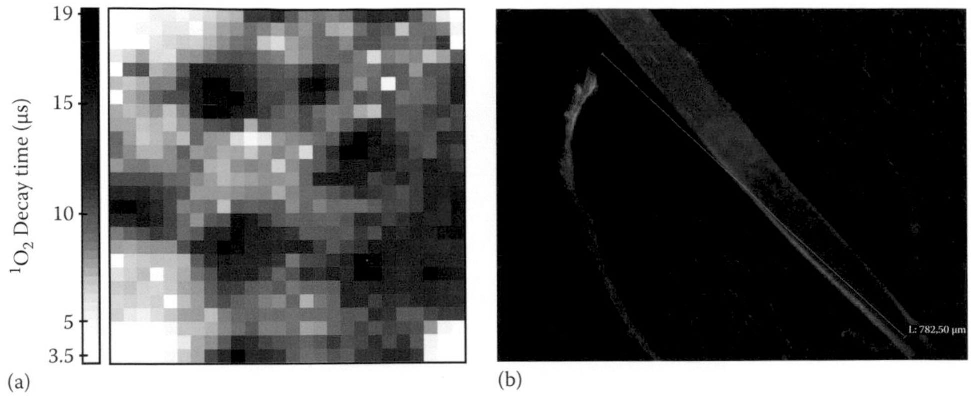

Figure 4.10 (a) Singlet oxygen decay times in μs of the scanned area in Figure 4.5. (b) Fluorescence microscopy image of a cryo-biopsy of pig ear skin prepared with pheophorbide-a in crème. The fluorescence of pheophorbide-a is shown in red and originates from within the stratum corneum as well as the hair follicle. (Reprinted from Schlothauer, J.C. et al., *J. Biomed. Opt.*, 18(11), 115001, 2013.)

skinfold window chamber model in mice in vivo offers the possibility to image the $^1O_2$ luminescence in blood vessels. BALB/c nude mice (male, 25–27 g) were purchased from Shanghai SLAC Laboratory Animal Co. Ltd., Shanghai, China. During surgery and imaging, the mice were anesthetized with sodium pentobarbital (80–100 mg/kg intraperitoneally). To image the blood vessels, a titanium window chamber (small dorsal kit SM100, APJ Trading Co., Ventura, USA) was mounted onto a dorsal skin fold, as previously described by Palmer et al. and Maurin et al.[77,78]

Two symmetric titanium frames with central holes (d = 10 mm) sandwich the double layer of skin, of which one layer is surgically excised to create an observation window that is then covered with a circular glass slide, allowing the subdermal microvasculature of the opposing skin layer to be visualized, as shown in Figure 4.11.

4.2.3.2 $^1O_2$ LUMINESCENCE IMAGE OF BLOOD VESSEL

The dorsal skinfold window chamber model in mice in vivo was used to image the $^1O_2$ luminescence in blood vessels. Luminescence images were taken before and immediately after the mice were intravenously injected

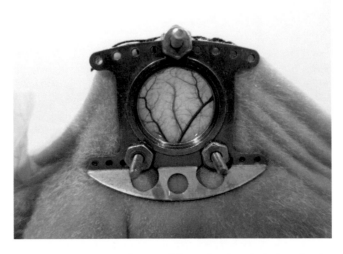

Figure 4.11 Pretreatment stereomicroscope image of the entire dorsal window chamber.

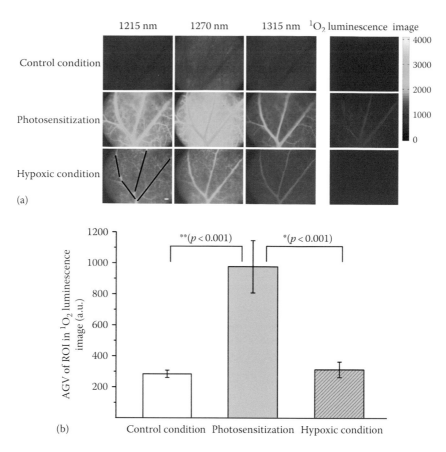

Figure 4.12 (a) Luminescence images of blood vessels in the dorsal skinfold window chamber model taken before (control condition) RB injection, immediately after injection, and 2 min after sacrifice (hypoxic condition). The ROIs are highlighted in black. Scale bar 500 μm. (b) Corresponding average grade values (AGVs) over the blood vessel ROIs in the calculated $^1O_2$ luminescence images. (From Lin, L. et al., *SPIE Photonics Europe*, SPIE, Brussels, Belgium, 2014, p. 91292.)

with RB solution (25 mg/kg body weight) at a laser intensity of 200 mW/cm². Representative luminescence images of blood vessels in the window chamber model are shown in Figure 4.12. For the control group, the blood vessels appear dark due to the strong absorption of the 532 nm irradiation light by oxyhemoglobin, as compared to the surrounding tissue.

Immediately after the mice were intravenously injected with PS RB, the intensities of the luminescence images were higher for measurements with all 3 BP filters, but were highest for the 1270 nm filter, as expected. After background subtraction, the image of $^1O_2$ luminescence in the blood vessels can be clearly seen. To verify that the 1270 nm signal was due to $^1O_2$ luminescence, its oxygen dependence was further investigated: For this, the imaging was repeated 2 min after euthanasia by anesthetic overdose. The NIR signal significantly decreased due to the reduced oxygen level in the blood vessels, so that the $^1O_2$ luminescence image no longer shows the vasculature. This is in agreement with previous observations using PMT-based $^1O_2$ luminescence detection. As illustrated in Figure 4.12b, significant differences ($p < 0.001$) in the AGV in the $^1O_2$ luminescence images were found between the photosensitization condition and the control and hypoxic conditions, respectively.

In summary, the novel configuration of an NIR-sensitive InGaAs camera and optimized light collection enables direct imaging of the $^1O_2$ luminescence generated in blood vessels during PDT, with a 2 s image integration time, which makes it practical for many in vivo studies. We are currently investigating the dependence of the $^1O_2$ luminescence images under varying PDT treatment conditions, such as PS type and concentration, oxygen concentration, and light dose, in order to better understand the mechanisms of $^1O_2$ generation during PDT. In parallel, we are also investigating the quantitative correlation between the intensities of $^1O_2$ luminescence images of blood vessels and the corresponding vasoconstriction after PDT, which holds the potential for establishing $^1O_2$ luminescence-based dosimetry in clinical treatments targeting the vasculature.

4.2.3.3 CHICKEN CHORIOALLANTOIC MEMBRANE MODEL

The chicken chorioallantoic membrane (CAM) model is a widely used, robust experimental platform for investigations in the fields of transplant biology, cancer research, drug development, and other biomedical topics.[79] It is a very convenient model for preclinical in vivo studies due to its accessibility and tissue composition. A comprehensive review about its diverse usage has been written by Nowak-Sliwinska et al.[79] Hornung et al. performed fluorescence measurements and presented a method of producing tumor growth on the CAM.[80] In 2007, Chin et al. also presented fluorescence investigations of the CAM model and showed the effectiveness of a Ce6-based photodynamic therapy of lung carcinoma xenografts in this model.[81] More recently, detailed investigations regarding the usage of the CAM model as an alternative to rodents for drug toxicity testing were carried out.[82] Therein, it was concluded that the CAM model allows quick screening of large numbers of pharmacological samples with comparable results to that performed on mice.

Hereinafter, the CAM model is used as a model for an organism with easily accessible blood vessels. It allows IV injection of a PS and $^1O_2$ luminescence and PS fluorescence scanning of the vascular system. The vascular changes after PDT treatment can be easily observed using a binocular microscope.

On egg development day (EDD)-9, the vascular system is sufficiently developed to inject PS intravenously.[83] Like the dorsal window chamber model, the CAM model is another suitable model for investigations of PDT effects on blood vessels. With a custom-made multifurcated fiber, $^1O_2$ luminescence kinetics as well as fluorescence spectra were acquired 30 min after IV injection of Ce6. In Figure 4.13, one can see a white light image of the CAM model overlaid by the fitted $^1O_2$ luminescence amplitude. The image was taken after the scanning procedure and shows that several blood vessels have already deteriorated. Signals measured in the blood vessels display the typical $^1O_2$ luminescence kinetics. In contrast, the luminescence intensity measured above areas without vacuoles is significantly lower.

The luminescence signal shown in Figure 4.13 could not be fitted according to Equation 4.1 or 4.2, indicating another source of NIR luminescence. For this reason, data were fitted using the biexponential model with an additional decay time according to Equation 4.3. Fitting the data at the location with most signal counts yields decay times of 5.4 and 2.3 µs as well as an additional decay time of 19.2 µs. Since $^1O_2$ decay times longer than in water are not likely for in vivo conditions, one could assign the 5.4 µs to the PS triplet decay time and the 2.3 µs to the $^1O_2$ decay time. A more detailed discussion of decay times can be found in the chapter "Photosensitizer activity imaging on the microscopic scale" *(This book chapter 15 by St. Hackbarth)*.

Even though a correlation between the vascular system and the $^1O_2$ luminescence intensity can clearly be seen, the assignment of decay kinetics to physical processes remains a difficult aspect. Possibly, intrinsic NIR luminescence contributes to the measured signal. For a more detailed analysis of decay times and therefore a deeper understanding of PDT processes, further research is necessary.

4.2.4 SOLID TUMOR MODELS

Mice are a commonly used model organism for tumor research.[84] The laboratory mouse is considered one of the best systems for cancer investigations in vivo.[85] The first successful transplantation of human tumor tissue to mice was already reported in 1969.[86] Nowadays, studies are mostly performed on genetically engineered mice or mice with xenografted tumors. Up to now, the comprehensive mouse tumor biology database holds already over 70,000 tumor frequency records.

The mouse was the first mammal whose genome was sequenced even before completion of the human genome project. Genome sequencing of mice and many other mammals reveals the extent of

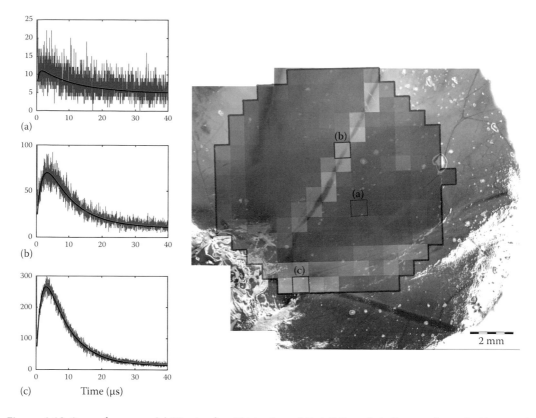

Figure 4.13 Scan of cam model 30 min after IV injection of Ce6 (2.5 mg/kg). Scan performed with a mode resulting in a circular area, overlaying a white light microscopic image (consisting of four single images), which was taken after the $^1O_2$ scan. One sees already some damage to the blood vessels due to the photodynamic treatment. (a) Spot without blood vessels and a very weak $^1O_2$ luminescence signal, (b) spot with a medium thick blood vessel, and (c) with a large blood vessel and the biggest luminescence signal.

cross-species genomic similarity.[87] This greatly increased the value of animal models for research on cancer and many other human disorders.

Most investigations regarding $^1O_2$ detection in the context of tumor PDT were therefore performed on mice or, less frequently, on rats. The following examples give an overview about experiments performed, findings and remaining questions about the interpretation of the data. It should not be taken as an exhaustive review about performed investigations. Only a handful of research groups worldwide are able to perform such measurements. For this, knowledge about such systems is very limited. In the literature, no reports exist that go beyond the simple biexponential model for describing the data, even though speculations were made.[49]

Direct $^1O_2$ luminescence measurements on photosensitized rats were reported in 2002 by Niedre et al. Due to the low SNR and an unexplained signal, decaying in the first 10 µs, data were fitted monoexponentially for times greater than 10 µs, yielding a decay time of around 30 µs.[64] Subsequent experiments from this group indicated that for the best-fit results a model with six parameters representing different microenvironments is required.[49] Lee et al. showed the feasibility of diode lasers as excitation source for time-resolved $^1O_2$ luminescence measurements. The effects of very long excitation periods of around 10 µs were discussed for homogenous systems. Even though longer excitation periods increase the light dose, the SNR of in vivo measurements did not allow an analysis of decay times.[88]

Most recently, $^1O_2$ luminescence measurements by Pfitzner et al.[89] carried out on tumor-bearing nude mice showed kinetics with a sufficient SNR suitable for a more detailed analysis. These measurements were performed with a custom made fiber allowing the use of red laser diodes as an excitation source. The optimized design maximized the detection efficiency while providing an easy-to-handle fiber tip.

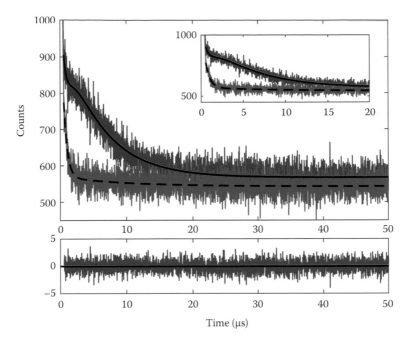

Figure 4.14 Luminescence signals at 1270 nm (red) and 1233 nm (blue) measured 16 h after IV injection of Ce6 dendrimer at the tumor area through the skin. The signal from the detection site (~7 mm²) was integrated for 50 s.

Figure 4.14 displays luminescence kinetics measured at the tumor location through the skin at 1270 nm (red) and 1233 nm (blue). At 1233 nm, the decaying signal with a decay time of about 0.5 µs is dominant. A second decay time of about 30 µs with a very low amplitude was observed. The short decay time can also be found in the data acquired at 1270 nm. In addition, at 1270 nm characteristic $^1O_2$ luminescence kinetics with decay times of 5.8 and 1 µs are observed.

However, the assignment to physical parameters, such as $^1O_2$ decay time or PS triplet decay time, remains a future task. From the literature, it can be concluded that the decay time of 5.8 µs in vivo is unlikely to be the $^1O_2$ decay time since it is expected to be shorter than in pure water.

4.3 CONCLUSIONS AND OUTLOOK

Singlet oxygen luminescence detection has been performed in many PDT-relevant biological systems, like skin, blood vessels, and even tumors. However, imaging in the strict sense has not yet been achieved in all of these systems due to technical or even physical limitations.

Time-resolved measurements require scanning procedures to gain spatial- and time-resolved $^1O_2$ luminescence data. These measurements are time-consuming and motion artifacts; the illumination due to the measurement as well as the duration of the measurement is still a serious concern. They may cause changes in the system, resulting in uncertainties of the $^1O_2$ kinetics. However, the illumination doses used for scanning of the skin and CAM samples as well as for measurements on the tumor were well below typical PDT treatment doses. Thus, it seems feasible to monitor PDT using time-resolved $^1O_2$ luminescence detection. Future detection devices with improved sensitivity like superconducting nanowire detectors may even improve such detection systems.[8]

Camera-based $^1O_2$ imaging requires significantly shorter measurement times but lack the crucial information about the $^1O_2$ luminescence kinetics. Therefore, this type of imaging lacks information about important parameters such as the amount of $^1O_2$ and oxygen or quencher depletion.

Table 4.2 Time-resolved vs. steady-state $^1O_2$ luminescence imaging

	Advantages	Disadvantages
Time-resolved imaging	Information about $^1O_2$-interaction with environment	Low spatial resolution
	Signal validation	Low speed
	Image with high SNR	
Steady-state imaging	High spatial resolution	No information about the $^1O_2$ interaction
	High speed	No signal validation
		Background discrimination

The main advantages and drawbacks of both methods are listed in Table 4.2. Since high-speed measurements are necessary in most biological environments and the kinetics may also not be omitted, it seems to be an expedient approach to combine the advantages of both time-resolved $^1O_2$ detection and wide-field steady-state imaging.

This way most information from the observed system can be gained, with the least interference due to the measurement. A rather rapid steady-state imaging of the area of interest should be performed. Based on this image, a limited amount of points can be chosen to acquire NIR luminescence kinetics to validate and extend information gained by the steady-state measurement.

This combination of both wide-field imaging and time-resolved spectroscopy for $^1O_2$ luminescence detection could be used in systems like the window chamber and CAM model where both methods individually have already been demonstrated. The implementation of such a technique for in vivo studies of, for example, skin and solid tumors is a challenging goal for the next stage in fundamental research to be performed in the future, likely resulting in new insights into PDT pathways.

ACKNOWLEDGMENTS

This work was supported in part by the Sino-German Symposium (GZ1140) and the National Natural Science Foundation of China (61520106015, 61275216).

M. Pfitzner thanks the LR Health and Beauty Systems GmbH for financial support.

For the possibility to perform the measurements on the CAM model, the authors thank Dr. Karin Kunzi-Rapp and Felicitas Genze (Institut für Lasermedizin und Meßtechnik an der Universität Ulm, Germany) for preparation.

The authors thank S. Pfitzner for last-minute textual revisions.

REFERENCES

1. B. Röder, Photodynamic therapy biomedical spectroscopy, in *Encyclopedia of Analytical Chemistry*, ed. R. A. Meyers, Wiley, New York, 2000, doi:10.1002/9780470027318.a0115.
2. S. Hackbarth, J. C. Schlothauer, A. Preuss, C. Ludwig, and B. Röder, *Laser Phys. Lett.*, 2012, **9**(6), 474, doi:10.7452/lapl.201110146.
3. J. C. Schlothauer, S. Hackbarth, L. Jäger, K. Drobniewski et al., *J. Biomed. Opt.*, 2012, **17**11, 115005, doi:10.1117/1.JBO.17.11.115005.
4. Y. Shen, H. Lin, Z. F. Huang, D. F. Chen et al., *Laser Phys. Lett.*, 2011, **8**(3), 232, doi:10.1002/lapl.201010113.
5. B. Hu, N. Zeng, Z. Liu, Y. Ji et al., *J. Biomed. Opt.*, 2011, **16**(1), 016003-1–016003-7, doi:16003, 10.1117/1.3528593.
6. S. Lee, M. E. Isabelle, K. L. Gabally-Kinney, B. W. Pogue, and S. J. Davis, *Biomed. Opt. Express*, 2011, **2**(5), 1233, doi:10.1364/BOE.2.001233.
7. J. F. B. Barata, A. Zamarrón, M. G. Neves, M. A. Faustino et al., *Eur. J. Med. Chem.*, 2015, **92**, 135, doi:10.1016/j.ejmech.2014.12.025.

8. J. C. Schlothauer, S. Hackbarth, and B. Röder, *Photon. Lasers Med.*, 2015, **4**(4), 303–306, doi:10.1515/plm-2015-0032.

9. J. C. Schlothauer, J. Falckenhayn, T. Perna, S. Hackbarth, and B. Röder, *J. Biomed. Opt.*, 2013, **18**(11), 115001, doi:10.1117/1.JBO.18.11.115001.

10. T. J. Dougherty, C. J. Gomer, B. W. Henderson, G. Jori et al., *J. Natl. Cancer Inst.*, 1998, **90**(12), 889, doi:10.1093/jnci/90.12.889.

11. B. C. Wilson, M. S. Patterson, and L. Lilge, *Lasers Med. Sci.*, 1997, **12**(3), 182.

12. H. Lin, Y. Shen, D. Chen, L. Lin et al., *J. Fluoresc.*, 2013, **23**(1), 41, doi:10.1007/s10895-012-1114-5.

13. C. Flors, M. J. Fryer, J. Waring, B. Reeder et al., *J. Exp. Bot.*, 2006, **57**(8), 1725, doi:10.1093/jxb/erj181.

14. A. Gollmer, J. Arnbjerg, F. H. Blaikie, B. W. Pedersen et al., *Photochem. Photobiol.*, 2011, **87**(3), 671, doi:10.1111/j.1751-1097.2011.00900.x.

15. S. K. Pedersen, J. Holmehave, F. H. Blaikie, A. Gollmer et al., *J. Org. Chem.*, 2014, **79**(7), 3079, doi:10.1021/jo500219y.

16. W. Bäumler, J. Regensburger, A. Knak, A. Felgentraeger, and T. Maisch, *Photochem. Photobiol. Sci.*, 2012, **11**(1), 107, doi:10.1039/c1pp05142c.

17. J. Moan and E. Wold, *Nature*, 1979, **279**(5712), 450.

18. R. F. Haseloff, B. Ebert, and B. Röder, *J. Photochem. Photobiol. B*, 1989, **3**(4), 593, doi:10.1016/1011-1344(89)80082-X.

19. B. Röder, *Biol. Rundsch.*, 1987, **25**, 273.

20. P. R. Crippa, A. Vecli, and C. Viappiani, *J. Photochem. Photobiol. B*, 1994, **24**(1), 3, doi:10.1016/1011-1344(93)06959-7.

21. J. Mosinger, K. Lang, J. Hostomský, J. Franc et al., *J. Phys. Chem. B*, 2010, **114**(48), 15773, doi:10.1021/jp105789p.

22. M. Geissbühler, T. Spielmann, A. Formey, I. Märki et al., *Biophys. J.*, 2010, **98**(2), 339, doi:10.1016/j.bpj.2009.10.006.

23. F. Anquez, I. El Yazidi-Belkoura, S. Randoux, P. Suret, and E. Courtade, *Photochem. Photobiol.*, 2012, **88**(1), 167, doi:10.1111/j.1751-1097.2011.01028.x.

24. A. A. Krasnovsky, *Biofizika*, 1976, **21**(4), 748.

25. A. A. Krasnovsky, *J. Photochem. Photobiol. A*, 2008, **196**(2–3), 210, doi:10.1016/j.jphotochem.2007.12.015.

26. L. K. Andersen, Z. Gao, P. R. Ogilby, L. Poulsen, and I. Zebger, *J. Phys. Chem. A*, 2002, **106**(37), 8488, doi:10.1021/jp021108z.

27. M. Scholz, R. Dědic, J. Valenta, T. Breitenbach, and J. Hála, *Photochem. Photobiol. Sci.*, 2014, **13**(8), 1203, doi:10.1039/C4PP00121D.

28. L. Lin, H. Lin, S. Xie, B. Li et al., *SPIE Newsroom*, 2014, doi:10.1117/2.1201406.005511.

29. M. J. Niedre, M. S. Patterson, A. Giles, and B. C. Wilson, *Photochem. Photobiol.*, 2005, **81**(4), 941.

30. W. Tian, L. Deng, S. Jin, H. Yang et al., *J. Phys. Chem. A*, 2015, **119**(14), 3393, doi:10.1021/acs.jpca.5b01504.

31. J. Arnbjerg, M. Johnsen, P. K. Frederiksen, S. E. Braslavsky, and P. R. Ogilby, *J. Phys. Chem. A*, 2006, **110**(23), 7375, doi:10.1021/jp0609986.

32. S. Hatz, J. D. C. Lambert, and P. R. Ogilby, *Photochem. Photobiol. Sci.*, 2007, **6**(10), 1106, doi:10.1039/b707313e.

33. J. R. Kanofsky, *Photochem. Photobiol.*, 2011, **87**(1), 14, doi:10.1111/j.1751-1097.2010.00855.x.

34. J. C. Schlothauer, M. Pfitzner, and B. Röder, *Singlet Oxygen: Applications in Biosciences and Nanosciences*, Royal Society of Chemistry, Cambridge, U.K., 2015, p. 41.

35. L. Lin, H. Lin, D. Chen, L. Chen et al., *SPIE Photonics Europe*, SPIE, Brussels, Belgium, 2014, p. 912920, doi:10.1117/12.2052033.

36. B. Li, L. Lin, Y. Gu, and B. C. Wilson, *Photon. Laser Med.*, 2015, **4**(4), 308, doi:10.1515/plm-2015-0032.

37. B. Li, L. Lin, H. Lin, and B. C. Wilson, *J. Biophoton.*, 2016, doi:10.1002/jbio.201600055.

38. S. Hackbarth, J. C. Schlothauer, A. Preuss, and B. Röder, *J. Photochem. Photobiol. B*, 2010, **98**(3), 173, doi:10.1016/j.jphotobiol.2009.11.013.

39. M. S. Patterson, S. J. Madsen, and B. C. Wilson, *J. Photochem. Photobiol. B*, 1990, **5**(1), 69, doi:10.1016/1011-1344(90)85006-I.

40. C. Schweitzer and R. Schmidt, *Chem. Rev.*, 2003, **103**(5), 1685, doi:10.1021/cr010371d.

41. T. Maisch, J. Baier, B. Franz, M. Maier et al., *Proc. Natl. Acad. Sci. USA*, 2007, **104**(17), 7223, doi:10.1073/pnas.0611328104.

42. S. Oelckers, *Singulett-Sauerstoff im Modellsystem photosensibilisierte Erythrozyten-Ghost-Suspensionen: Apparative Entwicklungen und zeitaufgelöste spektroskopische Untersuchungen*, Mensch-und-Buch-Verl., Berlin, Germany, 1999.

43. L. Chen, L. Lin, Y. Li, H. Lin et al., *J. Lumin.*, 2014, **152**, 98, doi:10.1016/j.jlumin.2013.10.034.

44. A. Preuß, I. Saltsman, A. Mahammed, M. Pfitzner et al., *J. Photochem. Photobiol. B Biol.*, 2014, **39**, 39–46, doi:10.1016/j.jphotobiol.2014.02.013.

45. M. H. Gold, *Photodynamic Therapy in Dermatology*, Springer, New York, 2011.

46. P. Babilas, M. Landthaler, and R.-M. Szeimies, *Eur. J. Dermatol.*, 2006, **16**(4), 340.

47. R.-M. Szeimies, A. Karrer, and W. Bäumler in *Licht und Gesundheit: Viertes Symposium 26. und 27. Februar 2004 ; eine Sondertagung der TU Berlin und der Deutschen Gesellschaft für Photobiologie*, ed. H. Kaase, Kistmacher, Berlin, Germany, 2004, p. 164.

48. T. Kiesslich, A. Gollmer, T. Maisch, M. Berneburg, and K. Plaetzer, *Biomed. Res. Int.*, 2013, **2013**, 840417, doi:10.1155/2013/840417.

49. M. T. Jarvi, M. J. Niedre, M. S. Patterson, and B. C. Wilson, *Photochem. Photobiol.*, 2006, **82**(5), 1198, doi:10.1562/2006-05-03-IR-891.

50. M. Rougee, R. V. Bensasson, E. J. Land, and R. Pariente, *Photochem. Photobiol.*, 1988, **47**(4), 485, doi:10.1111/j.1751-1097.1988.tb08835.x.

51. J. M. Allen, C. J. Gossett, and S. K. Allen, *Chem. Res. Toxicol.*, 1996, **9**(3), 605, doi:10.1021/tx950197m.

52. A. Beeby and A. E. Jones, *Photochem. Photobiol.*, 2000, **72**(1), 10, doi:10.1562/0031-8655(2000)0720010TPPOMA2.0.CO2.

53. U. Jacobi, M. Kaiser, R. Toll, S. Mangelsdorf et al., *Skin Res. Technol.*, 2007, **13**(1), 19, doi:10.1111/j.1600-0846.2006.00179.x.

54. J. de Lange, P. van Eck, G. R. Elliott, W. L. de Kort, and O. L. Wolthuis, *J. Pharmacol. Toxicol.*, 1992, **27**(2), 71, doi:10.1016/1056-8719(92)90024-U.

55. F. P. Schmook, J. G. Meingassner, and A. Billich, *Int. J. Pharm.*, 2001, **215**(1–2), 51, doi:10.1016/S0378-5173(00)00665-7.

56. B. Godin and E. Touitou, *Adv. Drug Deliv. Rev.*, 2007, **59**(11), 1152, doi:10.1016/j.addr.2007.07.004.

57. A. M. Barbero and H. F. Frasch, *Toxicol. In Vitro*, 2009, **23**(1), 1, doi:10.1016/j.tiv.2008.10.008.

58. A. Crovara Pescia, P. Astolfi, C. Puglia, F. Bonina et al., *Int. J. Pharm.*, 2012, **427**(2), 217, doi:10.1016/j.ijpharm.2012.02.001.

59. J. Lademann, H. Richter, M. Meinke, W. Sterry, and A. Patzelt, *Skin Pharmacol. Physiol.*, 2010, **23**(1), 47, doi:10.1159/000257263.

60. J. N. Silva, P. Filipe, P. Morlière, J.-C. Maziere et al., *Biomed. Mater. Eng.*, 2005, **16**(4 Suppl.), 147.

61. B. Liu, T. J. Farrell, and M. S. Patterson, *Phys. Med. Biol.*, 2010, **55**(19), 5913, doi:10.1088/0031-9155/55/19/019.

62. F. L. Primo, M. V. Bentley, and A. C. Tedesco, *J. Nanosci. Nanotechnol.*, 2008, **8**(1), 340.

63. S. Karrer, C. Abels, R.-M. Szeimies, W. Bäumler et al., *Arch. Dermatol. Res.*, 1997, **289**(3), 132, doi:10.1007/s004030050168.

64. M. J. Niedre, M. S. Patterson, and B. C. Wilson, *Photochem. Photobiol.*, 2002, **75**(4), 382, doi:10.1562/0031-8655(2002)0750382DNILDO2.0.CO2.

65. J. Baier, T. Maisch, M. Maier, M. Landthaler, and W. Bäumler, *J. Invest. Dermatol.*, 2007, **127**(6), 1498, doi:10.1038/sj.jid.5700741.

66. S. Nonell, M. García-Díaz, J. L. Viladot, and R. Delgado, *Int. J. Cosmet. Sci.*, 2013, **35**(3), 272, doi:10.1111/ics.12039.

67. J. C. Schlothauer, S. Hackbarth, and B. Röder, *Laser Phys. Lett.*, 2009, **6**(3), 216, doi:10.1002/lapl.200810116.

68. J. C. Schlothauer, B. Röder, S. Hackbarth, and J. Lademann, *Proc. SPIE*, 2010, **7551**, 755106, doi:10.1117/12.839851.

69. J. J. Thiele, S. N. Hsieh, K. Briviba, and H. Sies, *J. Invest. Dermatol.*, 1999, **113**(3), 335, doi:10.1046/j.1523-1747.1999.00693.x.

70. J. J. Thiele, *Skin Pharmacol. Physiol.*, 2001, **14**(Suppl. 1), 87, doi:10.1159/000056395.

71. A. Vogt, N. Mandt, J. Lademann, H. Schaefer, and U. Blume-Peytavi, *J. Investig. Dermatol. Symp. Proc.*, 2005, **10**(3), 252, doi:10.1111/j.1087-0024.2005.10124.x.

72. P. Agostinis, K. Berg, K. A. Cengel, T. H. Foster et al., *CA-Cancer J. Clin.*, 2011, **61**(4), 250, doi:10.3322/caac.20114.

73. A. Kawczyk-Krupka, K. Wawrzyniec, S. K. Musiol, M. Potempa et al., *Photodiagnosis Photodyn. Ther.*, 2015, **12**(4), 567, doi:10.1016/j.pdpdt.2015.10.001.

74. A. Kawczyk-Krupka, A. M. Bugaj, M. Potempa, K. Wasilewska et al., *Photodiagnosis Photodyn. Ther.*, 2015, **12**(2), 161, doi:10.1016/j.pdpdt.2015.03.007.

75. Z. Qiu, D. Chen, Y. Wang, G. Yao et al., *Photon. Laser Med.*, 2014, **3**(3), 273, doi:10.1515/plm-2014-0012.

76. H. Qiu, Y. Mao, Y. Gu, Y. Wang et al., *Photodiagnosis Photodyn. Ther.*, 2012, **9**(2), 109, doi:10.1016/j.pdpdt.2011.11.003.

77. G. M. Palmer, A. N. Fontanella, S. Shan, G. Hanna et al., *Nat. Protoc.*, 2011, **6**(9), 1355, doi:10.1038/nprot.2011.349.

78. M. Maurin, O. Stéphan, J.-C. Vial, S. R. Marder et al., *J. Biomed. Opt.*, 2011, **16**(3), 36001, doi:10.1117/1.3548879.

79. P. Nowak-Sliwinska, T. Segura, and M. L. Iruela-Arispe, *Angiogenesis*, 2014, **17**(4), 779, doi:10.1007/s10456-014-9440-7.

80. R. Hornung, M. J. Hammer-Wilson, S. Kimel, L.-H. Liaw et al., *J. Photochem. Photobiol. B*, 1999, **49**(1), 41, doi:10.1016/S1011-1344(99)00014-7.

81. W. W. L. Chin, P. W. S. Heng, and M. Olivo, *BMC Pharmacol.*, 2007, **7**, 15, doi:10.1186/1471-2210-7-15.

82. C. S. Kue, K. Y. Tan, M. L. Lam, and H. B. Lee, *Exp. Anim. Tokyo*, 2015, **64**(2), 129, doi:10.1538/expanim.14-0059.

83. D. Ribatti, B. Nico, A. Vacca, L. Roncali et al., *Anat. Rec.*, 2001, **264**(4), 317.

84. Z. S. Silva, S. K. Bussadori, K. P. S. Fernandes, Y.-Y. Huang, and M. R. Hamblin, *Biosci. Rep.*, 2015, **35**(6), 1–14, doi:10.1042/BSR20150188.

85. K. K. Frese and D. A. Tuveson, *Nat. Rev. Cancer*, 2007, **7**(9), 645, doi:10.1038/nrc2192.

86. J. Rygaard and C. O. Poulsen, *Acta Pathol. Microbiol. Scand.*, 1969, **77**(4), 758, doi:10.1111/j.1699-0463.1969.tb04520.x.

87. R. H. Waterston, K. Lindblad-Toh, E. Birney, J. Rogers et al., *Nature*, 2002, **420**(6915), 520, doi:10.1038/nature01262.

88. S. Lee, D. H. Vu, M. F. Hinds, S. J. Davis et al., *J. Biomed. Opt.*, 2008, **13**(6), 64035, doi:10.1117/1.3042265.

89. M. Pfitzner, J. C. Schlothauer, E. Bastien, S. Hackbarth et al., *Photodiagnosis Photodyn. Ther.*, 2016, **14**, 204–210, doi:10.1016/j.pdpdt.2016.03.002.

Microbial biofilms and antimicrobial photodynamic therapy

ANIL KISHEN

5.1 INTRODUCTION

Microbes persisting as biofilms have received major attention in recent times due to the difficulty they pose against their therapeutic measures. Antibiotics were dubbed as the "wonder drugs" of the twentieth century to curb the threat of infectious diseases [1]. In recent years, the expectations surrounding these drugs as the first line of choice for treating infectious diseases started to vanish due to the emergence and spread of antibiotic-resistant microbes. Drugs that were once lethal have now become ineffective against certain organisms that have evolved and developed the ability to survive therapeutic doses. Ranging from systemic disease conditions to localized oral infections, antimicrobial resistance shown by the bacteria is an area of

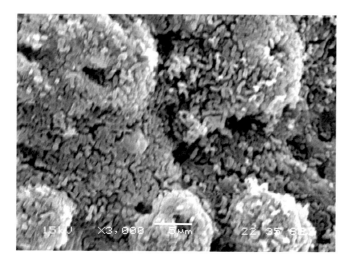

Figure 5.1 Scanning electron microscopic image showing the ultrastructure of a biofilm.

increasing concern. The epidemic of resistant bacteria has spurred renewed interest in the research community to develop alternative antimicrobial approaches [2].

Bacterial infection generally presents as a polymicrobial infection, in which communities of bacteria with different requirements (oxygen, nutrient, etc.), cell wall characteristics (Gram-positive and Gram-negative), are established as a biofilm [3]. Gram-positive and Gram-negative bacteria are different in their three-dimensional cellular architecture structure. The membrane barrier of a bacterium limits the diffusion of antimicrobials into the cytosol. The membrane barriers of Gram-positive bacteria consist of a relatively thick but porous, interconnected peptidoglycan layer surrounding a cytoplasmic membrane. The teichoic acid in the Gram-positive bacterial cell wall contributes to the negative charge and consequently serves as binding sites for cationic molecules. The cell envelope of Gram-negative bacteria is composed of an outer membrane, a thin peptidoglycan layer, and a cytoplasmic membrane. The transfer of molecules across a Gram-negative cell wall is strictly regulated at the outer membrane, which is rich in lipopolysaccharide (LPS). Consequently, the susceptibility of bacteria to antimicrobials will depend upon the type of cell wall. In addition to the inherent resistance of different bacterial species to antimicrobials, bacteria are observed to demonstrate further resistance to antimicrobials when they are in a biofilm mode [4,5]. Unfortunately, biofilm is the preferred mode for bacterial existence in most disease conditions [6] (Figure 5.1).

5.2 BIOFILM BACTERIA AS A THERAPEUTIC TARGET

Bacteria in a biofilm are protected from antimicrobials by unique mechanisms. These mechanisms are mostly due to certain factors associated with the growth and structure of a biofilm. Schematic diagrams of the hypothesized mechanisms of antimicrobial resistance in biofilm are shown in Figure 5.2. There is no single mechanism that accounts for the general resistance of biofilm bacteria to antimicrobials. Different mechanisms are known to act in a concerted manner within the biofilm and amplify the effect of small variations in susceptible phenotypes [6,7]. Some of these relevant mechanisms for antimicrobial resistance in bacterial biofilms are (1) resistance associated with the extracellular polymeric matrix, (2) resistance associated with growth rate and nutrient availability, and (3) resistance associated with the adoption of resistance phenotype.

A mature biofilm is composed of multiple layers of microbes embedded in a matrix, which is secreted by microbes and formed of extracellular polymeric substance (EPS). Thus, a biofilm is a community of bacteria that is irreversibly attached to a solid substrate and is protected by the EPS. The EPS has the potential to

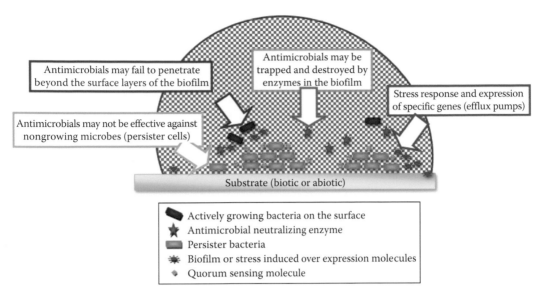

Figure 5.2 Different mechanisms for antimicrobial resistance in biofilm.

modify the response of resident bacteria to antimicrobials by acting as a barrier and deactivator against the chemical effects of antimicrobials. The highly charged and interwoven structure of EPS hinders the diffusion of antimicrobials. The constituents of the EPS will further augment the barrier effect of EPS [6,7].

A biofilm exhibits a high density of resident bacteria when compared to planktonic bacteria. The spatial arrangement of bacteria will expose the bacterium in the deeper layers of the biofilm to limited nutrients and redox potential than the bacterium on the surface of the biofilm. In addition, the bacteria in a biofilm experience different growth conditions. The slow growth and starvation has been linked with the resistance of resident bacteria within a biofilm. Since the degree of nutrient and gas gradients increases with thickness and maturity of a biofilm structure, the influence of growth rate and oxygen on the antimicrobial resistance is particularly marked in a mature biofilm [6,8].

The *persister cells* in a biofilm also contribute to the antimicrobial resistance of a biofilm. They are non-growing phenotypes of general cell population. They are specialized survivor cell population formed when bacteria are exposed to unfavorable growth conditions or low-level antimicrobials [9]. The persistent cell grows rapidly in the presence of nutrients following purging of unfavorable conditions. Biofilm population is rich in persistor cells, with capacities to survive treatment procedures and proliferate in the posttreatment phase. Due to reduced metabolic activity, these persistent cells easily escape the antibiotics, which are known to actively growing cells. Moreover, the bacteria in biofilms can upregulate the expression of stress-response genes, shock proteins, and multidrug efflux pumps, switching the bacteria to more resistant phenotypes, when compared to planktonic (free floating) bacteria [10]. In brief, the nature of biofilm structure and physiological characteristics of resident microbes offer the biofilm microbes, a marked resistance to antimicrobials.

5.3 THERAPEUTIC STRATEGIES AGAINST BIOFILMS

The therapeutic strategies against bacterial biofilms are generally said to focus on (1) inactivating the resident bacteria within the biofilm structure or (2) disrupting the biofilm structure and simultaneously kill the resident microbes (Figure 5.3). The aforementioned objectives are achieved by different antimicrobials and/or treatment strategies. It includes the application of antimicrobials that (1) produce slow destruction of the biofilm structure, (2) destroys persistent cell or quorums sensing signals in a biofilm, (3) diffuses agents into the biofilm structure producing resident bacterial killing, and (4) is used as combination strategy that

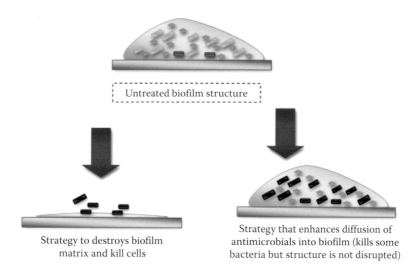

Figure 5.3 Two commonly employed antibiofilm strategies.

enhances the diffusion into the biofilm structure and destroy biofilm matrix [11]. Considering the potential challenges offered by in vivo environments and biofilms, a reliable therapeutic strategy should be to eliminate the biofilm structure and eradicate the resident bacteria, without causing any deleterious effect to the adjacent host tissues [3].

5.4 ANTIMICROBIAL PHOTODYNAMIC THERAPY

Photodynamic therapy applies a photosensitizer, that is, a light-sensitive chemical at extremely low-toxic and nontoxic concentration, which, when activated with a specific wavelength of light, produces activated oxygen radicals that causes toxic effects on the bacterial cells.

5.4.1 PHOTOSENSITIZERS

A photosensitizer is as a chemical species, which, when exposed to light at its peak absorption wavelength, produces highly reactive oxygen species, more specifically singlet oxygen. The reactive oxygen is responsible for bacterial cell death. Only the photosensitizer that undergoes efficient intersystem crossing to the excited triplet state, possesses a relatively long triplet state, and has few other competing pathways will produce high yields of singlet oxygen. Typically, photosensitizers display a triplet quantum yield of around 50%, with the singlet oxygen yield being slightly lower. The challenges during this process include the loss of energy by deactivation to ground state by fluorescence or internal conversion. However, in most cases a high yield of singlet oxygen is desirable [12–14].

Pharmacokinetics, stability, and degree of toxicity in vivo play critical roles as well. Toxicity can become an issue if high doses of photosensitizer are necessary for the therapeutic effect. Stability of the photosensitizer and the toxicity profile of the breakdown products may need to be evaluated prior to use in vivo. In spite of all these challenges, large numbers of photosensitizers are available with potential use in antimicrobial photodynamic therapy (APDT), several of which are currently in various stages of U.S. Food and Drug Administration approval. Some of the requirements of a photosensitizer are nontoxic to the host tissues; present local toxicity only after activation with light, high solubility in water; possess a mechanism of cell inactivation minimizing any induction of resistant microbial strains; maintain high quantum yield for the generation of long-lived triplet state and singlet oxygen, cost effectiveness, commercial availability; and possess storage and light stability [15,16].

Photosensitizers based on the phenothiazinium chromophore are emerging as promising candidates for use as photodynamic antimicrobial agents [12,13]. Methylene blue (MB) is generally accepted as the prototype of phenothiazinium-based photosensitizers [17]. A number of phenothiazinium-based photosensitizers have now been synthesized [18]. Generally, these are cationic molecules with a core structure composed of a planar tricyclic aromatic ring system that functions as a chromophore of these compounds [18]. In addition to phenothiazinium-based photosensitizers, cationic porphyrins [19], phthalocyanines [20], and chlorins [21] have also gained popularity as photosensitizer due to their abilities to inactivate both Gram-positive and Gram-negative bacteria.

5.4.2 LIGHT SOURCES

A limiting factor in APDT is the penetration of the activating light into tissue. Visible light in the red region of the electromagnetic spectrum commonly has a penetration depth $(1/\varepsilon)$ in the range of 2–6 mm, depending on the absorption wavelength and the tissue. However, the depth of the therapeutic effect achieved by APDT is generally found to occur at approximately twice this depth, which is 4–12 mm. Light propagation through a tissue involves the processes of reflection, absorption, scattering, and transmission. It is generally considered that 4%–6% of light energy tends to be reflected from biological tissues. Further, in a biological tissue, absorption of light energy is largely by the free-water molecules, proteins, pigments, and other macromolecules. In this case, the absorption coefficient will strongly depend on the wavelength of the applied light/laser irradiation. Scattering of light has the most prominent effect on the intensity and direction of light within biological tissue. Scattering and refraction of light would produce a widening of light beam, which in turn would produce a loss of fluence rate (power per unit area) and change in directionality of the light beam [12].

Light sources used for APDT can be coherent (lasers) or noncoherent (lamps). Laser provides monochromatic, coherent, and collimated light, offering wide range of output power [22]. Thus, lasers provide a very powerful source of light that can reduce the time necessary to deliver the final APDT dose. Among the different types of lasers that can be used for APDT, diode lasers are very attractive for clinical use as they are easy to operate and portable. Most often, the choice of light source can be dictated by the location, light dose delivered, and the choice of photosensitizer. Currently, low-level lasers are the light sources of choice to irradiate tissues sites that can be accessed only with an optical fiber. Typically, light coupled to a fiber-optic delivery system is used for precise clinical applications.

Incandescent light sources, on the other hand, are difficult to be used in combination with miniature fiber-optic cables, mainly because of their modest beam quality, sizable beam dimension, and small power density. These light sources also provide a broad range of wavelengths at lower fluence rates [23]. The broad emission of these lamps, however, allows the use of several photosensitizers with different absorption maxima within the emission spectrum of the lamp. In addition, compared to lasers, lamps are more cost effective and easier to maintain and use. Typically, light sources such as Nd:YAG, KTP, HeNe, GaAlAs, and diode lasers, light-emitting diodes (LEDs), and Paterson lamps have been utilized for APDT. The superiority of one type of light source over the other has not been demonstrated and hence the use of lasers or lamps depends on the specific application.

5.4.3 MECHANISMS

APDT comprises of two specific steps: Step 1 is for the photosensitization of the infected tissue. This stage allows the uptake of the photosensitizer by the bacterial cells. Step 2 is for the irradiation of the photosensitized tissue. This stage will result in the destruction of bacteria. Two types of photodynamic reactions ensue: (1) *type I reaction*, in which the photosensitizer triplet state can react with a target, other than oxygen by hydrogen or electron transfer resulting in radical ions that can react with oxygen, yielding cytotoxic species such as hydrogen peroxide, superoxide anion, and hydroxyl radicals, and (2) *type II reaction*, in which the photosensitizer triplet state can transfer the excitation energy to ground-state molecular oxygen to produce excited-state singlet oxygen ($^1O_2$) [21].

Singlet oxygen is a strong oxidizing agent that is highly reactive, with a lifetime of less than 4 μs in a biological environment. It has a radius of action of less than 0.02 μm [23]. The reactions of singlet oxygen with the cellular targets lead to cell death. The two basic mechanisms that have been proposed to account for the lethal damage to bacterial cell are DNA damage and cytoplasmic membrane damage. APDT on bacteria has displayed breakage in both single- and double-stranded DNA and loss of the plasmid supercoiled fraction [24,25]. Previous studies have shown that the photooxidative effect caused by phenothiazinium photosensitizer in bacteria could lead to damage of multiple targets in bacterial cells such as DNA [24], membrane integrity [26], protease activity, and LPS [27]. George and Kishen reported functional impairment of cell wall, extensive damage to chromosomal DNA, and degradation of membrane proteins following MB-mediated APDT of *Enterococcus faecalis* [28]. Thus, the mode of action of APDT is markedly different from that of most antibiotics and they can be suggested as a feasible alternative to antibiotics.

5.4.4 ANTIBIOFILM EFFICACY

Many in vitro experiments have highlighted the antimicrobial and antibiofilm efficacy of photodynamic therapy. They showed that monospecies bacteria/biofilms of bacterial strains such as *E. faecalis*, *Staphylococcus intermedius*, *Peptostreptococcus micros*, *Prevotella intermedia*, and *Fusobacterium nucleatum* could be effectively killed by APDT with photosensitizer such as MB and *Toluidine Blue O* (TBO) activated with red light [29–33]. Previous studies have highlighted the limitations associated with APDT to eliminate well-matured bacterial biofilms in vitro [34,35]. On similar lines, in vivo experiments have highlighted the efficacy of combining APDT with conventional topical antimicrobials and mechanical disruption to achieve significant antibiofilm efficacy [36–38], instead of APDT achieving antibiofilm efficacy alone. Some of the tissue-specific challenges prevailing in the infected tissue are suggested to compromise the antibiofilm efficacy of APDT in vivo.

The selectivity of APDT toward killing prokaryotic cells when compared to eukaryotic cells at the suggested photosensitization periods and light fluence presents itself as a preferable choice among antibacterial alternatives. Soukos et al. compared the effect of APDT using a combination of TBO and red light against *Streptococcus sanguis* and human gingival keratinocytes and fibroblasts. They reported no reduction in the human cell viability, whereas the bacteria were effectively killed [39]. Zeina et al. reported kill rates for human keratinocyte cell line (H103) to be 18–200-folds slower than for cutaneous microbial species following LAD with a combination of MB and white light [40]. Soncin et al. reported the selective killing of *Staphylococcus aureus* over human fibroblasts and keratinocytes (from four- to sixfold) when subjected to LAD using cationic phthalocyanine and relatively low light fluencies [41]. More recently, George and Kishen demonstrated a 97.7% killing of *E. faecalis* compared to a 30% human fibroblast dysfunction following MB-mediated LAD [42].

5.5 CHALLENGES IN APDT

5.5.1 DEPTH OF PHOTOSENSITIZER/LIGHT PENETRATION IN INFECTED TISSUES

Achieving optimum concentration of photosensitizer and light dose throughout the infected tissue is key to achieve ideal efficacy with APDT. Different groups have carried different modifications to photosensitizer formulation of light energy delivery to counter this issue. In an approach to improve the antimicrobial efficacy of APDT in root canal system (tissue-specific approach), George and Kishen dissolved MB in different formulations: water, 70% glycerol, 70% polyethylene glycol (PEG), and a mixture of glycerol:ethanol:water (MIX) in a ratio of 30:20:50. Then, they analyzed for the photophysical, photochemical, and photobiological characteristics [30]. They showed that aggregation of MB molecules was significantly higher in water when compared to other formulations. Other than this, the MIX-based MB formulation had effective penetration into dentinal tubules and enhanced singlet-oxygen generation, which in turn improved bactericidal action. A significantly higher impairment of bacterial cell wall and extensive damage to chromosomal DNA was observed when MB in a MIX-based formulation was used when compared to water [43]. The same group also showed that the incorporation of an oxidizer and oxygen carrier with photosensitizer formulation in the form of an emulsion would produce significant photooxidation capabilities, which in turn facilitated comprehensive disruption of matured endodontic biofilm structure [44].

Conjugating photosensitizer to various agents or chemical moieties can result in improved efficacy for APDT. These modified photosensitizers are expected to bind with greater affinity to the outer membrane of bacteria and upon activation generated reactive oxygen species, which then diffuse into the cells, resulting in cell death. Therefore, photo-generated oxidative species is confined to the cell wall and its vicinity, which is a highly susceptible domain for photodynamic action. Soukos and coworkers formed a hypothesis that by covalently conjugating a suitable photosensitizer to a *poly-l-lysine* chain, a bacteria-targeted photosensitizer delivery vehicle could be constructed that would efficiently inactivate both Gram-positive and Gram-negative species [27]. This was demonstrated by preparing a conjugate of chlorin (e6) and a *poly-l-lysine* chain (20 lysine residues), which, after 1 min incubation and illumination with red light, killed >99% of the Gram-positive *Actinomyces viscosus* and Gram-negative *Porphyromonas gingivalis* [44]. Photosensitizer conjugated with positively charged chitosan has also been shown to be highly effective in removing biofilms of Gram-positive and Gram-negative bacteria [45]. Shrestha et al. showed that the rose bengal–conjugated chitosan presented a synergistic effect of the antimicrobial polymer chitosan and singlet oxygen generated following photoactivation [46].

5.5.2 Influence of Inactivating Factors in Infected Tissues

Tissue remnants and serum products compromise the antimicrobial efficacy of commonly used topical antimicrobials [47] and APDT [48]. Most studies concerning the APDT of microbial pathogens use deionized water or phosphate-buffered saline to dissolve the photosensitizer. In some studies, photosensitizer was dissolved in brain–heart infusion broth wherein reduced bactericidal effect with the tested photosensitizer was reported. This reduction in antibacterial effect was attributed to the presence of serum proteins in the broth [49,50]. Constituents of the infected hard tissue such as tissue remnants, serum, and hard tissue constituents have also been shown to significantly reduce the APDT effect in vitro [51]. This is either due to cross-linking action or the compromised half-life of singlet oxygen in the presence of proteins. Moreover, limited availability of environmental oxygen in the certain infected tissues or locations may diminish the quantum yield of singlet oxygen and consequently the antimicrobial efficacy of APDT.

5.6 STEPS TO ENHANCE ANTIBIOFILM EFFICACY OF APDT

5.6.1 Pretreatments with Membrane-Permeabilizing Agents

Different approaches have been attempted in the past to enhance the efficacy of APDT using membrane-permeabilizing agents. Earlier studies have used polycationic polypeptide polymyxin B nanopeptide (PMBN), which increases the permeability of the Gram-negative outer membrane and allowed photosensitizer that are normally excluded from the cell to penetrate to a location where the ROS generated upon illumination can cause fatal damage [52]. PMBN does not release LPS from the cells but expands the membrane, allowing photosensitizer to penetrate and subsequently inactivation of *E. coli* and *Pseudomonas aeruginosa*. Another study showed that the susceptibility of Gram-negative *Yersinia pseudotuberculosis* and *E. coli* to APDT was increased following the addition of PMBN [53]. Yonei and Todo demonstrated enhanced sensitivity to the lethal and mutagenic effects of photosensitizing action of chlorpromazine in ethylenediaminetetraacetic acid (EDTA)-treated *E. coli* [54]. The application of EDTA and calcium chloride to potentiate APDT with RB and hematoporphyrin (Hp)/zinc phthalocyanine was also reported [55,56].

5.6.2 APPLICATION OF PHOTOSENSITIZER CONJUGATES

Conjugating photosensitizer to various agents may not only enhance the photosensitizer–cell wall interaction but also minimize the aggregation and toxicity effects of the photosensitizer. Bezman et al. [57] covalently bound RB to small polystyrene beads that were allowed to mix with bacteria in suspension. It was thought that the photosensitizer bound at the outer membrane had the ability to generate ROS that diffuses into the bacterial cells. Friedberg et al. [58] covalently bound photosensitizer to a monoclonal antibody (Mab) that binds to cell surface antigens expressed on *P. aeruginosa* and demonstrated specific killing of target bacteria after illumination not produced by a nonspecific Mab conjugate. In another study [59], a nonspecific IgG that was recognized by protein A expressed on *S. aureus* was conjugated to the photosensitizer. They reported that the phototoxic effect of a conjugated dye of bacteriochlorophyll-serine derivative with IgG (Bchl-IgG) is 30 times more efficacious than the unconjugated photosensitizer, although considerably lesser Bchl-IgG molecules were bound per bacterium. The higher efficacy of Bchl-IgG was explained by (1) its location proximal to the bacterial cell wall and (2) the reactive photoproducts generated by sensitization, which are likely to damage the cell wall.

Soukos and coworkers hypothesized that by covalently conjugating a suitable photosensitizer to a *poly-l-lysine* chain, a bacteria-targeted photosensitizer delivery vehicle could be synthesized that in turn would efficiently inactivate both Gram-positive and Gram-negative species [60]. This was demonstrated by the preparation of a conjugate between one molecule of chlorin (e6) and a *poly-l-lysine* chain of 20 lysine residues that, after 1 min incubation and irradiation with red light, killed >99% of the Gram-positive *A. viscosus* and Gram-negative *P. gingivalis* oral pathogens. A similar construct composed of one ce6 molecule and a 5 amino-acid lysine chain was subsequently used to kill several oral pathogens in the presence of 25% whole blood [61]. Polo et al. [62] used conjugates between *poly-l-lysine* chain and porphycenes with a significant phototoxic activity against Gram-negative bacteria. Hamblin et al. demonstrated the effectiveness of a *poly-l-lysine*-ce6 conjugate with a chain length of 37 lysines attached to one ce6 molecule against both Gram-positive and Gram-negative species [21].

5.6.3 PHOTOSENSITIZER CHARGE, STIMULATION, AND MODIFICATION

Photosensitizer molecule with an intrinsic cationic charge has been found to potentiate APDT. A typical example of this approach has been the application of phenothiazinium dye, such as TBO and MB for APDT against a large range of both Gram-positive and Gram-negative bacteria [28,42,63]. Kennedy and Pottier demonstrated the possibility to stimulate an increased synthesis of porphyrins in bacteria by the exogeneous supplement of 5-aminolevulinic acid (5-ALA) [64]. Although these approaches could readily show improvement in planktonic bacteria, it is essential to characterize them on appropriate biofilm models since photosensitizer charge would influence the degree of diffusion of photosensitizer, possibility of aggregation, and risk of inactivation within biofilm matrix.

One of the major issues with a number of photosensitizers such as MB, TBO, RB, chlorin (e6), and Hp has been investigated for APDT of microbial pathogens. However, these PS have been found to aggregate easily in aqueous medium or biofilm matrix, which may lead to a self-quenching effect on the excited state, thus reducing the yield of singlet-oxygen ($^1O_2$) formation [65]. Relatively high proportion of aggregated photosensitizer in water may favor the formation of radicals instead of singlet oxygen [22]. Hence, to improve the efficacy of APDT, it is preferable to prepare photosensitizers in its monomeric form prepared in suitable carriers. Generally, photosensitizer solutions for APDT are prepared in deionized water or buffered saline [66,67]. Photosensitizer solutions when prepared in Brain Heart Infusion (BHI) broth [49,50,66] have displayed a reduced bactericidal effect, which was attributed to the presence of serum proteins in the BHI broth.

George and Kishen dissolved photosensitizer in different formulations: water, 70% glycerol, 70% PEG, and a mixture of glycerol:ethanol:water in the specific ratio. Then, they studied the photophysical, photochemical, and photobiological characteristics [22]. They showed that aggregation of photosensitizer molecules was significantly higher in water when compared to other formulations. The glycerol:ethanol:water-based photosensitizer formulation showed effective penetration into dentin tissue and generated higher singlet oxygen, which in turn improved bactericidal action [22]. A subsequent study showed that there was a significantly higher impairment of the bacterial cell wall and extensive damage to chromosomal DNA when MB was used in an MIX-based formulation when compared to water [28]. In the following year, the same group showed that inclusion of an oxidizer and oxygen carrier in the PS formulation would facilitate comprehensive disinfection of a matured biofilm by APDT [68].

5.6.4 SPECIFIC PHOTOSENSITIZER DELIVERY SYSTEMS

Customized tissue-specific photosensitizer delivery systems are suggested to reduce the likelihood of aggregation of photosensitizing agents. Encapsulation techniques that have been applied for such purposes include liposomes [69], polymeric micelles [70], and nanoparticles [71]. Recently, Tsai et al. conducted a study to increase the efficacy of PS, in which Hp was used as a model drug and encapsulated in liposomes and micelles by a modified reversed-phase evaporation and extrusion method [72]. The bactericidal efficacy of the carrier-entrapped Hp was assessed against Gram-positive bacteria. They concluded that a photosensitizer entrapped in micelle exerts similar or better APDT efficacy than that of liposome, thus indicating that this formulation may be useful for the treatment of local infections in the future. In a recent study, a bioactive polymeric chitosan nanoparticles functionalized with rose bengal (photosensitizer) was developed to produce marked antibiofilm effects as well as to stabilize structural integrity of dental hard tissue by photo-cross-linking dentin collagen, leading to efficient elimination of bacterial biofilms and stabilization of dentin matrix simultaneously [46].

5.6.5 EFFLUX PUMP INHIBITORS

Prokaryotic and eukaryotic cells possess families of membrane proteins termed efflux pumps that act to remove amphiphilic molecules from within the cell. Since many drugs are amphiphilic in nature, efflux pumps can effectively remove these molecules from within the prokaryotic and eukaryotic cells. Efflux is the process in bacteria, which transports compounds that are potentially toxic such as drugs or chemicals outside the cell [73]. Many of these efflux pump systems have broad substrate profiles that allow structurally diverse drugs/chemicals (including photosensitizer) to be extruded, while there are specific pumps that have been characterized to have a very limited profile of agents to extrude. Expression of efflux pumps on bacteria is one of the many factors that contributed to increased antimicrobial resistance in biofilm bacteria. Therefore, inhibiting bacterial efflux with an efflux pump inhibitor would reestablish the efficacy of an antimicrobial. The feasibility of this strategy has been demonstrated in vitro and in vivo [74]. It has been suggested that amphipathic cations represent the existing natural substrates of MEP [75] and these molecules have been frequently used to study MEP-mediated efflux. It has been established that disabling MEP by employing either MEP mutants or synthetic EPI leads to a striking increase in the activity of a wide array of plant secondary metabolites, including natural MEP substrates [76]. Tegos and Hamblin showed that phenothiazinium dyes, which are structurally characterized as amphipathic cations, were substrates of MEP [77]. They showed that inhibitors of bacterial MEP when used in combination with phenothiazinium dyes potentiate LAD [78]. In vitro experiments on biofilm models have also demonstrated the advantage of a cationic phenothiazinium photosensitizer combined with an efflux pump inhibitor to inactivate biofilm bacteria and disrupt biofilm structure [79,80]. Despite much work on discovering and optimizing the activity of EPI, unacceptable toxicity of some of these compounds in vivo still remains to be a challenge.

5.7 CONCLUDING REMARKS

It is well established that microbial biofilms are common cause of most chronic infections in humans. Current therapeutic strategies thus aim to eliminate bacterial biofilm in the treatment of localized infections. In the haste to introduce newer antibacterial strategies, it is important not to neglect potential constraining factors associated with their application in vivo. The key to the successful application of topical antimicrobials for the treatment of biofilm-induced infection is to address all the challenges possessed by the tissue environment (tissue-specific approach). Although APDT is effective in eliminating most tested microbes in laboratory conditions, their clinical applications require certain tissue-specific modifications. The delivery of light, optimization of light fluence, diffusion depth of photosensitizer, and effective singlet-oxygen yield are of particular interest while using APDT to achieve an efficient strategy against microbial biofilms.

REFERENCES

1. Cowen LE. The evolution of fungal drug resistance: Modulating the trajectory from genotype to phenotype. *Nat Rev Microbiol* 2008; **6**(3):187–198.
2. Witte W. International dissemination of antibiotic resistant strains of bacterial pathogens. *Infect Genet Evol* 2004; **4**(3):187–191.
3. Kishen A. Advanced therapeutic options for endodontic biofilms. *Endod Topics* 2010; **22**(1):99–123.
4. Costerton JW, Lewandowski Z, DeBeer D, Caldwell D, Korber D, James G. Biofilms, the customized microniche. *J Bacteriol* 1994; **176**(8):2137–2142.
5. Dunne WM, Mason EO, Kaplan SL. Diffusion of rifampin and vancomycin through a *Staphylococcus epidermidis* biofilm. *Antimicrob Agents Chemother* 1993; **37**(12):2522–2526.
6. Costerton JW. Introduction to biofilm. *Int J Antimicrob Agents* 1999; 11(3–4):217–221; discussion 237–219.
7. Rosan B, Correeia F, DiRienzo J. Corncobs: A model for oral microbial biofilms. In: Busscher H, Evans L, eds. *Oral Biofilms and Plaque Control*. Harwood Academic Publishers Amsterdam, the Netherlands; 1999, pp. 145–162.
8. Brooun A, Liu S, Lewis K. A dose–response study of antibiotic resistance in *Pseudomonas aeruginosa* biofilms. *Antimicrob Agents Chemother* 2000; **44**(3):640–646.
9. Lewis K. Persister cells and the riddle of biofilm survival. *Biochemistry (Mosc)* 2005; **70**(2):267–274.
10. Al C, Rocky R, Phil S, Anne C, Paul S, John L et al. Biofilms: Hypertext book. [cited; Center for Biofilm engineering, Montana State University]. Available from: http://www.hypertextbookshop.com/biofilm-book/v004/r003/ (accessed on December 02, 2015).
11. del Pozo JL, Patel R. The challenge of treating biofilm-associated bacterial infections. *Clin Pharmacol Ther* 2007; **82**(2):204–209.
12. Upadya MH. Influence of bacterial growth modes on the susceptibility of light activated disinfection. MSc thesis. National University of Singapore, Singapore; 2010.
13. Wainwright M. Photodynamic antimicrobial chemotherapy (PACT). *J Antimicrob Chemother* 1998; **42**(1):13–28.
14. Malik Z, Hanania J, Nitzan Y. Bactericidal effects of photoactivated porphyrins—An alternative approach to antimicrobial drugs. *J Photochem Photobiol B* 1990; **5**(3–4):281–293.
15. Marino L. Antimicrobial therapy. In: Hagerstown M, ed. *The ICU Book*. Lippincott Williams & Wilkins, New York; 2007, p. 817.
16. Spikes MJ. The historical development of ideas on applications of photosentized reactions in health sciences. In: *Primary Photoprocesses in Biology and Medicine*. Springer, New York; 1985, pp. 209–227.
17. Wainwright M, Crossley KB. Methylene Blue—A therapeutic dye for all seasons? *J Chemother* 2002; **14**(5):431–443.
18. Wainwright M, Giddens RM. Phenothiazinium photosensitisers: Choices in synthesis and application. *Dyes Pigments* 2003; **57**(3):245–257.
19. Merchat M, Bertolini G, Giacomini P, Villanueva A, Jori G. Meso-substituted cationic porphyrins as efficient photosensitizers of gram-positive and gram-negative bacteria. *J Photochem Photobiol B* 1996; **32**(3):153–157.
20. Minnock A, Vernon DI, Schofield J, Griffiths J, Parish JH, Brown ST. Photoinactivation of bacteria. Use of a cationic water-soluble zinc phthalocyanine to photoinactivate both gram-negative and gram-positive bacteria. *J Photochem Photobiol B* 1996; **32**(3):159–164.

21. Hamblin MR, O'Donnell DA, Murthy N, Rajagopalan K, Michaud N, Sherwood ME et al. Polycationic photosensitizer conjugates: Effects of chain length and Gram classification on the photodynamic inactivation of bacteria. *J Antimicrob Chemother* 2002; **49**(6):941–951.

22. George S, Kishen A. Photophysical, photochemical, and photobiological characterization of methylene blue formulations for light-activated root canal disinfection. *J Biomed Opt* 2007; **12**(3):034029.

23. Brancaleon L, Moseley H. Laser and non-laser light sources for photodynamic therapy. *Lasers Med Sci* 2002; **17**(3):173–186.

24. Burns T, Wilson M, Pearson GJ. Killing of cariogenic bacteria by light from a gallium aluminium arsenide diode laser. *J Dent* 1994; **22**(5):273–278.

25. Williams JA, Pearson GJ, Colles MJ, Wilson M. The effect of variable energy input from a novel light source on the photoactivated bactericidal action of toluidine blue O on *Streptococcus* Mutans. *Caries Res* 2003; **37**(3):190–193.

26. Bevilacqua IM, Nicolau RA, Khouri S, Brugnera A, Teodoro GR, Zângaro RA et al. The impact of photodynamic therapy on the viability of Streptococcus mutans in a planktonic culture. *Photomed Laser Surg* 2007; **25**(6):513–518.

27. Soukos NS, Ximenez-Fyvie LA, Hamblin MR, Socransky SS, Hasan T. Targeted antimicrobial photochemotherapy. *Antimicrob Agents Chemother* 1998; **42**(10):2595–2601.

28. George S, Kishen A. Influence of photosensitizer solvent on the mechanisms of photoactivated killing of *Enterococcus faecalis*. *Photochem Photobiol* 2008; **84**(3):734–740.

29. Wilson M, Dobson J, Sarkar S. Sensitization of periodontopathogenic bacteria to killing by light from a low-power laser. *Oral Microbiol Immunol* 1993; **8**(3):182–187.

30. Haas R, Dörtbudak O, Mensdorff-Pouilly N, Mailath G. Elimination of bacteria on different implant surfaces through photosensitization and soft laser. An in vitro study. *Clin Oral Implants Res* 1997; **8**(4):249–254.

31. Haapasalo M, Ranta H, Ranta KT. Facultative gram-negative enteric rods in persistent periapical infections. *Acta Odontol Scand* 1983; **41**(1):19–22.

32. Peciuliene V, Reynaud AH, Balciuniene I, Haapasalo M. Isolation of yeasts and enteric bacteria in root-filled teeth with chronic apical periodontitis. *Int Endod J* 2001; **34**(6):429–434.

33. Portenier I, Waltimo TMT, Haapasalo M. *Enterococcus faecalis*—The root canal survivor and 'star' in post-treatment disease. *Endod Topics* 2003; **6**(1):135–159.

34. Lim Z, Cheng JL, Lim TW, Teo EG, Wong J, George S et al. Light activated disinfection: An alternative endodontic disinfection strategy. *Aust Dent J* 2009; **54**(2):108–114.

35. Upadya MH, Kishen A. Influence of bacterial growth modes on the susceptibility to light-activated disinfection. *Int Endod J* 2010; **43**(11):978–987.

36. Bonsor SJ, Nichol R, Reid TM, Pearson GJ. Microbiological evaluation of photo-activated disinfection in endodontics (an in vivo study). *Br Dent J* 2006; **200**(6):337–341; discussion 329.

37. Garcez AS, Nuñez SC, Hamblin MR, Ribeiro MS. Antimicrobial effects of photodynamic therapy on patients with necrotic pulps and periapical lesion. *J Endod* 2008; **34**(2):138–142.

38. Pourabbas R, Kashefimehr A, Rahmanpour N, Babaloo Z, Kishen A, Tenenbaum HC et al. Effects of photodynamic therapy on clinical and gingival crevicular fluid inflammatory biomarkers in chronic periodontitis: A split-mouth randomized clinical trial. *J Periodontol* 2014; **85**(9):1222–1229.

39. Soukos NS, Wilson M, Burns T, Speight PM. Photodynamic effects of toluidine blue on human oral keratinocytes and fibroblasts and Streptococcus sanguis evaluated in vitro. *Lasers Surg Med* 1996; **18**(3):253–259.

40. Zeina B, Greenman J, Corry D, Purcell WM. Cytotoxic effects of antimicrobial photodynamic therapy on keratinocytes in vitro. *Br J Dermatol* 2002; **146**(4):568–573.

41. Soncin M, Fabris C, Busetti A, Dei D, Nistri D, Roncucci G et al. Approaches to selectivity in the Zn(II)-phthalocyanine-photosensitized inactivation of wild-type and antibiotic-resistant *Staphylococcus aureus*. *Photochem Photobiol Sci* 2002; **1**(10):815–819.

42. George S, Kishen A. Advanced noninvasive light-activated disinfection: Assessment of cytotoxicity on fibroblast versus antimicrobial activity against *Enterococcus faecalis*. *J Endod* 2007; **33**(5):599–602.

43. Bhatti M, MacRobert A, Meghji S, Henderson B, Wilson M. Effect of dosimetric and physiological factors on the lethal photosensitization of *Porphyromonas gingivalis* in vitro. *Photochem Photobiol* 1997; **65**(6):1026–1031.

44. Dobson J, Wilson M. Sensitization of oral bacteria in biofilms to killing by light from a low-power laser. *Arch Oral Biol* 1992; **37**(11):883–887.

45. Shrestha A, Kishen A. Polycationic chitosan-conjugated photosensitizer for antibacterial photodynamic therapy. *Photochem Photobiol* 2012; **88**(3):577–583.

46. Shrestha A, Hamblin MR, Kishen A. Photoactivated rose bengal functionalized chitosan nanoparticles produce antibacterial/biofilm activity and stabilize dentin-collagen. *Nanomedicine* 2014; **10**(3):491–501.

47. Zanin IC, Lobo MM, Rodrigues LK, Pimenta LA, Höfling JF, Gonçalves RB. Photosensitization of in vitro biofilms by toluidine blue O combined with a light-emitting diode. *Eur J Oral Sci* 2006; **114**(1):64–69.

48. Wakayama Y, Takagi M, Yano K. Photosensitized inactivation of *E. coli* cells in toluidine blue-light system. *Photochem Photobiol* 1980; **32**(5):601–605.

49. Soukos NS, Chen PS, Morris JT, Ruggiero K, Abernethy AD, Som S et al. Photodynamic therapy for endodontic disinfection. *J Endod* 2006; **32**(10):979–984.

50. Foschi F, Fontana CR, Ruggiero K, Riahi R, Vera A, Doukas AG et al. Photodynamic inactivation of Enterococcus faecalis in dental root canals in vitro. *Lasers Surg Med* 2007; **39**(10):782–787.

51. Shrestha A, Cordova M, Kishen A. Photoactivated polycationic bioactive chitosan nanoparticles inactivate bacterial endotoxins. *J Endod* 2015; **41**(5):686–691.

52. Nitzan Y, Gutterman M, Malik Z, Ehrenberg B. Inactivation of gram-negative bacteria by photosensitized porphyrins. *Photochem Photobiol* 1992; **55**(1):89–96.

53. Walther J, Bröcker MJ, Wätzlich D, Nimtz M, Rohde M, Jahn D et al. Protochlorophyllide: A new photosensitizer for the photodynamic inactivation of Gram-positive and Gram-negative bacteria. *FEMS Microbiol Lett* 2009; **290**(2):156–163.

54. Yonei S, Todo T. Enhanced sensitivity to the lethal and mutagenic effects of photosensitizing action of chlorpromazine in ethylenediaminetetraacetate-treated *Escherichia coli*. *Photochem Photobiol* 1982; **35**(4):591–592.

55. Valduga G, Bertoloni G, Reddi E, Jori G. Effect of extracellularly generated singlet oxygen on gram-positive and gram-negative bacteria. *J Photochem Photobiol B* 1993; **21**(1):81–86.

56. Bertoloni G, Rossi F, Valduga G, Jori G, van Lier J. Photosensitizing activity of water- and lipid-soluble phthalocyanines on *Escherichia coli*. *FEMS Microbiol Lett* 1990; **59**(1–2):149–155.

57. Bezman SA, Burtis PA, Izod TP, Thayer MA. Photodynamic inactivation of *E. coli* by rose bengal immobilized on polystyrene beads. *Photochem Photobiol* 1978; **28**(3):325–329.

58. Friedberg JS, Tompkins RG, Rakestraw SL, Warren SW, Fischman AJ, Yarmush ML. Antibody-targeted photolysis. Bacteriocidal effects of Sn (IV) chlorin e6-dextran-monoclonal antibody conjugates. *Ann N Y Acad Sci* 1991; **618**:383–393.

59. Gross S, Brandis A, Chen L, Rosenbach-Belkin V, Roehrs S, Scherz A et al. Protein-A-mediated targeting of bacteriochlorophyll-IgG to *Staphylococcus aureus*: A model for enhanced site-specific photocytotoxicity. *Photochem Photobiol* 1997; **66**(6):872–878.

60. Soukos NS, Hamblin MR, Hasan T. The effect of charge on cellular uptake and phototoxicity of polylysine chlorin (e6) conjugates. *Photochem Photobiol* 1997; **65**(4):723–729.

61. Rovaldi CR, Pievsky A, Sole NA, Friden PM, Rothstein DM, Spacciapoli P. Photoactive porphyrin derivative with broad-spectrum activity against oral pathogens in vitro. *Antimicrob Agents Chemother* 2000; **44**(12):3364–3367.

62. Polo L, Segalla A, Bertoloni G, Jori G, Schaffner K, Reddi E. Polylysine-porphycene conjugates as efficient photosensitizers for the inactivation of microbial pathogens. *J Photochem Photobiol B* 2000; **59**(1–3):152–158.

63. Wilson M. Photolysis of oral bacteria and its potential use in the treatment of caries and periodontal disease. *J Appl Bacteriol* 1993; **75**(4):299–306.

64. Kennedy JC, Pottier RH. Endogenous protoporphyrin-IX, a clinically useful photosensitizer for photodynamic therapy. *J Photochem Photobiol B Biol* 1992; **14**(4):275–292.

65. Jang WD, Nakagishi Y, Nishiyama N, Kawauchi S, Morimoto Y, Kikuchi M et al. Polyion complex micelles for photodynamic therapy: Incorporation of dendritic photosensitizer excitable at long wavelength relevant to improved tissue-penetrating property. *J Control Release* 2006; **113**(1):73–79.

66. Fimple JL, Fontana CR, Foschi F, Ruggiero K, Song X, Pagonis TC et al. Photodynamic treatment of endodontic polymicrobial infection in vitro. *J Endod* 2008; **34**(6):728–734.

67. Usacheva MN, Teichert MC, Biel MA. Comparison of the methylene blue and toluidine blue photobactericidal efficacy against gram-positive and gram-negative microorganisms. *Lasers Surg Med* 2001; **29**(2):165–173.

68. George S, Kishen A. Augmenting the antibiofilm efficacy of advanced noninvasive light activated disinfection with emulsified oxidizer and oxygen carrier. *J Endod* 2008; **34**(9):1119–1123.

69. Chang CC, Yang YT, Yang JC, Wu HD, Tsai T. Absorption and emission spectral shifts of rose bengal associated with DMPC liposomes. *Dyes Pigments* 2008; **79**(2):170–175.

70. Rijcken CJ, Hofman JW, van Zeeland F, Hennink WE, van Nostrum CF. Photosensitiser-loaded biodegradable polymeric micelles: Preparation, characterisation and in vitro PDT efficacy. *J Control Release* 2007; **124**(3):144–153.

71. Konan YN, Berton M, Gurny R, Allémann E. Enhanced photodynamic activity of meso-tetra(4-hydroxyphenyl)porphyrin by incorporation into sub-200 nm nanoparticles. *Eur J Pharm Sci* 2003; **18**(3–4):241–249.

72. Tsai T, Yang YT, Wang TH, Chien HF, Chen CT. Improved photodynamic inactivation of gram-positive bacteria using hematoporphyrin encapsulated in liposomes and micelles. *Lasers Surg Med* 2009; **41**(4):316–322.

73. Ryan BM, Dougherty TJ, Beaulieu D, Chuang J, Dougherty BA, Barrett JF. Efflux in bacteria: What do we really know about it? *Expert Opin Investig Drugs* 2001; **10**(8):1409–1422.

74. Renau TE, Léger R, Flamme EM, Sangalang J, She MW, Yen R et al. Inhibitors of efflux pumps in *Pseudomonas aeruginosa* potentiate the activity of the fluoroquinolone antibacterial levofloxacin. *J Med Chem* 1999; **42**(24):4928–4931.

75. Lewis K. Multidrug resistance: Versatile drug sensors of bacterial cells. *Curr Biol* 1999; **9**(11):R403–R407.

76. Tegos G, Stermitz FR, Lomovskaya O, Lewis K. Multidrug pump inhibitors uncover remarkable activity of plant antimicrobials. *Antimicrob Agents Chemother* 2002; **46**(10):3133–3141.

77. Tegos GP, Hamblin MR. Phenothiazinium antimicrobial photosensitizers are substrates of bacterial multidrug resistance pumps. *Antimicrob Agents Chemother* 2006; **50**(1):196–203.

78. Tegos GP, Masago K, Aziz F, Higginbotham A, Stermitz FR, Hamblin MR. Inhibitors of bacterial multidrug efflux pumps potentiate antimicrobial photoinactivation. *Antimicrob Agents Chemother* 2008; **52**(9):3202–3209.

79. Lynch AS. Efflux systems in bacterial pathogens: An opportunity for therapeutic intervention? An industry view. *Biochem Pharmacol* 2006; **71**(7):949–956.

80. Kishen A, Upadya M, Tegos GP, Hamblin MR. Efflux pump inhibitor potentiates antimicrobial photodynamic inactivation of Enterococcus faecalis biofilm. *Photochem Photobiol* 2010; **86**(6):1343–1349.

High-content imaging for photosensitizer screening

GISELA M.F. VAZ, MATHIAS O. SENGE, SARAH-LOUISE RYAN, AND ANTHONY DAVIES

6.1 INTRODUCTION

Clinical applications of imaging methods are continuously advancing and new and optimized imaging agents are in high demand. Likewise, the underlying techniques are becoming more sensitive and numerous, and range from simple spectroscopic and luminescence modalities to photoacoustic, thermal, and magnetic methods, the use of nanomaterials, to emerging areas such as terahertz spectroscopy, to name only a few. Nevertheless, due to the ease and sensitivity of detection, fluorescent imaging dyes feature prominently in this area (Kobayashi et al., 2010). Additionally, such dyes are often easily prepared, cheap, and available as a myriad of different chemical entities. Furthermore, provided the excited singlet state can undergo intersystem crossing to yield long-lived triplet states, photosensitization, that is, energy transfer to a secondary molecule—potentially a biological intervention as PDT—becomes possible (Henderson and Dougherty, 1992).

6.1.1 PHOTOSENSITIZERS IN PDT

Photodynamic therapy (PDT) is a selective cancer treatment, which can be used as an alternative or in addition to classical therapies, for example, surgery, radiation, or chemotherapy. It involves the administration of a tumor-localizing photosensitizing agent, followed by activation of the agent by light of a specific wavelength.

This approach generates a sequence of photochemical and photobiological processes involving reactive oxygen species, resulting in irreversible photodamage to tumor tissue. PDT as a modality holds many advantages over traditional cancer treatments such as radiation therapy, chemotherapy, and surgery as PDT is a relatively noninvasive treatment that has the potential to selectively destroy tumor cells while sparing healthy tissue (Henderson and Dougherty, 1992).

The principal characteristic of any PDT sensitizer is its capacity to preferentially accumulate in malignant tissue and, via the production of cytotoxic species, induce a desired biological effect. For a molecule to be considered a viable candidate as a photosensitizer, it must meet a number of requirements. Generally, molecules should exhibit a strong absorption in the near-infrared region of the electromagnetic spectrum (600–850 nm), which allows for a deeper penetration of light and should show no dark toxicity. Typically, they are pure dye compounds with a stable shelf life and constant composition and have a high quantum yield of singlet-oxygen production (Nyman and Hynninen, 2004; Wilson and Patterson, 2008; Rogers and Senge, 2014).

Historically speaking, the first photosensitizer (PS) to be used in a clinical setting was psoralen, still used today in psoriasis treatment (PUVA, psoralene and ultraviolet A radiation) (Figure 6.1). However, most commonly, photosensitizers are porphyrin derivatives due to not only their high absorption in the red–near-infrared region of light (significantly increasing the depth at which PDT can be used in tissue), but they are also naturally occurring compounds and/or can be chemically synthesized and modified using "simple" chemical synthetic approaches (Juzeniene and Moan, 2007). With regard to porphyrins, hematoporphyrin derivative (HpD) was the first to be developed for clinical use and is generally considered a first-generation PS. Attempts to improve on its poor light absorption, long tissue retention times, low tumor–tissue ratios, low water solubility, and prolonged photosensitization of patients led to so-called second-generation PS, typical examples being Visudyne, Temoporfin, and δ-aminolevulinic acid (ALA), the biosynthetic precursor of protoporphyrin IX (Juzeniene et al., 2007).

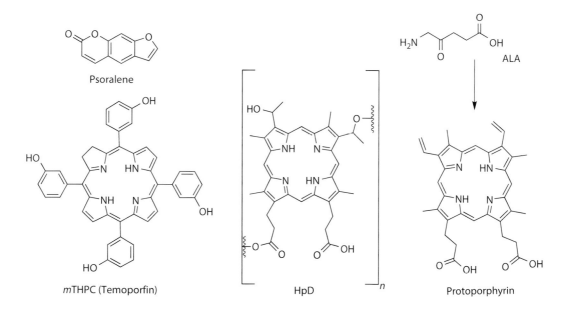

Figure 6.1 Selected first- and second-generation photosensitizers. ALA, δ-aminolevulinic acid; HpD, hematoporphyrin derivative; mTHPC = 5,10,15,20-tetrakis(3-hydroxyphenyl)porphyrin, Temoporfin. Although many new PSs have been developed for PDT (Nyman and Hynninen, 2004), many problems remain to be overcome. The selectivity of the PS agents for the target tissue must be improved and their pharmacokinetics and biodistribution must be tackled to provide a more beneficial course of treatment with fewer side effects.

With regard to the development of new PSs, specific characteristics apply to an "ideal" PS, which must be considered. It must be chemically pure and stable, fully characterized in terms of optimum absorption, distribution, metabolism, and excretion. Minimal dark toxicity should be observed and the PS should only be toxic when activated by light of specific wavelengths and not undergo photobleaching. Fast clearance from cells and the body would reduce severe side effects from skin photosensitization. Last but not least, solubility is often an issue as most PSs are organic dyes with limited water solubility. Thus, efforts to produce more soluble or amphiphilic PS feature prominently in contemporary syntheses.

6.1.2 THE QUEST FOR THIRD-GENERATION PHOTOSENSITIZERS

Ultimately, the success of PDT will depend on the development of PS with superior tissue localization and, ideally, as drug development mandates, identification of a specific cellular or tissue target that would improve the therapeutic action of that drug (Rogers and Senge, 2014). New PSs are required that exhibit significant selectivity for neoplastic tissue accumulation in such regions in high concentration, that is, target-specific dyes. Subcellular localization within organelles such as the mitochondria is beneficial to obtain apoptotic instead of necrotic cell death as the latter comes with a range of complex and dangerous side effects. The search for a novel PS that meets all the chemical, physical, and biological criteria is still ongoing.

Second-generation PSs coupled to carrier systems are now being evaluated as potential "third-generation" PS (Juzeniene et al., 2007); these are thought to accumulate more selectively in tumors, reducing even more the time for which the patient presents photosensitivity and could potentially reduce the amount of drug given to the patient. Novel carrier systems such as monoclonal antibodies, liposomes, antibody fragments, and nanoparticles are now under study (Paszko et al., 2011). In parallel, studies are continuing apace to optimize the basic tetrapyrrole framework structures in terms of absorption maxima (deeper tissue penetration), extension of the π-system (absorption and two-photon absorption), functional group chemistry (attachment of bioconjugate groups), formulation strategies, and solubility. Likewise, the use of known photosensitizers for different indications continues. Table 6.1 gives selected examples of such PDT agents in use and development.

Generally speaking, either relatively "simple" porphyrin molecules are used, which allow a quick entry into bioconjugate systems, for example, the A_x- or ABCD-type porphyrins (Senge, 2011), derivatives of protoporphyrin, or hydroporphyrins based on the natural phytochlorin or chlorin e_6 system with their superior absorption properties (Nyman and Hynninen, 2004; Figure 6.2). While many other tetrapyrrole-based systems are under scrutiny, only these two classes and the rapidly expanding number of BODIPY derivatives generate large enough numbers of compounds for QSAR-type screening approaches.

6.2 HIGH-CONTENT ANALYSIS

High-content analysis (HCA) is a convergence between cell-based assays, high-resolution fluorescent imaging, automation, and advanced image analysis by analysis software. It has been widely adopted by the pharmaceutical industry and academic centers for the validation of potential drugs and to elucidate the mechanisms of drug action at a cellular and subcellular level (Dove, 2003).

It is a powerful method that allows the simultaneous detection of multiple biological outputs, the preclinical toxicological evaluation of drugs, and can even be used (when coupled to an automated system) to screen for the effects of thousands of potential drugs within a relatively short amount of time. The technology is particularly valuable during the early stages of drug development as it provides a large-scale biological platform with significant potential for automation and miniaturization (Abraham et al., 2004). High-content screening (HCS) links various independent scientific disciplines from synthetic chemistry to biology (Figure 6.3) and from computational sciences to advanced microscopy (Johnston and Johnston, 2002). HCS has received much interest in the last decade, hence new "rules" for the use and development of relevant assays are now being established.

Table 6.1 Selected photosensitizers for photodynamic therapy, diseases treated, and their status of approval

PS	Trade name	Indication	λ_{max} (activation)
Drugs with regulatory approval			
mTHPC	Temoporfin	Head-and-neck cancers	652
BPD-MA	Verteporfin	Age-related macular degeneration	689
5-ALA	Ameluz	Actinic keratosis	635
5-ALA-methyl ester	Metvix	Actinic keratosis; basal cell carcinoma	635
Drugs in clinical development			
BPD-MA	Verteporfin	Basal cell carcinoma (BCC)	689
mTHPC	Temoporfin	BCC; prostate and pancreatic cancer	652
HpD	Photofrin	Brain tumors	630
SnEt2	Purlytin	Cutaneous metastatic breast cancer; BCC; Kaposi's sarcoma; prostate cancer	664
Lutetium texaphyrin	Lutex	Cervical, prostate, and brain cancers	732
Phthalocyanide-4	Pc4	Various cancers	670
AlPcS	Photosan	Head-and-neck cancers	670
Taporphin sodium	Talaporfin	Various solid tumors	664
Pd-Bacterio-pheophorbide	TOOKAD	Prostate cancer	763
5-ALA-hexyl ester	Hervix	Diagnosis of bladder cancer	~400
BPD-MA	Verteporfin	BCC	689
mTHPC	Temoporfin	BCC; prostate and pancreatic cancer	652
HpD	Photofrin	Brain tumors	630
SnEt2	Purlytin	Cutaneous metastatic breast cancer; BCC; Kaposi's sarcoma; prostate cancer	664
Lutetium texaphyrin	Lutex	Cervical, prostate, and brain cancers	732

HCS is based on the automated acquisition of images of fluorescently labeled cells. These images are then subsequently analyzed using automated analysis software allowing the quantification of numerous phenotypic characteristics of the assay cells (Smellie et al., 2005); this technique generates an enormous amount of data that need to be filtered in order to obtain biologically relevant information. To overcome this obstacle, data mining techniques have been developed linking biology to computer technologies. HCS is not only a robust technique but is also very versatile as many types of assays can be performed using the same platform, from toxicology to validation of targets, to RNAi experiments. The developers of assay technology have also made available a broad range of cellular platforms using microscopy slides to 394-well plates.

HCS owes its generalized acceptance and progress not only to its versatility, but also to the fact that phenotypic screens have yielded many commercially successful drugs in the past decade (Reisen et al., 2013). More powerful tools in the field of automated fluorescent imaging and a strong commercial interest from leading pharmaceutical companies also allowed for the rapid dissemination of HCS worldwide. They also sparked major advances on the technological side with evermore powerful hardware as well as an ever-increasing array of commercially available fluorophores such as Hoechst (a bis-benzimidazoline blue fluorescent dye used to stain DNA; Zanella et al., 2010).

In toxicology, HCS has been applied mainly in the prediction of hepatic toxicity of large libraries of compounds; however, novel phenotypic-based toxicity screens are increasingly used by pharma and academia alike (O'Brien et al., 2006; Bickle, 2010; Swinney and Anthony, 2011; Reisen et al., 2013). Central to the technique of fluorescent imaging (and consequently HCS technologies) lies a large range of molecules that are able to localize and accumulate in specific locations whether intracellularly or in a specific tissue and are fluorescent in nature (Table 6.2; Sergeeva et al., 2011).

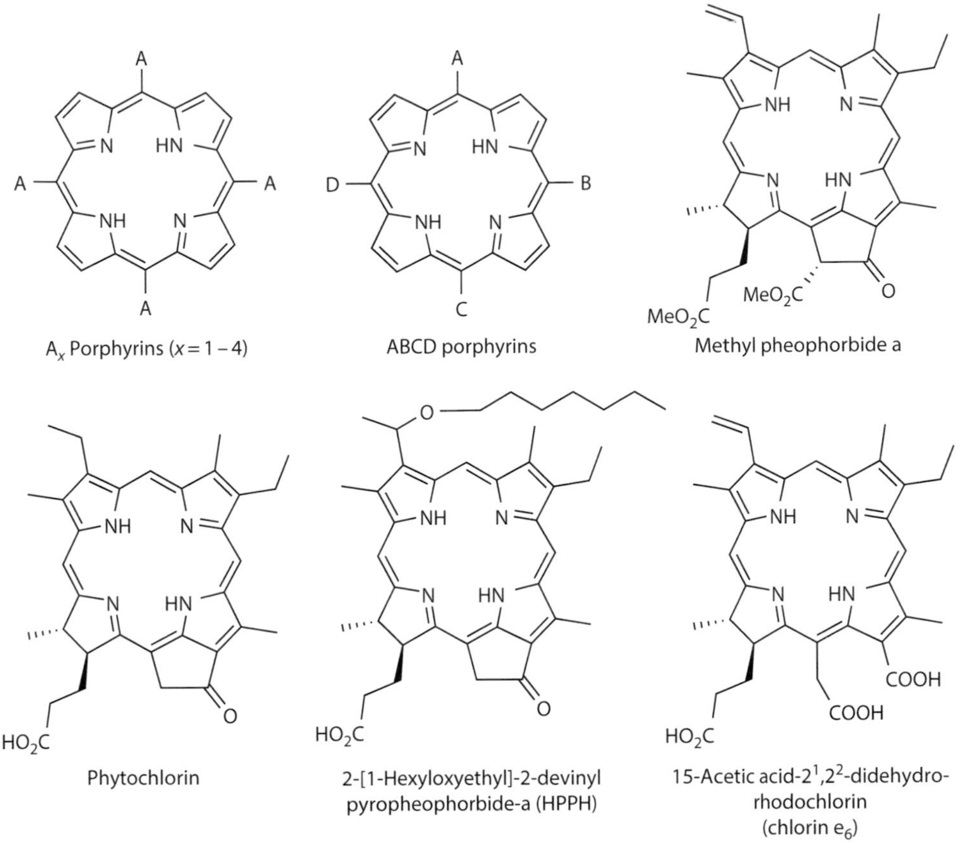

Figure 6.2 Molecular structures of porphyrin frameworks used for the development of lead compounds such as HPPH.

The study of the in vitro interactions of any naturally fluorescent molecule with cells, such as porphyrins and their derivatives, poses many difficulties. The following are the most prominent in the field of PDT assessment and development:

- When working with photoactive compounds, most experimental manipulations of living cellular material need to be carried out under special illumination conditions (because natural light activates these compounds and prematurely produces cellular damage).
- The fact that these compounds have been designed to convert light energy into cytotoxic-free radicals translates into easy photodegradation in the presence of any light.
- By their very nature, these compounds have an intrinsic fluorescence over a broad range of excitation and emission wavelengths. This makes analysis of these chemicals with techniques based on fluorescence analysis with various additional chromophores challenging to avoid spectral overlap.

Traditionally, a large number of methodologies are used for drug evaluation. A typical example is the MTT assay, an indirect method widely used to measure cell health, viability, and growth based on the principle that viable cells are able to metabolically reduce 3-(4,5-dimethylthiazol-2-yl)-2,5-diphenyltetrazolium bromide (MTT) into its insoluble form formazan inducing a color change (from yellow to purple); results are read as a measurement of absorbance (Mosmann, 1983). Other examples are the indirect measurement of drug efficacy with BrdU (5-bromo-2′-deoxyuridine), flow cytometry for the evaluation of fluorescent labeled cells, trypan blue exclusion, neutral comet or red assays, Raman spectroscopy, or confocal imaging (Bravery et al., 2013; Table 6.3).

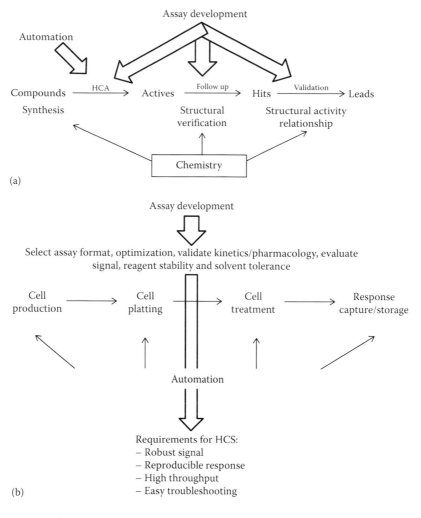

(a)

(b)

Figure 6.3 Summary of the two main strategies in the development of an HCS assay using potential toxic compounds. (a) Lead generation. A lead generation strategy must be developed for primary and secondary assays for the confirmation of HCS actives, hit assessment, lead validation, and lead optimization. (b) Cell-based assay development and additional challenges of the latter.

Table 6.2 Examples of commonly used DNA fluorescent probes

Dye name	Excitation (nm)	Emission (nm)	Live/fixed cell applications
Hoechst 33342	350	461	Live and fixed cell–based assays
DAPI	358	461	Fixed cell–based assays
Propidium iodide	530	625	Fixed, permeabilized, dead cell–based assays
Draq 5	647	670	Fixed, permeabilized, live cell–based assays
Draq 7	633	694	Fixed, permeabilized, dead cell–based assays
TOTO3	640	660	Fixed, permeabilized, dead cell–based assays

Source: Haney, S.A. et al., *Drug Discov. Today*, 11, 889, 2006.

Table 6.3 Summary of various methods traditionally used for determining efficacy of compounds in in vitro tests

Method	Suitable for large screen	Why
HCA	Yes	High-throughput, automatable, fast, multiple outputs, allows for spatial distribution of macromolecules
MTT	No	Overnight incubation needed before reading, single output, destructive
BrdU	No	Requires antibody and denaturation step, lengthy
Flow cytometry	No	Requires trypsinization, optimization needed, no drug parameters
Trypan blue exclusion	No	Manual, lengthy, automation not viable
Neutral comet assay	No	Requires lysis of cells, single output, no drug parameters
Neutral red assay	No	Read at 540 nm (maximum absorbance of porphyrins)
Raman spectroscopy	No	Labor intensive, single output, low throughput
Confocal imaging	No	Low throughput, not automatable

HCA has many advantages over the more traditional approaches. For example, it can be used as a one-step assay to screen a library of PDT compounds as its output may include parameters related to the effect of the PS on cells but also offers parameters related to the intracellular presence of the drug itself. However, all of these techniques pose issues when it comes to screening large libraries of compounds.

When determining toxicity, HCA is an ideal assay to screen a library of PDT compounds as its output may include parameters that relate directly to the potential PS (due to their inherent fluorescence) in the cells such as intensity and localization. It also allows for the study of live cells and results are obtained in intact cells (Abraham et al., 2004). Thus, the use of HCA techniques in a screening setting has evolved into its own field, HCS (Haney et al., 2006). This technique allows for the simultaneous detection of multiple biological pathways and the preclinical toxicological evaluation of pharmaceutical drugs. In vitro estimation of toxicity using HCS in cell lines has been used in recent years, particularly in predicting hepatic toxicity (Tolosa et al., 2015), but also to assess toxicity of anticancer agents (Liegg et al., 2010). Both HCA and HCS are, in essence, very simple methods. Based on in vitro evaluation of potentially therapeutic compounds, they enable simultaneous measurement of multiple features of cellular phenotype that are relevant to therapeutic and toxic activities of those compounds (Dove, 2003).

6.3 SAMPLE CASE: HCS FOR PDT OF ESOPHAGEAL CANCER

6.3.1 ASSAY DEVELOPMENT

Automated imaging has been available for the last 20 years and has significantly streamlined the process of in vitro drug screening in addition to decreasing the time needed both for high-quality image collection and analysis (Ramirez et al., 2011). Fluorescent drugs have, in the past, been evaluated by fluorescent microscopy (Frisoli et al., 1993). However, a phenotypic screen of toxicity in cells using naturally fluorescent compounds has seldom been attempted due to its inherent difficulties. To illustrate the concept, we offer a brief outline of the development of a high-content assay using fluorescent drugs in OE21 cells, a human esophageal squamous cell carcinoma cell line derived from a human carcinoma, and SKGT-4 cells, a human adenocarcinoma of the esophagus derived from a human adenocarcinoma caused by Barrett's esophagus (Vaz et al., 2013).

Figure 6.4 illustrates the general experimental protocol for these studies. In order to have a benchmark compound, we chose Temoporfin, an approved porphyrin PS (Senge and Brandt, 2011). Using classical assay techniques, for example, an MTT assay, we then ascertained that indeed a dose-dependent effect on cell proliferation is observed. In the case of PS, this naturally must involve the use of a dark control (to determine

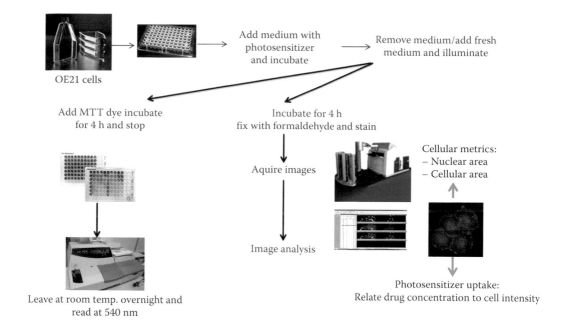

Figure 6.4 Flow scheme for the experimental protocol representing both MTT assay methodology and HCS protocol (method development).

dark cytotoxicity, if any) and illuminated samples. As PDT is dependent on the presence of the PS, oxygen, and the light conditions, the latter is crucial for assessing the overall effect and, for new compounds, must also include studies on optimum excitation wavelengths, light intensity and duration, etc. (Wilson and Patterson, 2008).

The next stage of the process is the use of an HCA platform to analyze the morphological changes that occur upon PDT treatment of the cells. Cell death results in many changes of characteristics of cellular morphology, and these may be used for HCA analysis. Figure 6.5 shows some examples of images collected using the HCA platform. Clearly, illumination in the presence of the photosensitizer results in dramatic changes to the cells compared to the dark control. The severity of these physical cell alterations increased with the concentration of Temoporfin.

The earliest phenotypic signs of cell toxicity are reflected by changes in nuclear size, cell fragmentation, and significant changes in the cell area and cell shape (Bortner and Cidlowski, 2002). Other phenotypic changes include cell membrane breakdown, leakage of cellular contents, and increased numbers of cytosolic, lysosomal vesicles. Thus, an automated approach to the quantification of these features can be useful during screening of a large number of compounds by taking advantage of these marked changes in cell morphology. Typically, changes in nuclear morphology are among the first effects seen during cell death (Dove, 2003). The next step is then the selection of appropriate criteria, which requires a strong correlation between the data from HCA and standard assays (for different drug concentrations). For example, the nuclear area in OE21 cells in fact reflected the phototoxicity of temoporfin in a dose-dependent fashion and followed this trend in the same fashion as seen in the cell proliferation assay. When both assay approaches give a strong statistical correlation, then the high-content approach can be considered to be validated.

In practical terms, this can be a laborious process as various cellular parameters, different drug concentrations, different cell media and growth conditions, illumination protocols, etc., need to be tested. The main advantage of HCS lies in the possibility to assess a large number of cellular parameters, with large libraries of compounds in a short time period and in a statistically reliable manner, once the high-content assay has been validated and developed.

	Untreated	3 μM temoporfin	0.5 μM temoporfin	5 μM temoporfin illuminated	0.5 μM temoporfin illuminated

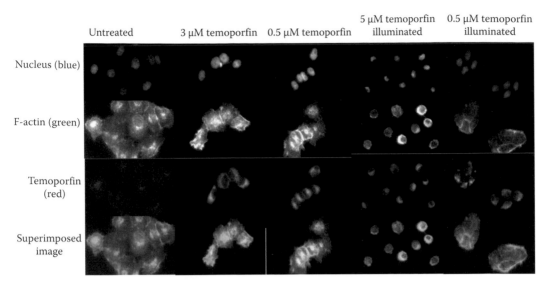

Nucleus (blue)

F-actin (green)

Temoporfin (red)

Superimposed image

Figure 6.5 Examples of images collected with an InCell imaging system for the different treatments used with OE21 cells treated with 3 μM temoporfin for 24 h before illumination and fixed at 4 h post illumination in 4% paraformaldehyde. Cells were labeled with Hoechst–nucleus (blue at 345 nm excitation, 435 nm emission), phalloidin–F-actin (green at 475 nm excitation and 535 nm emission). mTHPC (red) was acquired at 560 nm excitation and 700 nm emission. Images were acquired by an InCell analyzer automated microscope using a 10× objective (image size 0.897 mm × 0.671 mm). (From Vaz, G.M.F. et al., *PLoS One*, 8, e70653, 2013.)

6.3.2 SCREENING AND APPLICATIONS

Ultimately, HCS has to prove its worth in the identification of new lead compounds. In the case of our studies on esophageal cancer cells, a rapid screen of a small library of compounds indeed quickly identified compounds that had photocytotoxicities comparable to Temoporfin (Vaz et al., 2013). The information obtained using this methodology allowed the evaluation of several biological parameters, such as nuclear and cellular area. Furthermore, the time needed to evaluate the effects of many chemical compounds developed by chemical synthesis was greatly reduced.

Subsequently, this approach was used to evaluate a range of different classes of porphyrin-type photosensitizers with regard to their in vitro PDT efficacy (Figure 6.6). One example was a series of 5,10,15,20-tetrakis(*m*-hydroxyphenyl)porphyrins (*m*THPP), where one or all four hydroxyl groups had undergone a Steglich esterification with nonsteroidal anti-inflammatory drugs (e.g., Ibuprofen) in order to potentially increase the cytotoxicity of the treatment modality by targeting the tumor microenvironment. However, these compounds exhibited diminished singlet-oxygen production and no phototoxicity (Rogers et al., 2015). Similar results were obtained with porphyrin bile acid conjugates (Rogers et al., 2013). Bile acids, which are known to selectively bind to or be readily taken up by cancer cells, were chosen as the targeting moieties. The conjugates were synthesized via selective nucleophilic monofunctionalization of *m*THPP with propargyl bromide, followed by Cu(I)-mediated cycloaddition with bile acid azides (Click chemistry) in good yields. The compounds were readily taken up by esophageal cancer cells but showed no PDT activity, probably a result of the linker type. In the same context, significant numbers of glycoporphyrins were screened as well (Daly et al., 2012). The latter are prime examples of contemporary porphyrin bioconjugates with which increased water solubility and/or amphiphilic character (Moylan et al., 2015) is hoped to give improved PDT results.

Nevertheless, our studies also identified a new type of porphyrin lead compound for PDT. One of the major issues affecting the general use of porphyrins as PS in the clinic is solubility of the compound in aqueous mediums. A traditional chemical approach to overcome this is either by peripheral conjugation with soluble biological groups (e.g., the glycoporphyrins mentioned earlier) or the use of porphyrins with sulfonic or carboxylic acid functionalities (negative charge) or with alkylated nitrogen functionalities or phosphines

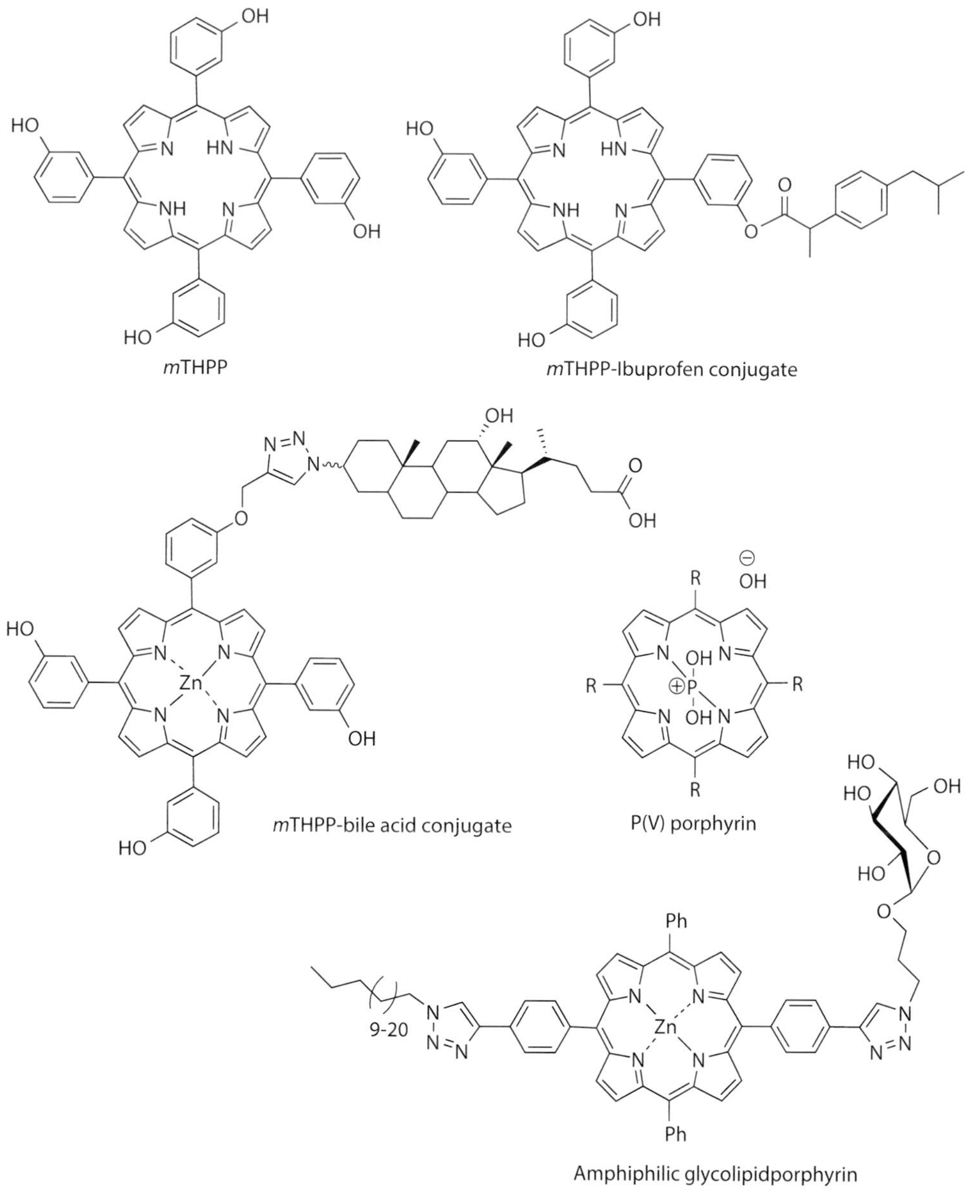

Figure 6.6 Molecular structures of porphyrin systems investigated with high-content techniques in esophageal cancer cells. Once established, an HCA protocol can also be used for the evaluation of different PS formulations. For example, we prepared polyethylene glycol grafted, transferrin-appended liposomes carrying temoporfin as the active PS (Paszko et al., 2013). The expression of transferrin (Tf) receptors (CD71) in the esophageal cancer cell line, OE21, was confirmed by immunoblot and confocal laser scanning microscopy and the antiproliferative effect of mTHPC liposomes was evaluated and compared with plain formulations (i.e., without attached Tf) as well as with free drug. The latter two gave comparable results with regard to photocytotoxicity. Surprisingly, MTT and HCS data demonstrated that Tf-modified liposomal formulations of temoporfin did not improve photocytotoxicity or intracellular accumulation of the photosensitizer in esophageal cancer cells. On the other hand, Tf-targeted drugs and drug delivery systems have improved the therapy of many other cancers. There are a number of possible explanations for this observation. The PS might have leaked from the Tf vehicles as a result of a membrane-destabilizing effect of Tf (Hefesha et al., 2011). Temoporfin is a highly lipophilic drug that can form aggregates in an aqueous environment, but might still be taken up by the cells, which would explain the lower intracellular temoporfin intensity as observed by HCA.

(positive charge) (Hudson et al., 2005). With this in mind, a series of simple, S_4 symmetric phosphorus(V) 5,10,15,20-tetraalkylporphyrins were prepared to yield amphiphilic systems (Ryan et al., 2014). Here, the periphery is lipophilic while the porphyrin core carries the charge.

Reasonable-to-good yields were obtained for all P(V) insertions, and all compounds underwent biological evaluation for their PDT activity in the esophageal cancer cell lines OE33 and SKGT-4. Three compounds displayed good uptake in the HCS assay, and, using the MTS cell proliferation assay, two compounds were shown to have photocytotoxicity on par with temoporfin, despite the different localization behavior of water-soluble versus non-water-soluble photosensitizers. These novel photosensitizing agents demonstrated significant toxicity after irradiation with light and minimal dark cytotoxicity, making them potential inexpensive candidates for PDT. While further improvements are necessary, the preliminary studies indicate that the "P(V) effect" methodology has the potential to enhance the PDT activity and cellular uptake of even the simplest of tetrapyrroles.

6.4 CURRENT DEVELOPMENTS IN HIGH-CONTENT IMAGING IN PDT

In parallel with the development of new HCS assays, general improvements of in vitro testing are required for new PDT drug development. While the general trend in lead identification points to the use of 3D cell systems as more appropriate tissue models, this is especially important in the context of PDT. In vivo tests have a high failure rate of "leads" identified with standard 2D cell culture monolayer in vitro screens, which fail to mimic the native tumor environment (Baker and Chen, 2012). Additionally, many aspects of PDT are tissue related. These include damage of the microvasculature via antiangiogenesis and antitumor immune responses. Additionally, PDT relies on the availability of oxygen in the target tissue, and thus tumor oxygenation and hypoxia impact the overall treatment effect (Castano et al., 2004). While none of this can be accurately modeled in 2D cell systems, the advent of 3D cell systems, for example, tissue explants, cellular spheroids, or self-assembling hydrogels as molecular scaffolds, offers significant improvements (Pampaloni et al., 2007).

Available data indicate that many drugs are significantly less effective in 3D models compared with monolayers, which is an indication of the significant effect that the tumor microenvironment has on the response to treatment. The use of high-content techniques with 3D cell cultures is nontrivial. Imaging of 3D systems has limitations, and the overall efficacy of PDT in 3D models can be difficult to assess. However, first screening models have been reported and applied to a variety of PDT-related projects (Rizvi et al., 2010). Two recent highlights are the specific optimization of PDT drugs for hypoxic tumor environments (Klein et al., 2012) and a microfluid-based breast cancer tissue model based on lab-on-a-chip technology (Yang et al., 2015).

6.5 COMBINATORIAL SYNTHESIS OF PORPHYRIN-BASED PHOTOSENSITIZERS

Finally, a word on the combinatorial synthesis of porphyrins. Combinatorial chemistry is often combined with HCA in drug development as it allows the generation of large libraries of potential leads and their rapid screening in a minimum amount of time. While established synthetic groups, such as ours, can prepare several hundreds of potential porphyrin lead compounds per year (Senge, 2011), this is still insufficient from the viewpoint of the pharmaceutical industry. Additionally, large-scale porphyrin synthesis is cumbersome and often only reaches gram scale at best.

Combinatorial approaches for the synthesis of porphyrin mixtures are easily accomplished; in a strategic sense, it only requires the use of different aldehydes (or pyrroles) in condensation reactions. Many different approaches have been reported and used for the preparation of dynamic combinatorial systems for use in coordination chemistry and investigations on the prebiotic biogenesis of tetrapyrroles (Drain and Singh, 2010; Taniguchi and Lindsey, 2012). Small combinatorial libraries of porphyrins have been used for biological testing, and libraries of up to 1540 members have been reported (Drain et al., 1999). Problematic is the low solubility of porphyrins and the very tedious chromatography required for the identification of leads. Solid-phase syntheses for porphyrin libraries have been reported as well and offer potential especially for the preparation of porphyrin bioconjugate libraries (Elgie et al., 2000).

ACKNOWLEDGMENT

The writing of this chapter and our studies described herein were supported by a grant from Science Foundation Ireland (IvP 13/IA/1894).

REFERENCES

Abraham VC, Taylor DL, Haskins, JR (2004) High content screening applied to large-scale cell biology. *Trends Biotechnol.*, **22**:15–22.

Baker BM, Chen CS (2012) Deconstructing the third dimension—How 3D culture microenvironments alter cellular cues. *J. Cell Sci.*, **125**:3015–3024.

Bickle M (2010) The beautiful cell: High-content screening in drug discovery. *Anal. Bioanal. Chem.*, **398**:219–226.

Bortner CD, Cidlowski JA (2002) Apoptotic volume decrease and the incredible shrinking cell. *Cell Death Differ.*, **9**:1307–1310.

Bravery CA et al. (2013) Potency assay development for cellular therapy products: An ISCT review of the requirements and experiences in the industry. *Cytotherapy*, **15**:9–19.

Castano AP, Demidova TN, Hamblin MR (2004) Mechanisms in photodynamic therapy: Part one-photosensitizers, photochemistry and cellular localization. *Photodiagn. Photodyn. Ther.*, **1**:279–293.

Daly R, Vaz G, Davies AM, Senge MO, Scanlan EM (2012) Synthesis and biological evaluation of a library of glycoporphyrin compounds. *Chem. Eur. J.*, **18**:14671–14679.

Dove A (2003) Screening for content—The evolution of high throughput. *Nat. Biotech.*, **21**:859–864.

Drain CM, Gong X, Ruta V, Soll CE, Chicoineau PF (1999) Combinatorial synthesis and modification of functional porphyrin libraries: Identification of new, amphipathic motifs for biomolecule binding. *J. Comb. Chem.*, **1**:286–290.

Drain CM, Singh S (2010) Combinatorial libraries of porphyrins: Chemistry and applications. In: *Handbook of Porphyrin Science* (Kadish KM, Smith KM, Guilard R, eds.), Vol. 3, pp. 485–537. Singapore: World Scientific.

Elgie KJ, Scobie M, Boyle RW (2000) Application of combinatorial techniques in the synthesis of unsymmetrically substituted 5,15-diphenylporphyrins. *Tetrahedron Lett.*, **41**:2753–2757.

Frisoli JK et al. (1993) Pharmacokinetics of a fluorescent drug using laser-induced fluorescence. *Cancer Res.*, **53**:5954–5961.

Haney SA, LaPan P, Pan J, Zhang J (2006) High-content screening moves to the front of the line. *Drug Discov. Today*, **11**:889–894.

Hefesha H, Loew S, Liu X, May S, Fahr A (2011) Transfer mechanism of temoporfin between liposomal membranes. *J. Control. Release*, **150**:279–286.

Henderson BW, Dougherty TJ (1992) How does photodynamic therapy work. *Photochem. Photobiol.*, **55**:145–157.

Hudson R, Savoie H, Boyle RW (2005) Lipophilic cationic porphyrins as photodynamic sensitisers—Synthesis and structure–activity relationships. *Photodiagn. Photodyn. Ther.*, **2**:193–196.

Johnston PA, Johnston, PA (2002) Cellular platforms for HTS: Three case studies. *Drug Discov. Today*, 7:353–363.

Juzeniene A, Moan J (2007) The history of PDT in Norway: Part one: Identification of basic mechanisms of general PDT. *Photodiagn. Photodyn. Ther.*, **4**:3–11.

Juzeniene A, Peng Q, Moan J (2007) Milestones in the development of photodynamic therapy and fluorescence diagnosis. *Photochem. Photobiol. Sci.*, **6**:1234–1245.

Klein OJ, Bhayana B, Park YJ, Evans CL (2012) In vitro optimization of EtNBS-PDT against hypoxic tumor environments with a tiered, high-content, 3D model optical screening platform. *Mol. Pharm.*, **9**:3171–3182.

Kobayashi H, Ogawa M, Alford R, Choyke PL, Urano Y (2010) New strategies for fluorescent probe design in medical diagnostic imaging. *Chem. Rev.*, **110**:2620–2640.

Liegg NT, Edvardsson A, O'Brien PJ (2010) Translation of novel anti-cancer cytotoxicity biomarkers detected with high content analysis from an in vitro predictive model to an in vivo cell model. *Toxicol. In Vitro*, **24**:2063–2071.

Mosmann T (1983) Rapid colorimetric assay for cellular growth and survival—Application to proliferation and cyto-toxicity assays. *J. Immunol. Methods*, **65**:55–63.

Moylan C, Sweed AMK, Shaker YM, Scanlan EM, Senge MO (2015) Lead structures for applications in photodynamic therapy 7. Efficient synthesis of amphiphilic glycosylated lipid porphyrin derivatives: Refining linker conjugation for potential PDT applications. *Tetrahedron*, **71**:4145–4153.

Nyman ES, Hynninen PH (2004) Research advances in the use of tetrapyrrolic photosensitizers for photodynamic therapy. *J. Photochem. Photobiol. B Biol.*, **73**:1–28.

O'Brien PJ et al. (2006) High concordance of drug-induced human hepatotoxicity with in vitro cytotoxicity measured in a novel cell-based model using high content screening. *Arch. Toxicol.*, **80**:580–604.

Pampaloni F, Reynaud EG, Stelzer EHK (2007) The third dimension bridges the gap between cell culture and live tissue. *Nat. Rev. Mol. Cell Biol.*, **8**:839–845.

Paszko E, Ehrhardt C, Senge MO, Kelleher DP, Reynolds JV (2011) Nanodrug applications in photodynamic therapy. *Photodiagn. Photodyn. Ther.*, **8**:14–29.

Paszko E, Vaz GMF, Ehrhardt C, Senge MO (2013) Transferrin conjugation does not increase the efficiency of liposomal Foscan during *in vitro* photodynamic therapy of oesophageal cancer. *Eur. J. Pharm. Sci.*, **48**:202–210.

Ramirez CN et al. (2011) Validation of a high-content screening assay using whole-well imaging of transformed phenotypes. *Assay Drug Dev. Technol.*, **9**:247–261.

Reisen F, Zhang X, Gabriel D, Selzer P (2013) Benchmarking of multivariate similarity measures for high-content screening fingerprints in phenotypic drug discovery. *J. Biomol. Screen.*, **18**:1284–1297.

Rizvi I et al. (2010) Synergistic enhancement of carboplatin efficacy with photodynamic therapy in a three-dimensional model for micrometastatic ovarian cancer. *Cancer Res.*, **70**:9319–9328.

Rogers L, Senge MO (2014) The translocator protein as a potential molecular target for improved treatment efficacy in photodynamic therapy. *Future Med. Chem.*, **6**:775–792.

Rogers L et al. (2013) Synthesis and biological evaluation of Foscan bile acid conjugates to target esophageal cancer cells. *Bioorg. Med. Chem. Lett.*, **23**:2495–2499.

Rogers L, Sergeeva NN, Paszko E, Vaz GMF, Senge MO (2015) Lead structures for applications in photodynamic therapy. 6. Temoporfin anti-inflammatory conjugates to target the tumor microenvironment for in vitro PDT. *PLoS One*, **10**:e0125372.

Ryan AA et al. (2014) Lead structures for applications in photodynamic therapy. 5. Synthesis and biological evaluation of water soluble phosphorus (V) 5,10,15,20-tetraalkylporphyrins for PDT. *Photodiagn. Photodyn. Ther.*, **11**:510–515.

Senge MO (2011) Stirring the porphyrin alphabet soup—Functionalization reactions for porphyrins. *Chem. Commun.*, **47**:1943–1960.

Senge MO, Brandt JC (2011) Temoporfin (Foscan®, 5,10,15,20-Tetra(*m*-hydroxyphenyl)chlorin—A second generation photosensitizer. *Photochem. Photobiol.*, **87**:1240–1296.

Sergeeva NN, Donnier-Marechala M, Vaz G, Davies AM, Senge MO (2011) Synthesis and evaluation of the europium(III) and zinc(II) complexes as luminescent bioprobes in high content cell-imaging analysis. *J. Inorg. Biochem.*, **105**:1589–1595.

Smellie A, Wilson CJ, Ng SC (2005) Visualization and interpretation of high content screening data. *J. Chem. Inf. Model.*, **46**:201–207.

Swinney DC, Anthony J (2011) How were new medicines discovered? *Nat. Rev. Drug Discov.*, **10**:507–519.

Taniguchi MM, Lindsey JS (2012) Enumeration of isomers of substituted tetrapyrrole macrocycles: From classical problems in biology to modern combinatorial libraries. In: *Handbook of Porphyrin Science* (Kadish KM, Smith KM, Guilard R, eds.), Vol. 23, pp. 1–80. Singapore: World Scientific.

Tolosa L, Gomez-Lechon MJ, Donato MT (2015) High-content technology for studying drug-induced hepatotoxicity in cell models. *Arch. Toxicol.*, **89**:1007–1022.

Vaz GMF, Paszko E, Davies AM, Senge MO (2013) High content screening as high quality assay for biological evaluation of photosensitizers *in vitro. PLoS One*, **8**:e70653.

Wilson BC, Patterson MS (2008) The physics, biophysics and technology of photodynamic therapy. *Phys. Med. Biol.*, **53**:R61–R109.

Yang Y, Yang X, Zou J, Jia C, Hu Y, Du H, Wang H (2015) Evaluation of photodynamic therapy efficiency using an in vitro three-dimensional microfluidic breast cancer tissue model. *Lab. Chip.*, **15**:725–744.

Zanella F, Lorens JB, Link W (2010) High content screening: Seeing is believing. *Trends Biotechnol.*, **28**:237–245.

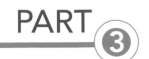

PART

IN VITRO MICROSCOPY OF CELL DAMAGE AND DEATH PROCESSES AFTER PDT

Enhanced efficacy of photodynamic therapy via an iron–lysosome–mitochondria connection
Studies with phthalocyanine 4

ANNA-LIISA NIEMINEN, HSIN-I HUNG, AND JOHN J. LEMASTERS

7.1 LOCALIZATION OF PHOTOSENSITIZERS: MITOCHONDRIA VERSUS LYSOSOMES

Most photosensitizers are highly hydrophobic molecules that preferentially accumulate in one or more cellular membranes. Even the photosensitizers that are water soluble still contain hydrophobic cores that tend to bind membranes. Photosensitizers usually target three main organelles: mitochondria, endoplasmic reticulum, and lysosomes (Oleinick et al., 2002). Photosensitizers that are effective in killing cancer cells tend to localize to mitochondria, suggesting that an effective means to kill cells is to deprive them of a primary energy source. Examples of mitochondria-targeted photosensitizers are porphyrins and porphyrin-related macromolecules that are hydrophilic and accumulate in cellular membranes (Roberts and Berns, 1989). Porphyrins are precursors in the biosynthetic pathway to heme, including the endogenous mitochondrial fluorescent photosensitizer protoporphyrin IX, which accumulates into mitochondria via the 18 kDa translocator protein in the mitochondrial outer membrane (Anholt et al., 1986). An example of a nonporphyrin mitochondria-targeted photosensitizer is phthalocyanine 4 (Pc 4), which binds preferentially to mitochondria, endoplasmic reticulum, and Golgi complex but not to plasma membrane as assessed by confocal microscopy (Trivedi et al., 2000; Lam et al., 2001).

Over the years, we have studied mechanisms underlying cell death induced by photodynamic therapy (PDT) with Pc 4 (Lam et al., 2001; Oleinick et al., 2002; Usuda et al., 2002, 2003a,b; Quiogue et al., 2009;

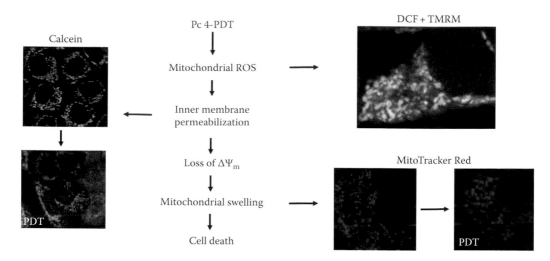

Figure 7.1 Events following photodynamic therapy with Pc 4. Pc 4-PDT induces initial mitochondrial ROS production detected by the conversion of nonfluorescent H$_2$DCF to fluorescent DCF. DCF fluorescence was colocalized with mitochondria-specific probe TMRM (upper right). Mitochondrial ROS further induce mitochondrial inner membrane permeabilization detected by release of mitochondrial calcein to the cytosol (left panels). Inner membrane permeabilization leads to mitochondrial depolarization (not shown) and mitochondrial swelling detected by MitoTracker Red fluorescence (right panels). Ultimately, cells die by apoptosis or necrosis.

Rodriguez et al., 2009; Hung et al., 2013; He et al., 2014). In human epidermoid carcinoma A431 cells, the initial response to Pc 4-PDT is production of mitochondrial reactive oxygen species (ROS) detected by confocal microscopy from conversion of nonfluorescent dichlorofluorescin (H$_2$DCF) to highly fluorescent DCF (Figure 7.1). Light activation of Pc 4 initially produces singlet oxygen ($^1O_2$) with a very short lifetime due to its reaction with a variety of other chemicals. H$_2$DCF itself does not detect $^1O_2$ but rather reacts with hydroperoxides (Taguchi et al., 1996), suggesting that $^1O_2$ formed during Pc 4-PDT initiates lipid peroxidation chain reactions resulting in conversion of DCF to green-fluorescing DCF. The iron chelator, desferal, strongly inhibited mitochondrial DCF conversion, suggesting that $^1O_2$ led to an iron-catalyzed Haber–Weiss reaction to form hydroxyl radical and subsequently lipid hydroperoxides.

Mitochondrial ROS formed during Pc 4-PDT further induced mitochondrial inner membrane permeabilization, as assessed with the fluorescent probe calcein. In untreated cells after ester loading of the fluorophore calcein in the presence of CoCl$_2$ to quench its cytosolic fluorescence, confocal microscopy revealed punctate calcein fluorescence localized to mitochondria (Figure 7.1; Lam et al., 2001). This finding indicated that mitochondria were retaining the ~600 Da calcein and hence were impermeable to low-molecular-weight solutes. After Pc 4-PDT, calcein fluorescence became diffuse, signifying release of calcein from mitochondria into the cytosol and onset of mitochondrial inner membrane permeabilization (Lam et al., 2001). Desferal almost completely blocked calcein release from mitochondria after Pc 4-PDT, which again suggested involvement of iron in the process of the mitochondrial inner membrane permeabilization. Inner membrane permeabilization was also accompanied by collapse of the mitochondrial membrane potential, as assessed by membrane potential–indicating probes like rhodamine 123 (Rh123) and tetramethylrhodamine methylester (TMRM). Inner membrane permeabilization was followed by mitochondrial swelling assessed by MitoTracker Red and ultimately cell death (Figure 7.1; Lam et al., 2001). Thus, early mitochondrial ROS formation plays a critical role in Pc 4-PDT-induced cell death.

Although direct targeting of photosensitizers to mitochondria produces an effective PDT response, one can argue that engaging other organelles in the killing pathway would produce even stronger PDT killing. This hypothesis has been tested in several experimental settings. In initial studies, Kessel's group showed that PDT sensitized by N-aspartyl chlorin e6, a photosensitizer that accumulates in lysosomes, also initiates the mitochondrial pathway of apoptosis through release of cytochrome c from mitochondria and subsequent activation of procaspases-9/3 (Kessel et al., 2002; Kessel and Reiners, 2014). The BH3-only protein Bid was cleaved at the time of cytochrome c release, presumably by proteases released from lysosomes. Thus, truncated Bid, an activated form of Bid, likely triggered the mitochondrial pathway of apoptosis. Interestingly, the kinetics of apoptotic death was slower than with photosensitizers directly targeted to mitochondria. Oleinick's group observed similar events with the Pc 4 analogs that preferentially bind to lysosomes as assessed by confocal microscopy (Rodriguez et al., 2009). The mechanism of one of these analogs, Pc 181, was studied in more detail. Compared with Pc 4, Pc 181 was taken up by cells more efficiently and produced greater photodynamic cell killing, as judged by a colony-formation assay (Rodriguez et al., 2009). Pc 181-PDT-induced lysosomal membrane damage triggered the mitochondrial cell death pathway mediated by cleavage and activation of Bid as a consequence of the release of proteases from lysosomes. Kessel's group has further extended the studies to examine whether sequential low dose of lysosomal and mitochondrial PDT enhances the overall PDT response (Kessel and Reiners, 2015). Indeed, synergistic killing resulted when the lysosomal-targeting photosensitizers 5-ethylamino-9-diethylaminobenzo [a]phenothiazinium chloride and galactose conjugate of 3-(1-hexyloxyethyl)-3-devinyl pyropeophorbide-α were each sequentially combined with a mitochondria-targeting benzoporphyrine derivative photosensitizer (Kessel and Reiners, 2015). Cell death ultimately involved lysosome-mediated loss of mitochondrial membrane potential, suggesting that lysosome-derived constituents were contributing to mitochondrial damage. Although the nature of these constituents was not determined, the observation that E-64d, an inhibitor of cysteine proteases, provided partial cytoprotection suggested at least partial involvement of such proteases in cell killing.

7.2 CONTRIBUTION OF IRON TO PDT

As discussed earlier, a number of studies indicate that photosensitizers localizing to lysosomes are effective in releasing lysosomal constituents that trigger mitochondrial damage after PDT. Lysosomes contain numerous hydrolytic enzymes, and some of these enzymes have been proposed to be involved in subsequent mitochondrial damage (Chiu et al., 2010; Kessel and Reiners, 2014, 2015). Lysosomes are also a source of chelatable iron that is redox-active and can participate in iron-mediated lipid peroxidation (Uchiyama et al., 2008).

7.2.1 CELLULAR IRON UPTAKE AND HOMEOSTASIS

Iron is an essential nutrient needed for oxygen-binding and redox-active prosthetic groups, such as heme and iron–sulfur clusters. Thus, a major manifestation of iron deficiency is microcytic anemia due to inadequate heme synthesis for hemoglobin in erythrocytes. After iron absorption by the gut, transferrin in the plasma distributes iron throughout the body (Levy et al., 1999). Transferrin has two binding sites for ferric iron (Fe^{3+}) and maintains the bound iron in a redox-inactive state. Transferrin is a very abundant protein whose concentration in serum is 30–40 μM. With iron occupancy of 30%–40% and two binding sites per transferrin molecule, the total serum transferrin–bound iron is 20–30 μM. Transferrin circulates until it encounters transferrin receptor 1 on the surface of plasma membranes (Aisen, 2004). Transferrin is then internalized by receptor-mediated endocytosis (de Figueiredo et al., 2001). As endosomes acidify due to the action of the proton-pumping vacuolar ATPase (V-ATPase) to a pH of ~6, transferrin releases its Fe^{3+} (Lee and Goodfellow, 1998). Transferrin and its receptor are then recycled to the cell surface. Subsequently, endosomes fuse with lysosomes that are even more acidic (pH ~4.5; Baravalle et al., 2005). Autophagy also recycles iron into the lysosomal compartment. Thus, lysosomes constitute the major cellular reservoir of mobilizable iron. In its ferric form, iron remains trapped inside lysosomes. However, cytosolic nicotinamide adenine dinucleotide phosphate (NADPH) reduces Fe^{3+} to Fe^{2+} by a ferrireductase in the lysosomal membrane called six-transmembrane epithelial antigen of prostate 3 (Lambe et al., 2009). Controlled release of Fe^{2+} into the cytosol then occurs through divalent metal transporter-1 also located in the lysosomal membrane (Tabuchi et al., 2000).

7.2.2 CHELATABLE AND NONCHELATABLE IRON

Intracellular iron exists in two pools. "Nonchelatable" iron is inaccessible to iron chelators like desferal and resides in ferritin, hemosiderin, and iron-containing prosthetic groups of proteins (e.g., heme, iron–sulfur complexes). In contrast, "chelatable" iron comprises free iron and iron loosely bound to anionic metabolites like ATP and citrate. Chelatable iron is accessible to desferal and other iron chelators. In hepatocytes, chelatable iron concentration is 5–15 µM (Petrat et al., 2001; Rauen et al., 2007). Chelatable iron can travel freely throughout the cell, whereas nonchelatable iron cannot. Chelatable iron also can promote oxidative stress by catalyzing the Fenton reaction, which produces highly reactive hydroxyl radical (OH$^{\bullet}$) from H_2O_2 and $O_2^{\bullet-}$ to damage DNA, proteins, and membranes (Kehrer, 2000).

7.2.3 LYSOSOMAL IRON ENHANCES PDT

Lysosomes are a source of rapidly mobilized chelatable iron that when released is taken up by mitochondria. After PDT using the mitochondria-targeted photosensitizer Pc 4, mitochondria are the major source of ROS formation leading to onset of the mitochondrial permeability transition (MPT), as assessed by increased mitochondrial DCF fluorescence and movement of calcein across the mitochondrial inner membrane (Lam et al., 2001). Increased mitochondrial iron can catalyze toxic ROS cascades. Therefore, we hypothesized that iron translocation from lysosomes to mitochondria enhances PDT-induced killing using mitochondria-targeted photosensitizers. Iron can be released from mitochondria pharmacologically using bafilomycin, which is a specific inhibitor of the V-ATPase (Uchiyama et al., 2008). Bafilomycin collapses acidic lysosomal and endosomal pH gradients, which results in release of lysosomal iron into the cytosol (Uchiyama et al., 2008). Bafilomycin greatly accelerated mitochondria-specific Pc 4-PDT-mediated cell killing, and this toxicity was mediated through mitochondrial depolarization and inner membrane permeabilization (Quiogue et al., 2009; Saggu et al., 2012; Hung et al., 2013). Similar results were obtained with chloroquine, which is another agent that causes lysosomal alkalinization (Saggu et al., 2012). Chloroquine is a weak base that increases pH of acidic lysosomal/endosomal vesicles (Poole and Ohkuma, 1981). Confocal microscopy showed that lysosomal membranes did not rupture after bafilomycin and Pc 4-PDT, as assessed by retention of 10 kDa Alexa 488 dextran in lysosomes (Figure 7.2; Saggu et al., 2012). Since Alexa 488 dextran fluorescence is pH-independent, loss of Alexa 488 dextran fluorescence would have indicated specific lysosomal disintegration rather than a change in lysosomal pH. By contrast, LysoTracker Red is a weak base that accumulates lysosomes in response to acidic pH (Griffiths et al., 1988). After bafilomycin, LysoTracker Red is released from lysosomes, as expected, confirming that bafilomycin was penetrating the cells (Figure 7.2; Saggu et al., 2012).

Ferrous iron (Fe^{2+}) reacts with H_2O_2 to form OH·, a highly reactive form of ROS (Halliwell, 2009). Desferal, an iron chelator, protected against PDT plus bafilomycin-induced mitochondrial depolarization and cell killing (Saggu et al., 2012). Desferal is poorly permeant across membranes, and therefore millimolar concentrations were required to protect. Some reports suggest that desferal may also be taken up by endocytosis, resulting in its accumulation in endosomes/lysosomes (Cable and Lloyd, 1999; Persson et al., 2003). Therefore, cytoprotection with desferal may partly be explained by chelation of redox-active iron inside lysosomes. To assess whether chelation of lysosomal iron is critical for bafilomycin plus Pc 4-PDT-induced toxicity, the effect of desferal conjugated to 10 kDa hydroxyethyl starch (starch-desferal, 1 mM desferal equivalency) was evaluated. Approximately 10 kDa starch-desferal only enters cells by endocytosis, resulting in lysosomal accumulation. Identically to desferal, starch-desferal also protected against bafilomycin plus Pc 4-PDT-induced mitochondrial depolarization and cell killing (Saggu et al., 2012). These results are consistent with the conclusion that lysosomes/endosomes release redox-active iron after bafilomycin and that desferal and starch-desferal prevent this release by chelating intraluminal iron of these organelles. The results also establish a link between lysosomal alkalinization and mitochondrial depolarization during PDT.

7.2.4 MITOCHONDRIAL IRON UPTAKE

Under physiological conditions, chelatable iron is mostly stored in lysosomes and therefore chelatable iron concentration in the cytosol is low. When lysosomal iron is released due to bafilomycin exposure or a pathological condition disrupting lysosomal pH or membrane integrity, then cytosolic iron concentration can increase to 200–300 µM (Uchiyama et al., 2008; Kurz et al., 2011). The question then is where does this iron go? Studies from nearly 40 years ago show that the classical mitochondrial calcium uniporter (MCU)

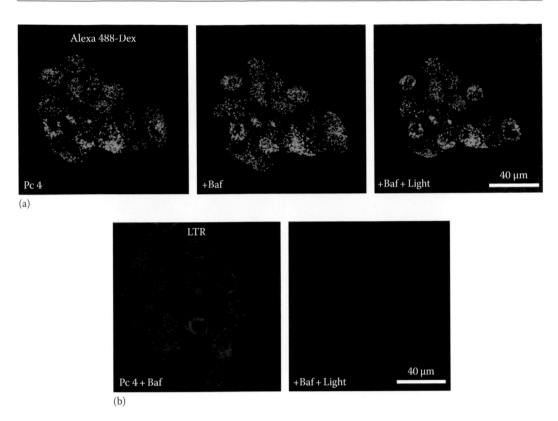

Figure 7.2 Bafilomycin collapses the lysosomal pH gradient but does not induce lysosomal membrane permeabilization. In (a), human epidermoid carcinoma A431 cells were loaded with 10 kDa Alexa 488-dextran (Alexa 488-Dex) and incubated with 25 nM Pc 4. Alexa 488-Dex is taken up by cells via endocytosis. Confocal images show retention of green Alexa 488-Dex fluorescence after treatment with 50 nM bafilomycin (+Baf) and even after Pc 4-PDT (+Baf + Light). In (b), cells were loaded with 500 nM LysoTracker Red (LTR), which accumulates into acidic compartments, and then incubated with Pc 4. Baf collapsed the lysosomal pH gradient as shown by virtually complete release of LTR from lysosomes (panel b). (Modified from Saggu, S. et al., *Photochem. Photobiol.*, 88, 461, 2012.)

catalyzes uptake of Fe^{2+} but not Fe^{3+} and that this uptake is driven by mitochondrial membrane potential (Flatmark and Romslo, 1975). Recently, the molecular identity of the core protein of the MCU was identified as the 40 kDa CCDC109A gene product called MCU that forms tetrameric or high-order oligomers in the mitochondrial inner membrane (Baughman et al., 2011; De Stefani et al., 2011). MCU has two highly conserved transmembrane domains and an intervening loop enriched in acidic residues that binds Ru360, a significant finding because Ru360 is a highly specific inhibitor that blocks electrogenic mitochondrial Ca^{2+} uptake at nanomolar concentrations and that does not inhibit plasmalemmal Ca^{2+} channels or sarcolemmal Ca^{2+} release pathways (Matlib et al., 1998; Zhou et al., 1998; Sanchez et al., 2001). Point mutation of the MCU (S259 A) prevents inhibitory action of Ru360 on MCU (Baughman et al., 2011). Interestingly, Ru360 protected UMSCC22A human head-and-neck squamous carcinoma cells against bafilomycin-enhanced PDT toxicity (Hung et al., 2013). In fact, Ru360 provided even greater protection than iron chelators desferal and starch-desferal (Hung et al., 2013). Desferal and starch-desferal-sensitive mitochondrial iron uptake through MCU also occurs in other pathological situations and contributes to cytotoxicity (Flatmark and Romslo, 1975; Uchiyama et al., 2008; Kon et al., 2010). These results indicate that Ru360 protection against bafilomycin toxicity during PDT is likely due to prevention of Fe^{2+} uptake into mitochondria through MCU.

Besides MCU, another mitochondrial protein, mitoferrin (Mfrn), mediates iron transport across the mitochondrial inner membrane (Shaw et al., 2006; Satre et al., 2007; Froschauer et al., 2009). Mfrn has two isoforms; Mfrn1 (SLC25A37) expressed primarily in erythroid cells and Mfrn2 (SLC25A28) expressed in nonerythroid tissues (Paradkar et al., 2009; Amigo et al., 2011; Troadec et al., 2011; Ren et al., 2012). No sequence homology is observed between MCU and Mfrn (De Stefani et al., 2011; Baughman et al., 2011). In what relative extent MCU and Mfrn contribute to mitochondrial iron uptake is still poorly understood.

Head-and-neck squamous carcinoma cell lines express very little Mfrn1 as expected for nonerythroid cells. Instead, the cell lines express predominantly Mfrn2. Cell lines expressing more Mfrn2 mRNA and protein were more sensitive to bafilomycin-enhanced PDT toxicity than lines expressing less Mfrn2 (Hung et al., 2013). In permeabilized cells, mitochondria of the sensitive cells also took up more Fe^{2+} compared with resistant cells.

To establish a link between Mfrn2 and mitochondrial membrane potential, Mfrn2 was silenced in high Mfrn2-expressing UMSCC22A head-and-neck cancer cells. Decreased expression of Mfrn2 decreased rates of mitochondrial Fe^{2+} uptake in permeabilized cells. Further, Mfrn2 silencing delayed mitochondrial depolarization and cell death after bafilomycin plus PDT (Figure 7.3; Hung et al., 2013).

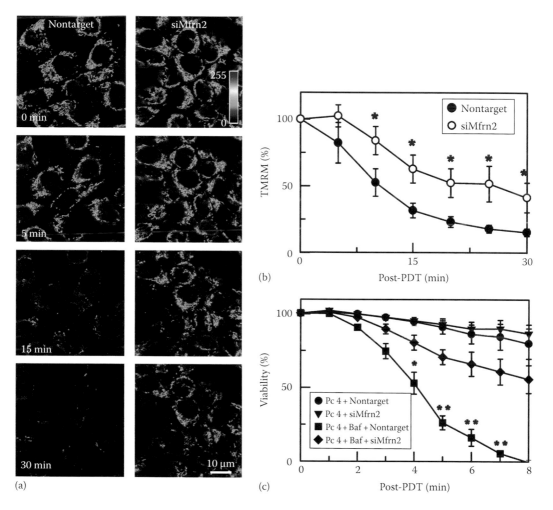

Figure 7.3 Mfrn2 knockdown confers resistance to mitochondrial depolarization and cell killing after PDT. UMSCC22A cells were transfected with siRNA against Mfrn2 and nontarget siRNA for 6 days followed by Pc 4-PDT in the presence of bafilomycin. In (a), mitochondrial membrane potential was monitored with TMRM by confocal microscopy. Image intensity was pseudocolored according to the reference bar. In (b), TMRM fluorescence after background subtraction was plotted as percentage of TMRM fluorescence at 0 min. *$p < 0.05$ compared to nontarget siRNA. In (c), cell viability under the same conditions as (a) was determined by propidium iodide fluorometry. *$p < 0.05$ compared to nontarget siRNA. (From Hung, H.I. et al., *J. Biol. Chem.*, 288, 677. Copyright 2013, American Society for Biochemistry and Molecular Biology.)

Our data support the conclusion that lysosomal iron release and mitochondrial iron uptake act synergistically to induce PDT-mediated and iron-dependent mitochondrial dysfunction and subsequent cell killing. Pc 4 localized to mitochondria is activated by light to produce intramitochondrial ROS. Iron released from lysosomes by bafilomycin is taken up by mitochondria in an Mfrn2-dependent fashion, where it participates in iron-mediated Fenton reaction and further enhances ROS-mediated cell death. Lysosomal iron chelation protects against mitochondrial depolarization and cell death. Knockdown of Mfrn2 by decreasing mitochondrial iron uptake also delays mitochondrial depolarization and cell death after PDT. Mfrn2-dependent mitochondrial iron uptake may also involve MCU since Ru360, a specific inhibitor of MCU, blocks Mfrn2-dependent iron uptake and protects against PDT toxicity (Hung et al., 2013). However, Mfrn2 does not have any known binding site for Ru360, suggesting that Ru360 does not directly inhibit Mfrn2. Thus, it is possible that Mfrn2 is a regulator of MCU and part of a larger MCU-containing Ca^{2+} and Fe^{2+}-transporting complex. In this way, silencing of Mfrn2 and inhibition of MCU with Ru360 both inhibit mitochondrial Fe^{2+} uptake (Figure 7.4). Further studies are needed to resolve this issue.

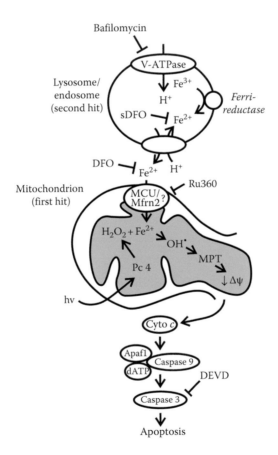

Figure 7.4 Mfrn2 contributes to PDT-induced cell death. Pc 4-PDT induces mitochondrial ROS production, resulting in apoptotic cell death. The photosensitizer Pc 4 localizes to mitochondria and is activated by light (hv) to produce formation of intramitochondrial ROS, including H_2O_2. Iron released from lysosomes by bafilomycin is taken up by mitochondria in Mfrn2-dependent fashion. Iron inside mitochondria participates in Fenton chemistry to further enhance the ROS-mediated MPT, mitochondrial depolarization, cytochrome *c* release, and apoptotic cell death. Cytotoxicity is decreased by the iron chelators desferal and starch-desferal and by Ru360 that prevents mitochondrial iron uptake. Knockdown of Mfrn2 delays mitochondrial depolarization and cell death induced by bafilomycin during PDT. (From Hung, H.I. et al., *J. Biol. Chem.*, 288, 677, Copyright 2013, American Society for Biochemistry and Molecular Biology.)

7.3 DELIVERY OF PHOTOSENSITIZER TO LYSOSOMES VIA A NANOPARTICLE CARRIER

Efficacy of PDT is dependent on drug concentration, light exposure, and oxygenation of the tissue. For maximal treatment efficacy, optimization of photosensitizer concentration and selective targeting of the photosensitizer to diseased tissue (e.g., tumor cells) are important goals. One targeting strategy is to use nanoformulations, whereby the photosensitizer is packaged within biocompatible nanoparticle constructs that are selectively taken up by tumor cells. To enhance tumor-specific accumulation of the drug, nanoparticles can be designed to contain ligands for tumor-specific internalizing surface receptors. Photosensitizer-loaded nanoparticles surface-modified by receptor-specific ligands or antibodies bind to such receptors to undergo cellular internalization via receptor-mediated endocytosis. Subsequently, nanoparticles undergo degradation or destabilization inside endosomes/lysosomes, leading to the intracellular release of the photosensitizer cargo. The released photosensitizer then binds to its own target organelles to produce a selective therapeutic effect.

Numerous nanoformulations of the photosensitizers have been described. Chemistry and synthesis of many of those formulations are described in more detail elsewhere in this volume. For example, Pc 4 has been encapsulated in nanoparticles by a number of investigators (Cheng et al., 2002; Master et al. 2012a,b; He et al., 2014). Gupta group formulated Pc 4 in biocompatible poly(ethylene glycol)-poly(ε-caprolactone) co-polymer micelles. The micelles were further surface-modified with epidermal growth factor receptor (EGFR)–targeting GE11 peptides for targeting to EGFR-overexpressing cancer cells (Master et al. 2012a,b). Basilion's group used a similar strategy but formulated Pc 4 in epidermal growth factor peptide-targeted gold nanoparticles (Cheng et al., 2011). In most cases, the nanoparticles enhanced Pc 4 uptake into cultured cells and Pc 4 accumulation in tumors (Cheng et al., 2011; Master et al. 2012a,b; He et al., 2014). Expansile nanoparticles, which enlarge their size in response to acidic pH, have been utilized as drug carriers for controlled drug release at targeted sites for enhanced therapeutic effect (Griset et al., 2009; Liu et al., 2011, 2013; Zubris et al., 2013). Sigma-2 receptor is overexpressed in many types of cancers, including skin, lung, and breast tumors, and has been explored as a target for tumor-specific drug delivery (Mach et al., 1997; Kashiwagi et al., 2007; Chono et al., 2008; Yang et al., 2012). Human tissue array analysis revealed increased expression of sigma-2 receptor also in head-and-neck tumors compared to normal counterparts, making sigma-2 a valid target for these tumors also (He et al., 2014). Head-and-neck tumors are also well suited for PDT treatment because of the relative easy access of the laser beam to the tumor. Accordingly, Pc 4 was conjugated into expansile nanoparticles that contained sigma-2 receptor–targeted ligand. Pc 4–conjugated nanoparticles were taken up by cells via endocytosis. After incubation of cells with Pc 4–conjugated nanoparticles, confocal microscopy revealed that Pc fluorescence appeared in endosomes/lysosomes as assessed by colocalization with LysoTracker Green fluorescence (Figure 7.5; He et al., 2014). After longer incubation, Pc 4 fluorescence appeared more in mitochondria, as assessed by colocalization of Pc 4 fluorescence with the mitochondrial membrane potential–indicating probe TMRM. The results indicated that Pc 4 escaped from lysosomes and transferred to mitochondria (Figure 7.5; He et al., 2014). Incorporating sigma-2 targeting ligand to Pc 4-conjugated nanoparticles greatly enhanced cellular uptake and PDT toxicity in head-and-neck cancer cells (He et al., 2014). Indeed, translocation of Pc 4 from lysosomes to mitochondria prior to light exposure may provide additional toxicity since engaging mitochondria in the killing pathway generally enhances toxicity.

7.4 CONCLUSIONS

PDT is an effective way to kill cells. However, the mechanisms of cell killing vary depending on the site of initial damage within cells. Mitochondria are generally regarded as the most important site for photosensitizers to produce effective PDT responses. Specifically, light of appropriate wavelength activates photosensitizers localized in mitochondria to produce intramitochondrial ROS. However, engaging lysosomes in cell death pathways can enhance mitochondria-mediated cell killing. Collapse of lysosomal pH gradients

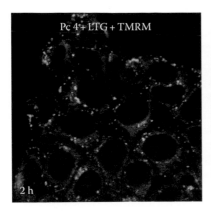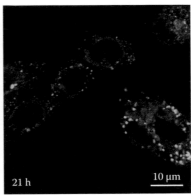

Figure 7.5 Subcellular localization of Pc 4–loaded nanoparticles in lysosomes and mitochondria. UMSCC22A cells were incubated with Pc 4–loaded nanoparticles (far red fluorescing shown in blue) for 2 and 21 h followed by co-loading with LysoTracker Green (LTG, green) and TMRM (red) to label lysosomes and mitochondria, respectively. Subsequently, images were collected by confocal microscopy. At 2 h after addition of the nanoparticles, small round green/light cyan spheres were observed in the cytoplasm representing colocalization of lysosome-specific LTR with Pc 4. At 21 h after nanoparticle addition, Pc 4 began to colocalize with mitochondria as shown by magenta representing colocalization of blue Pc 4 and red TMRM. (Modified from He, H. et al., *Biomaterials*, 35, 9546, 2014.)

without lysosomal membrane breakdown induces lysosomal iron release. Iron released from lysosomes is then taken up by mitochondria in an Mfrn2- and MCU-dependent fashion, where it catalyzes the Fenton reaction and further enhances ROS-mediated mitochondrial inner membrane permeabilization, mitochondrial depolarization, cytochrome c release, and both apoptotic and necrotic cell death. Therefore, agents that mobilize lysosomal iron could potentially be used clinically as adjuvants with mitochondria-targeted photosensitizers.

REFERENCES

Aisen P (2004) Transferrin receptor 1. *Int J Biochem Cell Biol* **36**:2137–2143.

Amigo JD, Yu M, Troadec MB, Gwynn B, Cooney JD, Lambert AJ, Chi NC et al. (2011) Identification of distal cis-regulatory elements at mouse mitoferrin loci using zebrafish transgenesis. *Mol Cell Biol* **31**:1344–1356.

Anholt RR, Pedersen PL, De Souza EB, Snyder SH (1986) The peripheral-type benzodiazepine receptor. Localization to the mitochondrial outer membrane. *J Biol Chem* **261**:576–583.

Baravalle G, Schober D, Huber M, Bayer N, Murphy RF, Fuchs R (2005) Transferrin recycling and dextran transport to lysosomes is differentially affected by bafilomycin, nocodazole, and low temperature. *Cell Tissue Res* **320**:99–113.

Baughman JM, Perocchi F, Girgis HS, Plovanich M, Belcher-Timme CA, Sancak Y, Bao XR et al. (2011) Integrative genomics identifies MCU as an essential component of the mitochondrial calcium uniporter. *Nature* **476**:341–345.

Cable H, Lloyd JB (1999) Cellular uptake and release of two contrasting iron chelators. *J Pharm Pharmacol* **51**:131–134.

Cheng G, Wessels A, Gourdie RG, Thompson RP (2002) Spatiotemporal and tissue specific distribution of apoptosis in the developing chick heart. *Dev Dyn* **223**:119–133.

Cheng Y, Meyers JD, Broome AM, Kenney ME, Basilion JP, Burda C (2011) Deep penetration of a PDT drug into tumors by noncovalent drug-gold nanoparticle conjugates. *J Am Chem Soc* **133**:2583–2591.

Chiu SM, Xue LY, Lam M, Rodriguez ME, Zhang P, Kenney ME, Nieminen AL, Oleinick NL (2010) A requirement for bid for induction of apoptosis by photodynamic therapy with a lysosome- but not a mitochondrion-targeted photosensitizer. *Photochem Photobiol* **86**:1161–1173.

Chono S, Li SD, Conwell CC, Huang L (2008) An efficient and low immunostimulatory nanoparticle formulation for systemic siRNA delivery to the tumor. *J Control Release* **131**:64–69.

de Figueiredo P, Doody A, Polizotto RS, Drecktrah D, Wood S, Banta M, Strang MS, Brown WJ (2001) Inhibition of transferrin recycling and endosome tubulation by phospholipase A2 antagonists. *J Biol Chem* **276**:47361–47370.

De Stefani D, Raffaello A, Teardo E, Szabo I, Rizzuto R (2011) A forty-kilodalton protein of the inner membrane is the mitochondrial calcium uniporter. *Nature* **476**:336–340.

Flatmark T, Romslo I (1975) Energy-dependent accumulation of iron by isolated rat liver mitochondria. Requirement of reducing equivalents and evidence for a unidirectional flux of Fe(II) across the inner membrane. *J Biol Chem* **250**:6433–6438.

Froschauer EM, Schweyen RJ, Wiesenberger G (2009) The yeast mitochondrial carrier proteins Mrs3p/Mrs4p mediate iron transport across the inner mitochondrial membrane. *Biochim Biophys Acta* **1788**:1044–1050.

Griffiths G, Hoflack B, Simons K, Mellman I, Kornfeld S (1988) The mannose 6-phosphate receptor and the biogenesis of lysosomes. *Cell* **52**:329–341.

Griset AP, Walpole J, Liu R, Gaffey A, Colson YL, Grinstaff MW (2009) Expansile nanoparticles: Synthesis, characterization, and in vivo efficacy of an acid-responsive polymeric drug delivery system. *J Am Chem Soc* **131**:2469–2471.

Halliwell B (2009) The wanderings of a free radical. *Free Radic Biol Med* **46**:531–542.

He H, Cattran AW, Nguyen T, Nieminen AL, Xu P (2014) Triple-responsive expansile nanogel for tumor and mitochondria targeted photosensitizer delivery. *Biomaterials* **35**:9546–9553.

Hung HI, Schwartz JM, Maldonado EN, Lemasters JJ, Nieminen AL (2013) Mitoferrin-2-dependent mitochondrial iron uptake sensitizes human head and neck squamous carcinoma cells to photodynamic therapy. *J Biol Chem* **288**:677–686.

Kashiwagi H, McDunn JE, Simon PO, Jr., Goedegebuure PS, Xu J, Jones L, Chang K et al. (2007) Selective sigma-2 ligands preferentially bind to pancreatic adenocarcinomas: Applications in diagnostic imaging and therapy. *Mol Cancer* **6**:48.

Kehrer JP (2000) The Haber-Weiss reaction and mechanisms of toxicity. *Toxicology* **149**:43–50.

Kessel D, Castelli M, Reiners JJ, Jr. (2002) Apoptotic response to photodynamic therapy versus the Bcl-2 antagonist HA14-1. *Photochem Photobiol* **76**:314–319.

Kessel D, Reiners JJ, Jr. (2014) Enhanced efficacy of photodynamic therapy via a sequential targeting protocol. *Photochem Photobiol* **90**:889–895.

Kessel D, Reiners JJ, Jr. (2015) Promotion of proapoptotic signals by lysosomal photodamage. *Photochem Photobiol* **91**:931–936.

Kon K, Kim JS, Uchiyama A, Jaeschke H, Lemasters JJ (2010) Lysosomal iron mobilization and induction of the mitochondrial permeability transition in acetaminophen-induced toxicity to mouse hepatocytes. *Toxicol Sci* **117**:101–108.

Kurz T, Gustafsson B, Brunk UT (2011) Cell sensitivity to oxidative stress is influenced by ferritin autophagy. *Free Radic Biol Med* **50**:1647–1658.

Lam M, Oleinick NL, Nieminen AL (2001) Photodynamic therapy-induced apoptosis in epidermoid carcinoma cells. Reactive oxygen species and mitochondrial inner membrane permeabilization. *J Biol Chem* **276**:47379–47386.

Lambe T, Simpson RJ, Dawson S, Bouriez-Jones T, Crockford TL, Lepherd M, Latunde-Dada GO et al. (2009) Identification of a Steap3 endosomal targeting motif essential for normal iron metabolism. *Blood* **113**:1805–1808.

Lee DA, Goodfellow JM (1998) The pH-induced release of iron from transferrin investigated with a continuum electrostatic model. *Biophys J* **74**:2747–2759.

Levy JE, Jin O, Fujiwara Y, Kuo F, Andrews NC (1999) Transferrin receptor is necessary for development of erythrocytes and the nervous system. *Nat Genet* **21**:396–399.

Liu R, Gilmore DM, Zubris KA, Xu X, Catalano PJ, Padera RF, Grinstaff MW, Colson YL (2013) Prevention of nodal metastases in breast cancer following the lymphatic migration of paclitaxel-loaded expansile nanoparticles. *Biomaterials* **34**:1810–1819.

Liu R, Khullar OV, Griset AP, Wade JE, Zubris KA, Grinstaff MW, Colson YL (2011) Paclitaxel-loaded expansile nanoparticles delay local recurrence in a heterotopic murine non-small cell lung cancer model. *Ann Thorac Surg* **91**:1077–1083.

Mach RH, Smith CR, al-Nabulsi I, Whirrett BR, Childers SR, Wheeler KT (1997) Sigma 2 receptors as potential biomarkers of proliferation in breast cancer. *Cancer Res* **57**:156–161.

Master AM, Livingston M, Oleinick NL, Gupta AS (2012a) Optimization of a nanomedicine-based silicon phthalocyanine 4 photodynamic therapy (Pc 4-PDT) strategy for targeted treatment of EGFR-overexpressing cancers. *Mol Pharm* **9**:2331–2338.

Master AM, Qi Y, Oleinick NL, Gupta AS (2012b) EGFR-mediated intracellular delivery of Pc 4 nanoformulation for targeted photodynamic therapy of cancer: In vitro studies. *Nanomedicine* **8**:655–664.

Matlib MA, Zhou Z, Knight S, Ahmed S, Choi KM, Krause-Bauer J, Phillips R, Altschuld R, Katsube Y, Sperelakis N, Bers DM (1998) Oxygen-bridged dinuclear ruthenium amine complex specifically inhibits Ca^{2+} uptake into mitochondria in vitro and in situ in single cardiac myocytes. *J Biol Chem* **273**:10223–10231.

Oleinick NL, Morris RL, Belichenko I (2002) The role of apoptosis in response to photodynamic therapy: What, where, why, and how. *Photochem Photobiol Sci* **1**:1–21.

Paradkar PN, Zumbrennen KB, Paw BH, Ward DM, Kaplan J (2009) Regulation of mitochondrial iron import through differential turnover of mitoferrin 1 and mitoferrin 2. *Mol Cell Biol* **29**:1007–1016.

Persson HL, Yu Z, Tirosh O, Eaton JW, Brunk UT (2003) Prevention of oxidant-induced cell death by lysosomotropic iron chelators. *Free Radic Biol Med* **34**:1295–1305.

Petrat F, de Groot H, Rauen U (2001) Subcellular distribution of chelatable iron: A laser scanning microscopic study in isolated hepatocytes and liver endothelial cells. *Biochem J* **356**:61–69.

Poole B, Ohkuma S (1981) Effect of weak bases on the intralysosomal pH in mouse peritoneal macrophages. *J Cell Biol* **90**:665–669.

Quiogue G, Saggu S, Hung HI, Kenney ME, Oleinick NL, Lemasters JJ, Nieminen AL (2009) Signaling from lysosomes enhances mitochondria-mediated photodynamic therapy in cancer cells. *Proc Soc Photo Opt Instrum Eng* **7380**:1–8.

Rauen U, Springer A, Weisheit D, Petrat F, Korth HG, De GH, Sustmann R (2007) Assessment of chelatable mitochondrial iron by using mitochondrion-selective fluorescent iron indicators with different iron-binding affinities. *Chembiochem* **8**:341–352.

Ren Y, Yang S, Tan G, Ye W, Liu D, Qian X, Ding Z et al. (2012) Reduction of mitoferrin results in abnormal development and extended lifespan in *Caenorhabditis elegans*. *PLoS One* **7**:e29666.

Roberts WG, Berns MW (1989) In vitro photosensitization I. Cellular uptake and subcellular localization of mono-L-aspartyl chlorin e6, chloro-aluminum sulfonated phthalocyanine, and photofrin II. *Lasers Surg Med* **9**:90–101.

Rodriguez ME, Zhang P, Azizuddin K, Delos Santos GB, Chiu SM, Xue LY, Berlin JC et al. (2009) Structural factors and mechanisms underlying the improved photodynamic cell killing with silicon phthalocyanine photosensitizers directed to lysosomes versus mitochondria. *Photochem Photobiol* **85**:1189–1200.

Saggu S, Hung HI, Quiogue G, Lemasters JJ, Nieminen AL (2012) Lysosomal signaling enhances mitochondria-mediated photodynamic therapy in a431 cancer cells: Role of iron. *Photochem Photobiol* **88**:461–468.

Sanchez JA, Garcia MC, Sharma VK, Young KC, Matlib MA, Sheu SS (2001) Mitochondria regulate inactivation of L-type Ca2+ channels in rat heart. *J Physiol* **536**:387–396.

Satre M, Mattei S, Aubry L, Gaudet P, Pelosi L, Brandolin G, Klein G (2007) Mitochondrial carrier family: Repertoire and peculiarities of the cellular slime mould *Dictyostelium discoideum*. *Biochimie* **89**:1058–1069.

Shaw GC, Cope JJ, Li L, Corson K, Hersey C, Ackermann GE, Gwynn B et al. (2006) Mitoferrin is essential for erythroid iron assimilation. *Nature* **440**:96–100.

Tabuchi M, Yoshimori T, Yamaguchi K, Yoshida T, Kishi F (2000) Human NRAMP2/DMT1, which mediates iron transport across endosomal membranes, is localized to late endosomes and lysosomes in HEp-2 cells. *J Biol Chem* **275**:22220–22228.

Taguchi H, Ogura Y, Takanashi T, Hashizoe M, Honda Y (1996) In vivo quantitation of peroxides in the vitreous humor by fluorophotometry. *Invest Ophthalmol Vis Sci* **37**:1444–1450.

Trivedi NS, Wang HW, Nieminen AL, Oleinick NL, Izatt JA (2000) Quantitative analysis of Pc 4 localization in mouse lymphoma (LY-R) cells via double-label confocal fluorescence microscopy. *Photochem Photobiol* **71**:634–639.

Troadec MB, Warner D, Wallace J, Thomas K, Spangrude GJ, Phillips J, Khalimonchuk O, Paw BH, Ward DM, Kaplan J (2011) Targeted deletion of the mouse Mitoferrin1 gene: From anemia to protoporphyria. *Blood* **117**:5494–5502.

Uchiyama A, Kim JS, Kon K, Jaeschke H, Ikejima K, Watanabe S, Lemasters JJ (2008) Translocation of iron from lysosomes into mitochondria is a key event during oxidative stress-induced hepatocellular injury. *Hepatology* **48**:1644–1654.

Usuda J, Azizuddin K, Chiu SM, Oleinick NL (2003a) Association between the photodynamic loss of Bcl-2 and the sensitivity to apoptosis caused by phthalocyanine photodynamic therapy. *Photochem Photobiol* **78**:1–8.

Usuda J, Chiu SM, Azizuddin K, Xue LY, Lam M, Nieminen AL, Oleinick NL (2002) Promotion of photodynamic therapy-induced apoptosis by the mitochondrial protein Smac/DIABLO: Dependence on Bax. *Photochem Photobiol* **76**:217–223.

Usuda J, Chiu SM, Murphy ES, Lam M, Nieminen AL, Oleinick NL (2003b) Domain-dependent photodamage to Bcl-2. A membrane anchorage region is needed to form the target of phthalocyanine photosensitization. *J Biol Chem* **278**:2021–2029.

Yang Y, Hu Y, Wang Y, Li J, Liu F, Huang L (2012) Nanoparticle delivery of pooled siRNA for effective treatment of non-small cell lung cancer. *Mol Pharm* **9**:2280–2289.

Zhou Z, Matlib MA, Bers DM (1998) Cytosolic and mitochondrial Ca^{2+} signals in patch clamped mammalian ventricular myocytes. *J Physiol* **507**(Pt 2):379–403.

Zubris KA, Liu R, Colby A, Schulz MD, Colson YL, Grinstaff MW (2013) In vitro activity of Paclitaxel-loaded polymeric expansile nanoparticles in breast cancer cells. *Biomacromolecules* **14**:2074–2082.

Role of cell death pathways in response to photodynamic therapy in gliomas

LEONARDO BARCELOS DE PAULA, FERNANDO LUCAS PRIMO, AND ANTONIO CLAUDIO TEDESCO

8.1 INTRODUCTION

8.1.1 GLIOBLASTOMA

Identifying new therapeutic targets for the treatment of solid and hematopoietic neoplasms has been a focus within the scientific community. Solid neoplasms include glioblastomas, which are tumors originating from malignant transformations of cells of the astrocytic lineage (Mercer et al., 2009). These neoplasms are classified as grade IV astrocytomas by the World Health Organization and are the most common malignant brain tumors (Cohen and Weller, 2007; Mercer et al., 2009). Glioblastoma multiforme (GBM) is considered a very aggressive type of brain cancer, invasive and with few therapeutic alternatives (Koukourakis et al., 2009; Eljamel, 2015). The mean survival rate of the patients is only 12 months (Koukourakis et al., 2009; Sathornsumetee and Reardon, 2009; Eljamel, 2015). The classical treatment for glioblastoma includes surgical removal of the tumor mass followed by total cranial radiotherapy with concomitant and adjuvant alkylating chemotherapy (Mercer et al., 2009). For patients diagnosed early, the addition of alkylating chemotherapy improves the survival rate, between 24 and 60 months, compared to radiotherapy alone. However, patients with delayed diagnosis show a shorter survival rate of 14 months (Krakstad and Chekenya, 2010). The severity of this prognosis is the result of several factors that render GBMs complex and difficult to treat.

The current standard treatment for GBM is neurosurgical resection of the tumor followed by radiotherapy and chemotherapy combination. The maximal resection for each tumor is based on case-specific tumor size and shape, angiogenesis process, or sensitive brain regions affected by the diseases. Neurosurgical resection is generally classified as gross resection and subtotal resection when the tumor is not completely removed (Carlsson et al., 2014). Thus, it is essential to improve tumor resection techniques in order to increase the survival rate of patients with GBM (Orringer et al., 2012; Carlsson et al., 2014). However, the infiltrative nature of the tumor renders complete resection difficult. Thus, local progression is common, resulting in a poor prognosis (Pardridge, 2012).

The role of chemotherapy in addition to postoperative radiotherapy remains unclear (Chintagumpala and Gajjar, 2015). Temozolomide (TMZ) is a DNA alkylating agent (chemotherapeutic agent) used in the routine treatment of patients with malignant glioma. While TMZ provides overall survival benefits for patients with gliomas, the degree of effectiveness is greatly influenced by the O-methyltransferase 6-methylguanine-DNA (MGMT) gene promoter methylation status. MGMT methylation occurs in 35%–45% of these tumors (Serwer and James, 2012) and confers drug resistance to the tumor.

Deeper characterization of signaling pathways important in glioma growth is needed and may enable the development of new pharmacological agents, which could be utilized in new therapies for patients who do not respond to conventional antitumor therapies. Protein kinase B (PKB/Akt) and the transcription factor, nuclear factor kappa B (NF-kappaB), have garnered attention as potential targets for cell death induction and sensitization to chemotherapy in many tumor cell types such as lung cancer, ovarian cancer, and glioblastoma (Aggarwal, 2004; Kapoor et al., 2004; Sethi et al., 2007; Wu et al., 2008; Xu et al., 2009; Koul et al., 2010; Zanotto-Filho et al., 2010).

GBM is highly resistant to the chemotherapeutic treatment since cancer cells have a high capacity for DNA repair and cells can be at levels different stages of the cell cycle (not only at the G2/M phase) and the tumors have different areas of hypoxia containing chemoresistant cells. Moreover, the blood–brain barrier (BBB) impedes the delivery of drugs to the central nervous system (CNS). Together, all of these obstacles can be an important mechanism for the survival of cancer stem cells after treatment (Selbo et al., 2012).

The major limiting factor in developing new drugs directed to the CNS is the BBB. The BBB limits the brain penetration of most drug candidates for the treatment of CNS disorders. Essentially, 100% of large drug molecules, including peptides, recombinant proteins, monoclonal antibodies, drugs based on RNA interference, and gene therapy, do not cross the BBB (Pardridge, 2007).

Therefore, the combined use of different components of therapy—cellular, photodynamic, and nanotechnology—can bring increased benefits to patients who suffer from this disease.

The main idea is to design a drug delivery system (DDS) to allow the uptake in the brain of the active or photoactive compounds during the early stage of treatment, where the chemotherapeutic drug will shrink the tumor mass. After a period of time, the neoplastic tissue and the surrounding area will be impregnated by the photosensitizer's (PS's) molecules.

After resection of the tumor, the resection cavity can be treated by photodynamic therapy (PDT), to allow destruction of residual tumor cells. This is the basic idea of synergistic treatment for GBM using chemotherapy and PDT treatment at the same time. The same approach could also be used with the combination of hyperthermia treatment, where a nanocomposite containing PSs could be applied and hyperthermia and PDT light treatment could be used together with excellent results as already proved in previous studies (de Paula et al., 2012, 2015; Feuser et al., 2015).

8.1.2 PKB/Akt

PKB/Akt is a serine-/threonine-specific protein kinase. Three isoforms of α PKB (Akt 1), β PKB (Akt 2) (Jones et al., 1991; Cheng et al., 1992), and γ PKB (Akt 3) (Brodbeck et al., 1999) have been identified in mammals. Activation of the PKB/Akt pathway occurs in response to stimuli consisting of hormonal, growth factors, and extracellular matrix components (Nicholson and Anderson, 2002). The signaling cascade involves the activation of PKB/Akt by PI3K class 1 A and 1B, which are activated by tyrosine kinase receptors and G-protein-coupled receptors, respectively. Once activated, PI3Ks can promote the activation of various cellular proteins and transcription factors, including BAD, CREB, IkB kinase, α and β GSK3, and mTOR, which are involved in many processes such as metabolism, proliferation, differentiation, and antiapoptotic stimuli (Nicholson and Anderson, 2002).

In gliomas, overactivation of the PI3K/Akt pathway has been demonstrated in more than 60% of the tumors as a result of mutations, which lead to the inhibition of PTEN, a negative modulator of PI3K. Due to this antiapoptotic and proliferative modulation, PKB/Akt has been considered an important factor in the development of gliomas (Hill and Hemmings, 2002). Therefore, PKB/Akt inhibition could act as a tumor cell sensitization mechanism, facilitating the activation of the pro-apoptotic machinery and representing a possible target in cancer therapy (Hill and Hemmings, 2002).

Evidence indicates that PI3K/Akt pathway is involved in the expression of HIF-1α-induced hypoxia (Wan et al., 2015). This pathway contributes to maintenance of the malignant phenotype of tumor cells (Befani et al., 2012; Wan et al., 2015). The expression of HIF-1α through PI3K/Akt pathway is associated with tumor microenvironment (Filippi et al., 2014; Wan et al., 2015). However, the relationship of this pathway in regulating the ability of tumor to escape immune surveillance remains unclear.

PDT is reported to cause trauma in tumor tissue through cytotoxicity mediated by oxidative stress of light-activated PSs. PDT as an antitumor therapy has been validated in the clinic (Wan et al., 2015). However, a study has shown that a low-dose PDT did not inhibit tumor growth as expected and tumor-bearing mice undergoing low-dose PDT showed shorter survival times. These results show that the Lewis lung cell carcinoma cells (LLCs) showed greater capacity for immune evasion by upregulation of HIF-1α expression through PI3K/Akt in response to a low-dose PDT (Wan et al., 2015). Furthermore, our data show that low-dose PDT can contribute to immune evasion of LLC cells suppressing the population of cytotoxic T lymphocytes (CTLs) in splenic T cells and induce apoptosis of CTLs. This process also depends on the regulation of HIF-1α and PI3K/Akt and may be blocked by HIF-1α siRNA, as well as a specific inhibitor of PI3K (Wan et al., 2015).

8.1.3 TRANSCRIPTION FACTOR: NF-KAPPAB

Besides PI3K/Akt, studies have reported that the transcription factor NF-kappaB is a key component in glioma growth and antiapoptotic resistance, although the mechanisms involved in the activation of this factor have not yet been elucidated (Aggarwal, 2004; Kapoor et al., 2004; Sethi et al., 2007; Zanotto-Filho et al., 2010). NF-kappaB is a transcription factor consisting of members of a protein family combined into homo- and heterodimers (mainly heterodimers of p65 and p50 proteins). The complex p65/p50 is recruited into the cytosol in the form of a ternary complex bound to an inhibitory subunit called IkB. Under the action of stimuli such as inflammatory cytokines and reactive oxygen species (ROS), IkB is phosphorylated by IKK (IkB kinase) and is dissociated from NF-kappaB, and the pIkB is routed for proteasomal degradation. Among the NF-kappaB-regulated genes, some are antiapoptotic genes, BCL-xL, c-FLPI, and cIAP1/2. Others are antioxidants such as the mitochondrial superoxide dismutase 2 or involved in invasion (ICAM-1, VCAM-1, MMP2, and MMP9), angiogenesis (VEGF), proliferation (cyclin D1 and MYC), and metastasis (TWIST and CXCR4), which are related to the inhibition of the apoptosis machinery. Due to its antiapoptotic/antioxidant role, NF-kappaB has been considered as a transcription factor directly related to proliferation, metastasis, and tumor resistance to chemotherapeutic agents and to the immune system (Xie et al., 2010; Zanotto-Filho et al., 2010).

The exacerbated activation of the NF-kappaB pathway also contributes to the uncontrolled proliferation and resistance to anticancer agents in patients with tumors that are refractory to chemotherapy protocols (Furman et al., 2000; Masuko-Hongo et al., 2003; Jost and Ruland, 2007). The hyperactivation of NF-kappaB in response to chemotherapy has been correlated with therapy failure associated with classic drugs such as taxol, etoposide (Morotti et al., 2006; Kuo and Chen, 2015), vincristine, and vinblastine (García et al., 2005), as well as with the new generation of drugs such as imatinib (Cilloni et al., 2006). In this context, studies suggested that the combined use of NF-kappaB inhibitors and classical antitumor cell death could enhance or even break the cell resistance to these compounds.

NF-kappaB is known to control the cell death induced by PDT (Matroule et al., 2006; Uzdensky et al., 2015). A study shows that NF-kappaB-mediated necrosis induced PDT apoptosis of neurons and glial cells. On the other hand, glial cells are protected from photodynamic necrosis. In fact, activation of NF-kappaB by betulinic acid levels led to increased necrosis induced by PDT in mechanoreceptor neurons and caused apoptosis of glial cells. NF-kappaB has also exerted an antinecrotic action in glial cells (Uzdensky et al., 2015).

8.1.4 Cell death

Cell death can be classified according to the cell morphological appearance (which may be apoptotic, necrotic, or autophagic associated with mitosis), enzymatic criteria (with or without the involvement of different classes of nucleases or proteases such as caspases, calpain, cathepsin, and transglutaminases), functional aspects (planned or accidental, physiological or pathological characteristics), or immunological (immunogenic or nonimmunogenic) (Kroemer et al., 2009).

8.1.4.1 APOPTOSIS

Cell death by apoptosis is of great importance for the development of the embryonic organism, as well as in regulating the immune system and defense against diseases. Morphologically, apoptosis is characterized by nuclear changes such as chromatin condensation and fragmentation as well as the formation of membrane blebs and changes in shrinking organelles and whole cells. Two general apoptosis mechanisms have been described, an extrinsic pathway and an intrinsic pathway. These mechanisms differ, but are partially interconnected. The extrinsic pathway is activated by external signals to the cell through transmembrane death receptors that propagate the signal to the cytoplasm. These death receptors belong to the tumor necrosis factor receptors superfamily. After receptor activation, the caspase cascade is activated by dimerization of caspase 8, which cleaves and activates caspases 3 and 7 to execute apoptosis (Mahmood and Shukla, 2010; Tait and Green, 2010). The intrinsic signaling pathway is not mediated by receptors, but by changing the permeability of the mitochondria. Stimuli that initiate the intrinsic pathway produce positive or negative intracellular signals. Negative signals involve the absence of certain growth factors, hormones, and cytokines that can lead to failure of suppression of death programs, hence leading to apoptosis. Positive signals include radiation, toxins, hypoxia, hyperthermia, viral infections, and free radicals (Elmore, 2007).

All these stimuli induce changes in the inner mitochondrial membrane that result in an opening of the permeability transition pores, loss of mitochondrial membrane potential, and release of cytochrome c, Smac/DIABLO, and serine protease HtrA2/Omi into the cytosol (Du et al., 2000; Garrido et al., 2005). Cytosolic cytochrome c binds to and activates apoptotic protease activating factor 1, which in turn activates caspase-9, forming an apoptosome, which will promote a signaling cascade subsequently activating caspases 3 and 7 (Hill et al., 2004; Tait and Green, 2010; Galluzzi et al., 2012). The control and regulation of these events occur through mitochondrial apoptotic members of the Bcl-2 protein family (Cory and Adams, 2002). The tumor suppressor p53 plays a critical role in the regulation of Bcl-2; however, the exact mechanisms have not yet been fully elucidated (Schuler and Green, 2001). The Bcl-2 family of proteins regulates mitochondrial membrane permeability and can be both pro- and antiapoptotic. To date, a total of 25 genes belonging to the Bcl-2 family have been identified. The antiapoptotic proteins include Bcl-2, Bcl-xL, Bcl-XL, Bcl-XS, Bcl-w, and BAG, while Bcl-10, Bax, Bak, Bid, Bad, Bim, Bik, and Blk are pro-apoptotic. These proteins play a critical role in determining whether a cell undergoes apoptosis or not. It is believed that Bcl-2's primary mechanism of action is to regulate the release of cytochrome c from mitochondria by altering the permeability of the mitochondrial membrane. The expression of both Bcl-2 and Bax is regulated by the $p53$ tumor suppressor gene (Demuth and Berens, 2004; de la Iglesia et al., 2008; Tu et al., 2014). Therapeutic strategies targeting the death receptor pathways would help in reducing the resistance of glioblastoma to chemotherapeutic agents.

8.1.4.2 NECROSIS

Necrosis occurs when a cell loses the ability to die by apoptosis (i.e., due to a low level of ATP). Cells can undergo necrosis due to extreme stress such as oxidative stress, high temperature, contact with toxins, and mechanical shock with varying intensities based on the cell type (Syntichaki and Tavernarakis, 2003). Necrosis was long considered to be a process of uncontrolled, unplanned cell death, resulting in irreversible dramatic changes in cellular parameters essential for metabolism and cellular structure (Cilloni et al., 2006). In recent years, many studies demonstrated that cell death by necrosis can be controlled and some markers of this process have been discovered. The term "programmed necrosis" or "necroptosis" was assigned to a type of nonaccidental death in which caspases are inhibited and cell death occurs without uncontrolled release of cell contents, emphasizing a degree of regulation of this death process. Necroptosis especially depends on the activity of receptor interacting protein kinase-1, RIPK3, caspase inhibitors, ubiquitin E3 ligase enzymes, poly (ADP-ribose) polymerase-1(PARP-1), ROS, bioenergetic reactions involving members of the Bcl-2 family, cytosolic hydrolases, and permeabilization of lysosomal and plasma membrane (Galluzzi and Kroemer, 2008; Vandenabeele et al., 2010). TNF is a key activator of necrosis, which induces the formation of mitochondrial ROS and activates PARP-1, leading to ATP depletion (Skulachev, 2006). ROS formation induces DNA damage and the subsequent activation of PARP-1, which is a nuclear enzyme involved in DNA repair and stability as well as in transcriptional regulation (Leist and Jäättelä, 2001; Los et al., 2002). PARP-1 activation consumes a large amount of NAD+ and induces a massive consumption of ATP. The rapid depletion in ATP favors necrosis and the subsequent inhibition of cell death by apoptosis, which is dependent on energy (Los et al., 2002).

8.1.4.3 AUTOPHAGY

Autophagy is a highly conserved degradation pathway, which includes macroautophagy, microautophagy, and chaperone-mediated autophagy (Mizushima and Komatsu, 2011). Microautophagy involves the engulfment of the cytoplasm by invagination of the lysosomal membrane (Rodriguez-Rocha et al., 2011). Autophagy is related to many physiological and pathological processes, including cell survival, death, metabolism, development, infection, immunity, and aging (Mehrpour et al., 2010). This type of programmed death is intimately involved in the etiology of many important human diseases, including cancer, neurodegenerative diseases, and metabolic disorders (Meijer and Codogno, 2009). It is characterized by the formation of autophagosomal double membranes, which fuse with lysosomes to generate a functional structure, which recycles and degrades cellular components in an acidic environment containing lysosomal hydrolases (Kroemer et al., 2005).

Autophagy is mainly a mechanism of cell survival, through its role in suppressing cell death by necrosis such as necroptosis and cell death mediated by PARP-1. Autophagy is regulated by a family of autophagy genes, called *Atg*, *Atg5*, *Atg7*, *Atg8*, *Atg10*, and *Atg12*, which are the first to be recruited during the autophagy process and are responsible for the formation of the autophagosome. Atg8, also known as light chain-3 (LC3), exists in two forms, LC3-I, located in the cytosol, and its proteolytic form LC3-II, located in the autophagosome (Kogel et al., 2010). LC3 is an ubiquitin protein ligase that can be conjugated to phosphatidylethanolamine (PE). LC3 is initially synthesized in an unprocessed form, proLC3, which is cleaved at the C-terminal carbon, resulting in LC3-I, which is subsequently conjugated to PE, forming LC3-II. LC3-II is the only protein marker associated with autophagosomes (Klionsky et al., 2012).

Besides these proteins, Atg6 is an essential regulator of the autophagic process and a component of the PI3K class III complex. It is involved in the autophagosome trafficking. *Atg6* is a tumor suppressor gene, which is deleted in multiple tumor types such as breast, ovarian, and prostate cancers. In gliomas, *Atg6* expression levels are inversely proportional to the tumor grade. Thus, patients with low levels of *Atg6* present a worse prognosis, suggesting that the autophagic process may amplify the response to therapy, improving the clinical outcome (Pirtoli et al., 2009).

Typically, activation of the insulin receptor results in the activation of PI3K, which, in turn, activates AKT. Autophagy can be suppressed through the PI3K pathway, which can be influenced by PTEN inhibition and PI3K/Akt interaction. Activated Akt can inhibit apoptosis and autophagy through mTOR. This signaling cascade is crucial for the formation of autophagosomes through interaction of the Atg family members (Baehrecke, 2005).

8.2 PHOTODYNAMIC THERAPY

PDT was the first drug-light device combination approved by the U.S. Food and Drug Administration for over four decades and is used in clinical trials and treatment around the world (Tapajós et al., 2008; Passos et al., 2011, 2013; Primo and Tedesco, 2013; Bolfarini et al., 2014; Castagnos et al., 2014; Heinrich et al., 2014). The success of this therapeutic modality is linked to the fact that, while commonly used, classical therapies lead to the massive destruction of tumor tissues and induce immunosuppression (Triesscheijn et al., 2006) and several undesirable side effects for the patients.

PS drug can be administered systemically, topically, or intratumorally, followed by a biodistribution period of 0–72 h (depending on the PS kinetics) so that the PS drug accumulates in tumor tissues. The lesions are then exposed to light at the wavelength of maximum absorption of the PS drug (600–800 nm). The main objective of PDT is to induce the death of neoplastic cells by the PS drug (Figure 8.1) with regression of the tumor, while minimizing the damage to healthy cells and, therefore, the side effects associated with the apoptosis or necrosis process. PDT has been increasingly used in cancer treatment due to a series of physical, chemical, and biological events (Tapajós et al., 2008; Plaetzer et al., 2009; Bacellar et al., 2015; Broekgaarden et al., 2015; Chen et al., 2015; Rapozzi et al., 2015; Uzdensky et al., 2015).

PDT involves oxidative damage to cellular components by the generation of ROS, especially singlet oxygen ($^1O_2$). After intravenous injection or topical application, the PS drug accumulates in the tumor tissue pathway internalization (Triesscheijn et al., 2006). At this stage, the PS drug is in its ground state (S_0) and stable. Once the tissue is irradiated at a specific wavelength, typically red or infrared region of the electromagnetic

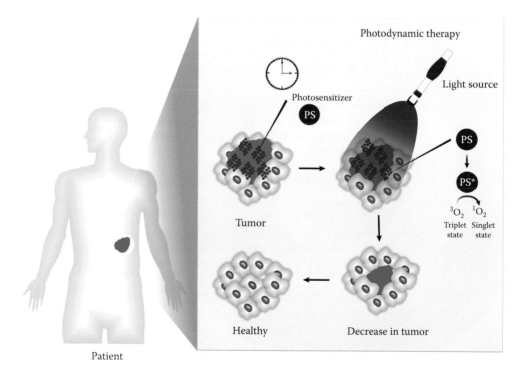

Figure 8.1 Principles of photodynamic therapy. A photosensitizer (PS) is administered systemically or topically. After a period of systemic PS distribution, it selectively accumulates in the tumor. Irradiation activates the PS and, in the presence of molecular oxygen, triggers a photochemical reaction that culminates in the production of singlet oxygen ($^1O_2$). Irreparable damage to cellular macromolecules leads to tumor cell death via an apoptotic, necrotic, or autophagic mechanism, accompanied by the induction of an acute local inflammatory reaction that participates in the removal of dead cells, restoration of normal tissue homeostasis, and, sometimes, in the development of systemic immunity.

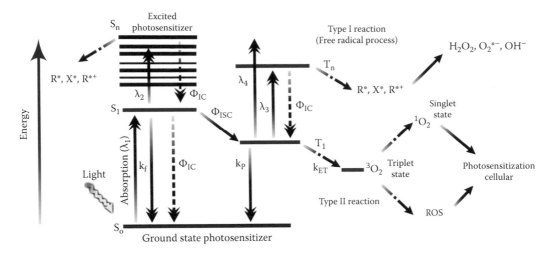

Figure 8.2 Jablonski diagram for the photosensitization process: λ = light absorption appropriate wavelength; S_0 = ground state; S_1 = first excited singlet state; S_n = higher singlet excited state; T_1 = first excited state triplet; T_n = higher triplet excited state; Φ_{IC} = internal quantum efficiency of conversion; Φ_{ISC} = quantum efficiency of intersystem crossing; k_f = fluorescence constant speed; k_p = phosphorescence constant speed; k_{ET} = constant energy transfer.

spectrum (600–800 nm), the PS drug that accumulated in tumor cells absorbs the energy provided by the light source in the form of photons, reaching a singlet excited state of higher energy (S_n), rapidly declining to the lowest singlet excited state (S_1). During the conversion to the triplet state through intersystem crossing, according to the Jablonski diagram (Lakowicz and Masters, 2008; Figure 8.2), the same sequence can induce a series of reactions that generate ROS. Meanwhile, the PS can very quickly undergo two types of reactions (Arumainayagam et al., 2010).

PDT mechanisms of action are classified into types I and II and are derived from a combination of physical (light interaction with the molecule), chemical (production of ROS), and biological phenomena (tumor destruction; Plaetzer et al., 2009).

Type I involves hydrogen atom abstraction or electron transfer reactions between the excited states of the PS and a biological substrate, resulting in the production of free radicals and radical ions. These radicals are highly reactive and react with molecular oxygen, generating superoxide anions or hydroxyl radicals that cause irreparable damage to tumor tissues (Plaetzer et al., 2009).

Type II results from the energy transfer between the excited triplet state of the PS and molecular oxygen, generating the first excited state of oxygen ($^1O_2$). The reactive molecule causes damage to cell structures, including breaches of genomic DNA and destruction of the plasmatic membrane, liposomes, and mitochondria (Ficheux, 2009).

Both types of reaction can occur simultaneously, and the ratio between these processes is dependent upon the PS used and the concentration of substrates and oxygen present in the environment. Due to the high reactivity and short half-life of singlet oxygen ($^1O_2$) and hydroxyl radicals, only molecules that are next to the PS location areas are directly affected by PDT (Castano et al., 2004; Robertson et al., 2009).

The massive generation of ROS triggers many cellular mechanisms, resulting in direct cell death via apoptosis or necrosis depending on the cell type, the PS concentration employed, the dose of energy provided, and the PS intracellular localization (Agostinis et al., 2011). The PS intracellular localization dictates the cell death pathway. PS accumulation in mitochondria is associated with induction of apoptosis by cytochrome *c* release and the induction of the caspase cascade. Drugs located in organelles such as lysosomes membranes tend to cause necrosis due to loss of membrane integrity as well as the rapid depletion in intracellular ATP. Reports indicate that a cell viability rate lower than 70% is predictive of apoptosis, while necrosis is detected with cytotoxicity rates over 90% (Mroz and Hamblin, 2011).

In addition to direct cellular damage, PDT also promotes damage to the tumor vasculature, resulting in lack of oxygen and nutrient supply to the tumor cells in the tumor microenvironment, thereby promoting cell death associated with secondary tissue necrosis. A study showed that shorter intervals of time between administration of the PS and tumor radiation favor the occurrence of vascular injury since there is no complete dissipation of the PS to the tumor cells and some PS remains in the tumor blood vessels, increasing the efficiency of treatment and leading to greater tumor reduction, providing the desired effect in this treatment modality (Barnes et al., 2009).

8.3 PS USED IN PDT

PSs are the active agents in the PDT process. A large number of studies described the development of new compounds, which are potentially more active and more specifically retained and distributed in carcinogenic tissues. In recent years, PDT research focused on developmental studies investigating the administration and biodistribution of possible PS candidates usable in the photochemical treatment of tumor tissues (Allison et al., 2004).

The appropriate PSs were developed from the first-generation PS, Photofrin, to the second- (chlorine PS or derivatives and phthalocyanines (PCs)) and third (conjugated PS on carrier)-generation PSs to overcome undesired disadvantages and to increase selective tumor accumulation and excellent targeting (Yoon et al., 2013). The first-generation PS mainly includes porphyrins and their derivatives and its main representative is Photofrin (Ethirajan et al., 2011).

The second-generation of PS was established in order to circumvent the limiting effects of the first-generation drugs. The main second-generation drugs are the PCs, chlorins, and some dyes. Among the chlorins, the most often used is Foscan (Bonnett, 1995), which is a potent PS activated at a wavelength of 652 nm. It presents faster tissue elimination than Photofrin. Despite its effectiveness, Foscan triggers high cutaneous photosensitivity that may last for several weeks after treatment (O'Connor et al., 2009). PCs are second-generation PSs and are stable PSs with improved photochemical abilities. They are effective inducers of cell death in various neoplastic models. Metallated PCs localize in critical cellular organelles and are better inducers of cell death than previous generation PSs as they favor mainly apoptotic cell death events (Mfouo-Tynga and Abrahamse, 2015).

The third-generation PSs refer to second-generation PS conjugates coupled to carriers such as cholesterol, antibodies, and liposomes for selective accumulation and targeting within the tumor tissue (Yoon et al., 2013). Several nanomaterials have been synthetized to increase the therapeutic activity of PSs. Some dyes have limitations on the solubility, biocompatibility, and cell internalization. Thus, it is necessary to combine the PS molecules and nanomaterials to improve the targeting and controlled release of drug (Simioni et al., 2011). Nanotechnology has led to increase of intracellular drug accumulation with minimal side effects for biological target. The main nanomaterials applied in PDT protocols are based in the synthesis of nanoparticles from copolymer and biopolymer molecules. Nanoshells are obtained in controlled conditions to promote the drug entrapment into nanodevices. Polymeric nanoemulsions, nanocapsules, and nanospheres have been widely used in PDT assays due to the great potential of lipophilic encapsulation (Siqueira-Moura et al., 2010; Primo et al., 2011; Simioni et al., 2011).

In vitro studies have used nanoemulsions as a DDS combined with PSs and PDT in human glioblastoma cells (Chakrabarti et al., 2013; Fisher et al., 2013; Miki et al., 2014). Glioblastoma cells (T98G and U87MG) used were incubated with nanoemulsion chloroaluminum-PC (NE/ClAlPc: 0.5 mol/L) over 3 h. Activation of the PS delivered intracellularly by the NE was accomplished by laser excitation of ClAlPc at 670 nm; subsequent cell death could be measured by cell viability assays (Figure 8.3).

T98G and U87MG cells were treated with three steps: (1) NE/ClAlPc in the absence of visible light (dark assay), (2) exposure to visible light at a dose of 700 mJ/cm^2 in the absence of NE/ClAlPc, or (3) exposure to visible light at doses of 100, 200, and 700 mJ/cm^2. After 3 h of incubation, the accumulation of NE/ClAlPc-PDT in T98G cells showed cell death by 77%, 59%, and 60% presence to visible light at doses of 100, 200, and 700 mJ/cm^2, respectively, when U87MG cells showed 64%, 65%, and 41% compared to dark assay (Figure 8.4).

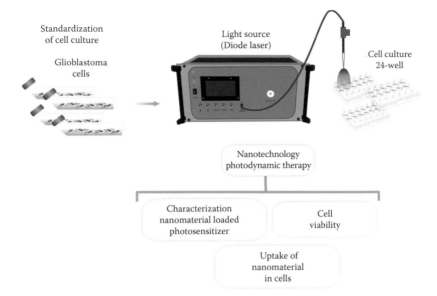

Figure 8.3 Schematic representation of in vitro assay of nanotechnology and photodynamic therapy using glioma monolayer culture and diode laser for photoactivation.

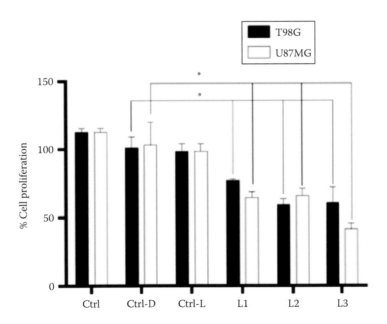

Figure 8.4 Effect of nanoemulsion chloroaluminum-phthalocyanine (NE/ClAlPc: 0.05 mol/L) and different irradiation conditions. Glioblastoma grade IV (T98G and U87MG). Ctrl: control samples cultured cells with 3% fetal bovine serum; ctrl-D: control samples with NE/ClAlPc in the absence of visible light (darkness); ctrl-L: control samples that were subjected to visible light at a dose of 700 mJ/cm² in the absence of NE/ClAlPc; L1: samples with NE/ClAlPc subjected to visible light at a dose of 100 mJ/cm²; L2: samples with NE/ClAlPc subjected to visible light at a dose of 200 mJ/cm²; L3: samples with NE/ClAlPc subjected to visible light at a dose of 700 mJ/cm². Statistical analysis was performed by two-way (ANOVA) followed by Tukey's test. Statistical significance was expressed as *p < 0.05. All data were expressed as the mean ± SEM of three independent experiments.

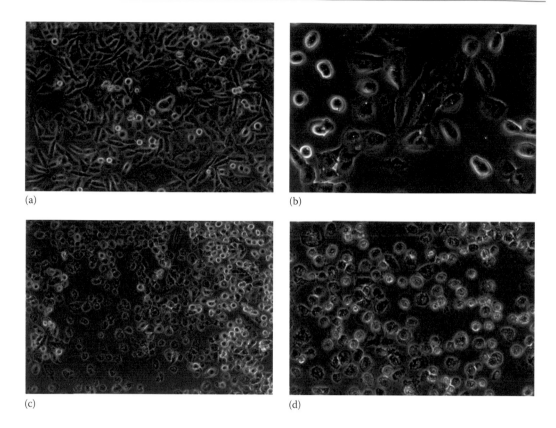

Figure 8.5 T98G cells control in Dulbecco's modified eagle medium and supplemented with 10% fetal bovine serum at confluent stage (a) 10× and (b) 20×. T98G cells incubated with NE/ClAlPc containing 0.5 mg/mL ClAlPc in DMEM/FBS 3% treated with the diode laser at 700 mJ/cm² (c) 10× and (d) 20×. Cell micrography obtained using a Carl Zeiss microscope Axiovert 40-CFL coupled with a digital high-resolution camera Axiocam MRC.

Figure 8.5 illustrates T98G cells at the typical confluent stage (Figure 8.5a and b) and the NE/ClAlPc after incubation for 3 h at 37°C. Then, we carried out the PDT treatment (Figure 8.5c and d). The results suggested that the after 24 h of treatment is possible to observe to cell death due to the drastic morphological changes of NE/ClAlPc-PDT-treated T98G cells. When T98G cells were irradiated with laser of 700 mJ/cm² and NE/ClAlPc-pretreated cells (0.05 mol/L), incidence of membrane-blebbing, cell shrinkage, and nuclear fragmentation, a defining characteristic of apoptosis, while these cells completely have lost cell adhesion making them nonviable.

These data indicated that, while NE/ClAlPc-PDT effectively induced cell death in T98G and U87MG cells, NE/ClAlPc in the absence of visible light (dark assay) and exposure to visible light at a dose of 700 mJ/cm² in the absence of NE/ClAlPc alone did not cause such cytotoxicity. The confocal studies developed with two cell culture of GBM, T98G and U87MG, help to precisely address where is the subcellular localization of the ClAlPc in the designed DDS. T98G and U87MG cells internalized NE/ClAlPc after incubation for 3 h at 37°C (Figure 8.6). The results indicated that NE/ClAlPc-PDT are predominantly localized at the cytoplasmic level with an distribution was homogenous. This cellular uptake for NE as a nanocarriers was also observed by mesenchymal stem cells (de Paula et al., 2015) and in the tissue of human glioblastomas (Trylcova et al., 2015). Muehlmann et al. (2014) also found that ClAlPc internalization was concentrated in the cytosol of cancerous and noncancerous cells. These results also reinforce the propose of the use of PDT in the design of a GBM treatment in late stages.

All these findings point to the potential of a multifunctional DDS associated with PTD, to target malignant tumor cells mainly glioblastoma and reduce untoward PS cytotoxicity within the surrounding milieu.

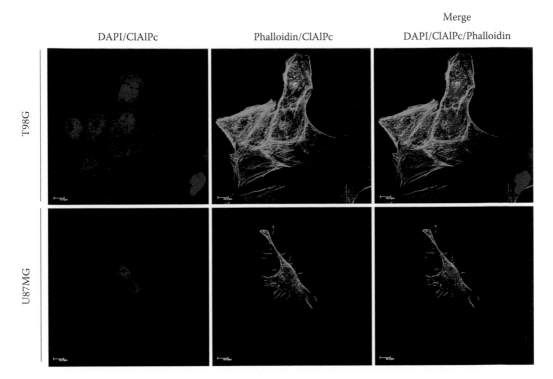

Figure 8.6 Subcellular localization of nanoemulsion loaded with photosensitive drug (NE/ClAlPc) of in vitro in T98G and U87MG cells. DAPI (blue): nuclear staining; Phalloidin (green): labeling actin filaments; ClAlPc (red): labeling nanoemulsion loaded with chlorine-aluminum PC.

8.4 FUTURE PROSPECTS

Current GBM treatments have not significantly improved patient survival rates to the levels achieved for other brain tumors. From the basic science viewpoint, there is an essential need to understand how GBM occurs or derives from earlier gliomas. Specific therapies may prove to present a limited efficacy as GBM might arise from a variety of mutations. Early diagnosis can be the key to improving patient survival rates through prevention of tumor growth and, therefore, the identification of early biomarkers is critical. Noninvasive blood monitoring, for instance, using tumor microvesicles that are released from tumors could provide quick, accurate, and early detection of GBM. The combination of treatment approaches might provide an effective regimen for the treatment of GBM tumors. Surgery for GBM is partially efficient because of the inability to perform wide tumor resection without injury to the surrounding normal nervous tissue and because of the high infiltration of glioma into the normal tissues. PDT has been proven to be extremely effective, especially in combination with other treatment modalities for different types of tumors such as breast, lung, ovarian, and skin cancer, but has not yet been employed for GBM treatment. Studies demonstrated that the combination of PDT, radiotherapy, and chemotherapy provided better effects during the treatment of patient than the classical single treatments.

Despite the use of PDT as the first-line treatment especially for skin cancer, PDT is still not considered as an important modality for the treatment of several solid tumors because of heterogeneity in the cellular responses to PDT. The experimental evidence on the molecular signaling leading to the activation NF-kappaB discussed in this perspective indicates that tumor cells respond to PDT in many ways based on the PS used, its intracellular localization, and its physicochemical properties.

Analysis of the molecular pathways leading to NF-kappaB activation by PDT revealed that this transcription factor is situated at the crossroad between tumor biology and the immune system. NF-kappaB is important for the immune cell attraction to the tumor and, therefore, to establish an immune response to prevent recurrence. Moreover, it also protects the tumor from death through both apoptosis and necrosis. The pharmacological inhibition of NF-kappaB during PDT should therefore be performed with caution and only after verifying that tumor cells eradication is improved without interfering with the immune response.

REFERENCES

Aggarwal BB (2004) Nuclear factor-kappaB: The enemy within. *Cancer Cell* **6**:203–208.

Agostinis P, Berg K, Cengel KA, Foster TH, Girotti AW, Gollnick SO, Hahn SM, Hamblin MR, Juzeniene A, Kessel D (2011) Photodynamic therapy of cancer: an update. *CA: A Cancer Journal for Clinicians* **61**:250–281.

Allison RR, Downie GH, Cuenca R, Hu X-H, Childs CJ, Sibata CH (2004) Photosensitizers in clinical PDT. *Photodiagnosis and Photodynamic Therapy* **1**:27–42.

Arumainayagam N, Moore C, Ahmed HU, Emberton M (2010) Photodynamic therapy for focal ablation of the prostate. *World Journal of Urology* **28**:571–576.

Bacellar IO, Tsubone TM, Pavani C, Baptista MS (2015) Photodynamic efficiency: From molecular photochemistry to cell death. *International Journal of Molecular Sciences* **16**:20523–20559.

Baehrecke EH (2005) Autophagy: Dual roles in life and death? *Nature Reviews Molecular Cell Biology* **6**:505–510.

Barnes LD, Giuliano EA, Ota J, Cohn LA, Moore CP (2009) The effect of photodynamic therapy on squamous cell carcinoma in a murine model: Evaluation of time between intralesional injection to laser irradiation. *The Veterinary Journal* **180**:60–65.

Befani CD, Vlachostergios PJ, Hatzidaki E, Patrikidou A, Bonanou S, Simos G, Papandreou CN, Liakos P (2012) Bortezomib represses HIF-1a protein expression and nuclear accumulation by inhibiting both PI3K/Akt/TOR and MAPK pathways in prostate cancer cells. *Journal of Molecular Medicine* **90**:45–54.

Bolfarini GC, Siqueira-Moura MP, Demets GJ, Tedesco AC (2014) Preparation, characterization, and in vitro phototoxic effect of zinc phthalocyanine cucurbit [7] uril complex encapsulated into liposomes. *Dyes and Pigments* **100**:162–167.

Bonnett R (1995) Photosensitizers of the porphyrin and phthalocyanine series for photodynamic therapy. *Chemical Society Reviews* **24**:19–33.

Brodbeck D, Cron P, Hemmings BA (1999) A human protein kinase B? With regulatory phosphorylation sites in the activation loop and in the C-terminal hydrophobic domain. *Journal of Biological Chemistry* **274**:9133–9136.

Broekgaarden M, Kos M, Jurg FA, van Beek AA, van Gulik TM, Heger M (2015) Inhibition of NF-κB in tumor cells exacerbates immune cell activation following photodynamic therapy. *International Journal of Molecular Sciences* **16**:19960–19977.

Carlsson SK, Brothers SP, Wahlestedt C (2014) Emerging treatment strategies for glioblastoma multiforme. *EMBO Molecular Medicine* **6**:1359–1370.

Castagnos P, Siqueira-Moura M, Goto PL, Perez E, Franceschi S, Rico-Lattes I, Tedesco A, Blanzat M (2014) Catanionic vesicles charged with chloroaluminium phthalocyanine for topical photodynamic therapy. In vitro phototoxicity towards human carcinoma and melanoma cell lines. *RSC Advances* **4**:39372–39377.

Castano AP, Demidova TN, Hamblin MR (2004) Mechanisms in photodynamic therapy: Part one—Photosensitizers, photochemistry and cellular localization. *Photodiagnosis and Photodynamic Therapy* **1**:279–293.

Chakrabarti M, Banik NL, Ray SK (2013) Photofrin based photodynamic therapy and miR-99a transfection inhibited FGFR3 and PI3K/Akt signaling mechanisms to control growth of human glioblastoma in vitro and in vivo. *PloS One* **8**:e55652.

Chen J-J, Hong G, Gao L-J, Liu T-J, Cao W-J (2015) In vitro and in vivo antitumor activity of a novel porphyrin-based photosensitizer for photodynamic therapy. *Journal of Cancer Research and Clinical Oncology* **141**:1553–1561.

Cheng JQ, Godwin AK, Bellacosa A, Taguchi T, Franke TF, Hamilton TC, Tsichlis PN, Testa JR (1992) AKT2, a putative oncogene encoding a member of a subfamily of protein-serine/threonine kinases, is amplified in human ovarian carcinomas. *Proceedings of the National Academy of Sciences* **89**:9267–9271.

Chintagumpala M, Gajjar A (2015) Brain tumors. *Pediatric Clinics of North America* **62**:167–178.

Cilloni D, Messa F, Arruga F, Defilippi I, Morotti A, Messa E, Carturan S, Giugliano E, Pautasso M, Bracco E (2006) The NF-κB pathway blockade by the IKK inhibitor PS1145 can overcome imatinib resistance. *Leukemia* **20**:61–67.

Cohen N, Weller RO (2007) *Who Classification of Tumours of the Central Nervous System*, p. 312. Wiley Online Library.

Cory S, Adams JM (2002) The Bcl2 family: Regulators of the cellular life-or-death switch. *Nature Reviews Cancer* **2**:647–656.

de la Iglesia N, Konopka G, Lim K-L, Nutt CL, Bromberg JF, Frank DA, Mischel PS, Louis DN, Bonni A (2008) Deregulation of a STAT3–interleukin 8 signaling pathway promotes human glioblastoma cell proliferation and invasiveness. *The Journal of Neuroscience* **28**:5870–5878.

de Paula L, Primo F, Jardim D, Morais P, Tedesco A (2012) Development, characterization, and in vitro trials of chloroaluminum phthalocyanine-magnetic nanoemulsion to hyperthermia and photodynamic therapies on glioblastoma as a biological model. *Journal of Applied Physics* **111**:07B307.

de Paula LB, Primo FL, Pinto MR, Morais PC, Tedesco AC (2015) Combination of hyperthermia and photodynamic therapy on mesenchymal stem cell line treated with chloroaluminum phthalocyanine magnetic-nanoemulsion. *Journal of Magnetism and Magnetic Materials* **380**:372–376.

Demuth T, Berens ME (2004) Molecular mechanisms of glioma cell migration and invasion. *Journal of Neuro-Oncology* **70**:217–228.

Du C, Fang M, Li Y, Li L, Wang X (2000) Smac, a mitochondrial protein that promotes cytochrome *c*–dependent caspase activation by eliminating IAP inhibition. *Cell* **102**:33–42.

Eljamel S (2015) 5-ALA fluorescence image guided resection of glioblastoma multiforme: A meta-analysis of the literature. *International Journal of Molecular Sciences* **16**:10443–10456.

Elmore S (2007) Apoptosis: A review of programmed cell death. *Toxicologic Pathology* **35**:495–516.

Ethirajan M, Chen Y, Joshi P, Pandey RK (2011) The role of porphyrin chemistry in tumor imaging and photodynamic therapy. *Chemical Society Reviews* **40**:340–362.

Feuser PE, Santos-Bubniak L, Silva MCS, Viegas ADC, Fernandes AC, Ricci-Junior E, Nele M, Tedesco AC, Sayer C, de Araújo PHH (2015) Encapsulation of magnetic nanoparticles in poly(methyl methacrylate) by miniemulsion and evaluation of hyperthermia in U87MG cells. *European Polymer Journal* **68**:355–365.

Ficheux H (2009). Photodynamic therapy: Principles and therapeutic indications. *Annales Pharmaceutiques Francaises* **67**:32–40.

Filippi I, Morena E, Aldinucci C, Carraro F, Sozzani S, Naldini A (2014) Short-term hypoxia enhances the migratory capability of dendritic cell through HIF-1a and PI3K/Akt pathway. *Journal of Cellular Physiology* **229**:2067–2076.

Fisher CJ, Niu CJ, Lai B, Chen Y, Kuta V, Lilge LD (2013) Modulation of PPIX synthesis and accumulation in various normal and glioma cell lines by modification of the cellular signaling and temperature. *Lasers in Surgery and Medicine* **45**:460–468.

Furman RR, Asgary Z, Mascarenhas JO, Liou H-C, Schattner EJ (2000) Modulation of NF-κB activity and apoptosis in chronic lymphocytic leukemia B cells. *The Journal of Immunology* **164**:2200–2206.

Galluzzi L, Kroemer G (2008) Necroptosis: A specialized pathway of programmed necrosis. *Cell* **135**:1161–1163.

Galluzzi L, Vitale I, Abrams J, Alnemri E, Baehrecke E, Blagosklonny M, Dawson T, Dawson V, El-Deiry W, Fulda S (2012) Molecular definitions of cell death subroutines: Recommendations of the Nomenclature Committee on Cell Death 2012. *Cell Death and Differentiation* **19**:107–120.

García MG, Alaniz L, Lopes EC, Blanco G, Hajos SE, Alvarez E (2005) Inhibition of NF-κB activity by BAY 11-7082 increases apoptosis in multidrug resistant leukemic T-cell lines. *Leukemia Research* **29**:1425–1434.

Garrido G, Blanco-Molina M, Sancho R, Macho A, Delgado R, Muñoz E (2005) An aqueous stem bark extract of *Mangifera indica* (Vimang (R)) inhibits T cell proliferation and TNF-induced activation of nuclear transcription factor NF-kB. *Phytotherapy Research* **19**:211–215.

Heinrich TA, Tedesco AC, Fukuto JM, da Silva RS (2014) Production of reactive oxygen and nitrogen species by light irradiation of a nitrosyl phthalocyanine ruthenium complex as a strategy for cancer treatment. *Dalton Transactions* **43**:4021–4025.

Hill MM, Adrain C, Duriez PJ, Creagh EM, Martin SJ (2004) Analysis of the composition, assembly kinetics and activity of native Apaf-1 apoptosomes. *The EMBO Journal* **23**:2134–2145.

Hill MM, Hemmings BA (2002) Inhibition of protein kinase B/Akt: Implications for cancer therapy. *Pharmacology and Therapeutics* **93**:243–251.

Jones PF, Jakubowicz T, Hemmings BA (1991) Molecular cloning of a second form of rac protein kinase. *Cell Regulation* **2**:1001–1009.

Jost PJ, Ruland J (2007) Aberrant NF-kappaB signaling in lymphoma: Mechanisms, consequences, and therapeutic implications. *Blood* **109**:2700–2707.

Kapoor GS, Zhan Y, Johnson GR, O'Rourke DM (2004) Distinct domains in the SHP-2 phosphatase differentially regulate epidermal growth factor receptor/NF-κB activation through Gab1 in glioblastoma cells. *Molecular and Cellular Biology* **24**:823–836.

Klionsky DJ, Abdalla FC, Abeliovich H, Abraham RT, Acevedo-Arozena A, Adeli K, Agholme L, Agnello M, Agostinis P, Aguirre-Ghiso JA (2012) Guidelines for the use and interpretation of assays for monitoring autophagy. *Autophagy* **8**:445–544.

Kogel D, Fulda S, Mittelbronn M (2010) Therapeutic exploitation of apoptosis and autophagy for glioblastoma. *Anti-Cancer Agents in Medicinal Chemistry (Formerly Current Medicinal Chemistry-Anti-Cancer Agents)* **10**:438–449.

Koukourakis GV, Kouloulias V, Zacharias G, Papadimitriou C, Pantelakos P, Maravelis G, Fotineas A, Beli I, Chaldeopoulos D, Kouvaris J (2009) Temozolomide with radiation therapy in high grade brain gliomas: Pharmaceuticals considerations and efficacy; a review article. *Molecules* **14**:1561–1577.

Koul N, Sharma V, Dixit D, Ghosh S, Sen E (2010) Bicyclic triterpenoid Iripallidal induces apoptosis and inhibits Akt/mTOR pathway in glioma cells. *BMC Cancer* **10**:328.

Krakstad C, Chekenya M (2010) Review survival signalling and apoptosis resistance in glioblastomas: Opportunities for targeted. *Molecular Cancer* **9**:135.

Kroemer G, El-Deiry W, Golstein P, Peter M, Vaux D, Vandenabeele P, Zhivotovsky B, Blagosklonny M, Malorni W, Knight R (2005) Classification of cell death: Recommendations of the Nomenclature Committee on Cell Death. *Cell Death and Differentiation* **12**:1463–1467.

Kroemer G, Galluzzi L, Vandenabeele P, Abrams J, Alnemri E, Baehrecke E, Blagosklonny M, El-Deiry W, Golstein P, Green D (2009) Classification of cell death: Recommendations of the Nomenclature Committee on Cell Death 2009. *Cell Death and Differentiation* **16**:3–11.

Kuo Y-C, Chen Y-C (2015) Targeting delivery of etoposide to inhibit the growth of human glioblastoma multiforme using lactoferrin-and folic acid-grafted poly (lactide-*co*-glycolide) nanoparticles. *International Journal of Pharmaceutics* **479**:138–149.

Lakowicz JR, Masters BR (2008) Principles of fluorescence spectroscopy. *Journal of Biomedical Optics* **13**:9901.

Leist M, Jäättelä M (2001) Triggering of apoptosis by cathepsins. *Cell Death and Differentiation* **8**:324–326.

Los M, Mozoluk M, Ferrari D, Stepczynska A, Stroh C, Renz A, Herceg Z, Wang Z-Q, Schulze-Osthoff K (2002) Activation and caspase-mediated inhibition of PARP: A molecular switch between fibroblast necrosis and apoptosis in death receptor signaling. *Molecular Biology of the Cell* **13**:978–988.

Mahmood Z, Shukla Y (2010) Death receptors: Targets for cancer therapy. *Experimental Cell Research* **316**:887–899.

Masuko-Hongo K, Shang Z, Kato T, Nakamura H, Nishioka K (2003) 15-Deoxy-delta12, 14-prostaglandin J2 induces apoptosis in human articular chondrocytes. *Arthritis Research and Therapy* **5**:1.

Matroule JY, Volanti C, Piette J (2006) NF-κB in photodynamic therapy: Discrepancies of a master regulator. *Photochemistry and Photobiology* **82**:1241–1246.

Mehrpour M, Esclatine A, Beau I, Codogno P (2010) Overview of macroautophagy regulation in mammalian cells. *Cell Research* **20**:748–762.

Meijer AJ, Codogno P (2009) Autophagy: Regulation and role in disease. *Critical Reviews in Clinical Laboratory Sciences* **46**:210–240.

Mercer RW, Tyler MA, Ulasov IV, Lesniak MS (2009) Targeted therapies for malignant glioma. *BioDrugs* **23**:25–35.

Mfouo-Tynga I, Abrahamse H (2015) Cell death pathways and phthalocyanine as an efficient agent for photo-dynamic cancer therapy. *International Journal of Molecular Sciences* **16**:10228–10241.

Miki Y, Akimoto J, Hiranuma M, Fujiwara Y (2014) Effect of talaporfin sodium-mediated photodynamic therapy on cell death modalities in human glioblastoma T98G cells. *The Journal of Toxicological Sciences* **39**:821–827.

Mizushima N, Komatsu M (2011) Autophagy: Renovation of cells and tissues. *Cell* **147**:728–741.

Morotti A, Cilloni D, Pautasso M, Messa F, Arruga F, Defilippi I, Carturan S, Catalano R, Rosso V, Chiarenza A (2006) NF-kB inhibition as a strategy to enhance etoposide-induced apoptosis in K562 cell line. *American Journal of Hematology* **81**:938–945.

Mroz P, Hamblin MR (2011) The immunosuppressive side of PDT. *Photochemical and Photobiological Sciences* **10**:751–758.

Muehlmann LA, Ma BC, Longo JPF, Santos MdFMA, Azevedo RB (2014) Aluminum–phthalocyanine chloride associated to poly (methyl vinyl ether-*co*-maleic anhydride) nanoparticles as a new third-generation photosensitizer for anticancer photodynamic therapy. *International Journal of Nanomedicine* **9**:1199.

Nicholson KM, Anderson NG (2002) The protein kinase B/Akt signalling pathway in human malignancy. *Cellular Signalling* **14**:381–395.

O'Connor AE, Gallagher WM, Byrne AT (2009) Porphyrin and nonporphyrin photosensitizers in oncology: Preclinical and clinical advances in photodynamic therapy. *Photochemistry and Photobiology* **85**:1053–1074.

Orringer D, Lau D, Khatri S, Zamora-Berridi GJ, Zhang K, Wu C, Chaudhary N, Sagher O (2012) Extent of resection in patients with glioblastoma: Limiting factors, perception of resectability, and effect on survival: Clinical article. *Journal of Neurosurgery* **117**:851–859.

Pardridge WM (2007) Blood–brain barrier delivery. *Drug Discovery Today* **12**:54–61.

Pardridge WM (2012) Drug transport across the blood–brain barrier. *Journal of Cerebral Blood Flow and Metabolism* **32**:1959–1972.

Passos SK, De Souza PE, Soares PK, Eid DR, Primo FL, Tedesco AC, Lacava ZG, Morais PC (2013) Quantitative approach to skin field cancerization using a nanoencapsulated photodynamic therapy agent: A pilot study. *Clinical, Cosmetic and Investigational Dermatology* **6**:51.

Passos SK, Tedesco AC, Macedo Eid DR, Marques Lacava ZG (2011) Bowen disease treated with PDT using ALA in nanostructured vehicle and two light deliveries: A case report. *Journal of the American Academy of Dermatology* **64**:AB141–AB141.

Pirtoli L, Cevenini G, Tini P, Vannini M, Oliveri G, Marsili S, Mourmouras V, Rubino G, Miracco C (2009) The prognostic role of Beclin 1 protein expression in high-grade gliomas. *Autophagy* **5**:930–936.

Plaetzer K, Krammer B, Berlanda J, Berr F, Kiesslich T (2009) Photophysics and photochemistry of photodynamic therapy: fundamental aspects. *Lasers in Medical Science* **24**:259–268.

Primo FL, da Costa Reis MB, Porcionatto MA, Tedesco AC (2011) In vitro evaluation of chloroaluminum phthalocyanine nanoemulsion and low-level laser therapy on human skin dermal equivalents and bone marrow mesenchymal stem cells. *Current Medicinal Chemistry* **18**:3376–3381.

Primo FL, Tedesco AC (2013) Combining photobiology and nanobiotechnology: A step towards improving medical protocols based on advanced biological models. *Nanomedicine* **8**:513.

Rapozzi V, Della Pietra E, Bonavida B (2015) Dual roles of nitric oxide in the regulation of tumor cell response and resistance to photodynamic therapy. *Redox Biology* **6**:311–317.

Robertson C, Evans DH, Abrahamse H (2009) Photodynamic therapy (PDT): A short review on cellular mechanisms and cancer research applications for PDT. *Journal of Photochemistry and Photobiology B: Biology* **96**:1–8.

Rodriguez-Rocha H, Garcia-Garcia A, Panayiotidis MI, Franco R (2011) DNA damage and autophagy. *Mutation Research* **711**(1–2):158–166.

Sathornsumetee S, Reardon DA (2009) Targeting multiple kinases in glioblastoma multiforme. *Expert Opinion on Investigational Drugs* **18**(3):277–292.

Schuler M, Green D (2001) Mechanisms of p53-dependent apoptosis. *Biochemical Society Transactions* **29**:684–687.

Selbo PK, Weyergang A, Eng MS, Bostad M, Mælandsmo GM, Høgset A, Berg K (2012) Strongly amphiphilic photosensitizers are not substrates of the cancer stem cell marker ABCG2 and provides specific and efficient light-triggered drug delivery of an EGFR-targeted cytotoxic drug. *Journal of Controlled Release* **159**:197–203.

Serwer LP, James CD (2012) Challenges in drug delivery to tumors of the central nervous system: An overview of pharmacological and surgical considerations. *Advanced Drug Delivery Reviews* **64**:590–597.

Sethi G, Ahn K, Chaturvedi M, Aggarwal B (2007) Epidermal growth factor (EGF) activates nuclear factor-κB through IκBα kinase-independent but EGF receptor kinase dependent tyrosine 42 phosphorylation of IκBα. *Oncogene* **26**:7324–7332.

Simioni AR, Rodrigues M, Primo FL, Morais PC, Tedesco AC (2011) Effect of diode-laser and AC magnetic field of bovine serum albumin nanospheres loaded with phthalocyanine and magnetic particles. *Journal of Nanoscience and Nanotechnology* **11**:3604–3608.

Siqueira-Moura M, Primo F, Tedesco A (2010) Photochemotherapic effect of nanodevices containing chloro-aluminum phthalocyanine on oral cancer cell line. *Luminescence* **25**:208.

Skulachev V (2006) Bioenergetic aspects of apoptosis, necrosis and mitoptosis. *Apoptosis* **11**:473–485.

Syntichaki P, Tavernarakis N (2003) The biochemistry of neuronal necrosis: rogue biology? *Nature Reviews Neuroscience* **4**:672–684.

Tait SW, Green DR (2010) Mitochondria and cell death: Outer membrane permeabilization and beyond. *Nature Reviews Molecular Cell Biology* **11**:621–632.

Tapajós E, Longo J, Simioni A, Lacava Z, Santos M, Morais P, Tedesco A, Azevedo R (2008) In vitro photodynamic therapy on human oral keratinocytes using chloroaluminum-phthalocyanine. *Oral Oncology* **44**:1073–1079.

Triesscheijn M, Baas P, Schellens JH, Stewart FA (2006) Photodynamic therapy in oncology. *The Oncologist* **11**:1034–1044.

Trylcova J, Busek P, Smetana Jr K, Balaziova E, Dvorankova B, Mifkova A, Sedo A (2015) Effect of cancer-associated fibroblasts on the migration of glioma cells in vitro. *Tumor Biology* **36**:1–7.

Tu JB, Li QY, Jiang F, Hu XY, Ma RZ, Dong Q, Zhang H, Pattar P, Li SX (2014) Pingyangmycin stimulates apoptosis in human hemangioma-derived endothelial cells through activation of the p53 pathway. *Molecular Medicine Reports* **10**:301–305.

Uzdensky A, Berezhnaya E, Khaitin A, Kovaleva V, Komandirov M, Neginskaya M, Rudkovskii M, Sharifulina S (2015) Protection of the crayfish mechanoreceptor neuron and glial cells from photooxidative injury by modulators of diverse signal transduction pathways. *Molecular Neurobiology* **52**:811–825.

Vandenabeele P, Galluzzi L, Berghe TV, Kroemer G (2010) Molecular mechanisms of necroptosis: An ordered cellular explosion. *Nature Reviews Molecular Cell Biology* **11**:700–714.

Wan J, Wu W, Che Y, Kang N, Zhang R (2015) Low dose photodynamic-therapy induce immune escape of tumor cells in a HIF-1a dependent manner through PI3K/Akt pathway. *International Immunopharmacology* **28**(1):44–51.

Wu H, Cao Y, Weng D, Xing H, Song X, Zhou J, Xu G, Lu Y, Wang S, Ma D (2008) Effect of tumor suppressor gene PTEN on the resistance to cisplatin in human ovarian cancer cell lines and related mechanisms. *Cancer Letters* **271**:260–271.

Xie T-X, Xia Z, Zhang N, Gong W, Huang S (2010) Constitutive NF-κB activity regulates the expression of VEGF and IL-8 and tumor angiogenesis of human glioblastoma. *Oncology Reports* **23**:725–732.

Xu C, Jin H, Shin J, Kim J, Cho M (2009) Roles of protein kinase B/Akt in lung cancer. *Frontiers in Bioscience (Elite Edition)* **2**:1472–1484.

Yoon I, Li JZ, Shim YK (2013) Advance in photosensitizers and light delivery for photodynamic therapy. *Clinical Endoscopy* **46**:7–23.

Zanotto-Filho A, Delgado-Cañedo A, Schröder R, Becker M, Klamt F, Moreira JCF (2010) The pharmacological NF?B inhibitors BAY117082 and MG132 induce cell arrest and apoptosis in leukemia cells through ROS-mitochondria pathway activation. *Cancer Letters* **288**:192–203.

In search of specific PDT photosensitizers
Subcellular localization and cell death pathways

TAYANA M. TSUBONE, CHRISTIANE PAVANI, ISABEL O.L. BACELLAR, AND MAURÍCIO S. BAPTISTA

9.1 INTRODUCTION

Biological tissues can be efficiently oxidized and damaged upon illumination with light at the appropriate wavelength when this light is absorbed by natural or synthetic photosensitizers (PSs). The photodynamic effect starts with electronic excitation of the PS to the singlet excited state, which is subsequently converted to a triplet excited state by intersystem crossing. Triplets are reactive species that live long enough to interact with nearby species, leading either to energy transfer to oxygen (type II process) or to direct reactions with biological substrates (type I process). In the former case, there is the formation of singlet oxygen ($^1O_2$), which is a highly electrophilic molecule. Type I processes are based on the reaction between excited states (usually triplets) and biomolecules that are in close proximity or contact, forming a variety of products, and usually starting radical chain reactions. Both type I and II processes cause oxidation of biomolecules, and depending on the extent of the damage, they also impair cell viability (Foote 1968; Halliwell 2009; Hamblin and Hasan 2014; Henderson and Dougherty 1992; Krinsky 1977). This phenomenon is the basis of the clinical treatment known as photodynamic therapy (PDT). In PDT, exogenous PSs are given to the patient, and the target of the treatment (tumors or diseases tissues sites with infected areas) is selectively irradiated.

There are many classes of PSs commonly employed in PDT, such as chlorins, phthalocyanines, porphyrins, and phenothiazines. PSs belonging to the same class can have very distinct properties, given the diversity of side groups that can be attached to the chromophore (Joshi et al. 2011; Pavani et al. 2009; Pereira et al. 2009, 2010; Uchoa et al. 2010; 2011; Zheng et al. 2001). These side groups can influence both photochemical and biological responses. The interactions of the PS with biomolecules affect substantially the kind of photooxidation reaction taking place. For example, protein binding usually favors type I over type II processes (Baptista and Indig 1998). Polarity, lipophilicity, and net charge regulate the extent of cellular uptake and subcellular localization. Increased lipophilicity, for example, is often correlated with higher cellular uptake and enhanced photodynamic efficiency (Engelmann et al. 2007; Pavani et al. 2009; Ricchelli et al. 2005). The effect of electrical charges is well illustrated by the accumulation of many positively charged PSs in mitochondria due to the negative mitochondrial electrochemical potential (Gabrielli et al. 2004; Hoye et al. 2008). It is noteworthy to say that the site of intracellular localization also affects the efficiency and photochemical mechanisms of the PS. For example, positively charged PS tend to aggregate on negatively charged surfaces, which are present in the mitochondrial internal membrane favoring dye–dye electron transfer reaction instead of energy transfer to oxygen (Gabrielli et al. 2004; Junqueira et al. 2002).

Although PDT has more than 30 years of age counting as a starting point to the early studies of Dougherty, and it has clearly shown to be the best choice of treatment for several diseases, it has not yet come to the point that is widely known and used by medical doctors (Dougherty et al. 1998). We believe that several steps of the photodynamic effect can be still improved in order to attract more medical doctors and consequently to benefit more people. This is somehow already happening in terms of the light sources, a field that was completely changed in the last decade (Philipp and Berlien 2006; Wilson et al. 2005). However, in terms of drug development we are falling behind probably because we have been always using the same paradigms for designing new drugs. In the last decades, hundreds of new PSs were designed and synthesized but only very few went to clinics (Jurič et al. 2014; Scwingel et al. 2012; Wong et al. 2013; Zhao et al. 2015).

The two parameters most used for the optimization of the PDT efficiency of new PSs are (Figure 9.1): (1) increase in PS absorption in the red since light in the far-red and near-infrared penetrates deeper in the skin. For example, by reducing porphyrins to chlorins and bacteriochlorins, there is a shift in the absorption band to the red, allowing better photoactivation in deeper layers of the skin, (Allison et al. 2004; Ormond and Freeman 2013). (2) Maximization in the generation of $^1O_2$ and/or of radical species of the PS, by optimizing the photophysical quantum yields, mainly triplets and singlet oxygen, as well as by designing structures that avoid aggregation and photobleaching of PSs. We can mention two important examples of very efficient PSs that are on different stages of clinical trials and that were developed by optimizing these parameters: the purpurin derivatives developed by Rav Pandey and coworkers at Buffalo, United States (Joshi et al. 2011; Zheng et al. 2001) and the halogenated bacteriochlorins developed by the group of Luis G Arnaut in Coimbra, Portugal (Pereira et al. 2009, 2010).

Although optimization of these parameters certainly allows the development of more efficient PSs, it is not clear that these parameters (mentioned earlier) can actually be used to obtain a breakthrough in terms of the PDT efficiency. We think that the recently developed PDT drugs are not substantially different from the hundreds of other PSs that had been already been developed and are today only mentioned in patents or papers. In fact, we propose a change in paradigm in terms of the search for new and more efficient PS. Recently published data indicated that the amount of $^1O_2$ generation is actually not the most important factor that affects

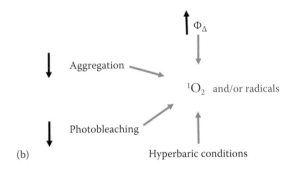

Figure 9.1 Usual strategies that have been used to optimize the performance of PDT PSs: (a) red shifting the absorption band; (b) maximizing the generation of singlet oxygen and/or ROS.

PDT efficiency. Oliveira and coworkers have shown that a PS with low photochemical and photophysical properties (crystal violet [CV]) becomes more efficient than an efficient PS (methylene blue [MB]) mainly for accumulating with 100% efficiency in mitochondria and for keeping its activity on such a strong reducing environment (Oliveira et al. 2011).

In fact, several authors have shown that subcellular localization is an important factor to be considered (perhaps the most important one, see later text) in terms of controlling the PDT efficiency of a PS (Castano et al. 2004), since it defines the site of photodamage. In the intracellular environment, $^1O_2$ diffuses less than ~100 nm (Mertins et al. 2014; Redmond and Kochevar 2006) from its site of generation, which is a much smaller pathway compared with the average size of some intracellular organelles such as mitochondria. More important is the fact that the site and the amount of photooxidative damage will define the cell death mechanisms taking place (Deda et al. 2013; Mroz et al. 2011; Oleinick and Evans 1998; Rodriguez et al. 2009). For that reason, PDT protocols leading to generation of reactive species in specific places (even if in a smaller quantity) may be more efficient than those resulting in spatially unspecific generation (Oliveira et al. 2011). Another strategy to obtain improved PDT efficiency in terms of cellular killing is to develop multifunctional PS. Albani and coworkers (2014) have shown the synergistic action of ruthenium-based PS that can generate $^1O_2$ as well as form DNA adducts after photoactivation.

Although this chapter is mostly covers the factors determining the improvement of PDT efficiency in terms of cellular killing, the final outcome of a PDT treatment in a patient that was given systemic PS is critically dependent on the pharmacodynamics and pharmaceutics of the drug. In fact, one of the most important factors is the targeting of the PS to specific diseased tissues in the organism being treated (Solban et al. 2006). We direct the interest reader of this subject to other reviews because it is out of the scope of this work (Celli et al. 2010; Chen et al. 2006; Pongue and Hasan 2003; Verma et al. 2007).

Earlier studies of induction of specific programed cell death pathways in PDT focused mostly on necrosis and apoptosis. More recently, autophagy has been shown to be a very efficient pathway to induce cell death as a consequence of photooxidative damage (Buytaert et al. 2006b, 2007; Xue et al. 2015a). Hence, unraveling ways to trigger autophagic cell death may lead to highly efficient PDT protocols (Ezzeddine et al. 2013; Kessel et al. 2003; Marchal et al. 2007; Rodriguez et al. 2009; Woodburn et al. 1991). We consider that the intracellular localization of PS is perhaps the most important parameter that could be controlled in order to allow the development of optimized PSs, which could maybe allow the desired breakthrough in terms of drug development for PDT.

Because of the unquestionable role of PS localization in the development of optimized PSs, microscopy techniques (light and electron) have become fundamental in this field of PDT research. Microscopy techniques can characterize the processes happening during PDT at the cellular level because cell responses to photooxidative damage usually involve morphological and biochemical changes. In this context, fluorescence microscopy is a powerful technique because it also provides information concerning the intracellular environments of the PS (most PS are fluorescent molecules). Besides, new microscopic fluorescent techniques were developed and made commercially available in recent years, that is, time resolved and high resolution. Fluorescent lifetime techniques, for example, allow one to directly sense diffusion and reactivity of the PS in the intracellular environment. Therefore, we suspect that fluorescence microscopy will continue to play an increasing role in the development of new and more efficient PS.

The classical experiment used to define the site of subcellular localization of a PS is based on the treatment of cells with both the PS and an organelle marker, followed by the comparison of the fluorescence image coming from the PS with that coming from the organelle-specific probe (Castano et al. 2004). Fluorescent probes can also be used to indirectly sense the presence of intermediate compounds or products, or to sense intracellular properties, such as pH and redox misbalance (e.g., singlet oxygen, radicals, or proteins) (Flors et al. 2006; Price et al. 2009; Winterbourn 2014). For example, probes that accumulate in acidic vacuoles, like acridine orange (AO), can be used to initially identify autophagy inhibition (Martins et al. 2013). Another important methodology concerning fluorescence microscopy is the use of antibodies in immunofluorescence assays. By targeting specific antigens, it is possible to acquire information on cellular processes and to define the cell death mechanisms. Given the great potential of fluorescence microscopy to investigate biological processes, in this chapter we will review the field of fluorescent microscopy in PDT, initially focusing on identifying the major sites of localization of the PS and posteriorly on cell death mechanisms, specially autophagic cell death.

9.2 SUBCELLULAR LOCALIZATION OF PS

There are three main sites of intracellular PS concentration (Table 9.1): mitochondria, lysosomes, and Golgi/ER. Most of the PSs have some formal charge, inhibiting direct crossing through membranes and consequently cellular internalization happens through endocytosis or crossing through other sorts of protein channels/pumps. Usually, PSs do not accumulate in cell nuclei of eukaryotic cells, and therefore, nuclear DNA is preserved from direct damage during PDT. Of course, this is beneficial for PDT because it avoids DNA oxidation and possible malignant transformation due to PDT (Castano et al. 2005; Evans et al. 1997; Oleinick and Evans 1998).

Mitochondria present a constant transmembrane potential ($\Delta\psi$) of around −180 mV generated by the ion proton pumps coupled to the respiratory electron transport chain (Hoye et al. 2008). The magnitude of $\Delta\psi$ is around six times higher than transmembrane potential present at the cytoplasmic membranes (Dessolin et al. 2002). Therefore, positively charged dyes are either electrophoretic driven to mitochondria or diffuse and accumulate at these organelles. A simple calculation based on the Nernst equation predicts that a single and positively charged dye will have a 10,000-fold accumulation in mitochondria (Lemasters and Ramshesh 2007). As a consequence, specific probes and PS with positive charge and the proper hydrophobic/hydrophilic balance will mainly localize in mitochondria (Barbieri et al. 2011; Dummin et al. 1997; Engelmann et al. 2007; Fernandez-Sanz et al. 2014; Oliveira et al. 2011; Pavani et al. 2009; Presley et al. 2003).

Table 9.1 Subcellular localization of PSs in vitro

Photosensitizer (PS)	Intracellular localization	References
mTHPC, Foscan®	Mitochondria/Golgi/ER	Teiten et al. (2003); Chen et al. (2000)
Photofrin®	Plasma membrane/mitochondria	Yeh et al. (2012); Wilson et al. (1997); Hsieh et al. (2003)
Cristal violet (CV)	Mitochondria	Oliveira et al. (2011)
Benzoporphyrins derivates (BPD)	Mitochondria	Glidden et al. (2012); Celli et al. (2011)
Hypericin	Endoplasmic reticulum (ER)	Buytaert et al. (2006a,b, 2007)
Cationic zinc (II) phthalocyanines	Mitochondria	Dummin et al. (1997)
Methylene blue (MB)	Mitochondria and lysosomes	Oliveira (2011)
Pc 4	Mitochondria/ER/Golgi	Singh et al. (1987)
TPPS$_{1-4}$	Lysosomes	Berg et al. (1990)
AlPcS$_{2-4}$	Lysosomes	Moan et al. (1992)
NPe6	Lysosomes	Reiners et al. (2002)
Lysyl chlorin p6	Lysosomes	Luo et al. (2010); Leach et al. (1993); Kessel et al. (2000)
Chlorophyllin e4	Mitochondria/lysosome	Lihuan et al. (2014)
Rose Bengal	Golgi	Soldani et al. (2004)
Cationic porphyrins	Mitochondria	Uchoa et al. (2010); Deda et al. (2013); Pavani et al. (2009)
9-Capronyloxytetrakis (methoxyethyl)porphycene (CPO)	ER	Kessel et al. (2005)

As an example, rhodamine 123 (Rh123) is a fluorescent dye with the ability to accumulate in mitochondria (Hoye et al. 2008). Some other probes (Mitotracker® family) not only accumulate but also covalently bind to mitochondrial proteins by reacting with free thiol groups of cysteine residues. These probes allow the calculation of the mitochondrial mass and/or the status of $\Delta\psi$ because the amount of remaining probe after a washing step depends on the two parameters mentioned earlier (Agnello et al. 2008; Barbieri et al. 2011; Cottet-Rousselle et al. 2011; Fernandez-Sanz et al. 2014; Presley et al. 2003). Therefore, mitochondrial $\Delta\psi$ offers a unique opportunity for selectively targeting these organelles (Hoye et al. 2008). Our group has reported some cationic PSs that localize almost 100% in mitochondria. Oliveira et al. demonstrated that the cationic PS (crystal violet) has a close to perfect localization within mitochondria since its fluorescence presented 99% overlap with the fluorescence of Rh123 (Figure 9.2a; Oliveira et al. 2011). Uchoa et al. synthesized a cationic amphiphilic porphyrin bearing quaternary ammonium groups, which accumulates 95% in mitochondria (Figure 9.2b; Uchoa et al. 2010).

Although most positively charged PSs have certain levels of accumulation in mitochondria, the quantitative values of accumulation may be considerably different. In fact, it is not easy to find compounds that localize solely in mitochondria (Table 9.1; Beckman et al. 1987; Dummin et al. 1997; Kandela et al. 2002; Oliveira et al. 2011; Oseroff et al. 1986; Pavani et al. 2009; Uchoa et al. 2010). Therefore, there should be other properties that affect the localization of positively charged dyes. For example, MB, which is known to accumulate in lysosomes (Table 9.1), also accumulates in mitochondria as can be seen by the efficient delocalization of Rh123 fluorescence on its presence (Figure 9.2c). The lack of emission from MB within mitochondria was explained by the reduction of MB in these organelles (Gabrielli et al. 2004; Oliveira et al. 2011; Wainwright et al. 1997). Another example is a single structural change, such as adding a zinc atom in the porphyrin ring, which substantially decreases the mitochondrial localization. In the example shown in Figure 9.2d, the co-localization value in mitochondria increased from 11.4% to 42.8% upon addition to zinc to the porphyrin. The presence of zinc increases the hydrophilic character of the porphyrin and reduces the interaction with the mitochondrial membrane or increase the concentration in other organelles. Despite the lower binding to mitochondria, we found that molecules containing zinc-chelated porphyrin at the center of PS are more efficient to cause cell killing because these molecules bind more efficiently membranes in general, an effect

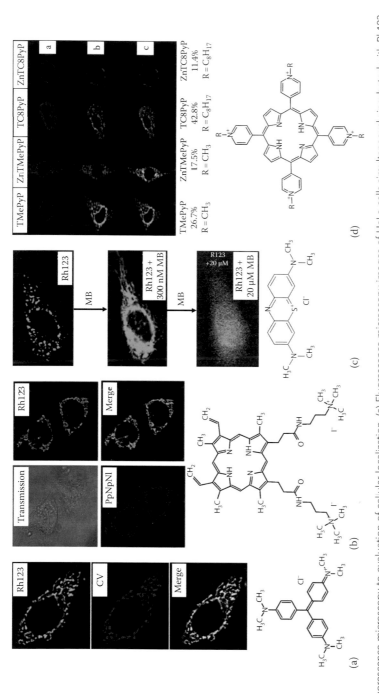

Figure 9.2 Fluorescence microscopy to evaluation of cellular localization. (a) Fluorescence microscopy images of HeLa cells simultaneously incubated with Rh123 and CV (both in 100 nM concentrations) and chemical structure of CV. On the top, fluorescence arising from Rh123 alone (green), fluorescence arising from CV alone (red), and the merge of the previous two images (yellow). (Reprinted from *Free Radic. Biol. Med.*, 51, Oliveira, C.S., Turchiello, R., Kowaltowski, A.J., Indig, G.L., and Baptista, M.S., Major determinants of photoinduced cell death: Subcellular localization versus photosensitization efficiency, 824–833. Copyright 2011, with permission from Elsevier.) (b) Chemical structure of porphyrin-PpNpNl and fluorescence microscopy images of HeLa cells simultaneously incubated with R123 and porphyrin-PpNpNl, including transmission image of cells, fluorescence of Rh123 alone (green), fluorescence from porphyrin-PpNpNl (red), and merge fluorescence images of the porphyrin and Rh123 images (yellow). (Republished from Uchoa, A.P. et al., *J. Porphyrins Phthalocyanines*, 14, 832, 2010. With permission of World Scientific Publishing.) (c) Fluorescence microscopy analysis of the subcellular localization of MB in HeLa cells and chemical structure of MB. Photomicrographs of HeLa cells incubated with Rh123 and MB at two different concentrations: 300 nM and 20 µM. (Reprinted from *Free Radic. Biol. Med.*, 51, Oliveira, C.S., Turchiello, R., Kowaltowski, A.J., Indig, G.L., and Baptista, M.S., Major determinants of photoinduced cell death: Subcellular localization versus photosensitization efficiency, 824–833. Copyright 2011, with permission from Elsevier.) (d) fluorescence microscopy, the percentage of mitochondrial localization, and chemical structure of PSs. On the top, fluorescence from porphyrins (red): TMePyP, ZnTMePyP, TC8PyP, ZnTC8PyP fluorescence of Rh123 alone (green), and overlay between porphyrins and Rh123 fluorescence (yellow). TMePyP: R = CH₃, ZnTMePyP: R = CH₃, TC8PyP: R = C₈H₁₇, ZnTC8PyP: R = C₈H₁₇. (Reproduced from Pavani, C., Uchoa, A.F., Oliveira, C.S., Iamamoto, Y., and Baptista, M.S., Effect of zinc insertion and hydrophobicity on the membrane interactions and PDT activity of porphyrin photosensitizers, *Photochem. Photobiol. Sci.*, 8(2), 233–240, 2009. Reproduced by the permission of The Royal Society of Chemistry (RSC) on behalf of the European Photochemistry Association and RSC.)

that the authors attributed to the chelating effect of zinc (Pavani et al. 2009). In terms of mitochondrial accumulation of PS, it is also important to mention the pro-drugs based on 5-aminilevulinic acid (ALA), which leads to the endogenous synthesis of protoporphyrin IX within mitochondria (Gardner et al. 1991). Some negatively charged and neutral PSs, such as photofrin® and silicon phthalocyanine (Pc 4), also tend to localize in mitochondria, possibly due to their binding to specific mitochondrial constituents (Singh et al. 1987).

Lysosomes are organelles that maintain a low pH within their interior via proton pumps. This low pH allows the activity of acid-dependent enzymes responsible for several intracellular digestion processes. One mechanism of dye accumulation in lysosomes is the gain of charge at low pH, that is, lysosomotropic agents freely diffuse across membranes in their uncharged form but become trapped in lysosomes and acidic vesicles once they become protonated. The term "lysosomotropic agents" is used to describe weak amine bases that attain concentrations ca. 100-fold higher within the lysosomes than in the cytosol (Boya and Kroemer 2008; Raben et al. 2009; Zong et al. 2014). LysoTracker® probes are supported by this principle and consist of a fluorophore linked to a weak base for labeling and tracking acidic organelles in live cells. Nonetheless, several amphiphilic negatively charged PSs are also known to accumulate in lysosomes. In fact, it has been reported that PS with net anionic character such as mono-L-aspartyl chlorin e6 (NPe6), $meso$-tetra-(p-sulphophenyl) porphine series (TPPS$_{1-4}$), aluminum phthalocyanine sulfonate series (AlPcS$_{2-4}$), lysyl chlorin p6, etiobenzochlorin, and other substituted $meso$-tetraphenylporphyrins usually localize in lysosomes (Berg and Moan 1994, 1997; Boyle and Dolphin 1996; Kessel and Morgan 1993; Leach et al. 1993; Moan et al. 1992; Mroz et al. 2009; Reiners et al. 2002; Tsai et al. 2015; Woodburn et al. 1991). Other examples that we can mention are the works of Reiners et al. and Wang et al., which demonstrated the co-localization between NPe6 and TPCS$_{2a}$ to Lucifer yellow (LY) and lysotracker®, respectively, indicating lysosome localization of both dyes (Figure 9.3a, b; Reiners et al. 2002; Wang et al. 2013). Interestingly, there are also some positively charged PSs that seem to accumulate in lysosomes. Some phenothiazines do not get further charged in the lysosomes but also accumulate there, MB being a clear example of this (Figure 9.3c; Oliveira et al. 2011).

This significant effect of charge in the intracellular localization of PS was also clearly reported by Woodburn and coworkers in the 1990s. Using a series of porphyrins with variable hydrophobicity and charge, it was shown that porphyrins with cationic side chains localize mainly in mitochondria, whereas those with a more anionic character tend to accumulate in lysosomes (Woodburn et al. 1991). However, not only the net charge but symmetry of charge distribution can also be an important parameter determining subcellular localization. Kessel et al. studied two meso-tetraphenylporphyrin derivatives bearing two cationic trimethylammonium groups in adjacent and opposite positions. The symmetrical compound localizes in the lysosomes, whereas the asymmetrical compound targets the mitochondria of murine leukemia cells (Ezzeddine et al. 2013; Kessel et al. 2003).

Plasma membrane is a relatively uncommon target in PDT, although it remains an interesting one due to its fast-response to the PDT effect (Caetano et al. 2007; Valenzeno 1987). Usually, very lipophilic PS can accumulate in the lipid bilayers and can cause extensive membrane damage as it was observed for modified hemato and protoporphyrins (Bronshtein et al. 2004; Lavi et al. 2002). The complexity of biomembranes and their crucial role for cell survival may explain the fast response to PDT. However, if one wants to escape necrotic cell death, membrane damage should be avoided (Kochevar et al. 2000).

Golgi apparatus and ER have been shown to be the major sites of localization for lipophilic PS (Linder and Shoshan 2005; Miller et al. 1995; Sibrian-Vazquez et al. 2007; Sun and Leung 2002). Both organelles are made of several lipid bilayers, which are associated with the protein synthesis and modifications. Therefore, damage in these organelles can drastically inhibit protein synthesis (Barr and Short 2003; Terasaki et al. 1984). Teiten et al. showed that Foscan® exhibits low localization in lysosomes and mitochondria, with preferential localization at Golgi apparatus and ER (Figure 9.4; Teiten et al. 2003). Zinc(II)-phthalocyanine included in dipalmitoyl-phosphatidylcholine liposomes also mainly localizes in Golgi apparatus (Soriano et al. 2014).

The mechanism of cellular uptake of the PSs also seems to affect its subcellular localization. The major entrance route of PS in the intracellular environment is endocytosis (Castano et al. 2004; Høgset et al. 2004). Endosomes follow an intracellular inward trafficking of membranes that ends up fusing with lysosomes. Therefore, if the molecule does not have a large tendency to be directed to a specific intracellular site, it will end up in lysosomes. Negatively charged amphiphilic porphyrins are examples of molecules that do not have

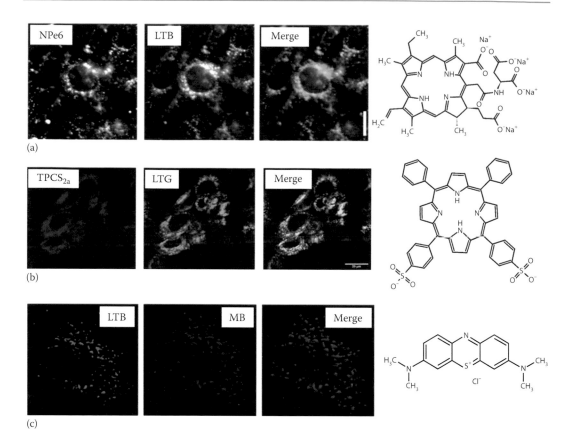

Figure 9.3 Subcellular localization of PSs that tend to accumulate in lysosomes. (a) Fluorescence microscopy images of 1c1c/ cells simultaneously incubated with LysoTracker and NPe6 and chemical structure of NPe6. Panels represent fluorescence of NPe6, LysoTracker blue (LTB) and merged image of NPe6 and LTB. (Reprinted by permission from Macmillan Publishers Ltd. *Cell Death Differ.*, Reiners, J.J., Caruso, J.A., Mathieu, P., Chelladurai, B., Yin, X.-M., and Kessel, D., Release of cytochrome c and activation of pro-Caspase-9 following lysosomal photodamage involves bid cleavage, 9(9), 934–944. Copyright 2002.) (b) Fluorescence microscopy images and chemical structure of TPCS$_{2a}$. Red fluorescence of TPCS$_{2a}$ (0.1 μg/mL), green fluorescence of LysoTracker green (LTG) and merge image of TPCS$_{2a}$ and LTG. (From Wang, J.T.-W., Berg, K., Høgset, A., Bown, S.G., and MacRobert, A.J., Photophysical and photobiological properties of a sulfonated chlorin photosensitiser TPCS(2a) for photochemical internalisation (PCI), *Photochem. Photobiol. Sci.*, 12, 519–526, 2013. Reproduced by permission of The Royal Society of Chemistry.) (c) Photomicrographs of HeLa cells incubated with LysoTracker blue (LTB) and MB and overlap. Chemical structure of MB. (Reprinted from *Free Radic. Biol. Med.*, 51, Oliveira, C.S., Turchiello, R., Kowaltowski, A.J., Indig, G.L., and Baptista, M.S., Major determinants of photoinduced cell death: Subcellular localization versus photosensitization efficiency, 824–833. Copyright 2011, with permission from Elsevier.)

a tendency to accumulate in mitochondria and are not lipophilic enough to accumulate in Golgi and RE. Therefore, accumulation in lysossomes occur and they are able to cause specific damage in their membranes. This has been shown to occur for several amphiphilic negatively charged PSs such as meso-tetraphenyl porphyrin disulfonate (TPPS$_{2a}$), meso-tetraphenyl chlorin disulfonate (TPCS$_{2a}$), and aluminum phthalocyanine disulfonate (AlPcS$_{2a}$) (Berg and Moan 1994, 1997; Boyle and Dolphin 1996; Kessel and Morgan 1993; Kessel et al. 2000; Leach et al. 1993; Moan et al. 1992; Mroz et al. 2009; Reiners et al. 2002; Tsai et al. 2015; Woodburn et al. 1991). These properties have been used to induce the release of endocytosed therapeutic agents after a photochemically induced rupture of the endosomes/lysosomes vesicles, a technique called photochemical internalization (PCI) (Berg et al. 2007; Norum et al. 2009).

Fluorescence lifetime imaging microscopy (FLIM) has also provided interesting data concerning PS intracellular localization. Fluorescence lifetimes are sensitive to intermolecular interactions and changes on the

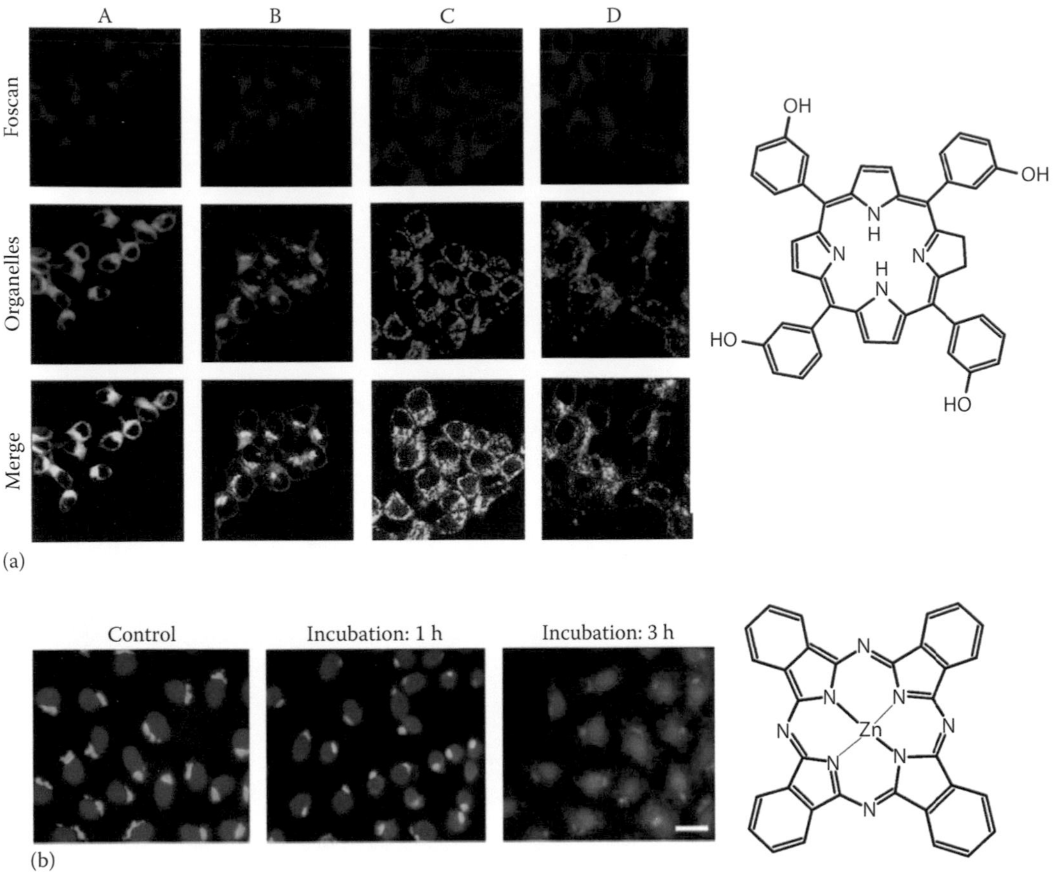

(a)

(b)

Figure 9.4 Fluorescence images of PSs that accumulate in Golgi and RE. (a) Chemical structure of Foscan® and subcellular localization in MCF-7 cells. 1 μg/mL Foscan® (red, column A, B, C, and D) with 125 μg/mL Lucifer yellow (green, column A) which staining lysosomes, 5 μM Rh123 (green, column B), which label mitochondria, 4 μM BODIPY® FL C_5-ceramide (green, column C) that stain Golgi apparatus and 2 μg/mL DiOC6 (green, column D) for ER labeling. (Reprinted by permission from Macmillan Publishers Ltd. *Br. J. Cancer*, Teiten, M.-H., Bezdetnaya, L., Morlière, P., Santus, R., and Guillemin, F., Endoplasmic reticulum and Golgi apparatus are the preferential sites of Foscan® localisation in cultured tumour cells, 88(1), 146–152. Copyright 2003.) (b) Chemical structure and localization in HeLa cells of zinc-phthalocyanine (ZnPc). Photomicrographs of HeLa cells processed for indirect immunofluorescence for golgin-130 (GM130) with Hoechst-33258 (H-33258) under UV and blue excitation light (overlay image). (Republished from Soriano, J. et al., *Int. J. Mol. Sci.*, 15(12), 22772, 2014. With permission of Multidisciplinary Digital Publishing Institute [MDPI].)

microenvironment of the excited state. For that reason, the image profile of PS fluorescence lifetime allows to monitor the binding states of PS and their microenvironments. For example, Yeh et al. followed the fluorescence lifetime of Photofrin® as a function of the incubation time and were able to observe localization in different intracellular components in MatLyLu (MLL) cell line (Figure 9.5a). They observed that Photofrin® is located at the cell membrane after a short-term incubation (1 h), showing a short fluorescence lifetime. With longer incubation times (2 h), other localization sites are accessible (cytoplasm and mitochondria) and longer lifetimes arise (Yeh et al. 2012). Other works have also reported that PS fluorescence lifetime significantly changes when the PS is bound to intracellular components. As examples, Photofrin®, 5-ALA, and Foscan® fluorescence lifetimes are all shortened in vitro compared to those in solution (Connelly et al. 2001; Kress et al. 2003; Lassalle et al. 2008; Russell and Diamond 2008). A similar experiment was performed by Wang and coworkers with TPCS$_{2a}$, obtaining lifetime values compatible with its localization environment, that is, lysosome membranes (Figure 9.5b).

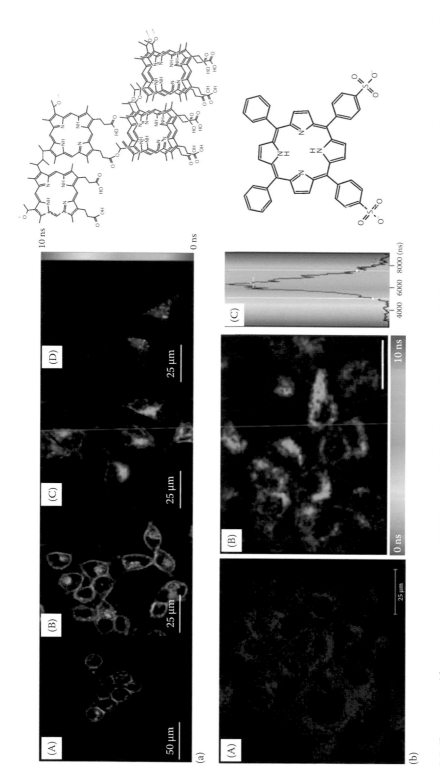

Figure 9.5 Fluorescence lifetime imaging microscopy (FLIM) to investigation of subcellular localization. (a) Chemical structure of Photofrin® and time-lapse average lifetime images of Photofrin® (20 μg/mL) uptake by MLL cells between 1 and 18 h. (A) The image shows Photofrin® uptake by the cell membrane at 1 h of incubation; (B) 2–4 h of incubation, (C) Photofrin® has localized at the perinuclear region after 6 h of incubation and (D) after 18 h of incubation. (Republished from Yeh, S.-C.A. et al., *Theranostics*, 2(9), 817, 2012. With permission of Theranostics.) (b) TPCS$_{2a}$ in HN5 cells after 18 h incubation. (A) Two-photon fluorescence confocal image ($\lambda_{excitation}$ = 840 nm); (B) color-coded FLIM image of same field as (a); (C) lifetime histogram (ns) measured from FLIM image (B). Scale bars represent 25 μm. Structure of TPCS$_{2a}$ is represented at the bottom. (From Wang, J.T.-W., Berg, K., Høgset, A., Bown, S.G., and MacRobert, A.J., Photophysical and photobiological properties of a sulfonated chlorin photosensitiser TPCS(2a) for photochemical internalisation (PCI), *Photochem. Photobiol. Sci.*, 12, 519–526, 2013. Reproduced by permission of The Royal Society of Chemistry.)

9.3 PS LOCALIZATION AND CELL DEATH MECHANISMS

The fact that PSs are able to localize in specific organelles and that this restricts photoinduced damage to the sub-microenvironment where the PS is localized indicates that it may be possible to identify differences in the cell responses depending on the PS structure. We have organized this part of the chapter by initially defining the consequences of causing specific damage in each of the main three main sites of intracellular location, that is, mitochondria, lysosome, and ER/Golgi. Afterward, we will discuss the methods that have been used to identify and study the main types of cell death, that is, necrosis, apoptosis, and autophagy. We have not considered the cytoplasmic membrane among these organelles because, as mentioned earlier, damage on this membrane will simply end up causing cells to die by necrosis. Necrosis is also the major type of cell death when there is extensive damage in any intracellular organelle because cells cannot keep up with the ATP production in order to engage in programed mechanisms of cell death (Figure 9.6).

In spite of being well accepted that mitochondria are key organelles to trigger apoptotic cell death, it is noteworthy that mitochondrial photodamage can induce not only cell death by apoptosis but also can trigger necrosis or autophagy (Figure 9.6a). When high PDT doses (PS and light) are applied, the onset of mitochondrial permeability can arise in virtually all cellular mitochondria, causing ATP levels to plum. Under these conditions, neither autophagy nor apoptosis can progress, and the cell will perish in an uncontrolled manner (Pavani et al. 2012). Apoptotic cell death can be triggered when the photodamage causes partial membrane permeabilization, but high enough to allow the dissipation of the inner membrane transmembrane potential ($\Delta\psi$) and the release of apoptosis-related proteins, such as cytochrome c, apoptosis-inducing factor,

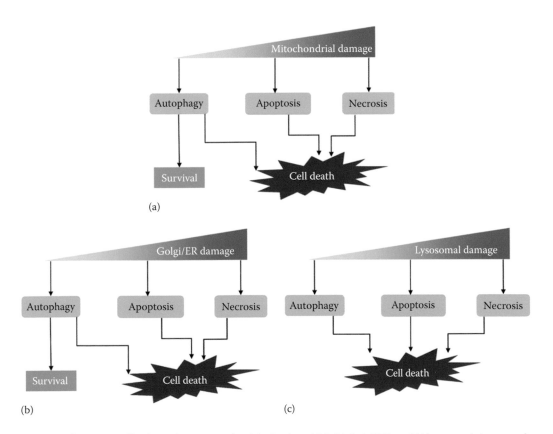

Figure 9.6 Illustration of biological response after (a) mitochondrial, (b) Golgi/ER, and (c) lysosomal damage after PDT at different doses.

second mitochondria-derived activator of caspases, and certain procaspases from the intermembrane space (Oleinick et al. 2002). Although direct mitochondria damage can clearly trigger apoptosis (Deda et al. 2013; Luo and Kessel 1997), signals from other photodamaged sites can also converge to mitochondria, leading to permeabilization of mitochondrial membranes (Oleinick et al. 2002).

With low PDT doses, limited mitochondrial permeability may also trigger autophagy (in this case, mitophagy) to protect cells by recycling damaged mitochondria as a repair mechanism. This protection system can fail and cause an opposite effect: autophagic cell death. Interventions that modulate the extent of mitochondrial permeability thus affect the relative amount of necrosis, apoptosis, and autophagy (Kim et al. 2007; Lemasters et al. 1998; Malhi et al. 2006; Scherz-Shouval and Elazar 2007).

The impact of PDT on the Golgi/ER apparatus has been less considered than the damage in mitochondria, but can also trigger controlled mechanisms of cell death if the damage is not too large (Figure 9.6a; Fabris et al. 2001; Matroule et al. 1999; Morlière et al. 1998; Teiten et al. 2003). PSs such as hypericin and that 9-capronyloxytetrakis-(methoxyethyl)-porphycene (CPO), which localize mainly in the ER, photodamage this organelle causing release of Ca^{2+} from the ER and initiation of apoptotic mechanism (Agostinis et al. 2004; Almeida et al. 2004; Buytaert et al. 2006a, 2007; Kessel et al. 2005; Oleinick et al. 2002). For example, hypericin and pheophorbide-a methyl ester PDT mediates caspase-dependent apoptosis, respectively, in mouse myeloma and nasopharyngeal carcinoma cells. None of these PSs have been shown to specifically localize in mitochondria (Xu and Leung 2006; Zhang et al. 2015). In fact, it was shown that ER damage by PDT can also trigger intrinsic apoptosis by accumulation of misfolded proteins and the breakage of calcium homeostasis (Marchal et al. 2007). A recently synthesized PS, chlorin-PEG-folate conjugate, primarily localizes in mitochondria and ER and triggers apoptosis after PDT (Li et al. 2015). Agostinis's group reported that ER photodamage by PDT with hypericin can also trigger autophagic cell death in Bax$^{-/-}$ Bak$^{-/-}$ double-knockout cells (Buytaert et al. 2006a,b, 2007a). As in mitochondria, depending on the intensity ER damage, it is also possible to induce reticulophagy to protect cells from the ER damaged or trigger autophagic cell death.

Lysosomes are also susceptible to be damaged by PSs that accumulate on it (Figure 9.6c). A direct consequence of lysosome photodamage is the rupture of its membrane and the release of proteolytic enzymes to the cytosol. High PDT doses cause massive lysosomal breakdown, which may induce cytosolic acidification, resulting in necrotic cell death (Boya and Kroemer 2008; Guicciardi et al. 2004), whereas low PDT doses can induce apoptosis and/or autophagy. Protease release from lysosomal lumen can cleave proapoptotic proteins such as procaspase-3 and Bid, thus activating the apoptotic pathway (Guicciardi et al. 2004; Kessel and Luo 2001; Kessel et al. 1997; Stoka et al. 2001). Also, there are some controversial proposals about the consequences of the autophagical process when PSs causes partial or selective photodamage in lysosomes. The proposal of Hung et al., which they named lysophagy, implies that damage to lysosomes induced by PDT activates autophagic processes to remove these damaged organelles (Hung et al. 2013), while Racoma et al. showed that thymoquinone selectively inhibits the clonogenicity of glioblastoma cells as compared to normal human astrocytes by inducing lysosome membrane permeabilization and subsequent translocation of lysosomal hydrolases to the cytosol (Racoma et al. 2013). It has also been reported that damage in lysosomes can cause the interruption of the autophagic flux since these organelles provide suitable environment (acidic organelles and specific enzymes in the digestion process) for autophagy (Inguscio et al. 2012).

Later, we will describe the microscopic techniques that can be used to identify and study necrosis, apoptosis, and autophagy. We will provide just a brief description on the techniques that can be used for necrosis and apoptosis and direct the reader to other reviews (Castano et al. 2005; Mroz et al. 2011; Oleinick and Evans 1998). In terms of autophagy, we will provide more in-depth description of the techniques, given that reviews providing this information for PDT-induced cell death are still missing.

9.3.1 NECROSIS AND APOPTOSIS

Cell death by necrosis presents some specific characteristics: lack of capacity to maintain ATP steady-state concentration, cell and organelle swelling, and loss of the plasma membrane integrity (Buytaert et al. 2007b; Festjens et al. 2006; Golstein and Kroemer 2007). Necrosis is usually considered accidental or uncontrolled though recent evidences indicate the existence of sequential steps that could characterize necrosis as a programed cell death mechanism under certain circumstances (Duprez et al. 2009; Golstein and Kroemer 2007).

In order to define cells that suffered enough to engage in necrosis, several authors used the permeabilization of the cytoplasmic membrane just after the photodamage as a reliable way to quantify the amount of necrosis (Deda et al. 2013; Pavani et al. 2009, 2012). Several dyes can be used to evaluate the cytoplasmic membrane permeabilization, such as propidium iodide (PI) and trypan blue. For example, Deda and coworkers showed that 5,10,15-triphenyl-20-(3-*N*-methylpyridinium-yl)porphyrin when delivered to the cell in a DMSO solution accumulates mainly in the cytoplasmic membrane, causing a quick damage to cell membrane and, consequently, necrotic cell death (Figure 9.7a(A); Deda et al. 2013). Interestingly, when the same porphyrin is delivered to cells encapsulated in polymeric nanocapsules, the PS no longer localizes in the cytoplasmic membrane, but instead the particle is internalized by endocytosis and the PS is directly delivered to intracellular environment. Under this condition, light irradiation causes apoptosis with exposition of phosphatidylserine in the cytoplasmic membrane, which can be quantified by the reaction with Annexin, Figure 9.7a(B); Deda et al. 2013).

Apoptosis is a complex ATP-requiring controlled mechanism of cell death. It can be initiated by external (extrinsic) and internal (intrinsic) signals. A signaling cascade results in mounting of protein complexes, the apoptosomes, which are responsible to disassemble several cellular structures. The important point of no return is the activation of caspases (cysteine-dependent aspartate-directed proteases). A series of morphological and biochemical changes is characteristic of this process and can be used to identify and quantify the apoptotic

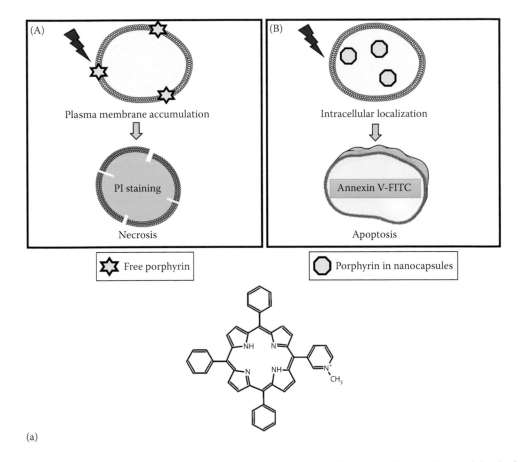

(a)

Figure 9.7 Characterization of necrosis and apoptosis process. (a) (A) cells labeled with propidium iodide 3 h after PDT mediated by 3MMe-DMSO; (B) cells labeled with annexin V-FITC 3 h after incubation with porphyrin encapsulated in nanocapsules. Chemical structure of porphyrin represented bottom. (Republished from Deda, D.K. et al., *J. Biomed. Nanotechnol.*, 9(8), 1307, 2013. With permission of American Scientific Publishers.)   (*Continued*)

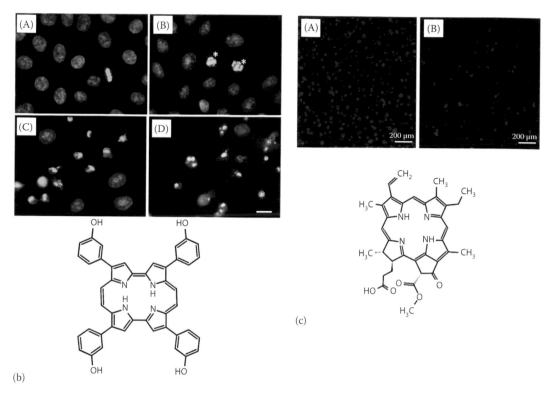

Figure 9.7 (Continued) Characterization of necrosis and apoptosis process. (b) H-33258 staining. (A) Control cells (without any treatment), (B) cells stained immediately after treatment (5 μM liposomal m-THPPo, 3.5 J/cm²), *aberrant mitosis. (C) Cells stained 6 h after treatment and (D) cells stained 24 h after treatment. On the bottom, chemical structure of m-THPPo. (Reprinted from *Biochim. Biophys. Acta—General Subjects*, 1830, Soriano, J., García-Díaz, M., Mora, M., Sagristá, M.L., Nonell, S., Villanueva, A., Stockert, J.C., and Cañete, M., Liposomal temocene (m-THPPo) photodynamic treatment induces cell death by mitochondria-independent apoptosis, 4611–4620. Copyright 2013, with permission from Elsevier.) (c) Collapse of mitochondrial membrane potential indicated with Rh123. (A) untreated PC-3 cells; (B) 30 min after PDT treatment with PhA. On the bottom, chemical structure of PhA. (Reprinted from *Photodiagn. Photodyn. Ther.*, 10, Xu, D.D., Lam, H.M., Hoeven, R., Xu, C.B., Leung, A.W.N., and Cho, W.C.S., Photodynamic therapy induced cell death of hormone insensitive prostate cancer PC-3 cells with autophagic characteristics, 278–287. Copyright 2013. with permission from Elsevier.)

process of cell death (Neves and Brindle 2014). The most common morphological changes are DNA fragmentation, chromatin condensation, phosphatidylserine exposure in the plasma membrane (as exemplified by the work of Deda et al. 2013), membrane blebbing though with maintenance of its integrity until the final stages of the process, and pyknosis and phagocytosis by neighboring cells (Buytaert et al. 2007b; Koff et al. 2015; Mroz et al. 2011). Fluorescence microscopy with Hoechst 33258 for nuclear staining can show the presence of apoptotic nuclei (Soriano et al. 2013; Xu and Leung 2006; Zhou et al. 2012). For example, by using Hoechst 33258, Soriano et al. showed normal nuclei, apoptotic cells, and apoptotic bodies at 0, 6, and 24 h, respectively, after a m-tetra (hydroxyphenyl) porphycene (m-THPPo)-PDT protocol (Soriano et al. 2013). Note that normal cells display weak fluorescence while apoptotic cells show increased bright fluorescence and some typical apoptotic bodies (Figure 9.7b). Another remarkable event on apoptosis process induced by PDT is the loss of mitochondrial transmembrane inner potential. As example, Figure 9.7c demonstrated the decrease of Rh123 fluorescence intensity after PDT treatment representing the collapse of mitochondrial membrane potential (Xu et al. 2013).

Biochemically, one can quantify different apoptotic markers by western blot or immunocytochemistry, such as presence of Bcl-2 and other antiapoptotic proteins, release of cytochrome *c*, and presence of APAF-1, procaspase-9, and other downstream caspases (Duprez et al. 2009; Mroz et al. 2011). There are also strong evidences that apoptosis can occur in complete absence of caspase activation, mainly by the action of other proteases such as cathepsins and calpains, being important to study this proteins as well (Foghsgaard et al. 2001; Johansson et al. 2010).

9.3.2 AUTOPHAGY

Autophagy is a catabolic process fundamental for the maintenance of cell homeostasis, in which lysosomes digest cellular contents, as organelles and proteins. Mechanistically, in a first step, a membrane surrounds the structure to be degraded, forming a structure called autophagosome. Next, fusion with a lysosome forms the autolysosome, where the autophagic content is degraded. The steady-state formation and degradation of these structures is called autophagic flux (Figure 9.8). Being a dynamic process, autophagy is subject to positive and negative modulation (Klionsky et al. 2008). Therefore, autophagosome accumulation can be a result of autophagy activation (increased autophagosome production) or inhibition (reduced autophagic flux, inhibition of the fusion of autophagosomes with lysosomes or loss of degradative function on lysosomes). Although autophagy acts in a basal level, driven by the Atg proteins (AuTophaGy-related), a variety of cell stressors can activate it (Shimizu et al. 2014). Depending on the extension of the autophagy activation, it can lead to cell death. This is still a controversial issue, and people publishing on this area may experience different opinions on this issue. Morphologically, autophagy in dying cells is characterized by accumulation of autophagic vacuoles, with a functional and intact cytoskeleton until the late steps (Sun and Peng 2009).

The classical autophagy induction by starvation starts with mTOR inhibition allowing Atg1 interactions with Atg13 and 17, followed by Bcl-2 phosphorylation and Beclin-1 release, causing both autophagy induction and autophagosome formation. Then, two ubiquitin-like conjugation systems are associated to membrane elongation and autophagosome completion. The most known autophagy ubiquitin-like conjugation systems involves Atg4 protein, which mediates microtubule-associated protein 1 light chain 3 (LC3) to be cleaved generating LC3-I, which mainly locates in cytosol and reacts with phosphatidylethanolamine to form the lipidated form of LC3, also called LC3-II. In this reaction, Atg7 and Atg3 proteins are catalysts and the Atg5-Atg12-Atg16 complex is responsible to control the specificity of the LC3-I site of lipidation. LC3-II associates with autophagosome membranes. The autophagosome maturation ends up with its fusion with lysosome, which is assisted by the lysosome receptor proteins lysosomal-associated protein LAMP1 and LAMP2. Therefore, LC3-II can be used as a reliable autophagic marker (Duprez et al. 2009; Inguscio et al. 2012; Kang et al. 2011; Mizushima 2004).

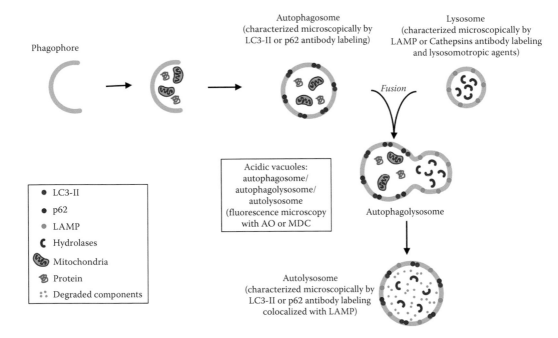

Figure 9.8 Main steps of the autophagic flux.

The other known autophagy ubiquitin-like conjugation system is the sequestration of damaged intracellular materials by autophagy, which is mainly driven by the protein P62, also known as sequestosome 1 (SQSTM1). When recruited, P62 aggregates the ubiquitinated substrates in larger units. Since p62 protein possesses a short LC3 interaction region, the direct interaction makes this protein to localize at the autophagosome and, consequently, the autophagosome membrane surrounds the aggregated substrate. During the lysosome digestion, p62 is also specifically degraded by autophagy (Johansen and Lamark 2011; Komatsu et al. 2007; Pankiv et al. 2007). The amount of p62/SQSTM1 increases when autophagy is inhibited and decreases when autophagy is induced. Therefore, accumulation of p62 has been used as a marker for inhibition of autophagy or defects in autophagic degradation (Bjørkøy et al. 2005; Klionsky et al. 2012; Komatsu et al. 2012; Mizushima and Yoshimori 2007; Rusten and Stenmark 2010).

The first observations of PDT causing cell death with autophagy were in apoptosis-deficient cells (Buytaert et al. 2006a; Dewaele et al. 2011; Kessel et al. 2006; Oleinick et al. 2009). In apoptosis-competent cells, Kessel and coworkers reported that PDT induced autophagy as a way to protect cells from photodamage (Kessel and Reiners 2007a). They also showed that the cytoprotective role of autophagy depends on the dose of PDT. At high PDT doses, inhibition of autophagosome formation occurs in both wild-type and Atg7 knockdown cells, showing apoptotic morphological features (Donohue et al. 2011). However, in low-dose PDT, it was observed that autophagy offers protection from the phototoxic effects of PDT (Andrzejak et al. 2011a; Kessel and Arroyo 2007). It was recently reported that PDT with rose bengal, Foscan®, or 9-capronyloxytetrakis(methoxyethyl)porphycene activates both apoptosis and autophagy at different time points by damaging different organelles (Kessel et al. 2006; Lihuan et al. 2014; Panzarini et al. 2011; Sasnauskiene et al. 2009).

There are other examples in the literature with different types of PSs leading to autophagy as cytoprotection mechanism after PDT (Andrzejak et al. 2011b; Kessel and Arroyo 2007; Kessel and Reiners 2007b). Nonetheless, Oleinick's group has found that blocking autophagy increased the survival of MCF-7 cells after low-dose PDT and increased the concentration needed to kill cells on the dose-response curve, indicating that autophagy favors cell death (Xue et al. 2015a). They also showed that the kinetic of apoptosis/autophagy switch depends on cell type, light dose, and PS type and concentration (Xue et al. 2015b).

PS that localizes in mitochondria, ER, and lysosomes are involved in PDT-induced autophagy (François et al. 2011; Kessel and Reiners 2007a). In general, ER and/or mitochondria photodamage triggers a pro-survival autophagic response (reticulophagy and/or mitophagy) to recycle injured organelles (Kessel and Arroyo 2007; Kessel and Reiners 2007a); conversely, PS localizing and damaging lysosomes block autophagosome processing, leading to autophagy inhibition. Lihuan et al. demonstrated that chlorophyllin e4 was located in both lysosome and mitochondria, and chlorophyllin e4-PDT induced autophagy in bladder cancer cells. In this case, photosensitized cells pretreated with the typical autophagy inhibitors, either 3-methyladenine or bafilomycin A1, exhibited much lower cell viability and higher apoptotic cell death, indicating that autophagy played a pro-survival role (Du et al. 2014; Lihuan et al. 2014).

Although PDT protocols employing lysosomal PS, such as NPe6 (Reiners et al. 2002), $TPPS_{1-4}$ (Berg et al. 1990), and $AlPcS_{2-4}$ (Moan et al. 1992), usually favor autophagic cell death, some authors described that lysosomes photodamage caused release of lysosomal proteases, which could either directly and/or indirectly activate caspases as a consequence of mitochondrial damage, resulting in apoptosis (Kessel et al. 2000). However, permeabilized or damaged lysosomes lead to the release of proteases and/or alkalinization of the organelle in such way that it would markedly affect autophagosome-lysosome fusion and/or degradation of the cargo contained in the autolysosomes (Reiners et al. 2002). PDT protocols with PSs that localize in lysosomes most likely inhibit autophagy, removing any kind of cytoprotection mechanism, and consequently collaborating to cell death (Berg and Moan 1994; Moan et al. 1992). The extent to which this blocking in autophagic flux is affected by the relative cytotoxicity of PS with accumulates in lysosomes is still unknown.

Autophagic cell death is a process that is still not well understood at the molecular level as apoptosis is, and therefore there are fewer options available to identify and study this process. Electron microscopy, fluorescence microscopy, western blot, and fluorescence-activated cell sorting are techniques commonly used to identify and to initially characterize autophagic flux. Although as many techniques as possible should be used to characterize autophagy induced by PDT, fluorescence microscopy itself offers the opportunity to perform a detailed evaluation. We propose a sequence of experimental work that starts by evaluating the accumulation of acidic vacuoles, characterizing specific proteins on these vacuoles and determining the pro-survival or the pro-death roles by using specific inhibitors.

Lysosomotropic agents such as AO and neutral red can be used to evaluate intracellular acidic vacuoles. AO is a metachromatic weak base that has green fluorescence in cytoplasmic environment, but when retained in acidic organelles become charged (AOH⁺), presenting red fluorescence. An example of visualization of acidic vacuoles stained by AO is presented in Figure 9.9a, where it is possible to observe the difference between untreated and PDT-treated cells. A significant increase in red/green fluorescence ratio was observed in cells after PDT treatment with hematoporphyrin (HP) compared to the control (Kim et al. 2014). Other authors also demonstrated similar observations using AO staining in cells after PDT treatment (Du et al. 2014; Kim et al. 2014; Krmpot et al. 2010; Lihuan et al. 2014; Xu et al. 2013).

Monodansylcadaverine (MDC) is a fluorescent compound proposed as a tracer for autophagic vacuoles (Biederbick et al. 1995). MDC is also a lysosomotropic dye, with green fluorescence when loaded to acidic compartments. Neutralization of these compartments leads to swift loss of MDC staining and/or lack of MDC uptake. Consequently, subcellular fractionation analyses demonstrated that MDC-positive structures contained lysosomal enzymes, but not early/late endosomal markers, proposing that MDC could be a specific marker for autophagic vacuoles (Biederbick et al. 1995; Mizushima 2004). Many authors have shown a significant increase in the number of MDC-labeled autophagic vacuoles after PDT treatment (Ahn et al. 2013; François et al. 2011; Kessel et al. 2006; Lihuan et al. 2014; Lin et al. 2015; Xue et al. 2015a,b). As an example, Figure 9.9b presents images of Ce6-PDT-treated cells showing a clear enhancement of punctuated vacuoles 8 h post PDT (Xue et al. 2015a).

The next step after observation of the accumulation of acidic vacuoles is their characterization. LC3-II is the most widely used among the several marker proteins for autophagosomes. LC3 can be marked by antibodies containing fluorescent probe or using green fluorescent protein (GFP) fused with LC3 protein (GFP-LC3), enabling observation of punctate signals under fluorescence microscopy. For example, Xu et al. used LC3-II primary antibody and characterized a significant increase of autophagic vacuoles formation after PhA-PDT treatment (Figure 9.9c; Xu et al. 2013). LC3 can also be co-localized with proteins found in mitochondria (e.g., CoxIV) or lysosome (LAMP II) in order to characterize the whole of the damage in this specific organelles (Kim et al. 2007; Rubio et al. 2012).

Although LC3 itself indicates the presence of autophagosomes, it does not provide information on kinetics of the autophagic flux. For example, accumulation of larger numbers of LC3 punctuation indicates either enhancement of autophagosome formation (induction) or a decrease in autophagosome turnover. If autophagosome-lysosome fusion is blocked, an elevated number of LC3 should be detected. In contrast, very rapid fusion of autophagosomes with lysosomes may result in a smaller number of LC3 dots, which would underestimate autophagic activity (Zhang et al. 2013).

The use of GFP-labeled cells has become more frequent in recent years. Similar to LC3-II, P62/SQSTM1 can either be marked by antibody containing fluorescent probes or by using GFP fused with p62 protein (GFP-p62). As an example, Donohue et al. showed elevated accumulation of P62 (Figure 9.10) in cells treated with bafilomycin and these punctuations co-localized with punctuation EGFP-LC3 as an indicative of undigested autophagosomes containing P62 cargo. By contrast, 4 h treatment with 10 μM verteporfin did not increase punctate P62 immunofluorescence, indicating that verteporfin does not induce P62 aggregate (Donohue et al. 2014). Oleinick's group used MCF-7 cells transfected with GFP-LC3 to determine the higher amount of GFP-LC3 punctuation after PDT treatment with phthalocyanine (Figure 9.10b; Xue et al. 2015b). Most of the scientists have been using LC3 proteins to characterize autophagy process in PDT protocols not only by using fluorescence microscopy, but also by western blot techniques (Bjørkøy et al. 2009; Dini et al. 2010; Lihuan et al. 2014; Luo et al. 2010; Palmeira-Dos-Santos et al. 2014; Xue et al. 2015a; Zhang et al. 2013).

The interaction between lysosomes and autophagosomes is crucial to complete the autophagic flux. This means that if fusion between the lysosome and the autophagosome is inhibited then incomplete

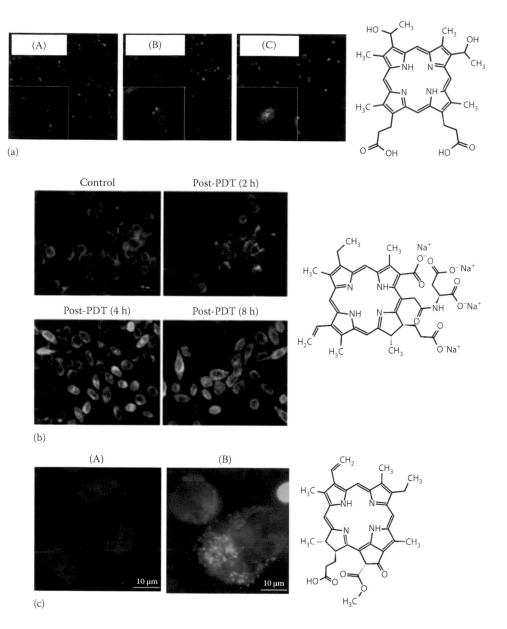

Figure 9.9 Autophagy investigation by fluorescence microscopy. (a) HP-PDT induced acidic vacuoles detection using acridine orange staining: (A) control, (B) 2 µM HP, and (C) 4 µM HP. On the right: Structure of HP. (From Kim, J., Lim, W., Kim, S., Jeon, S., Hui, Z., Ni, K., Kim, C., Im, Y., Choi, H., and Kim, O. Photodynamic therapy (PDT) resistance by PARP1 regulation on PDT-induced apoptosis with autophagy in head and neck cancer cells. *J. Oral Pathol. Med.* 2014. 43. 675–684. Copyright Wiley-VCH Verlag GmbH & Co. KGaA. Reproduced with permission.) (b) Staining of acidic vacuoles by MDC before and after (2, 4, and 8 h) PDT with chlorin-e6. On the right: Chemical structure of chlorin-e6. (Reprinted from *Photodiagn. Photodyn. Ther.*, 12, Xue, Q., Wang, X., Wang, P., Zhang, K., and Liu, Q., Role of p38MAPK in apoptosis and autophagy responses to photodynamic therapy with chlorin e6, 84–91. Copyright 2015b, with permission from Elsevier.) (c) Immunofluorescence analysis with LC3-II antibody. (A) Control; (B) PhA-PDT treatment. The labeled-LC3 are shown in green puncta fluorescence. On the right: chemical structure of PhA. (Reprinted from *Photodiagn. Photodyn. Ther.*, 10, Xu, D.D., Lam, H.M., Hoeven, R., Xu, C.B., Leung, A.W.N., and Cho, W.C.S., Photodynamic therapy induced cell death of hormone insensitive prostate cancer PC-3 cells with autophagic characteristics, 278–287. Copyright 2013, with permission from Elsevier.)

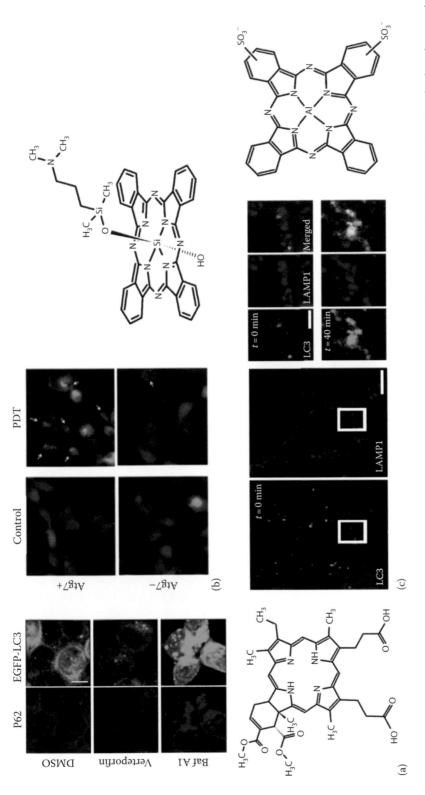

Figure 9.10 Observations of specific elements from the autophagic machinery. (a) Fluorescence images of MCF-7 EGFP-LC3 cells treated with p62 antibody and exposed to 0.1% DMSO, 10 µM verteporfin, or 100 nM bafilomycin A1. On the bottom: chemical structure of verteporfin. (Republished from Dougherty, T.J. et al., J. Natl. Cancer Instit., 90(12), 889, 1998. With authorization of the open access contract from Public Library of Science [PLoS].) (b) Cells were transiently transfected with GFP-LC3 construct, then treated with 150 nM pc 4 (under 200 mJ/cm²) and observed under microscopy. Arrows in a representative fluorescence micrograph indicate the autolysosomes/autophagosomes in PDT-treated cells. On the right: chemical structure of Pc 4. (Republished from Xue, L.-Y. et al., Autophagy, 6(2), 248, 2015a. With permission from Taylor & Francis.) (c) Photomicrographs of HeLa cell expressing EGFP-LC3-II and LAMP1-RFP after PDT-treatment with AlPcS$_{2a}$. White square region selected compare co-localization between LC3 and LAMP1 after 0 and 40 min of PDT-treatment. On the right: chemical structure of AlPcS$_{2a}$. (Reprinted by permission from Macmillan Publishers Ltd. Nat. Commun., Hung, Y.-H., Chen, L.M.-W., Yang, J.-Y., and Yang, W.Y., Spatiotemporally controlled induction of autophagy-mediated lysosome turnover, 4(2111), 1–7. Copyright 2013.)

autophagy would occur. While this scenario has not been extensively studied in PDT protocols, dysfunction in autophagosomal–lysosome fusion may prove to be a critical aspect of the autophagy process. For this reason, autophagy studies often employ probes that allow simultaneous visualization of autophagosomes and lysosomes within the same preparation. In order to visualize the fusion between autophagosomes and lysosomes, some reports use autophagosome markers such as LC3 and P62 (as mentioned earlier) in combination with lysosomal markers, such as fluorescent proteins that target lysosomes (Kim et al. 2008), antibodies against resident enzymes of the lysosome, such as cathepsins (Kim et al. 2008) or LAMP (Dolman et al. 2013; Pankiv et al. 2007). As an example, Hung et al. used images of co-localization between EGFP-LC3II and LAMP1-RFP after 40 min of AlPcS$_{2a}$-PDT treatment (Figure 9.10c) in order to demonstrate that autophagy induced by PDT matured into autolysosomes (Hung et al. 2013).

9.4 CONCLUSION AND FUTURE DIRECTIONS

PDT can mainly result in three cell death pathways: necrosis, apoptosis, and autophagy. It is known that the biological response of PDT is strongly related to the subcellular target of PS. It is common to associate PS localized in plasma membrane to necrosis as well as PS localized in mitochondria to apoptosis. However, parameters such as PDT dose also regulate how the PDT-treated cells respond. Necrosis and apoptosis are pathways well described for the cellular outcome after PDT, and recently autophagic cell death has also been characterized as a mode of cell death in PDT. Autophagy is defined as a protective mechanism to degrade and recycle damaged or aged organelles and proteins. However, it can also be a mechanism of cell death when it occurs in an unbalanced manner (too much induction or flux blocked), mainly in cells that are apoptosis-deficient. Considering that cancer cells are often resistant to death by apoptosis (Mohammad et al. 2015), autophagic cell death can be a good strategy to improve the efficiency of PDT to cancer treatment. It is also noteworthy that cancer cells have a higher level of autophagic flux if compared to normal cells (Mohammad et al. 2015; Racoma et al. 2013), so that impairing the balance of this protective mechanism in tumor cells (by excessive induction or inhibition) can lead to an efficient removal of unwanted cells. Despite the fact that the role of autophagy (cytoprotection or death induction) in clinical PDT is still in its "infancy", defining how to modulate autophagy toward cell death will hopefully result in the design of better PDT protocols, which could have wider applications as a cancer therapeutic modality. For this, it is necessary to understand which targets and PDT doses are necessary. Adding to the same principle of specifically-designed PDT protocols, we should keep in mind that because the intracellular location of the PS is not a very well-defined intrinsic property of the PS and may change with cell type and concentration, this also may happen with the cell death mechanism. Not only eukaryotic cells are involved in programed cell death but also prokaryotes, so that identifying ways to trigger one or the other mechanism of cell death may also work for antimicrobial PDT (Dai et al. 2009; Demidova and Hamblin 2004, 2005). We are confident that learning specific details of the interplay between the different mechanisms of programed cell death will allow our society to use light to trigger specifically programed ways to induce/force unwanted cells to die without causing damage to surrounding cells.

Fluorescence microscopy is a technique suitable to visualize organelles providing important subcellular information of PS localization and biological consequences of photodamage such as studying cell death mechanism. For this reason, different labeling methods can be used. In Section 9.5, we described selected fluorescence microscopy protocols as tool to evaluate subcellular localization and cell death mechanisms with focus on autophagy. All the methodologies are described according to the cited references.

9.5 EXPERIMENTAL PROTOCOLS

Next we describe protocols that can be used in the identification intracellular sites of localization of PSs, and in the initial studies of apoptotic and/or autophagic mechanisms of programed cell death.

9.5.1 SUBCELLULAR LOCALIZATION

9.5.1.1 INTENSITY-BASED FLUORESCENCE MICROSCOPY

PS and probes that target specific organelles of interest are incubated simultaneously in cells and the co-localization between their emission is evaluated. Rh123 or MitoTracker® can be used as mitochondria-specific fluorescent probes; LY or LysoTracker® as lysosome-specific probes, DAPI, Hoechst (33342 or 33258) as nucleus-specific probes, 3,3'-dihexyloxacarbocyanine iodide ($DiOC_6$) as a probe for ER, and N-((4-(4,4-difluoro-5-(2-thienyl)-4-bora-3a,4a-diaza-s-indacene-3-yl)phenoxy)acetyl)sphingosine (Bodipy® TR Ceramide) as a Golgi apparatus-specific probe. Cells are seeded (1×10^4 cells/mL) in culture medium as monolayers over 35 mm Petri dishes containing glass coverslips, which can be used for microscopy analysis. Cells are incubated with low concentration of PS (10^{-9} to 10^{-6} range) during several hours (typically 3 h), washed with phosphate-buffered saline (PBS) and then incubated with organelle-specific probes (hundreds of nanomolar to few micromolars) at 37°C and 5% CO_2. For staining mitochondria, incubation can be performed with Rh123 for 30 min; for Golgi apparatus, cells can be incubated with BODIPYs FL C5-ceramide for 15 min; for ER cells can be incubated with $DiOC_6$ for 15 min; and for lysosomes, cells can be incubated overnight with LY. At the end of double staining, cells are washed with culture medium containing 25 mM HEPES and samples are prepared for microscopic observation using an objective with 63× magnification or larger and numerical aperture of 1.3 (Teiten et al. 2003).

The co-localization can be presented both by an overlay image and by a calculation value. For example, in cells stained both with Rh123 (green emission) and a PS presenting red emission, the presence of yellow spots in the combined image is indicative of co-localization. The tool to obtain combined image is very common in image analysis software. Merged images produce the mixed color if the fluorescence intensity of both probes is similar (Dunn et al. 2011).

There are many different algorithms to calculate co-localization, and the algorithm must be chosen depending on the image to be analyzed. Generally, Pearson's correlation coefficient is widely applicable for well-calibrated images while Manders' overlap coefficient is more reliable to analyze co-localization if the fluorescence intensity is different between the fluorophores (Zinchuk et al. 2007). Background removal before calculation is essential since it can cause up to 30% co-localization overestimation, especially in case of weak fluorescence. Techniques like filtering, deconvolution, and background correction can be used for this purpose.

9.5.1.2 FLUORESCENCE LIFETIME

FLIM provides a more precise way to define location of a PS since not only emission intensity but also emission lifetime can be used to obtain microscopic contrasts. Protocols similar to those described earlier can be used, but the measurement must be performed in a time-resolved confocal microscope, which is not available as widely as the classical confocal microcopies (Yeh et al. 2012).

9.5.2 NECROTIC VERSUS APOPTOTIC CELL DEATH WITH ANNEXIN V/PI

The identification of the specific mechanism of cell death needs extensive investigation with the use of several protocols. However, an initial identification of the fraction of dying cell populations going through necrosis or apoptosis can be performed by double staining with Annexin V and PI. Annexin V detects exposition to phosphatidylserine. PI labels necrotic cells due to the loss of membrane integrity, which allows PI penetration inside cells and intercalation in nuclear DNA (Neves and Brindle 2014). An example of this assay was described by Deda et al. HeLa cells are incubated with PS during 3 h. Cells are then washed with PBS and irradiated. Three hours after irradiation, cells are labeled with Annexin V-FITC (12 µg/mL) and PI (PI, 2 µg/mL). Cells undergoing apoptosis are identified by Annexin V-FITC green fluorescence and necrotic cells are detected by PI red fluorescence. Images can be registered using an epifluorescence or a confocal fluorescence microscope (Deda et al. 2013). This protocol can also be used in flow cytometers, which enhances considerably the reliability of the assay, since the number of cells analyzed is increased by several orders of magnitude.

9.5.2.1 IDENTIFYING APOPTOTIC NUCLEI

Since one of the morphological hallmarks of apoptosis is chromatin condensation, DNA-binding stains like 4′,6-diamidino-2-phenylindole, Hoechst, and others allow for the visualization of chromatin condensation. As an example, Soriano et al. observed nuclear morphology of apoptotic cells. After a PDT protocol, cells are fixed in cold methanol for 5 min, stained with 5 μg/mL H-33258 in distilled water for 2 min, and washed with distilled water. Cells are observed by fluorescence microscopy under UV/blue excitation (Soriano et al. 2013, 2014).

9.5.3 DETECTION OF AUTOPHAGY BY FLUORESCENCE MICROSCOPY

9.5.3.1 STAINING ACIDIC VACUOLES WITH AO

One simple way to assess the involvement of autophagy during cell death is to observe the state of the acidic vacuoles, which can be stained by metachromatic weak bases such as AO and neutral red, or any lysosomotropic dye such as lysotracker® family. AO, for example, becomes charged ($pK_a = 10.3$) in acidic organelles and is retained by a proton trapping mechanism. On excitation with blue light, AO dimers (formed in lysosomes because of high AO concentration) exhibit red fluorescence and AO monomers (spread in cytoplasm and nucleus) present green fluorescence (Terman and Kurz 2013). For this purpose, cells are seeded to reach approximately 70% of confluence and subjected to PDT protocol with the correct controls. Usually, the PDT protocol consists of incubating cells with tenths of nanomolar to few micromolars of PS during the defined time that usually is of few hours. Low solubility PS may need longer incubation periods, such as HP, which requires 24 h incubation. Few hours after irradiation (usually 1–6 h), cells are incubated with 1 μg/mL AO in a serum-free medium for 15 min. Then, AO is removed, cells are washed, and AO emission profile is observed by fluorescence microscopy. Usually, excitation is performed at the 450–490 nm range and emission is observed in wavelengths above 515 nm. The cytoplasm and nucleus of the stained cells fluoresces bright green and acidic autophagic vacuoles fluoresces bright red. The observation of accumulation of acidic vacuoles indicates the involvement of autophagy, which can be activated or inhibited (Kim et al. 2014). Inhibition leads to a strong accumulation AO-stained vacuoles. Other more precise methods should be used to definitively define the status of the autophagic flux (Klionsky et al. 2008; Mizushima 2004).

9.5.3.2 ACIDIC VACUOLES STAINING BY MDC

As mentioned before, there are some studies reporting increased autophagic activity using MDC as an autophagic marker. Lihuan et al. used MDC to prove the involvement of autophagy on PDT-induced cell death. Cells are seeded with 2.5×10^4 cells/cm² and incubated with different concentrations of PS for 2 h at 37°C. After incubation, cells are washed and irradiated with 650 nm laser light. Two hours after irradiation, cells are labeled with 50 mM MDC in culture medium during 15 min at 37°C. MDC fluorescence is observed by fluorescence microscopy, with excitation at 335 nm and emission at 498 nm (Lihuan et al. 2014). Similar to AO data analysis, MDC also detects autophagic acidic vacuoles by monitoring the distribution of the fluorescent dye MDC in such a way that the increase in the number of MDC-labeled green autophagic vacuoles indicates formation of autophagosomes and decrease of MDC-green fluorescence is related to a lack of acidic vacuoles. There are examples of other protocols in the literature, leading to similar results (Ahn et al. 2013; François et al. 2011; Kessel et al. 2006; Lihuan et al. 2014; Lin et al. 2015; Xue et al. 2015a,b).

9.5.3.3 IMMUNOFLUORESCENCE TO IDENTIFY SPECIFIC PROTEINS PRESENT IN AUTOPHAGOSOMES

An important approach to prove the role of autophagy in cell death is to stain specific autophagosome proteins; LC3-II is lipidated and incorporated in the autophagosomal membrane both upon induction or late inhibition of autophagy. The subcellular distribution of LC3 can be followed by immunofluorescence microscopy. A characteristic pattern of LC3 punctuation can be observed in autophagic cells stained with anti-LC3 antibodies. Alternatively, cells can also be manipulated to express a recombinant form of LC3 fused with GFP or other fluorescent protein. This recombinant form of LC3 is processed in the same way than endogenous LC3, and hence when these cells are submitted to an autophagic stimulus, they exhibit a characteristic pattern of GFP–LC3 punctuation. The classical protocol for this is to fix treated and control cells with 2% paraformaldehyde at 4°C overnight. After fixation, cells are permeabilized with 0.1% Triton X-100 for 15 min at room temperature and blocked with 0.5% bovine serum albumine (BSA) and 0.5% glycine in PBS (BSA buffer) for 1 h at room temperature. Cells are then incubated with anti-LC3 (1:200 diluted in BSA buffer) antibody for 1 h at room temperature. After being washed with BSA buffer, cells are incubated with Alexa Fluor 488 conjugated anti-rabbit antibody (1:1000 diluted in BSA buffer) for 1 h at room temperature. Slides are mounted and examined using a fluorescence microscope (Li et al. 2010).

Ji et al. used GFP-LC3 transfected PC12 cells to evaluate whether 5-ALA-mediated PDT induces autophagic cell death. To produce GFP-LC3, transfected PC12 cells are transfected with pGFP-LC3 plasmid into subconfluent PC12 cells using the Lipofectamine 2000 transfection kit. Twenty-four hours after transfection, cells are PDT treated with 1 mM ALA for 3 h and then exposed to various doses of light. In order to detect the redistribution of GFP-LC3 after ALA-PDT, GFP-LC3-transfected PC12 cells are fixed and co-stained with Hoechst 33342 to label the nucleus. After that, cells are washed with PBS and observed under microscope. The fluorescence images of LC3-GFP are recorded upon excitation by a 488 nm laser and the emission measured at 525 ± 25 nm using the fluorescence confocal microscope. A diode UV laser (405 nm) is used to excite Hoechst 33342 and the emitted fluorescence is detected at 445 ± 15 nm (Ji et al. 2010). It is important to keep in mind that there are many protocols to identify others proteins from autophagosomes or autolysosomes such as P62, LAMP1, LAMP2, cathepsins, and others, which can be very similar to the described one, changing with respect to their respective antibodies and also therefore to the microscopy observation conditions.

9.5.3.4 CO-LOCALIZATION OF ORGANELLES AND AUTOPHAGOSOMES

Defining the co-localization of autophagosomes with proteins found in organelles such as mitochondria, ER or lysosome may provide information about the cell environment that suffers from ROS stress generation as well as the progression of the autophagic flux in terms of its different steps (lysosome fusion, for example). This can be studied by simultaneous staining ER and/or mitochondria with elements of the autophagic machinery, for example, LAMP, LC3, and P62 (Dolman et al. 2013). As an example of this experiment, we mention the work of Rubio et al., which showed autophagic degradation of oxidatively damaged organelles after PDT with hypericin. For this, cells are transfected with pBabe-EGFP-LC3. 24–72 h after viral transfection and filtered through a 0.45 μm filter and used to transduce cells. For reticulophagy and mitophagy experiments, cells overexpressing GFP-LC3 are fixed at 6 and 16 h after treatment with 4% paraformaldehyde at 37°C, permeabilized with 0.1% Triton X-100 at room temperature for 20 min and blocked with PBS containing 5% BSA and 1% goat serum. Cells are then incubated with anti-calreticulin and anti-TOMM20 primary antibodies followed by incubation with Texas Red and AlexaFluor 647 secondary antibodies, respectively. Cells are stained with DAPI Prolong Gold antifade reagent (1 μg/mL) and kept overnight. Fluorescence images are acquired using a confocal inverted microscope using a Plan APO VC 60× oil immersion objective. At the end, the co-localization of organelles and autophagosomes is evaluated in each image. The co-localization between autophagosomes and organelles revealed that hypericin-PDT induces an initial reticulophagy followed by morphological changes in mitochondria network, which preceded mitophagy (Rubio et al. 2012).

ACKNOWLEDGMENTS

The authors acknowledge FAPESP for financial support with scholarship grants (2013/16532-1 and 2013/11640-0) and research grants (2012/50680-5 and 2013/07937-8). The authors are also grateful for teh NAP-Phototech and CNPq (304071/2014-5) fellowships.

REFERENCES

Agnello, M, G Morici, and AM Rinaldi. 2008. A method for measuring mitochondrial mass and activity. *Cytotechnology* **56**(3): 145–149. doi:10.1007/s10616-008-9143-2.

Agostinis, P, E Buytaert, H Breyssens, and N Hendrickx. 2004. Regulatory pathways in photodynamic therapy induced apoptosis. *Photochemical and Photobiological Sciences* **3**(8): 721–729. doi:10.1039/B315237E.

Ahn, MY, H-E Yoon, S-M Kwon, J Lee, S-K Min, Y-C Kim, S-G Ahn, and J-H Yoon. 2013. Synthesized pheophorbide a-mediated photodynamic therapy induced apoptosis and autophagy in human oral squamous carcinoma cells. *Journal of Oral Pathology and Medicine: Official Publication of the International Association of Oral Pathologists and the American Academy of Oral Pathology* **42**(1): 17–25. doi:10.1111/j.1600-0714.2012.01187.x.

Albani, BA, B Pena, NA Leed, NA De Paula, C Pavani, MS Baptista, KR Dunbar, and C Turro. 2014. Marked improvement in photoinduced cell death by a new tris-heteroleptic complex with dual action: Singlet oxygen sensitization and ligand dissociation. *Journal of the American Chemical Society* **136**(49):17095–17101.

Allison, RR, GH Downie, R Cuenca, XH Hu, CJ Childs, and CH Sibata. 2004. Photosensitizers in clinical PDT. *Photodiagnosis and Photodynamic Therapy* **1**: 27–42. doi:10.1016/S1572-1000(04)00007-9.

Almeida, RD, BJ Manadas, AP Carvalho, and CB Duarte. 2004. Intracellular signaling mechanisms in photodynamic therapy. *Biochimica et Biophysica Acta* **1704**(2): 59–86.

Andrzejak, M, M Price, and DH Kessel. 2011a. Apoptotic and autophagic responses to photodynamic therapy in 1c1c7 murine hepatoma cells. *Autophagy* **7**(9): 979–984. doi:10.4161/auto.7.9.15865.

Andrzejak, M, M Santiago, and D Kessel. 2011b. Effects of endosomal photodamage on membrane recycling and endocytosis. *Photochemistry and Photobiology* **87**(3): 699–706.

Baptista, MS and GL Indig. 1998. Effect of BSA binding on photophysical and photochemical properties of triarylmethane dyes. *Journal of Physical Chemistry B* **102**(98): 4678–4688. doi:10.1021/jp981185n.

Barbieri, E, M Battistelli, L Casadei, L Vallorani, G Piccoli, M Guescini, AM Gioacchini et al. 2011. Morphofunctional and biochemical approaches for studying mitochondrial changes during myoblasts differentiation. *Journal of Aging Research* **2011**: 845379.

Barr, FA and B Short. 2003. Golgins in the structure and dynamics of the Golgi apparatus. *Current Opinion in Cell Biology* **15**(4): 405–413. doi:10.1016/S0955-0674(03)00054-1.

Beckman, WC, SK Powers, JT Brown, GY Gillespie, DD Bigner, and JL Camps. 1987. Differential retention of rhodamine 123 by avian sarcoma virus-induced glioma and normal brain tissue of the rat in vivo. *Cancer* **59**(2): 266–270.

Berg, K, M Folini, L Prasmickaite, PK Selbo, A Bonsted, BØ Engesaeter, N Zaffaroni et al. 2007. Photochemical internalization: A new tool for drug delivery. *Current Pharmaceutical Biotechnology* **8**(6): 362–372. doi:10.2174/138920107783018354.

Berg, K and J Moan. 1994. Lysosomes as photochemical targets. *International Journal of Cancer* **59**(6): 814–822. doi:10.1002/ijc.2910590618.

Berg, K and J Moan. 1997. Lysosomes and microtubules as targets for photochemotherapy of cancer. *Photochemistry and Photobiology* **65**(3): 403–409. doi:10.1111/j.1751-1097.1997.tb08578.x.

Berg, K, A Western, JC Bommer, and J Moan. 1990. Intracellular localization of sulfonated meso-tetraphenylporphines in a human carcinoma cell line. *Photochemistry and Photobiology* **52**(3): 481–487. doi:10.1111/j.1751-1097.1990.tb01789.x.

Biederbick, A, HF Kern, and HP Elsässer. 1995. Monodansylcadaverine (MDC) is a specific in vivo marker for autophagic vacuoles. *European Journal of Cell Biology* **66**(1): 3–14.

Bjørkøy, G, T Lamark, A Brech, H Outzen, M Perander, A Øvervatn, H Stenmark, and T Johansen. 2005. p62/SQSTM1 forms protein aggregates degraded by autophagy and has a protective effect on huntingtin-induced cell death. *Journal of Cell Biology* **171**(4): 603–614. doi:10.1083/jcb.200507002.

Bjørkøy, G, T Lamark, S Pankiv, A Øvervatn, A Brech, and T Johansen. 2009. Monitoring autophagic degradation of p62/SQSTM1. *Methods in Enzymology*, **452**:181–197. doi:10.1016/S0076-6879(08)03612-4.

Boya, P and G Kroemer. 2008. Lysosomal membrane permeabilization in cell death. *Oncogene* **27**(50): 6434–6451.

Boyle, RW and D Dolphin. 1996. Structure and biodistribution relationships of photodynamic sensitizers. *Photochemistry and Photobiology* **64**(3): 469–485. doi:10.1111/j.1751-1097.1996.tb03093.x.

Bronshtein, I, M Afri, H Weitman, AA Frimer, KM Smith, and B Ehrenberg. 2004. Porphyrin depth in lipid bilayers as determined by iodide and parallax fluorescence quenching methods and its effect on photosensitizing efficiency. *Biophysical Journal* **87**(2): 1155–1164. doi:10.1529/biophysj.104.041434.

Buytaert, E, G Callewaert, N Hendrickx, L Scorrano, D Hartmann, L Missiaen, JR Vandenheede, I Heirman, J Grooten, and P Agostinis. 2006a. Role of endoplasmic reticulum depletion and multidomain proapoptotic BAX and BAK proteins in shaping cell death after hypericin-mediated photodynamic therapy. *The FASEB Journal* **20**(6): 756–758. doi:10.1096/fj.05-4305fje.

Buytaert, E, G Callewaert, JR Vandenheede, and P Agostinis. 2006b. Deficiency in apoptotic effectors bax and bak reveals an autophagic cell death pathway initiated by photodamage to the endoplasmic reticulum. *Autophagy* **2**(3): 238–240. doi:10.4161/auto.2730.

Buytaert, E, M Dewaele, and P Agostinis. 2007. Molecular effectors of multiple cell death pathways initiated by photodynamic therapy. *Biochimica et Biophysica Acta (BBA)—Reviews on Cancer* **1776**(1): 86–107. doi:10.1016/j.bbcan.2007.07.001.

Caetano, W, PS Haddad, R Itri, D Severino, VC Vieira, MS Baptista, AP Schröder, and CM Marques. 2007. Photo-induced destruction of giant vesicles in methylene blue solutions. *Langmuir* **23**(17): 1307–1314. doi:10.1021/la061510v.

Castano, AP, TN Demidova, and MR Hamblin. 2004. Mechanisms in photodynamic therapy: Part one—Photosensitizers, photochemistry and cellular localization. *Photodiagnosis and Photodynamic Therapy* **1**(2004): 279–293. doi:10.1016/S1572-1000(05)00007-4.

Castano, AP, TN Demidova, and MR Hamblin. 2005. Mechanisms in photodynamic therapy: Part two—Cellular signaling, cell metabolism and modes of cell death. *Photodiagnosis and Photodynamic Therapy* **2**(1 Spec. iss.): 1–23. doi:10.1016/S1572-1000(05)00030-X.

Celli, JP, N Solban, A Liang, SP Pereira, and T Hasan. 2011. Verteporfin-based photodynamic therapy overcomes gemcitabine insensitivity in a panel of pancreatic cancer cell lines. *Lasers in Surgery and Medicine* **43**(7): 565–574. doi:10.1562/2006-xxxxxx.s1.Celli.

Celli, JP, BQ Spring, I Rizvi, CL Evans, KS Samkoe, S Verma, BW Pogue, and T Hasan. 2010. Imaging and photodynamic therapy: Mechanisms, monitoring, and optimization. *Chemical Reviews* **110**(5): 2795–2838. doi:10.1021/cr900300p.

Chen, B, BW Pogue, PJ Hoopes, and T Hasan. 2006. Vascular and cellular targeting for photodynamic therapy. *Critical Reviews in Eukaryotic Gene Expression* **16**(4): 279–305.

Chen, JY, NK Mak, CM Yow, MC Fung, LC Chiu, WN Leung, and NH Cheung. 2000. The binding characteristics and intracellular localization of temoporfin (mTHPC) in myeloid leukemia cells: Phototoxicity and mitochondrial damage. *Photochemistry and Photobiology* **72**(4): 541–547. doi:10.1562/0031-8655(2000)0720541TBCAIL2.0.CO2.

Connelly, JP, SW Botchway, L Kunz, D Pattison, AW Parker, and AJ MacRobert. 2001. Time-resolved fluorescence imaging of photosensitiser distributions in mammalian cells using a picosecond laser line-scanning microscope. *Journal of Photochemistry and Photobiology A: Chemistry* **142**(2–3): 169–175. doi:10.1016/S1010-6030(01)00511-1.

Cottet-Rousselle, C, X Ronot, X Leverve, and JF Mayol. 2011. Cytometric assessment of mitochondria using fluorescent probes. *Cytometry Part A* **79A**(6): 405–425. doi:10.1002/cyto.a.21061.

Dai, T, YY Huang, and MR Hamblin. 2009. Photodynamic therapy for localized infections-state of the art. *Photodiagnosis and Photodynamic Therapy* **6**(3–4): 170–188. doi:10.1016/j.pdpdt.2009.10.008.

Deda, DK, C Pavani, E Caritá, MS Baptista, HE Toma, and K Araki. 2013. Control of cytolocalization and mechanism of cell death by encapsulation of a photosensitizer. *Journal of Biomedical Nanotechnology* **9**(8): 1307–1317.

Demidova, TN and MR Hamblin. 2004. Photodynamic therapy targeted to pathogens. *International Journal of Immunopathology and Pharmacology* **17**(3): 245–254.

Demidova, TN and MR Hamblin. 2005. Effect of cell-photosensitizer binding and cell density on microbial photoinactivation. *Antimicrobial Agents and Chemotherapy* **49**(6): 2329–2235. doi:10.1128/AAC.49.6.2329.

Dessolin, J, M Schuler, A Quinart, F De Giorgi, L Ghosez, and F Ichas. 2002. Selective targeting of synthetic antioxidants to mitochondria: Towards a mitochondrial medicine for neurodegenerative diseases? *European Journal of Pharmacology* **447**(2–3): 155–161.

Dewaele, M, W Martinet, N Rubio, T Verfaillie, PA de Witte, J Piette, and P Agostinis. 2011. Autophagy pathways activated in response to PDT contribute to cell resistance against ROS damage. *Journal of Cellular and Molecular Medicine* **15**(6): 1402–1414. doi:10.1111/j.1582-4934.2010.01118.x.

Dini, L, V Inguscio, B Tenuzzo, and E Panzarini. 2010. Rose bengal acetate photodynamic therapy-induced autophagy. *Cancer Biology and Therapy* **10**(10): 1048–1056. doi:10.4161/cbt.10.10.13371.

Dolman, NJ, KM Chambers, B Mandavilli, RH Batchelor, and MS Janes. 2013. Tools and techniques to measure mitophagy using fluorescence microscopy. *Autophagy* **9**(11): 1653–1662. doi:10.4161/auto.24001.

Donohue, E, AD Balgi, M Komatsu, and M Roberge. 2014. Induction of covalently crosslinked p62 oligomers with reduced binding to polyubiquitinated proteins by the autophagy inhibitor verteporfin. *PLoS One* **9**(12): e114964. doi:10.1371/journal.pone.0114964.

Donohue, E, A Tovey, AW Vogl, S Arns, E Sternberg, RN Young, and M Roberge. 2011. Inhibition of autophagosome formation by the benzoporphyrin derivative verteporfin. *Journal of Biological Chemistry* **286**(9): 7290–7300. doi:10.1074/jbc.M110.139915.

Dougherty, TJ, CJ Gomer, BW Henderson, G Jori, D Kessel, M Korbelik, J Moan, and Q Peng. 1998. Photodynamic therapy. *Journal of the National Cancer Institute* **90**(12): 889–905.

Du, L, N Jiang, G Wang, Y Chu, W Lin, J Qian, Y Zhang, J Zheng, and G Chen. 2014. Autophagy inhibition sensitizes bladder cancer cells to the photodynamic effects of the novel photosensitizer chlorophyllin e4. *Journal of Photochemistry and Photobiology B: Biology* **133**: 1–10. doi:10.1016/j.jphotobiol.2014.02.010.

Dummin, H, Th Cernay, and HW Zimmermann. 1997. Selective photosensitization of mitochondria in HeLa cells by cationic Zn(II)phthalocyanines with lipophilic side-chains. *Journal of Photochemistry and Photobiology B: Biology* **37**(3): 219–229.

Dunn, KW, MM Kamocka, and JH McDonald. 2011. A practical guide to evaluating colocalization in biological microscopy. *American Journal of Cell Physiology* **300**(4): C723–C742. doi:10.1152/ajpcell.00462.2010.

Duprez, L, E Wirawan, T Vanden Berghe, and P Vandenabeele. 2009. Major cell death pathways at a glance. *Microbes and Infection* **11**(13): 1050–1062. doi:10.1016/j.micinf.2009.08.013.

Engelmann, FM, I Mayer, DS Gabrielli, HE Toma, AJ Kowaltowski, K Araki, and MS Baptista. 2007. Interaction of cationic meso-porphyrins with liposomes, mitochondria and erythrocytes. *Journal of Bioenergetics and Biomembranes* **39**(2): 175–185.

Evans, HH, MF Horng, M Ricanati, JT Deahl, and NL Oleinick. 1997. Mutagenicity of photodynamic therapy as compared to UVC and ionizing radiation in human and murine lymphoblast cell lines. *Photochemistry and Photobiology* **66**(5): 690–696. doi:10.1111/j.1751-1097.1997.tb03208.x.

Ezzeddine, R, A Al-Banaw, A Tovmasyan, JD Craik, I Batinic-Haberle, and LT Benov. 2013. Effect of molecular characteristics on cellular uptake, subcellular localization, and phototoxicity of Zn(II) N-alkylpyridylporphyrins. *The Journal of Biological Chemistry* **288**(51): 36579–36788. doi:10.1074/jbc.M113.511642.

Fabris, C, G Valduga, G Miotto, L Borsetto, G Jori, S Garbisa, and E Reddi. 2001. Photosensitization with zinc(II) phthalocyanine as a switch in the decision between apoptosis and necrosis. *Cancer Research* **61**: 7495–7500.

Fernandez-Sanz, C, M Ruiz-Meana, E Miro-Casas, E Nuñez, J Castellano, M Loureiro, I Barba et al. 2014. Defective sarcoplasmic reticulum–mitochondria calcium exchange in aged mouse myocardium. *Cell Death and Disease* **5**(12): e1573. doi:10.1038/cddis.2014.526.

Festjens, N, T Vanden Berghe, and P Vandenabeele. 2006. Necrosis, a well-orchestrated form of cell demise: Signalling cascades, important mediators and concomitant immune response. *Biochimica et Biophysica Acta—Bioenergetics* **1757**(9–10): 1371–1387. doi:10.1016/j.bbabio.2006.06.014.

Flors, C, MJ Fryer, J Waring, B Reeder, U Bechtold, PM Mullineaux, S Nonell, MT Wilson, and NR Baker. 2006. Imaging the production of singlet oxygen in vivo using a new fluorescent sensor, singlet oxygen sensor green. *Journal of Experimental Botany*, **57**: 1725–1734. doi:10.1093/jxb/erj181.

Foghsgaard, L, D Wissing, D Mauch, U Lademann, L Bastholm, M Boes, F Elling, M Leist, and M Jäättelä. 2001. Cathepsin B acts as a dominant execution protease in tumor cell apoptosis induced by tumor necrosis factor. *The Journal of Cell Biology* **153**(5): 999–1010.

Foote, CS 1968. Mechanisms of photosensitized oxidation. *Science* **162**(3857): 963–970.

François, A, S Marchal, F Guillemin, and L Bezdetnaya. 2011. mTHPC-based photodynamic therapy induction of autophagy and apoptosis in cultured cells in relation to mitochondria and endoplasmic reticulum stress. *International Journal of Oncology* **39**(6): 1537–1543. doi:10.3892/ijo.2011.1174.

Gabrielli, D, E Belisle, D Severino, AJ Kowaltowski, and MS Baptista. 2004. Binding, aggregation and photochemical properties of methylene blue in mitochondrial suspensions. *Photochemistry and Photobiology* **79**(3): 227–232. doi:10.1111/j.1751-1097.2004.tb00389.x.

Gardner, LC, SJ Smith, and TM Cox. 1991. Biosynthesis of delta-aminolevulinic acid and the regulation of heme formation by immature erythroid cells in man. *Journal of Biological Chemistry* **266**(32): 22010–22018.

Glidden, MD, JP Celli, I Massodi, I Rizvi, BW Pogue, and T Hasan. 2012. Image-based quantification of benzoporphyrin derivative uptake, localization, and photobleaching in 3D tumor models, for optimization of PDT parameters. *Theranostics* **2**(9): 827–839. doi:10.7150/thno.4334.

Golstein, P and G Kroemer. 2007. Cell death by necrosis: Towards a molecular definition. *Trends in Biochemical Sciences* **32**(1): 37–43. doi:10.1016/j.tibs.2006.11.001.

Guicciardi, ME, M Leist, and GJ Gores. 2004. Lysosomes in cell death. *Oncogene* **23**(16): 2881–2890. doi:10.1038/sj.onc.1207512.

Halliwell, B. 2009. The wanderings of a free radical. *Free Radical Biology and Medicine* **46**: 531–542. doi:10.1016/j.freeradbiomed.2008.11.008.

Hamblin, MR and T Hasan. 2014. Photodymamic therapy: A new antimicrobial approach to infectious disease? *Photochemical and Photobiological Sciences* **3**(5): 436–450. doi:10.1039/b311900a.Photodynamic.

Henderson, BW and TJ Dougherty. 1992. How does photodynamic therapy work? *Photochemistry and Photobiology* **55**(1): 145–157. doi:10.1111/j.1751-1097.1992.tb04222.x.

Høgset, A, L Prasmickaite, PK Selbo, M Hellum, B Engesæter, A Bonsted, and K Berg. 2004. Photochemical internalisation in drug and gene delivery. *Advanced Drug Delivery Reviews* **56**: 95–115. doi:10.1016/j.addr.2003.08.016.

Hoye, AT, JE Davoren, P Wipf, MP Fink, and VE Kagan. 2008. Targeting mitochondria. *Accounts of Chemical Research* **41**(1): 87–97.

Hsieh, YJ, CC Wu, CJ Chang, and JS Yu. 2003. Subcellular localization of photofrin determines the death phenotype of human epidermoid carcinoma A431 cells triggered by photodynamic therapy: When plasma membranes are the main targets. *Journal of Cellular Physiology* **194**(3): 363–375.

Hung, Y-H, LM-W Chen, J-Y Yang, and WY Yang. 2013. Spatiotemporally controlled induction of autophagy-mediated lysosome turnover. *Nature Communications* **4**(2111): 1–7. doi:10.1038/ncomms3111.

Inguscio, V, E Panzarini, and L Dini. 2012. Autophagy contributes to the death/survival balance in cancer photodynamic therapy. *Cells* **1**: 464–491. doi:10.3390/cells1030464.

Ji, H-T, L-T Chien, Y-H Lin, H-F Chien, and C-T Chen. 2010. 5-ALA mediated photodynamic therapy induces autophagic cell death via AMP-activated protein kinase. *Molecular Cancer* **9**: 91.

Johansen, T and T Lamark. 2011. Selective autophagy mediated by autophagic adapter proteins. *Autophagy* **7**(3): 279–296. doi:10.4161/auto.7.3.14487.

Johansson, AC, H Appelqvist, C Nilsson, K Kågedal, K Roberg, and K Öllinger. 2010. Regulation of apoptosis-associated lysosomal membrane permeabilization. *Apoptosis* **15**(5): 527–540.

Joshi, P, M Ethirajan, LN Goswami, A Srivatsan, JR Missert, and RK Pandey. 2011. Synthesis, spectroscopic, and in vitro photosensitizing efficacy of ketobacteriochlorins derived from ring-B and ring-D reduced chlorins via pinacol-pinacolone rearrangement. *Journal of Organic Chemistry* **76**(21): 8629–8640. doi:10.1021/jo201688c.

Junqueira, HC, D Severino, LG Dias, MS Gugliotti, and MS Baptista. 2002. Modulation of methylene blue photochemical properties based on adsorption at aqueous micelle interfaces. *Physical Chemistry Chemical Physics* **4**(11): 2320–2328.

Jurič, IB, V Plečko, DG Panduríć, and I Anić. 2014. The antimicrobial effectiveness of photodynamic therapy used as an addition to the conventional endodontic re-treatment: A clinical study. *Photodiagnosis and Photodynamic Therapy* **11**(4): 549–555. doi:10.1016/j.pdpdt.2014.10.004.

Kandela, RK, JA Bartlett, and GL Indig. 2002. Effect of molecular structure on the selective phototoxicity of triarylmethane dyes towards tumor cells. *Photochemical and Photobiological Sciences : Official Journal of the European Photochemistry Association and the European Society for Photobiology* **1**(5): 309–314.

Kang, R, HJ Zeh, MT Lotze, and D Tang. 2011. The Beclin 1 network regulates autophagy and apoptosis. *Cell Death and Differentiation* **18**(4): 571–580. doi:10.1038/cdd.2010.191.

Kessel, D and AS Arroyo. 2007. Apoptotic and autophagic responses to Bcl-2 and photodamage. *Photochemical and Photobiological Sciences* **6**(12): 1234–1245. doi:10.1039/b705461k.

Kessel, D, M Castelli, and JJ Reiners. 2005. Ruthenium red-mediated suppression of Bcl 2 loss and Ca(2+) release initiated by photodamage to the endoplasmic reticulum: Scavenging of reactive oxygen species. *Cell Death and Differentiation* **12**(5): 502–511. doi:10.1038/sj.cdd.4401579.

Kessel, D, M Graça H Vicente, and JJ Reiners. 2006. Initiation of apoptosis and autophagy by photodynamic therapy. *Autophagy* **2**(4): 289–290. doi:10.4161/auto.2792.

Kessel, D, R Luguya, M Graça, and H Vicente. 2003. Localization and photodynamic efficacy of two cationic porphyrins varying in charge distributions. *Photochemistry and Photobiology* **78**(5): 431–435.

Kessel, D and Y Luo. 2001. Intracellular sites of photodamage as a factor in apoptotic cell death. *Journal of Porphyrins and Phthalocyanines* **5**(2): 181–184.

Kessel, D, Y Luo, Y Deng, and CK Chang. 1997. The role of subcellular localization in initiation of apoptosis by photodynamic therapy. *Photochemistry and Photobiology* **65**(3): 422–426.

Kessel, D, Y Luo, P Mathieu, and JJ Reiners. 2000. Determinants of the apoptotic response to lysosomal photo-damage. *Photochemistry and Photobiology* **71**(2): 196–200. doi:10.1562/0031-8655(2000)0710196DOTART2.0.CO2.

Kessel, D and A Morgan. 1993. Photosensitization with etiobenzochlorins and octaethylbenzochlorins. *Photochemistry and Photobiology* **58**(4): 521–526.

Kessel, D and JJ Reiners Jr. 2007a. Apoptosis and autophagy after mitochondrial or endoplasmic reticulum. *Photochemistry and Photobiology* **83**: 1024–1028.

Kessel, D and JJ Reiners. 2007b. Initiation of apoptosis and autophagy by the Bcl-2 antagonist HA14-1. *Cancer Letters* **249**(2): 294–299.

Kim, I, S Rodriguez-Enriquez, and JJ Lemasters. 2007. Selective degradation of mitochondria by mitophagy. *Archives of Biochemistry and Biophysics* **462**: 245–253. doi:10.1016/j.abb.2007.03.034.

Kim, J, W Lim, S Kim, S Jeon, Z Hui, K Ni, C Kim, Y Im, H Choi, and O Kim. 2014. Photodynamic therapy (PDT) resistance by PARP1 regulation on PDT-induced apoptosis with autophagy in head and neck cancer cells. *Journal of Oral Pathology and Medicine* **43**: 675–684. doi:10.1111/jop.12195.

Kim, PK, DW Hailey, RT Mullen, and J Lippincott-Schwartz. 2008. Ubiquitin signals autophagic degradation of cytosolic proteins and peroxisomes. *Proceedings of the National Academy of Sciences of the United States of America* **105**(52): 20567–20574.

Klionsky, DJ, FC Abdalla, H Abeliovich, RT Abraham, A Acevedo-Arozena, K Adeli, L Agholme et al. 2012. Guidelines for the use and interpretation of assays for monitoring autophagy. *Autophagy* **8**(4): 445–544. doi:10.4161/auto.19496.

Klionsky, DJ, H Abeliovich, P Agostinis, DK Agrawal, G Aliev, DS Askew, M Baba et al. 2008. Guidelines for the use and interpretation of assays for monitoring autophagy in higher eukaryotes. *Autophagy* **4**(2): 151–175.

Kochevar, IE, MC Lynch, S Zhuang, and CR Lambert. 2000. Singlet oxygen, but not oxidizing radicals, induces apoptosis in HL-60 cells. *Photochemistry and Photobiology* **72**(4): 548–553.

Koff, J, S Ramachandiran, and L Bernal-Mizrachi. 2015. A time to kill: Targeting apoptosis in cancer. *International Journal of Molecular Sciences* **16**(2): 2942–2955. doi:10.3390/ijms16022942.

Komatsu, M, S Kageyama, and Y Ichimura. 2012. P62/SQSTM1/A170: Physiology and pathology. *Pharmacological Research* **66**(6): 457–462. doi:10.1016/j.phrs.2012.07.004.

Komatsu, M, S Waguri, M Koike, YS Sou, T Ueno, T Hara, N Mizushima et al. 2007. Homeostatic levels of p62 control cytoplasmic inclusion body formation in autophagy-deficient mice. *Cell* **131**(6): 1149–1163. doi:10.1016/j.cell.2007.10.035.

Kress, M, T Meier, R Steiner, F Dolp, R Erdmann, U Ortmann, and A Rück. 2003. Time-resolved microspectrofluorometry and fluorescence lifetime imaging of photosensitizers using picosecond pulsed diode lasers in laser scanning microscopes. *Journal of Biomedical Optics* **8**(1): 26–32. doi:10.1117/1.1528595.

Krinsky, NI. 1977. Singlet oxygen in biological systems. *Trends in Biochemical Sciences* **2**(2): 35–38. doi:10.1016/0968-0004(77)90253-5.

Krmpot, AJ, KD Janjetovic, MS Misirkic, LM Vucicevic, DV Pantelic, DM Vasiljevic, DM Popadic, BM Jelenkovic, and VS Trajkovic. 2010. Protective effect of autophagy in laser-induced glioma cell death in vitro. *Lasers in Surgery and Medicine* **42**(4): 338–347. doi:10.1002/lsm.20911.

Lassalle, HP, M Wagner, L Bezdetnaya, F Guillemin, and H Schneckenburger. 2008. Fluorescence imaging of Foscan® and foslip in the plasma membrane and in whole cells. *Journal of Photochemistry and Photobiology B: Biology* **92**(1): 47–53. doi:10.1016/j.jphotobiol.2008.04.007.

Lavi, A, H Weitman, RT Holmes, KM Smith, and B Ehrenberg. 2002. The depth of porphyrin in a membrane and the membrane's physical properties affect the photosensitizing efficiency. *Biophysical Journal* **82**(4): 2101–2110.

Leach, MW, RJ Higgins, SA Autry, JE Boggan, S-JH Lee, and KM Smith. 1993. Photodynamic effects of lysyl chlorin p6: Cell survival, localization and ultrastructural changes. *Photochemistry and Photobiology* **58**(5): 653–660.

Lemasters, JJ, AL Nieminen, T Qian, LC Trost, SP Elmore, Y Nishimura, RA Crowe et al. 1998. The mitochondrial permeability transition in cell death: A common mechanism in necrosis, apoptosis and autophagy. *Biochimica et Biophysica Acta* **1366**(1–2): 177–196. doi:10.1016/S0005-2728(98)00112-1.

Lemasters, JJ and VK Ramshesh. 2007. Imaging of mitochondrial polarization and depolarization with cationic fluorophores. *Methods in Cell Biology* **80**(06): 283–295. doi:10.1016/S0091-679X(06)80014-2.

Li, J, N Hou, A Faried, S Tsutsumi, and H Kuwano. 2010. Inhibition of autophagy augments 5-fluorouracil chemotherapy in human colon cancer in vitro and in vivo model. *European Journal of Cancer* **46**(10): 1900–1909. doi:10.1016/j.ejca.2010.02.021.

Li, D, L Li, P Li, Y Li, and X Chen. 2015. Apoptosis of HeLa cells induced by a new targeting photosensitizer-based PDT via a mitochondrial pathway and ER stress. *Onco Targets and Therapy* **8**: 703–711.

Lihuan, D, Z Jingcun, J Ning, W Guozeng, C Yiwei, L Wei, Q Jing, Z Yuanfang, and C Gang. 2014. Photodynamic therapy with the novel photosensitizer chlorophyllin F induces apoptosis and autophagy in human bladder cancer cells. *Lasers in Surgery and Medicine* **46**(4): 319–324. doi:10.1002/lsm.22225.

Lin, C-W, JR Shulok, SD Kirley, L Cincotta, and JW Foley. 1991. Lysosomal localization and mechanism of uptake of nile blue photosensitizers in tumor cells. *Cancer Research* **51**(10): 2710–2719.

Lin, H-Y, J-N Lin, J-W Ma, N-S Yang, C-T Ho, S-C Kuo, and T-D Way. 2015. Demethoxycurcumin induces autophagic and apoptotic responses on breast cancer cells in photodynamic therapy. *Journal of Functional Foods* **12**: 439–449. doi:10.1016/j.jff.2014.12.014.

Linder, S and MC Shoshan. 2005. Lysosomes and endoplasmic reticulum: targets for improved, selective anticancer therapy. *Drug Resistance Updates* **8**(4): 199–204. doi:10.1016/j.drup.2005.06.004.

Luo, S, D Xing, Y Wei, and Q Chen. 2010. Inhibitive effects of photofrin on cellular autophagy. *Journal of Cellular Physiology* **224**(2): 414–422. doi:10.1002/jcp.22137.

Luo, Y and D Kessel. 1997. Initiation of apoptosis versus necrosis by photodynamic therapy with chloroaluminum phthalocyanine. *Photochemistry and Photobiology* **66**(4): 479–483. doi:10.1111/j.1751-1097.1997.tb03176.x.

Malhi, H, GJ Gores, and JJ Lemasters. 2006. Apoptosis and necrosis in the liver: A tale of two deaths? *Hepatology* **43**(2 Suppl. 1): 31–44. doi:10.1002/hep.21062.

Marchal, S, A François, D Dumas, F Guillemin, and L Bezdetnaya. 2007. Relationship between subcellular localisation of foscan and caspase activation in photosensitised MCF-7 cells. *British Journal of Cancer* **96**(6): 944–951. doi:10.1038/sj.bjc.6603631.

Martins, WK, D Severino, C Souza, BS Stolf, and MS Baptista. 2013. Rapid screening of potential autophagic inductor agents using mammalian cell lines. *Biotechnology Journal* **8**: 730–737. doi:10.1002/biot.201200306.

Matroule, J-Y, G Bonizzi, P Morlie, N Paillous, V Bours, and J Piette. 1999. Activates transcription factor NF-B through the interleukin-1 receptor-dependent signaling pathway. *Biochemistry* **274**(5): 2988–3000.

Mertins, O, IOL Bacellar, F Thalmann, CM Marques, and R Itri. 2014. Physical damage on giant vesicles membrane as a result of methylene blue photoirradiation. *Biotechnology Journal* **106**: 162–171. doi:10.1016/j.bpj.2013.11.4457.

Miller, GG, K Brown, RB Moore, ZJ Diwu, J Liu, L Huang, JW Lown, DA Begg, V Chlumecky, and J Tulip. 1995. Uptake kinetics and intracellular localization of hypocrellin photosensitizers for photodynamic therapy: A confocal microscopy study. *Photochemistry and Photobiology* **61**(6): 632–638.

Mizushima, N. 2004. Methods for monitoring autophagy. *International Journal of Biochemistry and Cell Biology* **36**(12): 2491–2502. doi:10.1016/j.biocel.2004.02.005.

Mizushima, N and T Yoshimori. 2007. How to interpret LC3 immunoblotting. *Autophagy* **3**(6): 542–545. doi:10.4161/auto.4600.

Moan, J, K Berg, JC Bommer, and A Western. 1992. Action spectra of phthalocyanines with respect to photosensitization of cells. *Photochemical and Photobiology* **56**(2): 171–175.

Mohammad, RM, I Muqbil, L Lowe, C Yedjou, H-Y Hsu, L-T Lin, MD Siegelin et al. 2015. Broad targeting of resistance to apoptosis in cancer. *Seminars in Cancer Biology* **35**: 1–26. doi:10.1016/j.semcancer.2015.03.001.

Morlière, P, J-C Mazière, R Santus, CD Smith, MR Prinsep, CC Stobbe, MC Penning, JL Golberg, and JD Chapman. 1998. Tolyporphin : A natural product from cyanobacteria with potent photosensitizing activity against tumor cells in vitro and in vivo. *Cancer Research* **58**: 3571–3578.

Mroz, P, J Bhaumik, DK Dogutan, Z Aly, Z Kamal, L Khalid, HL Kee et al. 2009. Imidazole metalloporphyrins as photosensitizers for photodynamic therapy: Role of molecular charge, ccentral metal and hydroxyl radical production. *Cancer Letters* **282**(1): 63–76. doi:10.1016/j.canlet.2009.02.054.

Mroz, P, A Yaroslavsky, GB Kharkwal, and MR Hamblin. 2011. Cell death pathways in photodynamic therapy of cancer. *Cancers* **3**(2): 2516–2539. doi:10.3390/cancers3022516.

Neves, AA and KM Brindle. 2014. Imaging cell death. *Journal of Nuclear Medicine* **55**(1): 1–4. doi:10.2967/jnumed.112.114264.

Norum, OJ, PK Selbo, A Weyergang, KE Giercksky, and K Berg. 2009. Photochemical internalization (PCI) in cancer therapy: From bench towards bedside medicine. *Journal of Photochemistry and Photobiology B: Biology* **96**(2): 83–92. doi:10.1016/j.jphotobiol.2009.04.012.

Oleinick, NL and HH Evans. 1998. The photobiology of photodynamic therapy: Cellular targets and mechanisms. *Radiation Research* **150**: S146–S156.

Oleinick, NL, RL Morris, and I Belichenko. 2002. The role of apoptosis in response to photodynamic therapy: What, where, why, and how. *Photochemical and Photobiological Sciences* **1**: 1–21. doi:10.1039/b108586g.

Oleinick, NL, L-Y Xue, S-M Chiu, and S Joseph. 2009. Autophagy in response to photodynamic therapy: Cell survival vs. cell death. *Proceedings of SPIE* **7164**: 716403–716409. doi:10.1117/12.810933.

Oliveira, CS, R Turchiello, AJ Kowaltowski, GL Indig, and MS Baptista. 2011. Major determinants of photoinduced cell death: Subcellular localization versus photosensitization efficiency. *Free Radical Biology and Medicine* **51**(4): 824–833. doi:10.1016/j.freeradbiomed.2011.05.023.

Ormond, AB and HS Freeman. 2013. Dye sensitizers for photodynamic therapy. *Materials* **6**: 817–840. doi:10.3390/ma6030817.

Oseroff, AR, D Ohuoha, G Ara, D McAuliffe, J Foley, and L Cincotta. 1986. Intramitochondrial dyes allow selective in vitro photolysis of carcinoma cells. *Proceedings of the National Academy of Sciences of the United States of America* **83**(24): 9729–9733. doi:10.1073/pnas.83.24.9729.

Palmeira-Dos-Santos, C, GJS Pereira, CMV Barbosa, A Jurkiewicz, SS Smaili, and C Bincoletto. 2014. Comparative study of autophagy inhibition by 3MA and CQ on cytarabine-induced death of leukaemia cells. *Journal of Cancer Research and Clinical Oncology* **140**(6): 909–920. doi:10.1007/s00432-014-1640-4.

Pankiv, S, TH Clausen, T Lamark, A Brech, JA Bruun, H Outzen, A Øvervatn, G Bjørkøy, and T Johansen. 2007. p62/SQSTM1 binds directly to Atg8/LC3 to facilitate degradation of ubiquitinated protein aggregates by autophagy. *Journal of Biological Chemistry* **282**(33): 24131–24145. doi:10.1074/jbc.M702824200.

Panzarini, E, V Inguscio, and L Dini. 2011. Overview of cell death mechanisms induced by Rose Bengal acetate-photodynamic therapy. *International Journal of Photoenergy* **2011**: 1–11. doi:10.1155/2011/713726.

Pavani, C, Y Iamamoto, and MS Baptista. 2012. Mechanism and efficiency of cell death of type II photosensitizers: Effect of zinc chelation. *Photochemistry and Photobiology* **88**(4): 774–781.

Pavani, C, AF Uchoa, CS Oliveira, Y Iamamoto, and MS Baptista. 2009. Effect of zinc insertion and hydrophobicity on the membrane interactions and PDT activity of porphyrin photosensitizers. *Photochemical and Photobiological Sciences* **8**(2): 233–240. http://www.ncbi.nlm.nih.gov/pubmed/19247516.

Pereira, MM, CJP Monteiro, AVC Simões, SMA Pinto, AR Abreu, GFF Sá, EFF Silva et al. 2010. Synthesis and photophysical characterization of a library of photostable halogenated bacteriochlorins: An access to near infrared chemistry. *Tetrahedron* **66**(49): 9545–9551. doi:10.1016/j.tet.2010.09.106.

Pereira, MM, CJP Monteiro, AVC Simões, SMA Pinto, LG Arnaut, GFF Sá, EFF Silva, LB Rocha, S Simões, and SJ Formosinho. 2009. Synthesis and photophysical properties of amphiphilic halogenated bacteriochlorins: New opportunities for photodynamic therapy of cancer. *Journal of Porphyrins and Phthalocyanines* **13**(04n05): 567–573. doi:10.1142/S1088424609000553.

Philipp, CM and HP Berlien. 2006. The future of biophotonics in medicine—A proposal. *Medical Laser Application* **21**(2): 115–222. doi:10.1016/j.mla.2006.03.005.

Pongue, BW and T Hasan. 2003. Targeting in photodynamic therapy and photo-imaging. *Optics and Photonics News* **14**(8): 36–43.

Presley, AD, KM Fuller, and EA Arriaga. 2003. MitoTracker green labeling of mitochondrial proteins and their subsequent analysis by capillary electrophoresis with laser-induced fluorescence detection. *Journal of Chromatography B* **793**(1): 141–150. doi:10.1016/S1570-0232(03)00371-4.

Price, M, JJ Reiners, AM Santiago, and D Kessel. 2009. Monitoring singlet oxygen and hydroxyl radical formation with fluorescent probes during photodynamic therapy. *Photochemistry and Photobiology* **85**(5): 1177–1181. doi:10.1111/j.1751-1097.2009.00555.x.

Raben, N, L Shea, V Hill, and P Plotz. 2009. Monitoring autophagy in lysosomal storage disorders. *Methods in Enzymology* **453**: 417–449. doi:10.1016/S0076-6879(08)04021-4.Monitoring.

Racoma, IO, WH Meisen, QE Wang, B Kaur, and AA Wani. 2013. Thymoquinone inhibits autophagy and induces cathepsin-mediated, caspase-independent cell death in glioblastoma cells. *PLoS One* **8**(9): e72882. doi:10.1371/journal.pone.0072882.

Redmond, RW and IE Kochevar. 2006. Spatially resolved cellular responses to singlet oxygen. *Photochemical and Photobiology* **82**: 1178–1186. doi:10.1562/2006-04-14-1R-874.

Reiners, JJ, JA Caruso, P Mathieu, B Chelladurai, X-M Yin, and D Kessel. 2002. Release of cytochrome c and activation of pro-Caspase-9 following lysosomal photodamage involves bid cleavage. *Cell Death and Differentiation* **9**(9): 934–944.

Ricchelli, F, L Franchi, G Miotto, L Borsetto, S Gobbo, P Nikolov, JC Bommer, and E Reddi. 2005. Meso-substituted tetra-cationic porphyrins photosensitize the death of human fibrosarcoma cells via lysosomal targeting. *International Journal of Biochemistry and Cell Biology* **37**(2): 306–319. doi:10.1016/j.biocel.2004.06.013.

Rodriguez, ME, P Zhang, K Azizuddin, GB Delos Santos, SM Chiu, L-Y Xue, JC Berlin et al. 2009. Structural factors and mechanisms underlying the improved photodynamic cell killing with silicon phthalocyanine photosensitizers directed to lysosomes versus mitochondria. *Photochemistry and Photobiology* **85**(5): 1189–1200. doi:10.1016/j.biotechadv.2011.08.021.Secreted.

Rubio, N, I Coupienne, E Di Valentin, I Heirman, J Grooten, J Piette, and P Agostinis. 2012. Spatiotemporal autophagic degradation of oxidatively damaged organelles after photodynamic stress is amplified by mitochondrial reactive oxygen species. *Autophagy* **8**(9): 1312–1324. doi:10.4161/auto.20763.

Russell, J and K Diamond. 2008. Characterization of fluorescence lifetime of photofrin and delta-aminolevulinic acid induced protoporphyrin IX in living cells using single-and two-photon excitation. *IEEE Journal of Selected Topics in Quantum Electronics* **14**(1): 158–166.

Rusten, TE and H Stenmark. 2010. P62, an autophagy hero or culprit? *Nature Cell Biology* **12**(3): 207–209. doi:10.1038/ncb0310-207.

Sasnauskiene, A, J Kadziauskas, N Vezelyte, V Jonusiene, and V Kirveliene. 2009. Apoptosis, autophagy and cell cycle arrest following photodamage to mitochondrial interior. *Apoptosis* **14**(3): 276–286. doi:10.1007/s10495-008-0292-8.

Scherz-Shouval, R and Z Elazar. 2007. ROS, mitochondria and the regulation of autophagy. *Trends in Cell Biology* **17**(9): 422–427. doi:10.1016/j.tcb.2007.07.009.

Scwingel, AR, ARP Barcessat, SC Núñez, and MS Ribeiro. 2012. Antimicrobial photodynamic therapy in the treatment of oral candidiasis in HIV-infected patients. *Photomedicine and Laser Surgery* **30**(8): 429–432. doi:10.1089/pho.2012.3225.

Shimizu, S, T Yoshida, M Tsujioka, and S Arakawa. 2014. Autophagic cell death and cancer. *International Journal of Molecular Sciences* **15**(2): 3145–3153. doi:10.3390/ijms15023145.

Sibrian-Vazquez, M, TJ Jensen, and MGH Vicente. 2007. Porphyrin-retinamides: Synthesis and cellular studies. *Bioconjugate Chemistry* **18**(4): 1185–1193. doi:10.1021/bc0700382.

Singh, G, WP Jeeves, BC Wilson, and D Jang. 1987. Mitochondrial photosensitization by photofrin II. *Photochemistry and Photobiology* **46**(5): 645–649.

Solban, N, I Rizvi, and T Hasan. 2006. Targeted photodynamic therapy. *Lasers in Surgery and Medicine* **38**(5): 522–531. doi:10.1002/lsm.20345.

Soldani, C, MG Bottone, AC Croce, A Fraschini, G Bottiroli, and C Pellicciari. 2004. The Golgi apparatus is a primary site of intracellular damage after photosensitization with Rose Bengal acetate. *European Journal of Histochemistry* **48**(4): 443–448.

Soriano, J, M García-Díaz, M Mora, ML Sagristá, S Nonell, A Villanueva, JC Stockert, and M Cañete. 2013. Liposomal temocene (m-THPPo) photodynamic treatment induces cell death by mitochondria-independent apoptosis. *Biochimica et Biophysica Acta—General Subjects* **1830**(10): 4611–4620. doi:10.1016/j.bbagen.2013.05.021.

Soriano, J, A Villanueva, J Stockert, and M Cañete. 2014. Regulated necrosis in HeLa cells induced by ZnPc photodynamic treatment: A new nuclear morphology. *International Journal of Molecular Sciences* **15**(12): 22772–22785. doi:10.3390/ijms151222772.

Stoka, V, B Turk, SL Schendel, TH Kim, T Cirman, SJ Snipas, LM Ellerby et al. 2001. Lysosomal protease pathways to apoptosis: Cleavage of Bid, not pro-Caspases, is the most likely route. *Journal of Biological Chemistry* **276**(5): 3149–3157.

Sun, X and WN Leung. 2002. Photodynamic therapy with pyropheophorbide-a methyl ester in human lung carcinoma cancer cell: Efficacy, localization and apoptosis. *Photochemistry and Photobiology* **75**(6): 644–651. doi:10.1562/0031-8655(2002)075<0644:PTWPAM>2.0.CO;2.

Sun, Y and Z-L Peng. 2009. Programmed cell death and cancer. *Postgraduate Medical Journal* **85**(1001): 134–140.

Teiten, M-H, L Bezdetnaya, P Morlière, R Santus, and F Guillemin. 2003. Endoplasmic reticulum and Golgi apparatus are the preferential sites of foscan localisation in cultured tumour cells. *British Journal of Cancer* **88**(1): 146–152. doi:10.1038/sj.bjc.6600664.

Terasaki, M, J Song, JR Wong, MJ Weiss, and LB Chen. 1984. Localization of endoplasmic reticulum in living and glutaraldehyde-fixed cells with fluorescent dyes. *Cell* **38**(1): 101–108. doi:10.1016/0092-8674(84)90530-0.

Terman, A and T Kurz. 2013. Lysosomal iron, iron chelation, and cell death. *Antioxidants and Redox Signaling* **18**(8): 888–898. doi:10.1089/ars.2012.4885.

Tsai, S-R, R Yin, Y-Y Huang, B-C Sheu, S-C Lee, and MR Hamblin. 2015. Low-level light therapy potentiates NPe6-mediated photodynamic therapy in a human osteosarcoma cell line via increased ATP. *Photodiagnosis and Photodynamic Therapy* **12**(1): 123–130. doi:10.1016/j.pdpdt.2014.10.009.

Uchoa, AF, KT De Oliveira, MS Baptista, AJ Bortoluzzi, Y Iamamoto, and OA Serra. 2011. Chlorin photosensitizers sterically designed to prevent self-aggregation. *Journal of Organic Chemistry* **76**(21): 8824–8832. doi:10.1021/jo201568n.

Uchoa, AF, CS Oliveira, and MS Baptista. 2010. Relationship between structure and photoactivity of porphyrins derived from protoporphyrin IX. *Journal of Porphyrins and Phthalocyanines* **14**: 832–845. doi:10.1142/S108842461000263X.

Valenzeno, DP. 1987. Photomodification of biological membranes with emphasis on singlet oxygen mechanisms. *Photochemistry and Photobiology* **46**(1): 147–160. doi:10.1111/j.1751-1097.1987.tb04749.x.

Verma, S, GM Watt, Z Mai, and T Hasan. 2007. Strategies for enhanced photodynamic therapy effects. *Photochemistry and Photobiology* **83**(5): 996–1005. doi:10.1111/j.1751-1097.2007.00166.x.

Wainwright, M, DA Phoenix, L Rice, SM Burrow, and J Waring. 1997. Increased cytotoxicity and phototoxicity in the methylene blue series via chromophore methylation. *Journal of Photochemistry and Photobiology B: Biology* **40**(3): 233–239. doi:10.1016/S1011-1344(97)00061-4.

Wang, JT-W, K Berg, A Høgset, SG Bown, and AJ MacRobert. 2013. Photophysical and photobiological properties of a sulfonated chlorin photosensitiser TPCS(2a) for photochemical internalisation (PCI). *Photochemical and Photobiological Sciences : Official Journal of the European Photochemistry Association and the European Society for Photobiology* **12**: 519–526. doi:10.1039/c2pp25328c.

Wilson, BC, M Olivo, and G Singh. 1997. Subcellular localization of photofrin and aminolevulinic acid and photodynamic cross-resistance in vitro in radiation-induced fibrosarcoma cells sensitive or resistant to photofrin-mediated photodynamic therapy. *Photochemistry and Photobiology* **65**(1): 166–176.

Wilson, BC, VV Tuchin, and S Tanev. 2005. Photodynamic therapy. In *Advances in Biophotonics*, Wilson, BC, ed. Ottawa, Canada: IOS Press ISBN 1-58603-540-1.

Winterbourn, CC. 2014. The challenges of using fluorescent probes to detect and quantify specific reactive oxygen species in living cells. *Biochimica et Biophysica Acta* **1840**(2): 730–738. doi:10.1016/j.bbagen.2013.05.004.

Wong, SJ, B Campbell, B Massey, DP Lynch, EEW Cohen, E Blair, R Selle et al. 2013. A phase I trial of aminolevulinic acid-photodynamic therapy for treatment of oral leukoplakia. *Oral Oncology* **49**(9): 970–976. doi:10.1016/j.oraloncology.2013.05.011.

Woodburn, KW, NJ Vardaxis, JS Hill, AH Kaye, and DR Phillips. 1991. Subcellular localization of porphyrins using confocal laser scanning microscopy. *Photochemistry and Photobiology* **54**(5): 725–732.

Xu, CS and AWN Leung. 2006. Photodynamic effects of pyropheophorbide-a methyl ester in nasopharyngeal carcinoma cells. *Medical Science Monitor : International Medical Journal of Experimental and Clinical Research* **12**(8): R257–R262.

Xu, DD, HM Lam, R Hoeven, CB Xu, AWN Leung, and WCS Cho. 2013. Photodynamic therapy induced cell death of hormone insensitive prostate cancer PC-3 cells with autophagic characteristics. *Photodiagnosis and Photodynamic Therapy* **10**(3): 278–287. doi:10.1016/j.pdpdt.2013.01.002.

Xue, L-Y, S-M Chiu, and NL Oleinick. 2015a. Atg7 deficiency increases resistance of MCF-7 human breast cancer cells to photodynamic therapy. *Autophagy* **6**(2): 248–255.

Xue, Q, X Wang, P Wang, K Zhang, and Q Liu. 2015b. Role of p38MAPK in apoptosis and autophagy responses to photodynamic therapy with chlorin e6. *Photodiagnosis and Photodynamic Therapy* **12**(1): 84–91. doi:10.1016/j.pdpdt.2014.12.001.

Yeh, S-CA, KR Diamond, MS Patterson, Z Nie, JE Hayward, and Q Fang. 2012. Monitoring photosensitizer uptake using two photon fluorescence life-time imaging microscopy. *Theranostics* **2**(9): 817–826. doi:10.7150/thno.4479.

Zhang, J, L Shao, C Wu, H Lu, and R Xu. 2015. Hypericin-mediated photodynamic therapy induces apoptosis of myoloma SP2/0 cells depended on caspase activity in vitro. *Cancer Cell International* **15**(1): 58. doi:10.1186/s12935-015-0193-1.

Zhang, X-J, S Chen, K-X Huang, and W-D Le. 2013. Why should autophagic flux be assessed?. *Acta Pharmacologica Sinica* **34**(5): 595–599. doi:10.1038/aps.2012.184.

Zhao, M, F Zhang, Y Chen, H Dai, J Qu, C Dong, X Kang et al. 2015. A 50% vs 30% dose of verteporfin (photodynamic therapy) for acute central serous chorioretinopathy. *JAMA Ophthalmology* **133**(3): 333. doi:10.1001/jamaophthalmol.2014.5312.

Zheng, G, WR Potter, SH Camacho, JR Missert, G Wang, DA Bellnier, BW Henderson, MAJ Rodgers, TJ Dougherty, and RK Pandey. 2001. Synthesis, photophysical properties, tumor uptake, and preliminary in vivo photosensitizing efficacy of a homologous series of 3-(1′-alkyloxy)-ethyl-3-devinylpurpurin-18-N-alkylimides with variable lipophilicity. *Journal of Medicinal Chemistry* **44**(10): 1540–1559. doi:10.1021/jm0005510.

Zhou, Z, C Zhao, W Liu, Q Li, L Zhang, W Sheng, Z Li, Y Zeng, and R Zhong. 2012. Involvement of the mitochondria-caspase pathway in HeLa cell death induced by 2-ethanolamino-2-demethoxy-17-ethanolimino-hypocrellin B (EAHB)-mediated photodynamic therapy. *International Journal of Toxicology* **31**(5): 483–492.

Zinchuk, V, O Zinchuk, and T Okada. 2007. Quantitative colocalization analysis of multicolor confocal immunofluorescence microscopy images: pushing pixels to explore biological phenomena. *Acta Histochemica et Cytochemica* **40**(4): 101–111. doi:10.1267/ahc.07002.

Zong, D, K Zielinska-Chomej, T Juntti, B Mörk, R Lewensohn, P Hååg, and K Viktorsson. 2014. Harnessing the lysosome-dependent antitumor activity of phenothiazines in human small cell lung cancer. *Cell Death and Disease* **5**(3): e1111. doi:10.1038/cddis.2014.56.

THERANOSTIC AGENTS AND NANOTECHNOLOGY

Quantum dots in PDT

RIČARDAS ROTOMSKIS AND GIEDRE STRECKYTE

10.1 INTRODUCTION

Among the emerging cancer therapy methods, photodynamic therapy (PDT) is an improvement on the traditional methods (surgery, chemotherapy, and radiotherapy) because it is noninvasive in nature and has some selectivity for cancerous tissue compared with normal tissue (Spikes, 1997; Dolmans et al., 2003). Three key components are involved in the PDT process: photosensitizer (PS), light, and oxygen. In PDT, cancerous cells are locally killed by reactive oxygen species, mostly by the singlet oxygen produced by the PS under illumination and in the presence of oxygen. After injection into the organism, the PS selectively accumulates in the cancerous tissue, and a carefully regulated light dose at a selected wavelength initiates the photosensitization reaction that destroys the cancerous tissue (Figure 10.1). Activatable PSs, such as porphyrins, chlorins, phthalocyanines, and bacteriochlorin derivatives, have been demonstrated to possess simultaneous cancer imaging and therapy capabilities, and some of these PSs have been approved for clinical use (Lovell et al., 2010).

After absorption of light, the transfer of excitation energy from an excited PS to a nearby oxygen molecule occurs, resulting in the formation of singlet oxygen ($^1O_2$) or other reactive oxygen species (ROS), which can initiate cytotoxic reactions in cells and tissues (Figure 10.2). The cytotoxic processes induced by the generated ROS can destroy tumors by multifactorial mechanisms. They include direct cancer cell killing by necrosis or

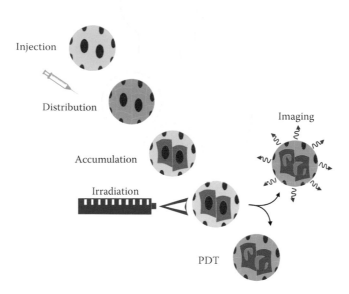

Figure 10.1 Principles of PDT.

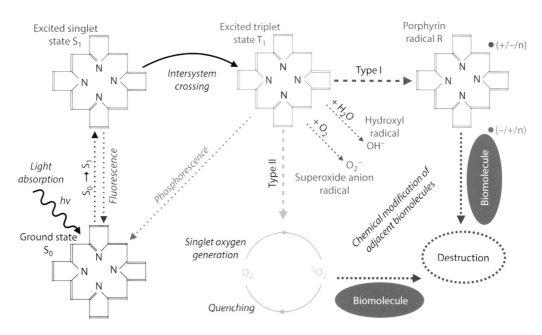

Figure 10.2 Photophysical and photochemical processes involved in PDT.

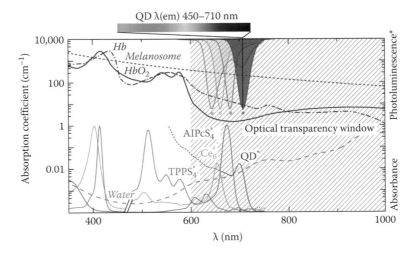

Figure 10.3 Tissue optical transparency window.

apoptosis (Oleinick et al., 2002; Agostinis et al., 2004), induction of antiangiogenesis resulting in the destruction of tumor vasculature (Dolmans et al., 2002; Michels and Schmidt-Erfurth, 2003), stimulation of immune system (De Vree et al., 1996; Cecic et al., 2005; Castano et al., 2006), and others. The main advantage of PDT over conventional chemotherapy and radiotherapy is that it can offer a selective therapeutic approach. This is due to possible site-specific photoactivation of targeted PSs using visible or near-infrared (NIR) light, leaving normal cells intact.

However, conventional PSs often have different drawbacks such as chemical impurities (Kessel and Thompson, 1987), poor water dispersibility, insufficient selectivity for cancer tissue (Moan, 1986; Moan and Berg, 1992), weak absorption in the spectral range of tissue transparency (Figure 10.3), low photostability (Rotomskis et al., 1996; Bonnett and Martinez, 2001), and prolonged phototoxicity, which lower the efficiency of the photosensitization process (Detty et al., 2004; Huang, 2005). To address these problems, new PSs are being sought together with improved drug carrier systems, including those based on nanoparticles. New opportunities could offer semiconductor nanoparticles—quantum dots (QDs). By varying the nanocrystal size and composition, QDs can be made to emit light over a wide range of wavelengths from UV-visible to near IR. The broad absorption window allows the simultaneous and efficient excitation of different color QDs at a single wavelength far from their respective emissions, which makes them very suitable for different applications (Chen, 2008). Distinctive properties of QDs such as a high photoluminescence (PL) quantum yield, broad absorption and narrow, symmetric emission spectra, very high molar extinction coefficients, as well as exceptional photostability form a basis for their use as a new class of fluorescent biological labels (Bruchez and Hotz, 2007). Due to their colloidal nature, QDs are larger than organic dye molecules and thanks to their spacious surface area that can offer multiple functionalization sites. Conjugation of biomolecules, such as antibodies, nucleic acids, peptides, etc., on the surface of QDs (Figure 10.4), can lead to their higher solubility, biocompatibility, and selectivity to tumor sites (Jamieson et al., 2007; Delehanty et al., 2009; Zhang et al., 2009). The ability to conjugate several biomolecules and/or PSs to a single QD may be particularly advantageous in certain situations, for instance, when QDs serve as a drug delivery platform (Probst et al., 2013) or as potential energy donors in conjugates with PSs (Medintz et al., 2005; Samia et al., 2006). Therefore, easily achievable surface functionalization of QDs with hydrophilic surface molecules and reactive functional groups as well as large two-photon absorption cross section (Biju et al., 2010; Rizvi et al., 2010) makes them applicable for different biomedical purposes including imaging and PDT.

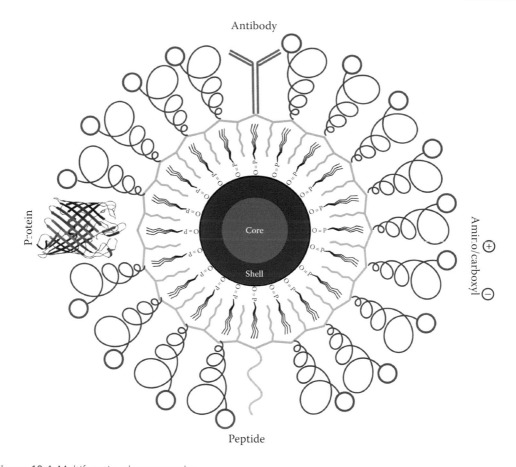

Figure 10.4 Multifunctional quantum dot.

10.2 PDT: SHORT HISTORY AND MAIN PRINCIPLES OF ACTION

Light has been employed in the treatment of disease since antiquity (Bonnett, 1999; Moan and Peng, 2003). Modern phototherapy was introduced by Niels Finsen, who found that sunlight or light from a carbon arc lamp with a heat filter could be used to treat *lupus vulgaris*, a tubercular condition of the skin (Finsen, 1901). This discovery was awarded the Nobel Prize in 1903 and marks the beginning of modern phototherapy. Almost at the same time it was also observed that light activation of a dye-induced lethal effect on bacteria (Raab, 1900). Von Tappainer in 1904 discovered that oxygen was essential for the process and introduced the term "photodynamic action" (Tappeiner and Jodlbauer, 1904). This is the fundamental photobiological process involved in PDT: it thus requires oxygen, a PS, and visible light.

The first report of fluorescent porphyrin localization in a malignant tumor appeared in 1924, when Polycard observed the characteristic red fluorescence of hematoporphyrin in an experimental rat sarcoma illuminated with ultraviolet light (Policard, 1924). In 1942, Auler and Banzer described the localization and fluorescence of exogenously administered porphyrins in malignant tumors (Auler and Banzer, 1942). The modern era of PDT began with the studies by Lipson and Schwartz at the Mayo Clinic (USA) in 1960. They observed that injection of crude preparations of hematoporphyrin led to fluorescence in neoplastic lesions. The emphasis was on diagnosis, leading to the development of fluorescence endoscopy (Lipson et al., 1961, 1967). This remains an important aspect that continues to be subject to new investigations.

The therapeutic application of PDT to cancer patients took a long time to develop. In 1975, Dougherty (Dougherty et al., 1975) reported successful PDT of induced and transplanted tumors in mice and rats. The next year the first human trials of PDT were initiated (Kelly and Snell, 1976). Later, it was demonstrated that crude hematoporphyrin contains a range of different porphyrins and, when converted to hematoporphyrin derivative (HpD) by sulfuric and acetic acids followed by hydrolysis, further porphyrins were produced. The active component of HpD comprised a mixture of porphyrin rings, between 5 and 8, linked by a number of ether and ester bonds. Partial purification of the most active of these oligomers led to the production of the drug Photofrin®, which has been approved in the clinic in several countries for the treatment of early- and late-stage lung cancer, superficial and advanced esophageal cancer, bladder cancer, superficial and early-stage gastric cancers, early-stage cervical cancer, and cervical dysplasia.

Although Photofrin is the most commonly used PS, it still has significant disadvantages. Therefore, major efforts have been invested in the development of new PSs. The desired features for the ideal PDT sensitizer are chemical purity, simplicity of synthesis, significant absorbance in the red spectral region (in optical transparency window of biological tissues (Figure 10.3), high quantum yield for generation of ROS produced by photochemical reactions, preferential tumor localization, minimal dark toxicity, and rapid clearance from normal tissue. So, more selective and potent sensitizers have been developed, some of them are introduced in clinics, others are under investigation in clinical trials.

The aim of PDT is to bring about a cytotoxic or modifying effect to cancerous tissue. Its great promise arises from its dual-selective mode of action: a PS of negligible dark toxicity is introduced into the body and accumulates preferentially in rapidly dividing cells. When the drug reaches an appropriate ratio of accumulation in diseased *versus* healthy tissue, light activates the drug only in the target tissue and elicits the toxic action (Figure 10.2). Upon illumination, PS is excited from the ground state (S_0) to the first excited singlet state (S_1), followed by conversion to the triplet state (T_1) via intersystem crossing. The longer lifetime of the triplet state enables the interaction of the excited PS with the surrounding molecules, and it is generally accepted that the generation of cytotoxic species produced during PDT occurs while in this state. The excited triplet state may react in two ways, defined as type I and type II mechanisms. A type I mechanism involves hydrogen atom abstraction or electron transfer reactions between the excited state of the PS and a substrate to yield free radicals and radical ions. These free radical species are generally highly reactive and can cause irreparable biological damage. A type II mechanism results from an energy transfer between the excited triplet state of the sensitizer and the ground state of molecular oxygen, generating the first excited state of oxygen, singlet oxygen. Singlet oxygen is an extremely reactive species and can interact with a large number of biological substrates, inducing oxidative damage and ultimately cell death. Singlet oxygen is generally accepted as the major damaging species in PDT (Weishaupt et al., 1976), and therefore photosensitization typically does not occur in anoxic areas of tissue. Because of the short half-life of $^1O_2$ (in biological systems <0.04 µs), only cells that are in close proximity to $^1O_2$ are affected (Moan and Berg, 1991); therefore, the selective damage of sensitized cells close to the PS is achieved. The ROS are responsible for irreversible damage to various cell membranes.

10.3 QDs IN PDT

The advent of nanotechnology opened up new possibilities for PDT, in which nanoparticles were used as highly sophisticated, multifunctional medicines. More specifically, nanoparticles have been employed as PSs; carriers of photosensitizing molecules; light antennas for photosensitizing molecules (up- and down-converters), and carriers of multiple functionalities, for example, targeting moieties or magnetic nanoparticles. Theoretically, nanoparticles have the potential to improve PDT beyond its current limitations (Cuenca et al., 2006; Chatterjee et al., 2008; Hild et al., 2008; Nann, 2011). Surfaces of nanoparticles can be modified with different functional moieties such as PSs and/or targeting molecules (e.g., antibodies against certain types of cancer cells). Thus, although administered systemically, the nanoparticles are expected to concentrate at the target site.

Several types of nanoparticles have been discussed as potential candidates for PDT, but only QDs demonstrably generate singlet oxygen (Samia et al., 2003). Besides, among various nanoparticles, proposed as promising materials for many biological and medical applications, QDs are most attractive due to their unique spectral properties and easy surface modification by binding different functional groups and biomolecules (Medintz et al., 2005).

Although QDs have great potential for biomedicine, there are some limitations restricting their usefulness. One of them is possible instability and the following toxicity of the individual components that may be released. A few reports suggest that QDs can exert deleterious effects on metabolic processes. QDs-induced toxicity was found to be correlated with a slow release of toxic Cd^{2+} and Te^{2-} ions (Lovric et al., 2005a,b; Yang et al., 2007; Karabanovas et al., 2008). Excitation by UV radiation induced degradation of QDs (Nel et al., 2006; Ramanavicius et al., 2009). Precipitation of the QDs caused by the ligands desorption from the surface was observed after 1–2 days in aqueous buffer (Kloepfer et al., 2005). Therefore, the stability and toxicity of QDs should be carefully considered when determining whether they could be used for in vivo applications. The detrimental effect of the highly toxic element cadmium (Matović et al., 2011), which is a component of the widely used CdSe QDs, might be avoided by using alternative materials such as InP (Xu et al., 2006, 2008, 2009).

The direct generation of singlet oxygen by CdSe QDs was first studied in 2003 (Samia et al., 2003). The authors found that the quantum yield of $^1O_2$ production was approximately 5%. Later, a quantum yield of about 1% for the direct generation of $^1O_2$ by CdTe QDs was observed (Ma et al., 2008). The same group using the same type of QDs declared the generation of ROS by a so-called type I mechanism (Chen et al., 2010). Quantum yields of the ROS generation have not been measured. It has to be noted that some wide band-gap semiconductor QDs such as ZnO (Li et al., 2010) and TiO_2 (Cai et al., 1992; Yamaguchi et al., 2010) have been tested as direct PSs too; however, no systematic studies as to the quantum yields and nature of the ROS have been performed yet. A principal limitation of wide band-gap QDs is that they have to be excited by UV light, which does not penetrate deep into tissue and may cause radiation damage.

It is reasonable to conclude that QDs themselves are no match for conventional molecular PSs. The quantum efficiencies for $^1O_2$ generation measured so far are far below figures suitable for clinical applications. However, the fact that QDs have a very high absorption cross section for excitation light makes them still interesting as light antennas for molecular PSs (Leatherdale et al., 2002; Osborne et al., 2004) if one ignores the possibility that the patients might suffer from subsequent heavy-metal poisoning.

In contrast to the unique optical properties of QDs, conventional PSs usually demonstrate relatively low absorption in the spectral region of good tissue transparency, they can have poor photostability and small two-photon absorption cross sections, yet the efficiency of ROS generation by PSs is up to 60%–70% while that of QDs is only about 5%. Nevertheless, it has been suggested to exploit QDs not only as diagnostic agents, but also as resonance energy donors to excite classical PSs. It is believed that using QD–PS systems could improve efficiency of PDT in many ways. The ability to control the QDs encapsulation and surface functionalization for better water solubility, biocompatibility, and targeting makes QDs favorable for PDT. Moreover, the optical properties of QDs such as a high extinction coefficient (10^5–10^6 M^{-1} cm^{-1}) and broad-absorption spectrum makes it easier to excite a PS in the QD–PS conjugate. Furthermore, due to the tunable emission spectrum that can be achieved by varying the QD size, the high emission quantum yield, and long lifetime, QDs can work simultaneously as fluorescent reporters for imaging as well as energy donors for PS. The energy transmitted from QD to PS could further be used for generation of ROS (Ipe et al., 2005; Lovric et al., 2005b; Shi et al., 2006; Cho et al., 2007). The scheme in Figure 10.5 illustrates these processes, which could be induced after photoexcitation of QD–PS conjugate during PDT. So, the unique spectral properties of QDs make them very suitable donors for the Förster resonance energy transfer (FRET) process. Therefore, it has been suggested that QDs conjugated with conventional PSs could form photosensitizing nanoparticles efficiently generating powerful oxidizing species, and such conjugates have been investigated as a possible new type of PSs in which the excited singlet and triplet states of PS are indirectly generated by nonradiative energy transfer from photoactivated QDs during the FRET process (Samia et al., 2003; Medintz and Mattoussi, 2009).

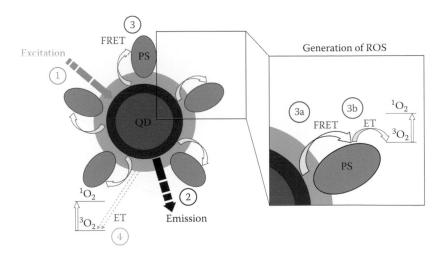

Figure 10.5 The processes induced after photoexcitation of QD in QD–PS conjugate. The absorbed energy by QD could be returned by emission, which is an advantage when QDs are used for imaging. The excitation energy could also be transferred to a bound PS molecule via FRET mechanism (3). PS excited by this indirect way can further pass the energy to surrounding oxygen molecules ($^3O_2$) by exciting them to a singlet state ($^1O_2$) (3b). The third possible way is when photoexcited QD directly generates singlet oxygen or other reactive species (4). These last two processes are desirable for PDT.

As indicated earlier, there are several advantages and limitations for both conventional PSs and for QDs when they are individually applied for PDT. The aim of QD–PS conjugates was to combine the advantages and limitations of both the QDs and PS so that they complement each other. Thus, in order to utilize the photostability of QDs and improve the production of $^1O_2$, conjugates of QDs and conventional PSs have been investigated as possible new-generation drugs for PDT. In such conjugated systems, the excited states of PSs are indirectly generated by nonradiative FRET from photoactivated QDs. Due to the indirect photoactivation, photobleaching of PSs can be minimized. The indirectly excited PSs transfer energy to $^3O_2$, and generate $^1O_2$ and other ROS.

10.3.1 FÖRSTER RESONANCE ENERGY TRANSFER

The experimental data of nonradiative energy transfer between QDs (donors—D) and PSs (acceptors—A) are excellently described by the formal Förster theory. FRET involves the nonradiative transfer of excitation energy from an excited state of a donor fluorophore molecule to a ground state of a proximal acceptor molecule; it is driven by dipole–dipole coupling between donor and acceptor (Förster, 1965).

FRET between organic molecules is quite a common process and has been widely exploited in a variety of biological studies (Lakowitcz, 1999). However, only recently has FRET been reported in hybrid nanomaterials composed of QDs and organic dyes. The first demonstration that QDs could efficiently transfer energy via FRET was reported in QDs systems between QDs of different sizes. In the pioneering experiments, it was shown that FRET occurs between closely packed QDs of two different diameters: smaller (38.5 Å diameter) serving as exciton donors and larger ones (62 Å) functioning as energy acceptors (Kagan et al., 1996). Further studies demonstrated that inorganic QDs could function perfectly as FRET donors for different organic fluorophores (Clapp et al., 2004; Medintz et al., 2004), including porphyrin-type PSs used for PDT (Samia et al., 2003).

The use of QDs as FRET donors for PS molecules is particularly attractive due to (1) the ability to tune the emission wavelength of QDs by either simple manipulation of the dimensions of the nanocrystal and/or modification of the composition of the inorganic core, which can allow a better spectral overlap with the acceptor absorption band; (2) high quantum yield and long lifetime of emission; (3) resistance to photobleaching; and (4) ease of surface modifications and subsequent possibilities of stable and controllable binding of donor molecules.

The primary conditions that need to be met in order for FRET to occur are relatively few.

1. The donor and acceptor molecules must be in close proximity to one another (typically 10–100 Å). The efficiency of the energy transfer (E) depends on the inverse sixth power of the distance between donor and acceptor:

$$E = \frac{R_0^6}{R_0^6 + r^6} \tag{10.1}$$

where

R_0 is a "Förster distance" at which the efficiency of transfer is 50%
r is the actual distance between donor and acceptor

In Equation 10.1, R_0 is determined by

$$R_0 = \left(\frac{9000 (\ln 10) Q_D \kappa^2}{128 N_A \pi^5 n^4} J \right)^{1/6} \tag{10.2}$$

where

Q_D is the quantum yield of the donor emission in the absence of acceptor
κ^2 is a dipole orientation factor describing the relative orientation of the transition dipoles of the donor and acceptor
n is the refractive index of the medium ($n = 1.33$ for water)
J is the spectral overlap integral of donor emission and acceptor absorbance.

From Equation 10.2, the Förster distance in angstroms becomes

$$R_0 = 0.211 \left(Q_D \kappa^2 n^{-4} J \right)^{1/6} \quad \left(\text{in } \overset{\circ}{A} \right) \tag{10.3}$$

The key requirement for the efficient energy transfer in conjugates is close proximity of the components— QD and PS. Therefore, when mixed in solutions QD and PS should be either covalently bound or a complex formed due to noncovalent interactions.

2. The absorption spectrum of the acceptor must overlap the emission spectrum of the donor (Figure 10.6). The overlap integral J is calculated from

$$J = \frac{\int F_D (\lambda) \varepsilon_A (\lambda) \lambda^4 d\lambda}{\int F_D (\lambda) d\lambda} \tag{10.4}$$

where

$F_D(\lambda)$ is the emission spectrum of donor
$\varepsilon_A(\lambda)$ is the molar extinction coefficient of acceptor
λ is the wavelength in nanometers

3. The process also strongly depends on the relative orientation of the donor and acceptor transition dipoles. The κ^2 is the donor (QDs) and acceptor (PS) dipole orientation factor ($\kappa^2 = 2/3$ is often assumed, considering that both donor and acceptor are isotropically oriented during the excited state lifetime).

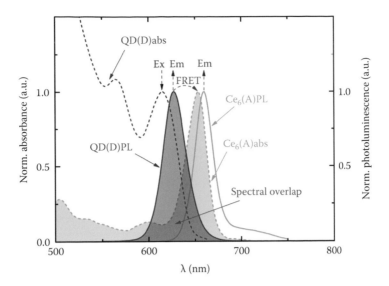

Figure 10.6 Normalized absorption and emission spectra of CdSe/ZnS QDs and Ce$_6$ in PBS of pH 7. Filled area indicates the overlap of donor QDs emission with the absorption spectrum of acceptor Ce$_6$.

Experimentally the FRET efficiency is estimated from

$$E = 1 - \frac{F_{DA}}{F_D} \tag{10.5}$$

where
F_{DA} is the integrated fluorescence intensity of the donor in the presence of the acceptor
F_D is the integrated fluorescence intensity of the donor alone (no acceptors present).

The quantum yield of donor fluorescence in Equation 10.3 is estimated by comparison with a reference fluorophore with a well-known quantum yield (Q_R):

$$Q = Q_R \frac{F}{F_R} \frac{OD_R}{OD} \frac{n^2}{n_R^2} \tag{10.6}$$

where F and F_R are the integrated emission intensities of donor and reference, respectively.

10.3.2 QD–PS CONJUGATES

The majority of studies on different noncovalent QD-PS systems reported to date have focused on assemblies in solution, based mostly either on electrostatic (Samia et al., 2003; Shi et al., 2006; Orlova et al., 2008a,b; Idowu and Nyokong, 2010; Keane et al., 2012) or coordinational (Zenkevich et al., 2005; Dayal et al., 2006a,b) interactions. Despite the rather efficient FRET in these conjugates, they tend to aggregate or may lose noncovalently bound PSs. Covalently coupled QD–PS systems (Tsay et al., 2007; Qi et al., 2011; Charron et al., 2012) meet the stability requirements in this respect; however, efficient FRET is hard to achieve because PS molecules are grafted at the interface between water and the QD coating, which is relatively far from the QD core. The first demonstration utilizing QD-based FRET to facilitate excitation of a PS to generate ROS was performed in the organic solvent toluene (Dayal et al., 2006a,b; Samia et al., 2006).

The formation of CdS/ZnS QDs capped with TOPO and nonspecific conjugates with pyridyl-substituted porphyrins in toluene solution was also demonstrated by Zenkevich et al. (2005, 2007). It was shown that the quenching efficiency of QDs emission by porphyrins was dependent on the number and position of pyridyl rings and on the position of nitrogen atom within the pyridyl ring. This was related to the manner and orientation of pyridyl groups having an effect on porphyrin attachment to the surface of QDs. It was concluded that pyridyl-substituted porphyrin molecules are anchored on the CdSe/ZnS surface in a nearly perpendicular fashion with two nitrogen lone pair orbitals forming coordination bonds with the surface. The authors stated that FRET is a good qualitative tool to identify formation of QD–PS conjugates (Zenkevich et al., 2005).

10.3.2.1 QD–PS CONJUGATES IN AQUEOUS MEDIUM

The first study on a QD-porphyrin conjugate in aqueous solution was reported by Shi et al. (2006). Water-soluble CdTe QDs coated with 2-aminoethanethiol (cysteamine) and meso-tetra(4-sulfonatophenyl)porphine (TSPP) as a PS were used. It was proposed that a QD–TSPP conjugate was formed via electrostatic interaction. The measurements in D_2O revealed that such conjugate was able to produce $^1O_2$ with the quantum yield of 0.43. Since QD–TSPP conjugate was excited at the wavelength where the absorption of free TSPP was minimal, the authors suggested that $^1O_2$ was produced via excitation of QDs followed by a FRET mechanism. No $^1O_2$ was generated when QDs were excited in the absence of TSPP; this was in contrast to results obtained by Samia et al. (2003) who observed a small amount (5%) of $^1O_2$ formed directly from excitation of CdSe QDs.

The investigations of energy transfer and $^1O_2$ generation were extended to a large number of QD-phthalocyanine (QD–Pc) conjugates as functions of donor–acceptor distance, relative numbers of QDs and Pcs, terminal functional group in Pc, bulkiness of spacers between donors and acceptors, the mode of binding between QD and Pc, and the size and surface states of QDs (Dayal et al., 2006a, 2008; Samia et al., 2006; Dayal and Burda, 2007). It was stated that functional groups in Pc played important roles in both QD–Pc bonding and quenching of the excited state of QDs. In particular, the energy transfer efficiency was found higher when Pc molecules were linked to QDs through two axial amine or thiol groups (Dayal et al., 2006a,b, 2008). Also, the authors found that functional groups such as amine and thiol in the Pc played important roles in both QD to Pc bonding and quenching of the excited state of QDs. In particular, the energy transfer efficiency was found higher when Pc molecules were linked to QDs through two axial amine or thiol groups.

Investigations on energy transfer from QD to Pc and the $^1O_2$ generation efficiency were extended into conjugates of CdTe QDs and tetrasulfonated aluminum Pc (AlTSPc) (Idowu et al., 2008; Moeno and Nyokong, 2008, 2009). The mixtures of CdTe–AlTSPc were prepared by adding solutions of AlTSPc of different concentrations to solutions of CdTe QDs with three different capping ligands (Idowu et al., 2008). In this mixture, the excited state of QDs was quenched and resulted in an increase in the triplet yield for AlTSPc along with fluorescence emission from AlTSPc. Further investigations were extended to energy transfer to various metallophthalocyanines linked to CdTe QDs through sulfonic acid, carboxylic acid, and pyridinium group (Moeno and Nyokong, 2009). By varying the metal ion and functional groups in Pc, conjugates of QD–Pc systems with exceptionally high triplet yields and energy transfer efficiencies (up to 80%) were obtained. The most important properties of these conjugates were their water solubility and ability to generate singlet oxygen.

10.3.2.2 SPECTROSCOPY OF THE QD–PS CONJUGATION PROCESS

To study conjugation occurring between QDs and PS molecules, water-soluble CdSe/ZnS QDs with a lipid-based coating-bearing terminal amine or carboxyl groups (Figure 10.4) were coupled to the second-generation PS chlorin e_6 (Ce$_6$) in aqueous solution at pH 7 and the process was investigated spectroscopically (Valanciunaite et al., 2010; Valanciunaite and Rotomskis, 2010; Rotomskis et al., 2013). It is well established that the CdSe nanocrystal core capped with ZnS shell (which not only increases the stability and emission quantum yield, but also reduces the toxicity of the core by shielding reactive Cd^{2+} ions from exposure to the environment) coated with a phospholipid block–copolymer micelle with attached poly(ethylene glycol) polymer and terminal carboxyl and amine groups have a high quantum yield of PL and display a great reduction of photobleaching and colloidal stability in a variety of bioenvironments (Dubertret et al., 2002). QDs were chosen in accordance with an emission maximum to fulfill the condition of spectral overlap between the emission of donor and absorption of acceptor for FRET (Figure 10.6). The absorption spectrum of QD is broad with gradual decrease in intensity toward the red spectral range, while the emission band is narrow with a maximum at 605 nm. The emission band of QDs partially overlaps with the last two absorption bands

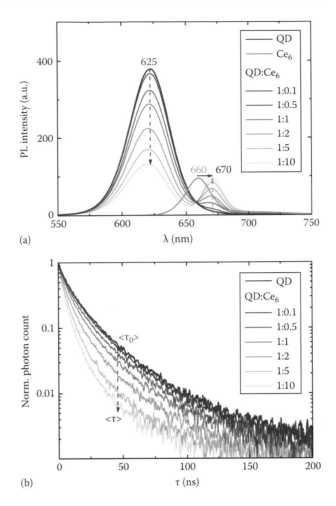

Figure 10.7 Emission spectra of QD, Ce_6, and mixed QD–Ce_6 solutions at increasing QD:Ce_6 molar ratio from 1:0.1 to 1:10, $\lambda_{ex} = 465$ nm (a). PL decay of QD and QD–Ce_6 solutions at increasing QD:Ce_6 molar ratio from 1:0.1 to 1:10 registered at $\lambda_{em} = 620$ nm (b).

of Ce_6. For FRET studies, the excitation wavelength ($\lambda_{ex} = 465$ nm) was selected to coincide with the minimum of Ce_6 absorption spectrum in order to reduce contributions resulting from the direct excitation of Ce_6.

Distinct changes in intensity were observed in the fluorescence spectra of mixed QD–Ce_6 solutions at different molar ratios of QDs and Ce_6 (Figure 10.7a). When Ce_6 was added to QDs solution, the fluorescence band of Ce_6 underwent a bathochromic shift from 660 to 670 nm. Upon increase in Ce_6 concentration, the intensity of QDs emission significantly decreased, while the intensity of Ce_6 fluorescence at 670 nm increased simultaneously. The formation of QD–Ce_6 conjugate and occurrence of FRET was confirmed by the measurements of the fluorescence lifetime performed in QD–Ce_6 mixtures in solution with different molar ratios of QDs and Ce_6 (Figure 10.7b). The results showed shortening of the QDs fluorescence lifetime at increasing Ce_6 concentration (Valanciunaite and Rotomskis, 2010; Valanciunate et al., 2010, 2014). The fluorescence decay of QDs in the absence as well as in the presence of Ce_6 could be satisfactorily fitted to a three-exponential decay model with respect to time. The average lifetime of the entire decay process of pure QDs was $<\tau> = 18.9$ ns ($\chi^2 = 1.01$), while in the presence of Ce_6 (QD:Ce_6 1:20) it shortened to $<\tau> = 4.9$ ns ($\chi^2 = 1.16$).

The fluorescence excitation spectra confirmed that part of the QDs energy was transferred to Ce_6 molecules since the spectrum of QD–Ce_6 solutions measured at $\lambda_{em} = 670$ nm displayed a spectral contribution from both QDs and Ce_6 (Valanciunaite et al., 2010). The intensity of contribution from the QDs spectrum was significantly higher than the intensity of fluorescence excitation spectrum of pure QDs in solution measured at this emission wavelength. These findings indicated that a self-assembled QD–Ce$_6$ conjugate was formed and the process of energy transfer from QDs to bound Ce$_6$ molecules occurred within it.

In the first approach, it was reasonable to expect that the electrostatic interaction between the positively charged amino groups of the QD coating and negatively charged carboxyl groups of Ce$_6$ might be a pivotal mechanism for QD–Ce$_6$ conjugate formation.

Attempts to produce stable QD–PS conjugates in aqueous solutions via electrostatic interaction have been reported (Idowu et al., 2008; Orlova et al., 2008a,b; Idowu and Nyokong, 2010; Jhonsi and Renganathan, 2010). However, in most of these studies the aggregation of the conjugates appeared to be the main cause of instability. For instance, aggregation was found during the formation of a complex between CdTe(TGA) QDs and metal-free tetra(p-trimethylamino) phenylporphyrin (Orlova et al., 2008a), as well as between CdTe(cysteamine) QDs and AlOH-tetrasulfophthalocyanine (Orlova et al., 2008b). Addition of CdTe(MPA) QDs also caused the aggregation of cationic zinc phthalocyanine in methanol–water solution (Idowu and Nyokong, 2010). Interesting results were obtained with TGA capped CdTe QDs and porphyrins with differently charged meso-substituents (Jhonsi and Renganathan, 2010). The quenching of QDs luminescence was observed upon increasing the concentration of both negatively and positively charged porphyrins; however, the intensity of emission from negatively charged (but not positively charged) porphyrins increased and became higher than that in the absence of QDs. The authors concluded that the negatively charged porphyrins interacted with QDs through an energy transfer mechanism, while positively charged porphyrin molecules interacted through a charge transfer mechanism (Jhonsi and Renganathan, 2010).

In a recent study of Orlova et al. (2013), conjugates were formed as a result of electrostatic interaction between QDs and some PSs widely used in PDT, AlOH-tetrasulfophthalocyanine (TSPC) and metal-free tetra(p-trimethylamino)phenylporphin, which is a positively charged substituted derivative of tetraphenyl-porphin. The authors stated that electrostatic (or another type) interaction occurred in the fabrication of QD–PS conjugates, in which FRET from QDs to PS molecules could occur, and stressed that the nature of the interaction between QDs and PS molecules is crucial for the stability, photophysical properties, and FRET efficacy.

To elucidate the actual nature of the QDs and PSs interaction and conjugate formation, spectroscopic measurements were performed with identical QDs, which were coated with terminal carboxyl (negatively charged) groups replacing amino (positively charged) groups (Valanciunaite et al., 2010). Interaction between QDs coated with either positively charged amino groups or negatively charged carboxyl groups and Ce$_6$ resulted in identical spectral positions of the fluorescence band of the latter, implying that electrostatic interaction was not responsible for the observed formation of a conjugate of QDs and Ce$_6$. The shifted position of this band in relation to that observed in PBS and its similarity with that of Ce$_6$ dissolved in chloroform (Valanciunaite et al., 2010) indicated that the spectral properties of Ce$_6$ are very sensitive to environmental polarity. Since chloroform solution is hydrophobic, it is reasonable to presume that upon binding to QDs, Ce$_6$ molecules are immersed in the hydrophobic part of the QD lipid coating. This presumption is in agreement with a report, demonstrating the localization of Ce$_6$ in most cellular membranes (Bachor et al., 1991). Another study using NMR spectroscopy of Ce$_6$ also demonstrated its localization in phospholipid bilayers, where molecules of Ce$_6$ were immersed in the vicinity of polar heads of phospholipids (Vermathen et al., 2010). On the basis of these considerations, it could be stated that Ce$_6$ molecules within the QD coating are situated in a hydrophobic microenvironment, most likely, the hydrophobic part of QD lipids. This was also confirmed by the absorption and fluorescence measurements of Ce$_6$ in the presence of 5% Triton-X 100, a well-known nonionic surfactant whose critical micelle concentration is above 0.02%. Addition of Triton-X 100 to aqueous solution of Ce$_6$ produced precisely the same red-shift in its absorption and fluorescence bands as was the case with QDs (Valanciunaite et al., 2014). The same bathochromic shift of the Ce$_6$ fluorescence maximum to 670 nm was also reported for Ce$_6$ in the presence of lipid bilayers (Frolov et al., 1990; Magde et al., 1999). Under excitation at 400 nm, where both QDs and free Ce$_6$ can be efficiently excited, this red-shifted emission was observed for the range of Ce$_6$/QD ratios 0.5–5, without any sign of unbound Ce$_6$ at 660 nm.

Meanwhile, the measurements performed with QDs, which did not have a lipid-based coating, but were capped with MUA or TGA, did not result in any changes in the Ce$_6$ spectrum. This finding suggested that lipid-based coating plays a major role in the formation of QD–Ce$_6$ conjugate. Indeed, a similar bathochromic

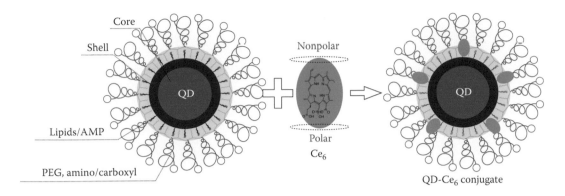

Figure 10.8 Model of QD–Ce$_6$ conjugate formation. Ce$_6$ bears polar carboxyl groups on one side of the porphyrin macro cycle whereas the opposite side is rather nonpolar. Most probably upon binding to QDs, the nonpolar part of Ce$_6$ molecule immerses in the hydrophobic part of lipid coating of QD, while carboxyl groups are exposed to water surroundings.

shift of fluorescence bands was observed upon binding of Ce$_6$ to plasma proteins, LDL and to DOPC unilamellar vesicles (Mojzisova et al., 2007), that is, when Ce$_6$ molecules localize in hydrophobic environment. Most probably, upon binding to QD, the nonpolar part of Ce$_6$ molecule is immersed in the hydrophobic part of lipid coating of QD. This is also in agreement with Ce$_6$ cellular localization studies, which demonstrated that Ce$_6$ molecules tend to localize in most cellular membranes (Bachor et al., 1991) and membrane models (Vermathen et al., 2000). Therefore, by summarizing these results, we proposed a model of QD–Ce$_6$ conjugate formation with a schematic illustration of how Ce$_6$ molecules might be arranged within it (Figure 10.8). Results of spectroscopic investigations (Valanciunaite and Rotomskis, 2010; Valanciunaite et al., 2010, 2014) imply that hydrophobic interactions might be a promising way for creating of QD–PS conjugates for PDT.

10.3.2.3 COVALENTLY LINKED QD–PS CONJUGATES

The first covalently linked QD–PS conjugates were created from peptide-coated CdSe/CdS/ZnS QDs and two PSs known to generate singlet oxygen with relatively high yield, rose bengal and Ce$_6$ (Tsay et al., 2007). The conjugates of Ce$_6$ with CdSe/CdS/ZnS QDs were linked noncovalently using an alkyl amine linker or covalently using a lysine-terminated peptide linker in this study. The authors found that the PL lifetime of QDs was decreased as a result of energy transfer from QDs to Ce$_6$, as well as that the energy transfer efficiency from QD to Ce$_6$ increased with increase in the number of Ce$_6$ molecules attached to a single QD.

The PSs were first coupled to a phytochelatin related peptide via an NHS ester linkage and then were used to cap the surface of CdSe–ZnS QDs. In such conjugates, the average number of PS molecules per QD conjugate was controlled by mixing with other unlabeled peptides (mixed surface conjugates) and changing the molar ratio of peptide-PS before assembly on the QDs. The dramatic increase in fluorescence intensity of both rose bengal as well as Ce$_6$ in comparison to the PSs alone was observed after such covalent attachment to QDs. This observation was accompanied by a decrease in emission intensity and lifetime of QDs. Moreover, it was shown that such conjugates were able to not only undergo FRET but also produce singlet oxygen. Detection of singlet oxygen generated from QD–PS conjugates was accomplished by measuring the singlet oxygen phosphorescence signal at 1270 nm, while excitation of the system (at either 532 or 355 nm) was provided by an Nd:YAG multiphoton laser. The highest quantum yield of singlet oxygen generation was obtained for QD–Ce$_6$ (0.31).

10.3.3 GENERATION OF SINGLET OXYGEN BY QD–PS CONJUGATES

Singlet oxygen and ROS are main inducers of damage to cellular components such as proteins, lipids, DNA, and carbohydrates, leading to cell death (Figure 10.2). Therefore, in the studies on the application of QD–PS conjugates in PDT, employing QDs as potential energy donors for PSs, researchers usually tested the most important requirement for PDT agents—the ability to generate $^1O_2$ as the main reactive intermediate in photosensitized cancer cell killing.

The concept of the production of $^1O_2$ by a QD–PS conjugate was tested by preparing a noncovalent mixture composed of CdSe QDs and a silicon phthalocyanine (Pc4), where the PS was linked to QD through an alkyl group on the axial substituent of Pc4 (Samia et al., 2003). The first report about water-soluble QD–PS conjugate capable of producing $^1O_2$ via FRET was presented by Shi et al. (2006). The authors used a QD–TSPP conjugate formed by electrostatic interaction. QDs were excited by Nd:YAG laser light of 355 nm. TSPP absorbs light at this wavelength relatively weakly, although the production of singlet oxygen was observed using NIR detection at 1270 nm. The CdTe-TSPP conjugate produced $^1O_2$ with 43% efficiency when photoactivated at 355 nm. It was stated that detectable levels of $^1O_2$ were produced only by QDs–TSPP conjugate. In the conjugates of CdSe/CdS/ZnS QDs and Ce_6, constructed noncovalently using an alkyl amine linker or covalently using a lysine-terminated peptide linker, a 31% efficiency of $^1O_2$ generation was obtained (Tsay et al., 2007).

In contrast to the generation of $^1O_2$ and other ROS by CdSe QDs (Samia et al., 2003; Anas et al., 2008), $^1O_2$ production was not detected for CdTe QDs alone, indicating that QD–PS conjugates were significantly more suitable for PDT compared with QDs alone. The generation of $^1O_2$ by thiol-capped CdTe QDs bound to a sulfonated aluminum phthalocyanine was investigated (Ma et al., 2008). Indirect excitation of the PS resulted in efficient $^1O_2$ generation with an overall quantum yield of approximately 0.15, whereas excitation of the pure QDs resulted in an insignificant $^1O_2$ generation with a yield of only 0.01.

It has been found that photoactivated QDs can directly transfer energy to nearby oxygen molecules and generate $^1O_2$ (Samia et al., 2003; Bakalova et al., 2004) and other ROS (Ipe et al., 2005), but the efficiency of this processes is poor (Samia et al., 2003; Lovric et al., 2005b; Anas et al., 2008; Yaghini et al., 2009). Although the QDs are superior to organic PSs in terms of photostability and water dispersability (Gao et al., 2004; Michalet et al., 2005; Resch-Genger et al., 2008), the clinical translation of these agents has been limited owing to their cytotoxicity and low ROS generation efficiency (Samia et al., 2003; Bakalova et al., 2004; Ye et al., 2012).

On the other hand, energy transfer processes from QDs to PS and from PS to oxygen, in QD–PS conjugates may provide a significantly higher efficiency for $^1O_2$ and ROS production compared with free PSs (Clarke et al., 2006; Hsieh et al., 2006; Shi et al., 2006; Tsay et al., 2007; Ma et al., 2008; Narband et al., 2008; Neuman et al., 2008; Duong and Rhee, 2011; Ishii, 2012). Therefore, approaches such as modifying semiconductor QDs with a traditional PDT agent (porphyrin derivative, Ce_6) and then coating them with a shell of peptides have been developed to reduce the cytotoxicity of these agents (Tsay et al., 2007). The conjugation of QDs with PS that is targeted for cancer might help to solve some of the excitation and selectivity problems of conventional tetrapyrroles, thus greatly enhancing their applicability and efficiency in PDT. A PDT agent with a high $^1O_2$ quantum yield and excellent photostability and biocompatibility is highly desirable.

In the studies on the possible application of QD-Ce_6 conjugates in PDT, the ability to generate $^1O_2$ was tested using the commercially available fluorescent reporter dye—singlet oxygen sensor green (SOSG). CdSe/ZnS (605 nm) QDs bearing lipid-based coating with terminal amine groups diluted to the concentration of 0.02 μM and Ce_6 diluted to the working 0.2 μM concentration were used for the preparation of conjugate (the QD:Ce_6 molar ratio 1:10 was obtained). All solutions were irradiated with a light beam at around 460 nm since the absorbance of Ce_6 at this wavelength is minimal. Thus, the stability of a QD-Ce_6 conjugate and generation of singlet oxygen were assessed in a way preventing the direct photoexcitation of Ce_6 (Rotomskis et al., 2013). Figure 10.9 shows changes in fluorescence intensity of SOSG in QDs, Ce_6, and QD–Ce_6 mixture solutions measured at 528 nm after various exposures to the light beam at about 460 nm. A significant increase of SOSG fluorescence intensity for about 30% was observed in QD–Ce_6 conjugate solution after exposure to 160 J/cm², and almost no fluorescence changes of SOSG were observed in solutions of QDs and Ce_6. This result indicates that upon irradiation in the region of QDs absorbance, $^1O_2$ is produced, and an increase in intensity of SOSG fluorescence measured at 528 nm is proportional to the detected amount of $^1O_2$.

So, it seems that a QD–Ce_6 conjugate irradiated by visible light that was almost completely not absorbed by the PS, is able to produce $^1O_2$ more efficiently than QDs or Ce_6 alone, and could be a potential candidate for PDT.

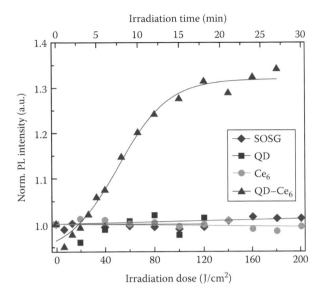

Figure 10.9 Fluorescence of SOSG measured at 528 nm after various exposures to light beam at about 460 nm. Intensities were normalized according to formulae $I_{irr}/I_{nonirr} \times A_{nonirr}/A_{irr}$.

10.3.4 PDT VIA FRET IN QD–PS CONJUGATES

There have been only a few reports to date about QDs being used as donors coupled to PSs acceptors with the idea to use the conjugates for photosensitization via FRET. For the effective functioning of such conjugates as singlet-oxygen generators, two conditions should be simultaneously fulfilled: (1) the ability of the PS molecules (usually tetrapyrroles) to generate singlet oxygen upon conjugation should be maintained and (2) the effective intraconjugate photoexcitation energy transfer should occur (Martynenko et al., 2013). So, close conjugation (Equation 10.1), typically within 10 nm, of PS to QD is necessary for efficient energy transfer and ROS production (Medintz and Mattoussi, 2009).

Following the first investigation of conjugated system (Samia et al., 2003), the attention of researchers was attracted to the energy transfer properties of covalent and noncovalent QD–PS systems composed of CdSe, CdSe/CdS/ZnS, CdSe/ZnS, and CdTe QDs as energy donors and various chromophores such as phthalocyanines, porphyrins, and other organic dyes as energy acceptors. One of the advantages of QD–PS conjugates over conventional PSs is possibility to photoactivate PS indirectly by using photostable QDs, which offers prolonged imaging and PDT without photobleaching. Most of PSs used in PDT are not photostable. In simple solutions as well as in complex environments, PSs undergo light-induced modification, resulting in a decrease of their initial absorption and fluorescence intensity. This phenomenon is called photobleaching and includes the following photoprocesses: (1) photodegradation—the conversion of sensitizer into products that do not absorb visible light appreciably (Spikes, 1992); (2) photorelocalization—the alteration of photophysical properties due to the light-induced migration of sensitizer from one binding site to another (Moan and Kessel, 1988); or (3) phototransformation—as in case of some porphyrins, leading to the formation of new red-absorbing photoproducts (Giniunas et al., 1991; Rotomskis et al., 1996, 1997a,b). Photobleaching has important consequences for PDT dosimetry. In clinical trials, PSs are generally illuminated by red light. Therefore, calculation of phototherapeutic dose requires additional information about the formation of red-absorbing photoproducts. Photodegradation of the PS results in a decrease in its initial concentration and, as a consequence, a lower sensitizing effect. This can be either an advantage or a disadvantage depending on the initial concentration of the sensitizer and its distribution in tumor and surrounding tissues (Mang et al., 1987). If the PS bleaches too rapidly, tumor destruction will not be complete but the use of appropriate illumination doses can protect normal tissues from irreversible damage.

Another advantage of these conjugates is the rather large surface area of QDs that can serve as space for binding PSs and corresponding binding ligands for targeted cancer imaging and PDT. QDs can be functionalized by conjugation to a number of biological molecules, such as avidin, biotin, oligonucleotides, peptides, antibodies, and DNA (Alivisatos et al., 2005), through surface reactive groups for specific targeted action. Methods of bioconjugation broadly fall into two categories: noncovalent and covalent conjugation (Xing et al., 2009). Covalent linkage is the most stable of all the bioconjugation methods and utilizes functional groups on the QD surface, such as primary amines, carboxylic acids, and thiols, to form a covalent bond with similar groups present on the biomolecules or through the use of crosslinker molecules (Alivisatos et al., 2005). With their large surface areas, QDs can also individually accommodate several PSs molecules simultaneously and in this way enhance the local concentration of sensitizer (Medintz et al., 2005).

Up to the present, a few reports on the primary photophysical properties of QD–PS conjugates in aqueous solutions (assembled mainly by electrostatic interaction) have been performed (Shi et al., 2006; Juzenas et al., 2008; Orlova et al., 2008a; Yaghini et al., 2009; Martynenko et al., 2013). These studies have demonstrated the possibility for effective FRET processes (Medintz and Mattoussi, 2009; Masilela and Nyokong, 2012; Orlova et al., 2013; Dworak et al., 2014; Thomas et al., 2014) in various QD–PS donor–acceptor systems. However, the stability, compatibility in biological media, singlet-oxygen generation, and phototoxicity in vitro and in vivo of these conjugates is still an active area for investigation. Although much effort has been focused on FRET studies in conjugates and the fundamental energy transfer mechanisms underlying such hybrid systems, biomedical application of this phenomenon has remained largely unexplored. Biological systems are significantly more complicated as compared with pure solutions. Therefore, the question whether the FRET-mediated PDT by QD–PS conjugates would be efficient in living systems remains to be answered. There are very few studies on the efficacy of QD–PS conjugates killing of cancer cells via FRET-mediated PDT.

Conjugates of CdSe/ZnS QDs with Ce$_6$ after QD-selective irradiation at 470 nm showed phototoxicity in MiaPaCa2 cells: a light-induced damage to cancer cells via energy transfer was achieved (Steponkiene et al., 2014). Sulfonated aluminum phthalocyanine conjugates with QDs easily penetrated into human nasopharyngeal carcinoma cells and carried out the FRET in cells with an efficiency around 80% (Li et al., 2012). However, QDs technology is still in its infancy and extensive research about their different toxicity effects requires to be performed before their safe application in clinical medicine. Recently, less toxic InP/ZnS QDs conjugated with PS Ce$_6$ were used for in vitro PDT of MDA-MB-231 breast cancer cells. Illumination with UV light resulted in a decrease in the viability of the cells (Charron et al., 2012). One of the latest studies (Martynenko et al., 2015) was devoted to PDT testing of Cd-free ZnSe/ZnS QDs and Ce$_6$ conjugates on Erlich acsite carcinoma cells in culture. The results obtained demonstrated a twofold enhancement of the cancer cell photodynamic destruction compared with that of free Ce$_6$ molecules. It was shown that the PDT effect was significantly increased due to the efficient QD–Ce$_6$ photoexcitation energy transfer.

10.3.5 Killing of cancer cells via FRET

The main condition for conjugate application in living cells is the ability to maintain their conjugation intact, which requires stable binding between QDs and PSs. Besides, QD–PS conjugates are also required to maintain their physical properties in the cellular environment in order to carry out the FRET. Sufficient accumulation of conjugates in cancer cells is also necessary.

Sulfonated aluminum phthalocyanine (AlPcS) (a commonly used PDT PS) was conjugated with amine-dihydrolipoic acid-coated QDs by electrostatic binding (Li et al., 2012). AlPcS–QD conjugates were stable not only in solution but also in cellular environments. They easily penetrated into human nasopharyngeal carcinoma cells and carried out the FRET in cells with an efficiency around 80%. Under irradiation with 532 nm laser light, which is at the absorption region of QDs but does not fit the absorption of AlPcS, the cellular AlPcS–QD conjugates could destroy most cancer cells via FRET-mediated PDT, showing the potential of this new strategy for PDT. Furthermore, the AlPcS–QD conjugates killed carcinoma cells under irradiation with 532 nm light with a typical light-dose-dependent PDT relationship, demonstrating a new way of excitation in PDT using FRET mediated by AlPcS–QD. In addition, the AlPcS–QD conjugates easily penetrated into cells, demonstrating that these conjugates are good carriers for AlPcS intracellular delivery because the cellular uptake rate for free AlPcS was very low. So, the results suggest that the new strategy of AlPcS–QD conjugates combined with the FRET could be a feasible modality for PDT, and this new model is worth investigating further to improve PDT effects in cancer treatments (Li et al., 2012).

The photoinactivation of cells incubated with a QD–Ce$_6$ conjugate under irradiation in the spectral region minimizing direct excitation of a PS provided clear evidence for conjugate capacity to induce FRET-mediated cell eradication (Valanciunaite et al., 2014). Two-photon fluorescence lifetime imaging microscopy on living HeLa cells revealed that, independently of QD surface functional groups, QD–Ce$_6$ conjugates localized within the plasma membrane and intracellular compartments and preserved 50% FRET efficiency. This exceptional stability in cellulo of noncovalent QD–Ce$_6$ conjugates can be explained by coordination of carboxyl groups of Ce$_6$ with the ZnS shell of the QD, in addition to hydrophobic interactions. The data suggest that a simple protocol without chemical conjugation can lead to QD–PS conjugates characterized by efficient FRET and excellent stability in cells (Valanciunaite et al., 2014).

The PDT testing of the QD–Ce$_6$ conjugate against the Erlich acsite carcinoma cell culture was performed by using confocal luminescence microscopy, and the trypan blue assay showed that the conjugate dramatically improved PDT cancer cell killing efficacy due to synergistic effect of photoexcitation energy transfer from QD to Ce$_6$ and the increased cellular uptake of Ce$_6$ delivered by QDs (Martynenko et al., 2015).

The uptake of a QD–Ce$_6$ conjugate in human pancreatic carcinoma cells MiaPaCa-2 was examined using laser confocal microscopy with an accessory for PL lifetime imaging (Steponkiene et al., 2014). In order to investigate whether Ce$_6$ can be delivered to cells via this nanoparticle vehicle approach, MiaPaCa-2 cells were incubated with QD–Ce$_6$ conjugate. For comparison, pure QDs and pure Ce$_6$ were also used for incubation. The results obtained after 3 hours of incubation showed that Ce$_6$, QDs, and QD–Ce$_6$ conjugate tended to accumulate inside the cells, but with different intracellular localization (Figure 10.10). Molecules of PS distribute diffusely along the whole cell (Figure 10.10a). The spectral analysis revealed that the PL band of Ce$_6$ in live cells is shifted to the red (Figure 10.10a, insert), which suggests strong interaction of PS with cell substrate. Distribution of QDs in cells has a more discrete pattern (Figure 10.10b). QDs localized in the plasma membrane and vesicles. Figure 10.10c presents accumulation of QD–Ce$_6$ conjugate in cells and shows that the distribution pattern of conjugate inside the cells resembles the pattern of QDs alone. Although cells were incubated with a solution of purified QD-Ce$_6$ conjugate, the presence of cell-bound Ce$_6$ molecules can be seen from the red areas inside the cells (Figure 10.10c), which suggests the partial disruption of the conjugate upon cellular uptake. Spectroscopically, it is impossible to distinguish between intracellular Ce$_6$ and Ce$_6$ bound to QDs. The PL peak of Ce$_6$ accumulated in cells is at 674 nm (Figure 10.10a, insert) and coincides with the PL peak of Ce$_6$ after formation of conjugate with QDs (Figure 10.10c, insert).

To determine whether cell incubation with a QD–Ce$_6$ conjugate can cause photosensitization and induce photochemical damage upon irradiation, the cells were exposed to a light dose of 17.5 J/cm^2 at 470 nm, which is predominantly absorbed by QDs. Following light exposure, the morphology of the MiaPaCa-2 cells incubated with a conjugate changed dramatically. The phase contrast microscopy image (Figure 10.11c) shows the presence of the randomly shaped, volume-increased cells.

When considering application of a QD–Ce$_6$ conjugate in PDT, it is very important to ascertain whether weak hydrophobic interaction between PS molecules and QDs is sufficient to induce cancer cell killing by using the FRET mechanism. The interference of various kinds of biomolecules in the cytoplasm with a QD–Ce$_6$ conjugate may not only weaken its stability, but also enhance nonradiative decays and lead to shortening of the PL lifetime (Zhang et al., 2008), thus creating problems for FRET-based photosensitization. However, comparative PL lifetime imaging measurements performed in the cells (Rotomskis et al., 2013) revealed that the PL lifetime of QDs in the absence of Ce$_6$ was two times longer than in its presence, confirming intracellular stability of the conjugate as well as FRET occurrence. The observed photoinactivation of cells (Figure 10.11) incubated with a QD–Ce$_6$ conjugate under irradiation in the spectral region minimizing direct excitation of a PS provided clear evidence for the capacity of conjugate to induce FRET-mediated cell eradication. This observation is evidence that such conjugates could induce FRET-mediated cell destruction, implying that they could be used to create selective innovative techniques for PDT.

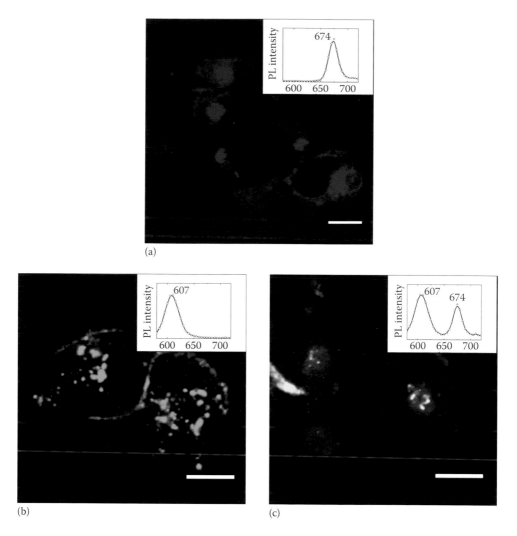

Figure 10.10 Intracellular distribution of Ce$_6$ (a), QDs (b), and QD–Ce$_6$ conjugate (c) in MiaPaCa2 cells under microscope (λ_{ex} = 488 nm). The yellow color seen in the cells (c) resulted from the merging of the red signal of Ce$_6$ and the green signal of QDs. Scale bar =10 μm.

10.4 CONCLUSION

Most of the authors of studies concerning different kinds of water-soluble QD–PS conjugates agree that this conjugation seems a potential way to increase the PDT efficiency. Additional surface modification and functionalization with targeting moieties could enhance the selective accumulation of the PS-loaded QDs at the target site. However, the mode of binding between QDs and different PSs, correlation between the quenching of QDs excited state and the formation of both the triplet and singlet states of PSs, toxicity due to cadmium and tellurium, as well as possibilities for QD–PS conjugates to really work in living systems need further attention. At all events, it is compelling that the studies from different authors clearly demonstrate the potential to enhance cancer PDT using potentially biocompatible QDs. It can be expected that QD conjugates with PSs could also be promising for further investigation in combination with other conventional therapeutic agents in human cancer theranostics since in recent years much effort has been channeled toward the development of multifunctional theranostic agents where a number of diverse diagnostic and therapeutic functionalities have been incorporated in a single nanoplatform for a "see and treat" approach.

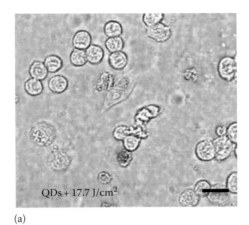

(a)

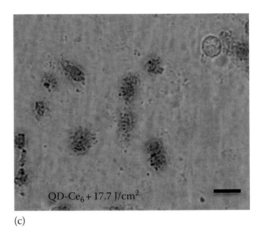

(b)   (c)

Figure 10.11 MiaPaCa2, a human pancreatic adenocarcinoma cells, after treatment with QDs, Ce_6, and QD–Ce_6 conjugate and irradiation at 17.7 J/cm² dose (470 nm) (a, b, and c, respectively). Under excitation by 470 nm, the fluorescence of nonconjugated Ce_6 is negligible; therefore, a minimal direct photosensitization by Ce_6 should be initiated. Photosensitizing properties of QD–Ce_6 conjugate was evaluated by propidium iodide (red) staining. Propidium iodide stains nuclei of dead cells, thus showing that viability of cells dramatically decreased only in the case when QD–Ce_6 conjugate was used. Scale bar = 10 μm.

REFERENCES

Agostinis P, Buytaert E, Breyssens H, Hendrickx N (2004) Regulatory pathways in photodynamic therapy induced apoptosis. *Photochem. Photobiol. Sci.* **3**: 721–729.

Alivisatos AP, Gu W, Larabell C (2005) Quantum dots as cellular probes. *Annu. Rev. Biomed. Eng.* **7**: 55–76.

Anas A, Akita H, Harashima H, Itoh T, Ishikawa M, Biju V (2008) Photosensitized breakage and damage of DNA by CdSe–ZnS quantum dots. *J. Phys. Chem. B* **112**: 10005–10011.

Auler H, Banzer G (1942) Untersuchungen uber die Rolle der Porphyrine bei geschwulstkranken Menschen und Tieren. *Z. Krebsforsch.* **53**: 65–68.

Bachor R, Shea CR, Gillies R, Hasan T (1991) Photosensitized destruction of human bladder-carcinoma cells treated with chlorin e6-conjugated microspheres. *Proc. Natl. Acad. Sci. USA* **88**: 1580–1584.

Bakalova R, Ohba H, Zhelev Z, Ishikawa M, Baba Y (2004) Quantum dots as photosensitizers? *Nat. Biotechnol.* **22**: 1360–1361.

Biju V, Mundayoor S, Omkumar RV, Anas A, Ishikawa M (2010) Bioconjugated quantum dots for cancer research: Present status, prospects and remaining issues. *Biotechnol. Adv.* **28**: 199–213.

Bonnett R (1999) Photodynamic therapy in historical perspective. *Rev. Contemp. Pharmacother.* **10**: 1–17.

Bonnett R, Martinez G (2001) Photobleaching of sensitizers used in photodynamic therapy. *Tetrahedron* **57**: 9513–9547.

Bos E, Boon P, Kaspersen F, McCabe R (1991) Passive immunotherapy of cancer: Perspectives and problems. *J. Control. Release* **16**: 101–112.

Bruchez MP, Hotz CZ (eds) (2007) *Quantum Dots: Applications in Biology.* Totowa, NJ: Humana Press.

Cai R, Kubota Y, Shuin T, Sakai H, Hashimoto K, Fujishima A (1992) Induction of cytotoxicity by photoexcited TiO_2 particles. *Cancer Res.* **52**: 2346–2348;

Castano AP, Mroz P, Hamblin MR (2006) Photodynamic therapy and anti-tumour immunity. *Nat. Rev. Cancer* **6**: 535–545.

Cecic I, Serrano K, Gyongyossy-Issa M, Korbelik M (2005) Characteristics of complement activation in mice bearing Lewis lung carcinomas treated by photodynamic therapy. *Cancer Lett.* **225**: 215–223.

Charron G, Stuchinskaya T, Edwards DR, Russell DA, Nann T (2012) Insights into the mechanism of quantum dotsensitized singlet oxygen production for photodynamic therapy. *J. Phys. Chem. C* **116**: 9334–9342.

Chatterjee DK, Fong LS, Zhang Y (2008) Nanoparticles in photodynamic therapy: An emerging paradigm. *Adv. Drug Deliv. Rev.* **60**: 1627–1637.

Chen JY, Lee YM, Zhao D, Mak NK, Wong RNS, Chan WH et al. (2010) Quantum dot-mediated photoproduction of reactive oxygen species for cancer cell annihilation. *Photochem. Photobiol.* **86**: 431–437.

Chen W (2008) Nanoparticle fluorescence based technology for biological applications. *J. Nanosci. Nanotechnol.* **8**: 1019–1051.

Cho SJ, Maysinger D, Jain M, Röder B, Hackbarth S, Winnik FM (2007) Long-term exposure to CdTe quantum dots causes functional impairments in live cells. *Langmuir* **23**: 1974–1980.

Clapp AR, Medintz IL, Mauro JM, Fisher BR, Bawendi MG, Mattoussi H (2004) Fluorescence resonance energy transfer between quantum dot donors and dye-labelled protein acceptors. *J. Am. Chem. Soc.* **126**: 301–310.

Clarke SJ, Hollmann CA, Zhang Z, Suffern D, Bradforth SE, Dimitrijevic NM et al. (2006) Photophysics of dopamine-modified quantum dots and effects on biological systems. *Nat. Mater.* **5**: 409–417.

Cuenca AG, Jiang H, Hochwald SN, Delano M, Cance WG, Grobmyer SR (2006) Emerging implications of nanotechnology on cancer diagnostics and therapeutics. *Cancer* **107**: 459–466.

Dayal S, Burda C (2007) Surface effects on quantum dot-based energy transfer. *J. Am. Chem. Soc.* **129**: 7977–7981.

Dayal S, Krolicki R, Luo Y, Qiu X, Berlin JC, Kenney ME et al. (2006a) Femtosecond time-resolved energy transfer from CdSe nanoparticles to phthalocyanines. *Appl. Phys. B* **84**: 309–315.

Dayal S, Li J, Li Y-S, Wu H, Samia ACS, Kenney ME et al. (2008) Effect of the functionalization of the axial phthalocyanine ligands on the energy transfer in QD-based donor-acceptor pairs. *Photochem. Photobiol.* **84**: 243–2499.

Dayal S, Lou YB, Samia ACS, Berlin JC, Kenney ME, Burda C (2006b) Observation of non-Forster-type energy-transfer behavior in quantum dot-phthalocyanine conjugates. *J. Am. Chem. Soc.* **128**: 13974–13975.

De Vree WJ, Essers MC, de Bruijn HS, Star WM, Koster JF, Sluiter W (1996) Evidence for an important role of neutrophils in the efficacy of photodynamic therapy in vivo. *Cancer Res.* **56**: 2908–2911.

Delehanty JB, Mattoussi H, Medintz IL (2009) Delivering quantum dots into cells: Strategies, progress and remaining issues. *Anal. Bioanal. Chem.* **393**: 1091–1105.

Detty MR, Gibson SL, Wagner SJ (2004) Current clinical and preclinical photosensitizers for use in photodynamic therapy. *J. Med. Chem.* **47**: 3897–3915.

Dolmans DEJGJ, Fukumura D, Jain RK (2003) Photodynamic therapy for cancer. *Nat. Rev. Cancer* **3**: 380–387.

Dolmans DEJGJ, Kadambi A, Hill JS, Waters CA, Robinson BC, Walker JP et al. (2002) Vascular accumulation of a novel photosensitizer, MV 6401, causes selective thrombosis in tumor vessels after photodynamic therapy. *Cancer Res.* **62**: 2151–2156.

Dougherty TJ, Grindey GB, Weishaupt KR, Boyle DG (1975) Photoradiation therapy II. Cure of animal tumours with haematoporphyrin and light. *J. Natl. Cancer Inst.* **55**: 115–121.

Dubertret B, Skourides P, Norris DJ, Noireaux V, Brivanlou AH, Libchaber A (2002) In vivo imaging of quantum dots encapsulated in phospholipid micelles. *Science* **298**: 1759–1762.

Duong HD, Rhee JI (2011) Singlet oxygen production by fluorescence resonance energy transfer (FRET) from green and orange CdSe/ZnS QDs to protoporphyrin IX (PpIX). *Chem. Phys. Lett.* **501**: 496–501.

Dworak L, Matylitsky VV, Ren T, Basché T Wachtveitl J (2014) Acceptor concentration dependence of Förster resonance energy transfer dynamics in dye–quantum dot complexes. *J. Phys. Chem. C* **118**: 4396–4402.

Finsen NF (1901) *Phototherapy*. London, U.K.: Arnold.

Förster T (1965) *Delocalized Excitation and Excitation Transfer*. Tallahassee, FL: Florida State University.

Frolov AA, Zenkevich EI, Gurinovich GP, Kochubeyev GA (1990) Chlorin e6-liposome interaction—Investigation by the methods of fluorescence spectroscopy and inductive resonance energy-transfer. *J. Photochem. Photobiol. B* **7**: 43–56.

Gao XH, Cui YY, Levenson RM, Chung LWK, Nie SM (2004) In vivo cancer targeting and imaging with semiconductor quantum dots. *Nat. Biotechnol.* **22**: 969–976.

Giniunas L, Rotomskis R, Smilgevicius V, Piskarskas A, Didziapetriene J, Bloznelyte L, Griciute L (1991) Activity of haematoporphyrin derivative photoproduct in photodynamic therapy in vivo. *Lasers Med. Sci.* **6**: 425–428.

Hild WA, Breunig M, Goepferich A (2008) Quantum dots—Nanosized probes for the exploration of cellular and intracellular targeting. *Eur. J. Pharm. Biopharm.* **68**: 153–168.

Hsieh JM, Ho ML, Wu PW, Chou PT, Tsai TT, Chi Y (2006) Iridium-complex modified CdSe/ZnS quantum dots; a conceptual design for bifunctionality toward imaging and photosensitization. *Chem. Commun.* **6**: 615–617.

Huang Z (2005) A review of progress in clinical photodynamic therapy. *Technol. Cancer Res. Treat.* **4**: 283–293.

Idowu M, Chen JY, Nyokong T (2008) Photoinduced energy transfer between water-soluble CdTe quantum dots and aluminium tetrasulfonated phthalocyanine. *New J. Chem.* **32**: 290–296.

Idowu M, Nyokong T (2010) Spectroscopic behavior of cationic metallophthalocyanines in the presence of anionic quantum dots. *Spectrochim. Acta Part A Mol. Biomol. Spectrosc.* **75**: 411–416.

Ipe BI, Lehnig M, Niemeyer CM (2005) On the generation of free radical species from quantum dots. *Small* **1**: 706–709.

Ishii K (2012) Functional singlet oxygen generators based on phthalocyanines. *Coord. Chem. Rev.* **256**: 1556–1568.

Jamieson T, Bakhshi R, Petrova D, Pocock R, Imanib M, Seifalian AM (2007) Biological applications of quantum dots. *Biomaterials* **28**: 4717–4732.

Jhonsi MA, Renganathan R (2010) Investigations on the photoinduced interaction of water soluble thioglycolic acid (TGA) capped CdTe quantum dots with certain porphyrins, *J. Colloid Interface Sci.* **344**: 596–602.

Juzenas P, Chen W, Sun YP, Coelho MA, Generalov R, Generalova N et al. (2008) Quantum dots and nanoparticles for photodynamic and radiation therapies of cancer. *Adv. Drug Deliv. Rev.* **60**: 1600–1614.

Kagan CR, Murray CB, Nirmal M, Bawendi MG (1996) Electronic energy transfer in CdSe quantum dot solids. *Phys. Rev. Lett.* **76**: 1517–1520.

Karabanovas V, Zakarevicius E, Sukackaite A, Streckyte G, Rotomskis R (2008) Examination of the stability of hydrophobic (CdSe)ZnS quantum dots in the digestive tract of rats. *Photochem. Photobiol. Sci.* **7**: 725–729.

Keane PM, Gallagher SA, Magno LM, Leising MJ, Clark IP, Greetham GM et al. (2012) Photophysical studies of CdTe quantum dots in the presence of a zinc cationic porphyrin. *Dalton Trans.* **41**: 13159–13166.

Kelly JF, Snell ME (1976) Haematoporphyrin derivative: A possible aid in the diagnosis and therapy of carcinoma of the bladder. *J. Urol.* **115**: 150.

Kessel D, Thompson P (1987) Purification and analysis of hematoporphyrin and hematoporphyrin derivative by gel exclusion and reverse phase chromatography. *Photochem. Photobiol.* **46**: 1023–1026.

Kloepfer JA, Bradforth SE. Nadeau JL (2005) Photophysical properties of biologically compatible CdSe quantum dot structures. *J. Phys. Chem. B* **109**: 9996–10003.

Lakowitcz JR (1999) *Principles of Fluorescence Spectroscopy*. New York: Springer Science and Business Media.

Leatherdale CA, Woo WK, Mikulec FV, Bawendi MG (2002) On the absorption cross section of CdSe nanocrystal quantum dots. *J. Phys. Chem. B* **106**: 7619–7622.

Li J, Guo D, Wang X, Wang H, Jiang H, Chen B (2010) The photodynamic effect of different size ZnO nanoparticles on cancer cell proliferation in vitro. *Nanoscale Res. Lett.* **5**: 1063–1071.

Li L, Zhao JF, Won N, Jin H, Kim S, Chen JY (2012) Quantum dot-aluminum phthalocyanine conjugates perform photodynamic reactions to kill cancer cells via fluorescence resonance energy transfer. *Nanoscale Res. Lett.* **7**: 386–393.

Lipson RL, Baldes EJ, Olsen AM (1961) The use of a derivative of haematoporphyrin in tumour detection. *J. Natl. Cancer Inst.* **26**: 1–11.

Lipson RL, Gray MJ, Baldes EJ (1967) Haematoporphyrin derivative for detection and management of cancer. *Cancer* **20**: 2255–2257.

Lovell JF, Liu TWB, Chen J, Zheng G (2010) Activatable photosensitizers for imaging and therapy. *Chem. Rev.* **110**: 2839–2857.

Lovric J, Bazzi HS, Cuie Y, Fortin GRA, Winnik FM, Maysinger D (2005a) Differences in subcellular distribution and toxicity of green and red emitting CdTe quantum dots. *J. Mol. Med.* **83**: 377–385.

Lovric J, Cho SJ, Winnik FM, Maysinger D (2005b) Unmodified cadmium telluride quantum dots induce reactive oxygen species formation leading to multiple organelle damage and cell death. *Chem. Biol.* **12**: 1227–1234.

Ma J, Chen JY, Idowu M, Nyokong T (2008) Generation of singlet oxygen via the composites of water-soluble thiol-capped CdTe quantum dots-sulfonated aluminum phthalocyanines. *J. Phys. Chem. B* **112**: 4465–4469.

Magde D, Rojas GE, Seybold PG (1999) Solvent dependence on the fluorescence lifetimes of dantene dyes. *Photochem. Photobiol.* **70**: 737–744.

Mang TS, Dougherty TJ, Potter WR, Boyle DG, Sommer S, Moan J (1987) Photobleaching of porphyrins used photodynamic therapy and implications in therapy. *Photochem. Photobiol.* **45**: 501–506.

Martynenko IV, Kuznetsova VA, Orlova AO, Kanaev PA, Maslov VG, Loudon A et al. (2015) Chlorin e6–ZnSe/ZnS quantum dots based system as reagent for photodynamic therapy. *Nanotechnology* **26**: 055102.

Martynenko IV, Orlova AO, Maslov VG, Baranov AV, Fedorov AV, Artemyev M (2013) Energy transfer in complexes of water-soluble quantum dots and chlorine e6 molecules in different environmetnts. *Beilstein J. Nanotechnol.* **4**: 895–902.

Masilela N, Nyokong T (2012) The photophysical and energy transfer behaviour of low symmetry phthalocyanine complexes conjugated to coreshell quantum dots: An energy transfer study. *J. Photochem. Photobiol. A* **247**: 82–92.

Matovic V, Buha A, Bulat Z, Đukic-Cosic D (2011) Cadmium toxicity focus on oxidative stress induction and interactions with zinc and magnesium. *Arh. Hig. Rada Toksikol.* **62**: 65–76.

Medintz IL, Konnert JH, Clapp AR, Stanish I, Twigg ME, Mattoussi H et al. (2004) A fluorescence resonance energy transfer-derived structure of a quantum dot-protein bioconjugate nanoassembly. *Proc. Natl. Acad. Sci. USA* **101**: 9612–9617.

Medintz IL, Mattoussi H (2009) Quantum dot-based resonance energy transfer and its growing application in biology. *Phys. Chem. Chem. Phys.* **11**: 17–45.

Medintz IL, Uyeda HT, Goldman ER, Mattoussi H (2005) Quantum dot bioconjugates for imaging, labelling and sensing. *Nat. Mater.* **4**: 435–446.

Michalet X, Pinaud FF, Bentolila LA, Tsay JM, Doose S, Li JJ et al. (2005) Quantum dots for live cells, in vivo imaging, and diagnostics. *Science* **307**: 538–544.

Michels S, Schmidt-Erfurth U. (2003) Sequence of early vascular events after photodynamic therapy. *Invest. Ophthalmol. Vis. Sci.* **44**: 2147–2154.

Moan J (1986) Porphyrin photosensitization and phototherapy. *Photochem. Photobiol.* **43**: 681–690.

Moan J, Berg K (1991) The photodegradation of porphyrins in cells can be used to estimate the lifetime of singlet oxygen. *Photochem. Photobiol.* **53**: 543–553.

Moan J, Berg K (1992) Photochemotherapy of cancer: Experimental research. *Photochem. Photobiol.* **55**: 931–948.

Moan J, Kessel D (1988) Photoproducts formed from Photofrin II in cells. *J. Photochem. Photobiol. B* **1**: 429–436.

Moan J, Peng Q (2003) An outline of the hundred-year history of PDT. *Anticancer Res.* **23**: 3591–3600.

Moeno S, Nyokong T (2008) The photophysical studies of a mixture of CdTe quantum dots and negatively charged zinc phthalocyanines. *Polyhedron* **27**: 1953–1958.

Moeno S, Nyokong T (2009) Interaction of water-soluble CdTe quantum dots with octacarboxy metallophthalocyanines: A photophysical and photochemical study. *J. Luminesc.* **129**: 356–362.

Mojzisova H, Bonneau S, Vever-Bizet C, Brault D (2007) The pH-dependent distribution of the photosensitizer chlorin e6 among plasma proteins and membranes: A physico-chemical approach. *Biochim. Biophys. Acta-Biomembr.* **1768**: 366–374.

Nann T (2011) Nanoparticles in photodynamic therapy. *Nano Biomed. Eng.* **3**: 137–143.

Narband N, Mubarak M, Ready D, Parkin IP, Nair SP, Green MA et al. (2008) Quantum dots as enhancers of the efficacy of bacterial lethal photosensitization. *Nanotechnology* **19**: 445102.

Nel A, Xia T, Madler L, Li N (2006) Toxic potential of materials at the nanolevel. *Science* **311**: 622–627.

Neuman D, Ostrowski AD, Mikhailovsky AA, Absalonson RO, Strouse GF, Ford PC (2008) Quantum dot fluorescence quenching pathways with Cr(III) complexes. Photosensitized NO production from *trans*-Cr(cyclam)(ONO)$_2$. *J. Am. Chem. Soc.* **130**: 168–175.

Oleinick NL, Morris RL, Belichenko I (2002) The role of apoptosis in response to photodynamic therapy: What, where, why and how. *Photochem. Photobiol. Sci.* **1**: 1–21.

Orlova AO, Martynenko IV, Maslov VG, Fedorov AV, Gun'ko YK Baranov AV (2013) Investigation of complexes of CdTe quantum dots with the alohsulphophthalocyanine molecules in aqueous media. *J. Phys. Chem. C* **117**: 23425–23431.

Orlova AO, Maslov VG, Baranov AV, Gounko I, Byrne S (2008a) Spectral-luminescence study of the formation of QD-sulfophthalocyanine molecule complexes in an aqueous solution. *Opt. Spektrosk.* **105**: 726–731.

Orlova AO, Maslov VG, Stepanov AA, Gounko I, Baranov AV (2008b) Formation of QD-porphyrin molecule complexes in aqueous solutions. *Opt. Spektrosk.* **105**: 889–895.

Osborne SW, Blood P, Smowton PM, Xin YC, Stintz A, Huffaker D et al. (2004) Optical absorption cross section of quantum dots. *J. Phys. Condens. Matter* **16**: S3749.

Policard A(1924) Etudes sur les aspects offerts par des tumeur experimentales examinee a la lumiere de woods. *C. R. Soc. Biol.* **91**: 1423–1428.

Probst CE, Zrazhevskiy P, Bagalkot V, Gao X (2013) Quantum dots as a platform for nanoparticle drug delivery vehicle design. *Adv. Drug Deliv. Rev.* **65**: 703–718.

Qi ZD, Li DW, Jiang P, Jiang FL, Li YS, Liu Y et al. (2011) Biocompatible CdSe quantum dot-based photosensitizer under two-photon excitation for photodynamic therapy. *J. Mater. Chem.* **21**: 2455–2458.

Raab O (1900) Uber die Wirkung fluorescierender Stoffe auf Infusorien. *Z. Biol.* **39**: 524–546.

Ramanavicius A, Karabanovas V, Ramanaviciene A, Rotomskis R (2009) Stabilization of (CdSe)ZnS quantum dots with polypyrrole formed by UV/VIS irradiation initiated polymerization. *J. Nanosci. Nanotechnol.* **9**: 1909–1915.

Resch-Genger U, Grabolle M, Cavaliere-Jaricot S, Nitschke R, Nann T (2008) Quantum dots versus organic dyes as fluorescent labels. *Nat. Methods* **5**: 763–775.

Rizvi SB, Ghaderi S, Keshtgar M, Seifalian AM (2010) Semiconductor quantum dots as fluorescent probes for in vitro and in vivo bio-molecular and cellular imaging. *Nano Rev.* **1**: 5161.

Rotomskis R, Bagdonas S, Streckyte G (1996) Spectroscopic studies of photobleaching and photoproduct formation of porphyrins used in tumour therapy. *J. Photochem. Photobiol. B* **33**: 61–67.

Rotomskis R, Streckyte G, Bagdonas S (1997a) Phototransformations of sensitizers: 1. The significance of the nature of the sensitizer for photobleaching and photoproduct formation in aqueos solution. *J. Photochem. Photobiol. B* **39**: 167–171.

Rotomskis R, Streckyte G, Bagdonas S (1997b) Phototransformations of sensitizers: 2. Photoproducts formed in aqueos solutions of porphyrins. *J. Photochem. Photobiol. B* **39**: 172–175.

Rotomskis R, Valanciunaite J, Skripka A, Steponkiene S, Spogis G, Bagdonas S et al. (2013) Complexes of functionalized quantum dots and chlorin e6 in photodynamic therapy. *Lithuanian J. Phys.* **53**: 57–68.

Samia AC, Chen X, Burda C (2003) Semiconductor quantum dots for photodynamic therapy. *J. Am. Chem. Soc.* **125**: 15736–15737.

Samia AC, Dayal S, Burda C (2006) Quantum dot-based energy transfer: Perspectives and potential for applications in photodynamic therapy. *Photochem. Photobiol.* **82**: 617–625.

Shi X, Hernandez B, Selke M (2006) Singlet oxygen generation from water-soluble quantum dot-organic dye nanocomposites. *J. Am. Chem. Soc.* **128**: 6278–6279.

Spikes JD (1992) Quantum yields and kinetics of the photobleaching of hematoporphyrin, photofrin II, tetra(4-sulfonatophenyl)-porphyrin and uroporphyrin. *Photochem. Photobiol.* **55**: 797–808.

Spikes JD (1997) Photodynamic action: From paramecium to photochemotherapy. *Photochem. Photobiol.* **12**: 142–147.

Steponkiene S, Valanciunaite J, Skripka A, Rotomskis R (2014) Cellular uptake and photosensitizing properties of quantum dot-chlorin e6 complex: In vitro study. *J. Biomed. Nanotechnol.* **10**: 679–686.

Tappeiner Hv, Jodlbauer A (1904) Ueber wirkung der photodynamischen (fluorescierenden) Stoffe auf Protozoan und Enzyme. *Dtsch. Arch. Klin. Med.* **80**: 127–187.

Thomas A, Nair PV, Thomas GK (2014) InP quantum dots: An environmentally friendly material with resonance energy transfer requisites. *J. Phys. Chem. C* **118**: 3838–3845.

Tsay JM, Trzoss M, Shi L, Kong X, Selke M, Jung ME et al. (2007) Singlet oxygen production by peptide-coated quantum dot-photosensitizer conjugates. *J. Am. Chem. Soc.* **129**: 6865–6871.

Valanciunaite J, Klymchenko AS, Skripka A, Richert L, Steponkiene S, Streckyte G et al. (2014) A non-covalent complex of quantum dots and chlorin e6: Efficient energy transfer and remarkable stability in living cells revealed by FLIM. *RSC Adv.* **4**: 52270–52278.

Valanciunaite J, Rotomskis R (2010) Quantum dots as energy donors for photosenstizers: Perspectives for photodynamic therapy of cancer. *Med. Phys. Baltic States* **2**: 44–49.

Valanciunaite J, Skripka A, Streckyte G, Rotomskis R (2010) Complex of water-soluble CdSe/ZnS quantum dots and chlorine e6: Interaction and FRET. *Proc. SPIE* **7376**: 737607.

Vermathen M, Louie EA, Chodosh AB, Ried S, Simonis U (2000) Interactions of water-insoluble tetraphenyl-porphyrins with micelles probed by UV visible and NMR spectroscopy. *Langmuir* **16**: 210–221.

Vermathen M, Marzorati M, Vermathen P, Bigler P (2010) pH-Dependent distribution of chlorin e6 derivatives across phospholipid bilayers probed by NMR spectroscopy. *Langmuir* **26**: 11085–11094.

Weishaupt KR, Gomer CJ, Dougherty TJ (1976) Identification of singlet oxygen as the cytotoxic agent in photoinactivation of a murine tumor. *Cancer Res.* **36**: 2326–2329.

Xing Y, Xia Z, Rao J (2009) Semiconductor quantum dots for biosensing and in vivo imaging. *IEEE Trans. Nanobioscience* **8**: 4–12.

Xu S, Klama F, Ueckermann H, Hoogewerff J, Clayden N, Nann T (2009) Optical and surface characterisation of capping ligands in the preparation of InP/ZnS quantum dots. *Sci. Adv. Mater.* **1**: 125–137.

Xu S, Kumar S, Nann T (2006) Rapid synthesis of high-quality InP nanocrystals. *J. Am. Chem. Soc.* **128**: 1054–1055.

Xu S, Ziegler J, Nann T (2008) Rapid synthesis of highly luminescent InP and InP/ZnS nanocrystals. *J. Mater. Chem.* **18**: 2653–2656.

Yaghini E, Seifalian AM, MacRobert AJ (2009) Quantum dots and their potential biomedical applications in photosensitization for photodynamic therapy. *Nanomedicine* **4**: 353–363.

Yamaguchi S, Kobayashi H, Narita T, Kanehira K, Sonezaki S, Kubota Y et al. (2010) Novel photodynamic therapy using water-dispersed TiO_2–polyethylene glycol compound: Evaluation of antitumor effect on glioma cells and spheroids in vitro. *Photochem. Photobiol.* **86**: 964–971.

Yang RH, Chang LW, Wu JP, Tsai MH, Wang HJ, Kuo YC et al. (2007) Persistent tissue kinetics and redistribution of nanoparticles, quantum dot 705, in mice: ICP-MS quantitative assessment. *Environ. Health Perspect.* **115**: 1339–1343.

Ye L, Yong KT, Liu LW, Roy I, Hu R, Zhu J et al. (2012) A pilot study in non-human primates shows no adverse response to intravenous injection of quantum dots. *Nat. Nanotechnol.* **7**: 453–458.

Zenkevich E, Cichos F, Shulga A, Petrov EP, Blaudeck T, von Borczyskowski C (2005) Nanoassemblies designed from semiconductor quantum dots and molecular arrays. *J. Phys. Chem. B* **109**: 8679–8692.

Zenkevich EI, Blaudeck T, Shulga AM, Cichos F, von Borczyskowski C (2007) Identification and assignment of porphyrin-CdSe hetero-nanoassemblies. *J. Luminesc.* **122**: 784–788.

Zhang H, Zeng X, Li Q, Gaillard-Kelly M, Wagner CR, Yee D (2009) Fluorescent tumour imaging of type I IGF receptor in vivo: Comparison of antibody-conjugated quantum dots and small-molecule fluorophore. *Br. J. Cancer* **101**: 71–79.

Zhang Y, Mi L, Wang PN, Lu SJ, Chen JY, Guo J et al. (2008) Photoluminescence decay dynamics of thiol-capped CdTe quantum dots in living cells under microexcitation. *Small* **4**: 777–780.

Tetrapyrrole-based theranostic combinations of photodynamic action and magnetic resonance imaging

DUYGU AYDIN TEKDAŞ, DEVRIM ATILLA, VEFA AHSEN, AND AYŞE GÜL GÜREK

Theranostics is one of the promising ways to personalized medicine, more especially against cancer, combining diagnostic and therapeutic effects. The third generation of photosensitizers (PSs) combines imaging agents and PSs in order to benefit from a see and treat process for the patient, and theranostics became quickly established in the photodynamic therapy (PDT) field. Among the different types of PSs, consisting mainly of molecular tetrapyrroles of well-defined structures and tailorable properties, porphyrins and phthalocyanines are particularly employed. The porphyrins and phthalocyanines as tetrapyrrole derivatives have a unique theranostic role in disease therapy as third-generation PSs; they have been used to image, detect and treat a number of different cancer types. The current focus is on the clinical imaging of tumor tissue, targeted delivery of PSs, and the potential of PSs in theranostic platforms. The roles of tetrapyrrole derivatives in imaging and PDT, along with research into improving their selective uptake in diseased tissue and their utility in theranostic applications, will be highlighted in this chapter.

11.1 INTRODUCTION TO THE CONCEPT OF THERANOSTICS

A theranostic is defined as a material that combines the modalities of therapy and diagnostic imaging. Thus, theranostics deliver therapeutic drugs and diagnostic imaging agents at the same time within the same dose (Kelkar and Reineke, 2011). A theranostic can be broadly defined as a viable drug that incorporates some form of marker for the imaging of that drug in vitro, ex vivo, and, most importantly, in vivo (Rai et al., 2010; Lovell et al., 2011; Ng et al., 2011; Huang et al., 2012b). The field of theranostics research is the area of science trying to integrate therapeutic applications with diagnostic imaging (Kelkar and Reineke, 2011). The term "theranostic" is formed by the combination of therapy and diagnostics—for the right drug at the right dose and moment. This term has been expanded to define drugs that are developed for personalized medicine. Theranostics agents play an important role especially in the field of cancer as it is important to comprehend the location of the tumor, define the type of cancer, its frontiers, and whether the disease has spread locally or systemically before beginning any treatment of cancer. When the nature of the disease is clarified, efficient treatment options can be found so as to control the spread of the disease and diminish the primary tumor. A key factor of cancer detection and therapy is to deliver therapeutic agents selectively to tumors at effective concentrations. Present treatment processes include the use of diagnostic as well as therapeutic agents separately. The goal of the field of theranostics is to have the capability to image, identify, and monitor the disease prior to and after the treatment so as to optimize the treatment parameters and providing long-term tumor cure. A schematic illustration of theranostics contents is presented in Figure 11.1.

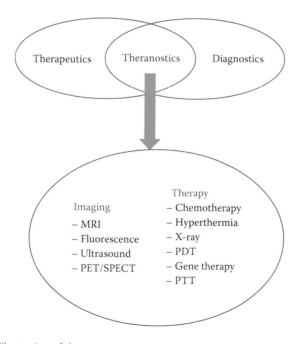

Figure 11.1 Schematic illustration of theranostics scopes.

11.1.1 BASICS OF PDT

PDT is still considered to be a new and promising antitumor strategy. Classical cancer therapies including surgical intervention, radiation therapy, and chemotherapy result in serious side effects, causing damage on normal cells and tissues. PDT is clinically approved and deemed as a minimally invasive procedure that can exert a selective activity toward malignant cells (Lovell et al., 2010; Agostinis et al., 2011; Ethirajan et al., 2011). This procedure has several advantages over other classical therapies: (1) it can be applied to tissues where surgery cannot be carried out, (2) correlated with low morbidity, (3) selectivity to cancer cells, (4) the lack of side effect, and (5) it can treat patients with repeated doses without initiating resistance or exceeding total dose limitations (Lovell et al., 2010; Ethirajan et al., 2011). The application of PDT is not only limited to cancer treatments, but can also be used for the treatment of cardiovascular, ophthalmic, and infectious diseases. Owing to the tumor targeting ability of appropriately designed PS agents, as well as the selective light irradiation of the lesion region, phototherapies exhibit remarkably reduced side effects and improved selectivity compared with traditional remedies.

PDT requires three elements for an effective treatment: a nontoxic drug or dye known as a PS, appropriate light, and molecular oxygen. A PS is administered systemically, locally, or topically. After the PS selectively accumulates by a period of its systemic distribution in the tumor, selective illumination with appropriate wavelength and power of light activates the PS. The activated PS transfers the absorbed photon energy to surrounding oxygen molecules, generating highly reactive oxygen species (type I photosensitization) or singlet oxygen (type II photosensitization) (Figure 11.2; Konan et al., 2002). This excited oxygen form then attacks cellular targets to damage, leading to tumor cell death via an apoptotic, necrotic or autophagy mechanism, combined by the induction of an acute local inflammatory reaction that participates in the removal of dead cells, restoration of normal tissue homeostasis, and sometimes in the development of systemic immunity. Most of the photosensitization reactions are type II processes.

11.1.2 PSS IN PDT

PSs are the key component in PDT. After the approval of Photofrin® for the PDT treatment, researchers from all over the world got actively involved in developing an efficient PS (Agostinis et al., 2011; Ethirajan et al., 2011). First of all, an ideal PS agent should be a pure compound with low-cost manufacturing, have good stability in storage, and be easy to solve in injectable solvents. It should be able to produce singlet oxygen efficiently

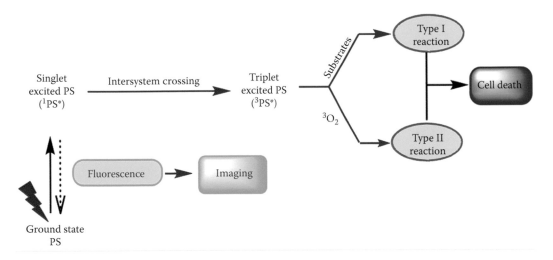

Figure 11.2 Schematic illustration of a typical photodynamic reaction. (Reprinted from *J. Photochem. Photobiol. B*, 66, Konan, Y.N., Gurny, R., Allémann, E., State of the art in the delivery of photosensitizers for photodynamic therapy, 89–106. Copyright 2002, with permission from Elsevier.)

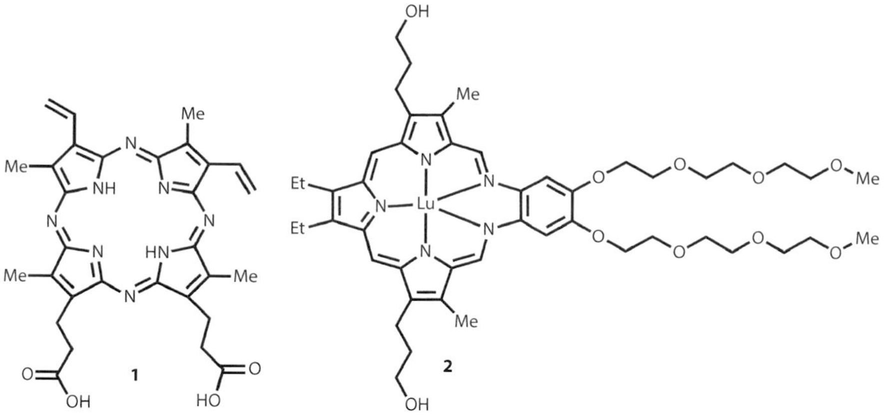

Figure 11.3 Structure of some of the clinically treated PSs.

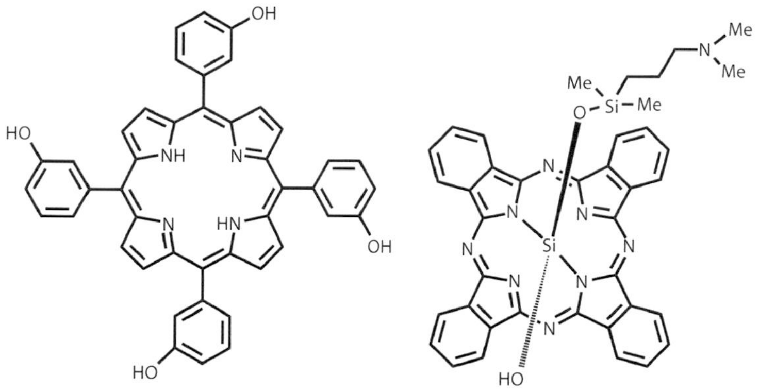

because singlet oxygen is a cytotoxic agent responsible for the destruction of tumors by PDT. It should have a high absorption peak in the long wavelength region (600–800 nm) because the penetration of light into tissue increases with its wavelengths. It should have no dark toxicity, minimal skin photosensitivity, and the important issue of selectively accumulation of PS in tumor tissue (Allison and Sibata, 2010; Agostinis et al., 2011; Ethirajan et al., 2011). PS can be classified into five groups according to their chemical structure. Most of the PSs used in cancer therapy are based on a tetrapyrrole structure, porphyrins, phthalocyanines, chlorins, bacteriochlorins, texaphyrins, and porphycenes (Dumoulin, 2012). Among these PSs (Figure 11.3), 5-aminolevulinic acid (ALA)-induced protoporphyrin IX (1), lutetium texaphyrin (LuTx) (2), *meta*-tetra (hydroxyphenyl) chlorin (Foscan®) (3), and silicon phthalocyanine (Pc4) (4) are some of the clinically treated PSs. BODIPY (for boron-dipyrromethene), ALA, phenotthiazinium, and hypericin are other groups of PSs. Table 11.1 is a partial list of the porphyrin-based PSs that are currently approved for clinical applications or are in human trials.

Another way to classify the PSs has a more historical perspective. The first developed PSs, hematoporphyrin derivatives (HPD), were designed as the first-generation PS. Following the development of new strategies such as selective accumulation of the PS in the targeted tissue and photophysical and photochemical optimization of singlet oxygen generation, second- and third-generation PSs have been developed.

11.1.3 IMAGING AND DIAGNOSTICS

Molecular imaging is an emerging technology that allows the visualization of interactions between molecular probes and biological targets (Herschman, 2003; Sosnovik and Weissleder, 2007; Wester, 2007; Mankoff et al., 2008; Josephs et al., 2009; Hilderbrand and Weissleder, 2010). Molecules that either direct

Table 11.1 Clinical indications treated with various porphyrin-based photosensitizers

PS	Indications and approval status[a]
ALA (5-aminolevulinic acid)	*Approved*: Actinic keratosis, basal cell carcinoma. *Clinical trials*: Bladder cancer, penile cancer, gliomas, acne vulgaris.
Foscan (*meta*-tetra(hydroxyphenyl) chlorin)	*Approved*: Palliative head and neck cancer.
Lu-Tex (lutetium texaphyrin)	*Clinical trials*: Prostate cancer and coronary artery disease.
Metvix (5-aminolevulinic acid methyl ester)	*Approved*: Actinic keratosis, superficial basal-cell carcinoma, and basal-cell carcinoma.
NPe6 (mono-L-aspartyl chlorin-e6)	*Approved*: Early lung cancer.
Pc4 (silicon phthalocyanine)	*Clinical trials*: Cutaneous T-cell lymphoma, cutaneous skin cell lesions, sterilization of blood products.
Photochlor (hexyl ether pyropheophorbide-*a* derivative)	*Clinical trials*: Lung carcinoma, basal cell carcinomas, Barrett's esophagus.
Photofrin (hematoporphyrin derivatives)	*Approved*: Advanced and early lung cancer, superficial gastric cancer, esophageal adenocarcinoma, cervical cancer and dysplasia, superficial bladder cancer, Barrett's esophagus. *Clinical trials*: Intraperitoneal cancer, cholangiocarcinoma, restenosis.
Photolon (chlorin-e6-polyvinylpyrrolidone)	*Approved*: Malignant skin and mucosa tumors, myopic maculopathy, central choroidal neovascularization.
Photosens (aluminum phthalocyanine)	*Clinical trials*: Age-related macular degeneration.
Purlytin (tin ethyl etiopurpurin)	*Clinical trials*: Prostate cancer, metastatic breast cancer, Kaposi's sarcoma (in AIDS patients).
Tookad (palladium-bacteriopheophorbide)-*a*	*Clinical trials*: Prostate cancer.
Visudyne (benzoporphyrin derivative monoacid ring A)	*Approved*: Age-related macular degeneration, subfoveal choroidal, neovascularization.

Source: Reprinted with permission from Lovell, J.F., Liu, T.W., Chen, J., Zheng, G., Activatable photosensitizers for imaging and therapy, *Chem. Rev.*, 110, 2839–2857. Copyright 2010 American Chemical Society.
[a] Approval status varies regionally. Consult references for further details (Brown et al., 2004; Huang, 2005; Triesscheijn et al., 2006; Juzeniene et al., 2007; Josefsen and Boyle, 2008; Juarranz et al., 2008; O'Connor et al., 2009).

or are subject to homeostatic controls in biological systems could be labeled with the appropriate radioisotopes for the quantitative measurement of selected molecular interactions during normal tissue homeostasis and again after perturbations of the normal state. Imaging plays an essential role at every stage of PDT, from disease detection to treatment planning, dosimetry, therapy monitoring, and outcome assessment. Ultimately, multimodality imaging combined with PDT will be most useful where both structural and functional images may be obtained. Molecular imaging is particularly relevant to PDT as the fluorescent entity can be the same as the therapeutic one and any molecular targeting that is done for therapy can also be exploited for imaging. The choice of molecular targets becomes critical, and perhaps the best results will be achieved when the molecular expression of host tissue is maximally different from the disease being monitored or treated.

Imaging is the other aspect of a theranostic agent that allows for visualization of a target before treatment. Molecular imaging is an area that provides both anatomical and functional information. In a literal sense, molecular imaging agents provide images of molecules. The idea of imaging is to determine the characteristics of the tumor to develop a treatment regimen so as to get the best possible outcome for the patient. Imaging also allows visualizing the margins of the tumor, whether the tumor has spread to other sites in the body;

it is also used for early detection of tumors, and finally, imaging is a powerful tool for real-time monitoring of the treatment (Pysz et al., 2010). Imaging modalities include a variety of techniques using a number of different characteristics ranging from anatomical, physiological and molecular properties of tumors. Targeted delivery is a promising strategy to improve the diagnostic imaging and therapeutic effect of cancers (Wang et al., 2015). Various imaging methods are used for medical imaging, including positron emission tomography (PET), single-photon emission computed tomography (SPECT), magnetic resonance imaging (MRI), magnetic resonance spectroscopy (MRS), ultrasound (US), and computed tomography (CT).

11.1.4 THERAPEUTICS

The development of agents for the simultaneous detection and treatment of disease has recently gained significant attention. These multifunctional theranostic agents possess a number of advantages over their monofunctional counterparts as they potentially allow for the concomitant determination of agent localization, release, and efficacy. The combination of diagnostic and therapeutic entities into one drug delivery vehicle yields agents that are capable of simultaneous diagnosis and treatment of disease. The theranostic agents have unique applications as they not only promote the diagnosis and therapy of disease, but allow for feedback mechanisms to determine the localization, release, and therapeutic efficacy of treatments. The ability to deliver contrast or therapeutic agents selectively to tumors at effective concentrations is a key factor for the efficacy of cancer detection and therapy. Current treatment methodologies involve the use of diagnostic as well as therapeutic agents separately. This leads to the problem of selectivity with respect to tumors, differences in the biodistribution of the agents within the body. The goal of therapeutics is to have the capability to image, identify, and monitor the disease prior to and after the treatment, which should help in optimizing the treatment parameters and provide long-term tumor cure.

The therapeutics comprise of chemotherapeutic drugs, radioactive compounds, and antibodies targeting the vasculature of the tumor or targeting key pathways required for the growth of the tumor. Gene therapy involving delivery of siRNA, plasmids, antisense oligonucleotides, ribozymes, DNAzymes, and viral vectors delivering DNA and RNA to tumor cells are also currently under research for theranostic applications. Nanoparticles such as gold nanorods and nanoshells (Aurolase®) are therapeutic in nature by themselves. These particles can lead to tumor destruction by photothermal effect (Panchapakesan et al., 2011). This effect is seen wherein light activation of the nanoparticles leads to generation of heat, which causes tumor ablation. Similar effect is also seen by use of magnetic nanoparticles as well. Das et al. (2009) have shown that the use of magnetic nanoparticles loaded with a fluorescence dye (RITC) along with methotrexate and folate moiety to target tumors overexpressing the folate receptor.

Theranostic agents are generally classified into two groups based on their mode of design. The first approach is the use of nanoparticles that can be functionalized with a variety of imaging and therapeutic moieties for use as theranostic particles. The properties offered by nanoparticles allow for their use as agents to carry both imaging and therapeutic drugs. The main advantages of using nanoparticles include their size (in 10–100 nm), which limits their clearance from the body allowing for increased circulation time. Nanoparticles are easily customizable and allow for surface functionalization with targeting ligands for increased tumor specificity and can be surface coated with polymers such as polyethylene glycol (PEG) (Jokerst et al., 2011) or poly(lactic-co-glycolic acid) (PLGA) (Danhier et al., 2009, 2012) for increased circulation times. Nanoparticles also allow for efficient loading of imaging as well as therapeutic agents. It is possible to control the ratio of the imaging agent to the therapeutic agent using nanoparticle chemistry. In the field, it has been shown that it is possible to have a single nanoparticle formulation carrying high payload of the therapeutic drug and a lower dose of the imaging agent. Also, theranostic nanoparticles can be modulated to release the drug at the site of tumor based on tumor microenvironment conditions, for example, peptide linkages that can be cleaved by matrix metalloproteinases (MMPs) (Van de Wiele and Oltenfreiter, 2006; Scherer et al., 2008a,b), which are normally abundant in a variety of tumors.

In spite of all the advantages provided by nanoparticles, they are still lacking some properties, which will allow their application in the clinic for treatment of patients. The use of nanoparticles for the development of theranostics has mainly focused on improving the sensitivity or increasing the image resolution.

Macrophages and other phagocytes readily engulf most nanoparticles. This leads to accumulation with the liver, the spleen, and the lymphatic system. The long-term safety of nanoparticles, their clearance from the various organs, is still not well understood. There have been issues with the toxicity induced by nanoparticles after administration. Quantum dots, which are comprised of cadmium salts, might induce toxicity if released in serum after injection (Bentolila et al., 2005; Michalet et al., 2005; Cai et al., 2006; Chen et al., 2012). There have been cases of renal toxicity with use of gadolinium chelates used in a variety of MRI agents. Another concern is that the shape and size of the nanoparticles can induce adverse effects on various types of the cells. Different types of nanoparticles have been shown to be cytotoxic to human cells, induce oxidative stress, or elicit an immune response. Lastly, there have been few nanoparticles that have been approved by the United States Food and Drug Administration (FDA) for use within the clinic, and most notably Abraxane is the only NP formulation approved for treatment (Elsadek and Kratz, 2012). There have been far and few nanoparticles that have found use within the clinic either as therapeutic drugs or for imaging purposes.

The other approach to developing theranostic agents involves synthesizing single agents that offer both therapeutic and imaging capabilities. The number of single agents that can serve this purpose is far and few in the literature. Most of the chemotherapeutic agents are not good candidates for synthesis of theranostic agents as the amount of drug required is far higher than imaging dose. Antibodies are class of molecules that have shown promise as agents for developing theranostic but antibodies are expensive and do not exhibit multiple killing effects as they have single target. They have poor penetration into tumors, often generate anti-immune responses from the host, and developing theranostic agents for using antibodies cost prohibitive. PSs, which are the drugs used in PDT, offer a chance for developing effective theranostic agents. PDT is a popular mode of treatment for a variety of malignant tumors. Porphyrin-based compounds that are well-established drugs for use in PDT allow for the development of a single theranostic agent as they can be modified to develop agents for multimodal tumor imaging and therapy by PDT. Most PSs have the ability to fluoresce when excited by light. This provides the opportunity for tumor imaging prior to therapy. Tetrapyrrole-based structures such as porphyrins also allow for attachment of tumor targeting and other imaging moieties for developing tumor-specific theranostic agents. The present review focuses on the theranostic agents involving synthesizing single agents, mainly tetrapyrrole-based derivatives such as porphyrins, phthalocyanines, porphyrazines (Pz), etc., for tumor imaging and therapy by PDT.

11.2 MOLECULAR IMAGING

Molecular biology and natural chemistry have experienced dramatic advances in the comprehension of the disease and the procedures that go before the unusual conditions. There has been an expansive push to create treatments that are aimed at specific cellular or molecular targets in an attempt to terminate the inflicting disease. There has been an increment in therapeutics in the past 20 years; however, the ability to visualize the effects of these therapies has not kept up. Imaging on the cellular scale would like to solve this problem by monitoring mechanisms of cell growth, multiplication, and cell death, as well as other processes that trigger or arrest disease, and the effects of medicines on these mechanisms (Hengerer and Grimm, 2006). Molecular and cellular imaging is the in vivo visualization of intact animals that intends to picture and/or quantify cellular processes and molecular events (Weissleder and Mahmood, 2001). In addition to cellular and molecular imaging in pharmaceuticals, visualization of biological events in the area of developmental biology to accomplish cell lineage and fate mapping will be important fields. Diagnostic imaging modalities are currently one of the most rapidly expanding areas in the field of medicine, with several methods for imaging internal structures and functions of the body, including X-ray, CT, PET, SPECT, US, and MRI. Each method has its advantages and disadvantages according to the physical phenomena that are being employed to create imaging information. Major preclinical imaging modalities are given in Table 11.2 with their advantages and disadvantages. In addition, fusion systems (PET–CT, SPECT–CT, and PET–MRI) are playing an increasingly essential role in molecular imaging by combining the high sensitivity of PET and SPECT with the high resolution of CT and MRI (Pysz et al., 2010). The choice of imaging modality depends on the spatiotemporal resolution, sensitivity, and depth of penetration required for the specific application.

Table 11.2 Major preclinical imaging modalities used with their advantages and disadvantages

Modality	Advantages	Disadvantages	Contrast agents	Radiation
Computed tomography (CT)	Unlimited tissue depth penetration	Radiation exposure	Krypton	X-rays
	High spatial resolution	Poor soft tissue contrast	Xenon	
	Can be used for whole body imaging		Iodine	
	Low acquisition time		Barium	
	Anatomical imaging			
Positron emission tomography (PET)	Unlimited tissue depth penetration	Radiation exposure	^{11}C	High-energy γ-rays
	Can be used for whole body imaging	Low spatial resolution and long acquisition time	^{18}F	
	Detailed anatomical information can be obtained when combining with CT or MRI	Expensive	^{64}Cu	
Single photon emission computed tomography (SPECT)	Unlimited tissue depth penetration	Radiation exposure	^{99}Tc	High-energy γ-rays
	High sensitivity	Low spatial resolution and long acquisition time	^{111}In	
		Expensive	^{123}I	
Magnetic resonance imaging (MRI)	Unlimited tissue depth penetration	Expensive	Gd^{3+}	Radio waves
	Nonionizing radiation	Long acquisition time and limited sensitivity	SPIO, USPIO	
	High spatial resolution and excellent soft tissue contrast			
	Whole body imaging is possible			
Ultrasound	High spatial resolution	Cannot be used for whole body imaging	Microbubbles	High-frequency sound
	Real-time imaging with low acquisition time			
	Highly sensitive and inexpensive			
Optical imaging	High spatial resolution	Cannot be used for whole-body imaging	Fluorescence dyes and molecules	Visible or NIR light
	Real-time imaging with low acquisition time	Limited tissue depth penetration	Light-sensitive NPs	
	Highly sensitive and inexpensive			

11.2.1 OPTICAL IMAGING AND NIRF IMAGING PROBES
FOR CANCER DIAGNOSIS AND TREATMENT

Optical imaging is one of the most preferred modality for tumor imaging. Molecular information that is related to the pathophysiological change is obtained by the light signals emitted from biological tissues. Among the optical imaging technologies, near-infrared fluorescence (NIRF) imaging is an adorable modality for early tumor detection with its high sensitivity and multidetection capability. This approach fundamentally depends on a fluorescence probe with emissions in the NIR region. In this region (650–900 nm), lower tissue autofluorescence and less fluorescence extinction enhance deep tissue penetration with minimal background interference (Yi et al., 2014). Nanoparticles including NIRF dyes and anticancer agents provide to the collegial treatment of cancer. Furthermore, novel NIRF dyes can be employed as effective agents for photothermal and PDT.

In the last two decades, phthalocyanines and porphyrin derivatives are among the most commonly used dyes in bioimaging and therapeutics as NIRF probes. These dyes can calmly be conjugated with various moieties such as nucleotides, DNA, DNA primers, amino acids, small molecules, proteins and antibodies to achieve specific targeting capacity (Luo et al., 2011). Porphyrins and expanded porphyrins consist of four or more pyrrole or heterocyclic rings. This kind of macrocyclic structures demonstrates the benefits of superior chemical stability and great photophysical properties at the point when used as new platforms for NIRF probe design. Their new derivatives are also encouraging in clinical application for cancer theranostics. Karunakaran and coworkers developed a hydrophilic porphyrin (THPP) and its derivative (Zn-THPP). They demonstrate superior quantum yield and excellent free radical generation rates. THPP displayed higher photodynamic activity compared to the clinical drug Photofrin. Moreover, THPP rapidly permeated into cells and localized in the nucleus, indicating its potential application as an NIR probe for PDT as well as nucleus imaging (Karunakaran et al., 2013).

Fluorescent molecules could be dyes targeted to specific biological events or could be generated in genetically modified tumor cells. Fluorescence is limited by tissue depth and has to deal with the natural fluorescence of some biological molecules. This method is inexpensive and has high sensitivity (picomolar–nanomolar) and resolution (approximately 1–2 mm in vivo). Although this technique is at the cutting edge of imaging developmental biology, it has serious limitations in the clinical scene due to low penetration depth.

11.2.2 PET AND SPECT

Nuclear medicine or nuclear imaging uses the decay of radionucleotides to visualize biological processes in vivo. There are two main techniques clinically used: PET and SPECT. The radioisotopes are linked with biologically active compounds to form radiopharmaceuticals, which are targeted to specific biochemical events (Cassidy and Radda, 2005). The basic advantages of radioactive assays are their high sensitivity and the ability of radiation detection systems to supply quantitative analysis of radioactivity concentrations deep inside tissue (Cherry, 2004). Nuclear imaging has been utilized for many years for imaging biological processes due to high sensitivity, availability, specificity of contrast agents (CAs), and fast acquisition times. Unfortunately, the use of radioactivity inside organisms possesses health complications, and spatial resolution is poor (millimeter rather than micrometer), and radiotracers are synthetically hard to produce.

PET CAs are radiolabeled with positron-emitting radionuclides. PET imaging is almost new in PDT and is still in its beginning; however, it exhibits promise in the ability to visualize real-time changes in treatment parameters, allowing an optimal therapeutic outcome to be accomplished. While PET is capable of following the change of radiolabeled synthetic molecules, it is not appropriate for radiolabeling biomolecules, such as peptides, antibodies, and hormones (Meikle et al., 2005).

SPECT is another CA–dependent technique using radioactive tracers to yield a signal. SPECT uses radioisotopes that emit only a single high-energy (gamma) photon from gamma-emitting isotopes such as ^{133}Xe, ^{99m}Tc, and ^{123}I. The main advantage of SPECT is the longer half-lives (hour to day time scale) of the radioisotopes used, which makes assessment of slowly diffusing macromolecules possible. However, the sensitivity of SPECT (~10^{-10} M) is lower than PET due to the use of mechanical collimators (which absorb photons), whereas PET sparkle is done electronically.

11.2.3 MRI

MRI has become one of the significant imaging modalities in today's ever-developing therapeutic field (Huang et al., 2012; Liu et al., 2014). In comparison to other imaging methods, for example, CT, the advantages of MRI involve better soft tissue differentiation, absence of radioactive materials, high resolution, and the ability to visualize organism temporally, allowing for developments of three-dimensional images without sacrificing the organism (Yan et al., 2011; Liang et al., 2014). Sensitivity with MRI is innately low, but CAs (generally a Gd(III) chelate) can be utilized to overcome this obstacle; MRI in biological systems is based on the nuclear magnetic resonance (NMR) signal from water protons. The paramagnetic ion most widely used in this view is gadolinium [Gd(III)] because of its seven unpaired electrons and large paramagnetic moment (Krzystek et al., 1999). The Gd(III)-based CAs approved by the FDA are Magnevist, Omniscan, and Prohances, and all these are carboxylate-containing water-soluble complexes.

11.2.3.1 MRI CONTRAST AGENTS

To overcome some of the disadvantages such as low sensitivity and long acquisition time in MRI, CAs can be employed. CAs usually exist in two main forms: either small molecule chelates or large macromolecules. Frequently the two are combined by adding a small molecule chelate to a macromolecule, like a protein.

Even though MRI offers high-resolution anatomical images with superior soft tissue contrast, it has limited ability to differentiate between pathological and healthy tissues that are magnetically similar but histologically apparent. Synthetic chemists desire to solve this complication by designing CAs that interact with a biological/pathological appropriate target, such as ions, enzymes, pH, or metabolites. In this manner, these agents can give specific information about a biochemical event or reflect a pathological situation. Usually, CAs are designed to have an increased relaxivity upon interaction with the targets by manipulating parameters such as q, τ_r, and T_{1e} (of T_1 CAs) or local magnetic field inhomogeneity (of T_2 CAs).

11.2.3.1.1 Overview of MRI CAs

More than 35% of MRI scans in clinical diagnosis utilize CAs (Caravan et al., 1999; Caravan, 2006; Chan and Wong, 2007). CAs can improve MRI signal-to-noise ratio through the interaction of a paramagnetic metal ion with surrounding water protons by decreasing the T_1 and T_2. In a given imaging acquisition time, a shorter relaxation rate means nuclei spins repeat the relaxation process many more times, leading to higher signal intensity. Depending on the effects, CAs can be classified as T_1 agents and T_2 agents. T_1 agents, such as paramagnetic ions Gd^{3+}, Mn^{2+}, and Fe^{3+}, make a positive effect on a T_1-weighted image and increase the brightness of affected regions. T_2 agents, such as superparamagnetic iron oxide nanoparticles (SPIONs), cause a negative effect on a T_2-weighted image and decrease the brightness. T_1 CAs are generally approved because an increased brightness is more readily visible than decreased intensity. Gd^{3+} complexes are the most commonly used CAs for MRI in T_1-weighted images. Gd^{3+} ion, with seven unpaired electrons, creates a high magnetic moment and a long electronic relaxation time so Gd^{3+} shows the strongest effect in reducing the longitudinal relaxation time of water protons compared to all the other paramagnetic ions. In solution, thousands of water molecules coordinate and disassociate with the octodentate Gd^{3+} rapidly on the MRI time scale and then diffuse to the surrounding bulk water pool. Thus, the paramagnetic enhanced relaxation effect can be widely spread.

11.2.3.1.2 Hyperpolarized MRI CAs

MRI is based on the measurements of water ^1H nuclei. Signal intensity relies on proton density and relaxation times T_1 and T_2. The main disadvantages of this technique are the limited sensitivity because of long acquisition times and only uses of water protons. Together with proton (^1H), other nuclei are also employed for MRI. Encouraging candidates for the improvement of MRI are hyperpolarized ^{129}Xe, ^3He, ^{13}C, and a few other nuclei. The use of hyperpolarized substances as CAs can intensely reduce the acquisition times as long as the strong signal enhancement, and allows the detection of nuclei other than protons, producing high-intensity images without background signal. During the use of hyperpolarized CAs, images are created by observing the CA hyperpolarized nuclei directly. The higher the polarization or the concentration, the higher the signal that will be detected. Various hyperpolarization methods have been developed, including dynamic nuclear polarization (DNP; Abragam and Goldman, 1978), spin-exchange optical pumping (SEOP; Walker and Happer, 1997), and para-hydrogen and synthesis allow dramatically enhanced net alignment (PASADENA; Bowers and Weitekamp, 1986). DNP includes transfer of polarization from the electronic spins to coupled nuclear spins. When the free radical doped material containing the nuclei to be hyperpolarized is subjected to low temperature and high magnetic fields, the unpaired electrons of the free radical are polarized. During irradiation, this polarization is transferred to the nuclei of interest. The material is rapidly dissolved into an injectable liquid to be used for imaging (Ardenkjær-Larsen et al., 2003).

11.3 MRI IN PDT

11.3.1 DEVELOPMENT OF THERANOSTIC AGENTS FOR PDT AND MRI

PDT is based on the cytotoxic effect of sensitizing drugs photoactivated in the presence of oxygen. Most of the clinical work on PDT has used either HPD or PhotofrinB; both preparations contain a large number of porphyrin derivatives. New, pure sensitizing drugs are being developed with several design objectives in mind such as enhanced photodynamic effect, reduction of *drug* retention time in the patient, and tissue specificity (Kessel, 1992). The most generally accepted mechanism of PDT activity in vivo for a number of sensitizers, including Photofrin, phthalocyanines, and chlorins, is cellular and vascular damage. In experimental tumor systems, transient vasoconstriction, vasodilation, and eventual complete blood stasis and hemorrhage occur after light exposure (Henderson and Dougherty, 1992; Pass, 1993; van Geel et al., 1996).

MRI and MRS are excellent techniques for the noninvasive, in vivo evaluation of tissue damage after PDT (Boesch, 2007; De Stefano et al., 2007; Soares and Law, 2009; van der Graaf, 2010). The intrinsic properties of water in normal, necrotic, and viable tumor tissue can be used in proton, ^{1}H, MR experiments to identify discrete regions within the tissue anatomy. Conjugating probes that are detectable by different techniques create agents of multimodality. For example, covalent attachment of a fluorescent probe to an MR agent results in a conjugate that reports cellular and subcellular localization via fluorescence while providing deep anatomical information by MRI (Frullano and Meade, 2007; Modo et al., 2007). Diethylene triamine pentaacetic acid (DTPA) Gd complexes are the most widely used ones, as is the commercially available Magnevist, Omniscan being a bismethylamide substituted DTPA Gd complex (Tamada et al., 2009). The efficacy of these CAs depends on the interchanging of water between the bulk solvent and the coordination sphere. The swapping scale of bound water relies upon the nature of the ligand and the metal ion. Complexes made with the chelator 1,4,7,10-tetraazacyclododecane-1,4,7,10-tetraacetic acid (DOTA) exhibit the fastest rate of bound water.

In particular, protein cages have been utilized as nanometer-sized carriers of covalently attached Gd(III)-based CAs (Caravan et al., 1999) for MRI (Allen et al., 2005; Anderson et al., 2006; Hooker et al., 2007; Liepold et al., 2007, 2009; Prasuhn et al., 2007; Datta et al., 2008; Garimella et al., 2011; Pokorski et al., 2011; Lucon et al., 2012) of porphyrins (Prasuhn et al., 2008; Stephanopoulos et al., 2009, 2010; Rhee et al., 2012) and Pcs (Brasch et al., 2011) as near-infrared light-absorbing molecules with potential applications in biomedicine. Chelates of the Gd(III) ion represent the predominantly used MRI CAs, while Pc derivatives are well-known chromophores with different biomedical applications. The synergy of MRI CAs and photoactive organic molecules into biocompatible nanoparticles is indeed highly desirable, yet it is not an easy task from the synthetic point of view. While virus capsids are excellent alternative nanosized scaffolds for achieving high loading of CAs (Werner et al., 2008), their covalent modification often requires extensive synthetic procedures (Millan et al., 2014).

In addition to being MRI probes, over the last several years, magnetic nanoparticles (MNPs) have been extensively explored for other nanomedicine applications due to their unique magnetic behaviors (Son et al., 2005; Sokolova and Epple, 2008; Namiki et al., 2009; Huang et al., 2010; Lee et al., 2010a, 2011; Thomas et al., 2010; Di Corato et al., 2011; Sanson et al., 2011; Song et al., 2011; Bilalis et al., 2012; Cho et al.,

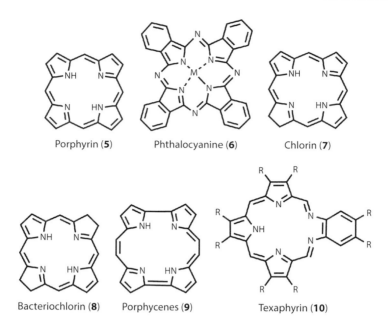

Porphyrin (**5**)   Phthalocyanine (**6**)   Chlorin (**7**)

Bacteriochlorin (**8**)   Porphycenes (**9**)   Texaphyrin (**10**)

Figure 11.4 Basic structure of the examples of tetrapyrrole-based PSs.

2012; Pernia Leal et al., 2012). These applications enabled inorganic MNPs not only to be used as MRI CAs, but also potentially as theranostic (diagnostic and therapeutic) agents (Yoo et al., 2011; Peng et al., 2015).

Imaging is the other aspect of a theranostic agent, which allows for visualization of a target before treatment. Molecular imaging is an area that provides both anatomical and functional information. In a literal sense, molecular imaging agents provide images of molecules.

Pc (**6**), porphyrins (**5**), and other related tetrapyrrolic derivatives as chlorins (**7**), bacteriochlorins (**8**), porphycenes (**9**), and texaphyrins (**10**) (Figure 11.4) are of interest as PSs for PDT and fluorescence probes due to their suitable physical and biocompatible chemical properties (Ali and van Lier, 1999, 2010; Aratani and Osuka, 2010; Balaban, 2010; Lim et al., 2010). Porphyrins are 18π-electron aromatic macrocycles that exhibit characteristic optical spectra with a strong π–π^* transition around 400 nm (Soret band) and usually four Q bands in the visible region. Two of the peripheral double bonds in opposite pyrrolic rings are cross-conjugated and are not required to maintain aromaticity. Thus, reduction of one or both these cross-conjugated bonds maintains much of the aromaticity (chlorin and bacteriochlorin, respectively). A change in symmetry results in red shifted Q-bands (640–800 nm) with high extinction coefficient. Pcs are a class of tetrapyrroles in which the C- at *meso*-positions (5-, 10–15 and 20) is replaced by N. The longest wavelength absorption in this class of compounds falls near 700 nm. The Pcs are of particular interest since they exhibit high photo- and chemical stability that is desirable for chemical modifications as well as in vitro and in vivo applications. They show near-infrared absorbance where tissues are optimal transparent, high extinction coefficients and good quantum yield for singlet oxygen production. They can be synthesized in a straightforward manner and modified to alter hydrophobicity, absorption, and emission wavelengths for different applications. Combination of these properties makes them attractive theranostic agents, for example, as PS for PDT and probes for fluorescence and MRI (Ethirajan et al., 2011).

11.3.2 DIFFERENT TYPES OF TETRAPYRROLE-BASED STRUCTURES

11.3.2.1 PHTHALOCYANINES

Among the tetrapyrrolic derivatives, phthalocyanines exhibit properties particularly suitable for PDT, especially their maximum absorption wavelength centered approximately at 680 nm but tailorable by adapting the substitution pattern. Besides, their easy functionalization allows one to obtain asymmetrically substituted compounds, with functional moieties and other substituents providing the desired solubility. Several phthalocyanines are in advanced clinical trial stages, such as Photosens, mixture of sulfonated aluminum phthalocyanines in Russia (Filonenko, 2015) or Pc 4 in the United States (Kinsella et al., 2011). Numerous experiments have been done to follow by MRI the outcome of a photodynamic treatment based on phthalocyanine PSs: ZnPc (Winsborrow et al., 1997), Pc4 (Fei et al., 2007), and MRI agents are gadolinium-T_1 CAs such as DTPA. The action of AlPcS$_2$ either for PDT (Mathews et al., 2011) or related photochemical internalization (Norum et al., 2009) treatments was followed in the same manner.

Nevertheless, there are only a very few combinations of MRI and PDT agents that are real theranostics. Only one molecular combination of a photosensitizing phthalocyanine with an MRI agent is reported so far (Aydin Tekdas et al., 2014). It was designed to be water-soluble and regioisomerically pure. Click chemistry was used to graft a known alkynyl Gd-DOTA moiety (11) (Figure 11.5). The resulting conjugate exhibited slightly lower relaxivity than clinically used DOTA. Preliminary biological tests confirmed that it is a promising MRI/PDT molecular theranostic.

Other theranostic combinations of MRI agents and photosensitizing phthalocyanines are all nanoparticles. Two examples of upconverting nanoparticles (UCNPs) are reported, hence added a third property—luminescence imaging—to MRI and photodynamic effect. Dihydroxylated SiPc was covalently grafted to the mesoporous silica shell layer coating upconverting NaGdF$_4$:Yb,Er@CaF$_2$ nanophosphors, which is shown in Figure 11.6 (Qiao et al., 2012). NIR illumination at 980 nm gives an emission at 660 nm suitable for the phthalocyanine excitation, and a second emission at 550 nm for fluorescence imaging. Gd ions in the core of the nanoparticles provided the MRI property close to commercial Gd-DTPA. These nanoparticles were able to generate singlet oxygen but biological investigations of the photodynamic efficiency demonstrated that fine adjustments of light doses are necessary.

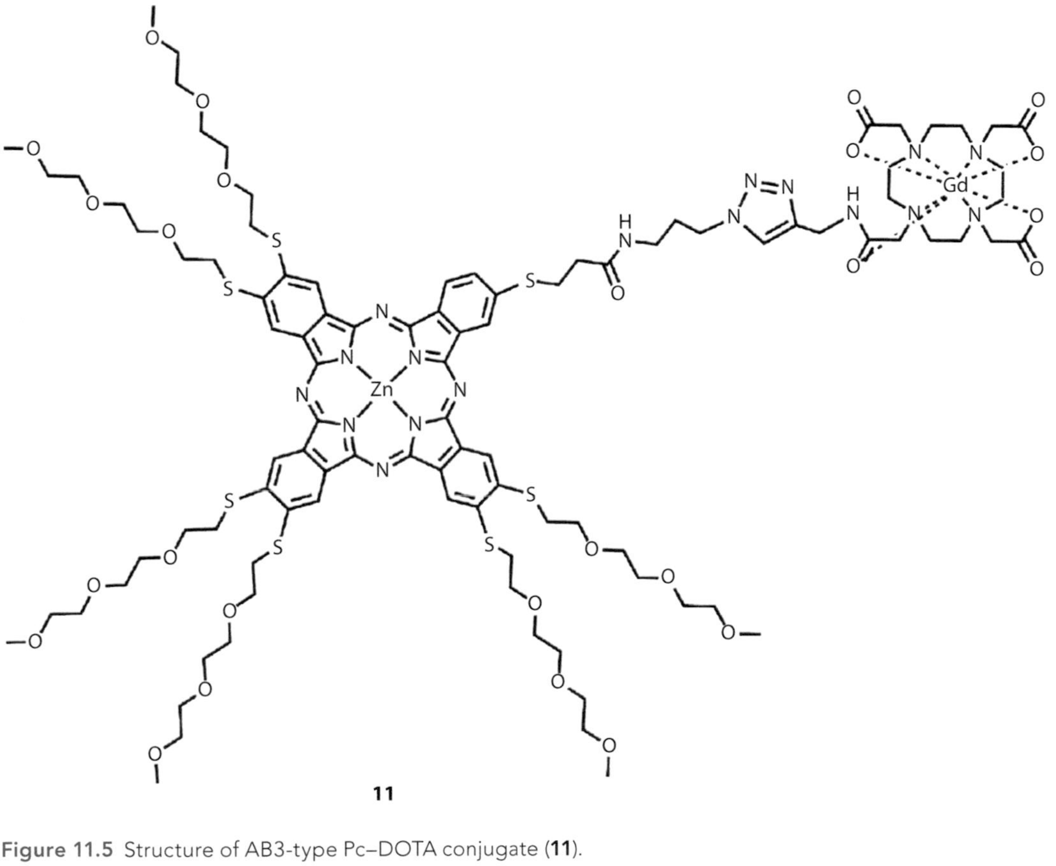

11

Figure 11.5 Structure of AB3-type Pc–DOTA conjugate (**11**).

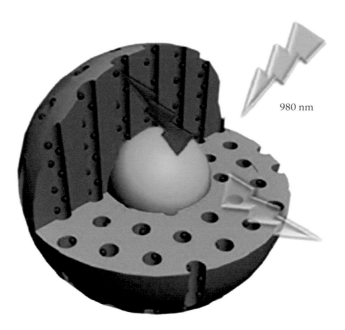

980 nm

Figure 11.6 Core–shell structured (NaGdF$_4$:Yb,Er@CaF$_2$@SiO$_2$-PS) nanomaterial. It consists of the NaGdF$_4$:Yb,Er@CaF$_2$ nanoparticle (green sphere) as the core and mesoporous silica (brown sphere) covalently grafted with PS (small pink sphere) as the shell. Under excitation at 980 nm (gray arrowhead), the nanomaterial gives luminescence emissions at 550 and 660 nm. The former is used for fluorescence imaging (green arrowhead), and the latter is used for energy absorption of PS to generate singlet oxygen (red arrowhead). (From Qiao, X.F., Zhou, J.C., Xiao, J.W., Wang, Y.F., Sun, L.D., Yan, C.H., Triple-functional core-shell structured upconversion luminescent nanoparticles covalently grafted with photosensitizer for luminescent, magnetic resonance imaging and photodynamic therapy in vitro, *Nanoscale*, 4, 4611–4623, 2012. Reproduced by permission of The Royal Society of Chemistry.)

In another example (Zeng et al., 2013), a Fe$_3$O$_4$ core with type 2 MRI properties was coated firstly by Y/Yb/Er ions, then by PEG units. AlPcS4 was then conjugated by electrostatic interactions. Irradiation at 980 nm of these nanoparticles significantly decreased the viability of MCF-7 cells while no serious dark toxicity was observed. Porous silica-coated γ-Fe$_2$O$_3$ nanoparticles were used as a drug carrier accommodating hydrophobic Zn(II) phthalocyanine (Xuan et al., 2012). These microspheres exhibited very good in vitro r$_2$ relaxivity, and high phototoxicity against HT29 cells.

Another type of NP based on the self-assembly of a virus protein was reported (Millan et al., 2014). The MRI agent is an amphiphilic ligand 1,4,7,10-tetraaza-1-(1-carboxymethylundecane)-4,7,10-triacetic acid cyclododecane (DOTAC10) complexing a Gd^{3+} cation and forming paramagnetic micelles together with an amphiphilic Zn(II) phthalocyanine (ZnPc). These micelles are then incorporated inside capsids of the cowpea chlorotic mottle virus protein (Figure 11.7). These original controlled stepwise self-assemblies led to capsides highly loaded in both phthalocyanine and MRI agents.

11.3.2.2 PORPHYRINS

Porphyrin is a key functional life molecule that exists ubiquitously in plants and animals. Heme derivatives have been used for cancer imaging as early as the 1920s, and they have been utilized as MR CAs since the 1980s. Heme has kept up its use in new imaging methods as the basic molecule that allows functional MRI. Porphyrins have been pioneering agents for modern theranostics. As expected, porphyrins have produced a clinical label on modern theranostics in the form of PDT. Most porphyrins can be used for therapeutic applications because of their capability to generate singlet oxygen upon irradiation. Over decades, porphyrins have been examined as florescent probes or radioactive tracers for tumor detection. Porphyrin dyes have great photophysical properties such as chemical and photochemical stability, high absorption coefficients

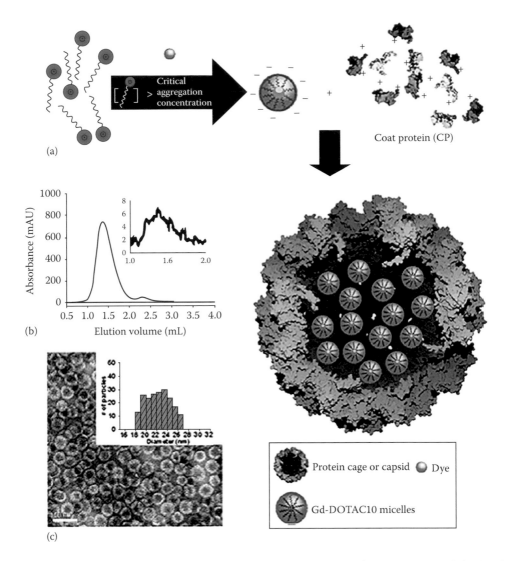

Figure 11.7 (a) Schematic representation of the self-assembly process toward PCNs containing Gd-DOTAC10/ ZnPc micelles. The ZnPc localization within micelles (depicted by yellow spheres) is only schematic, and multiple site-isolated dye molecules can actually be encapsulated in each micelle. (b) Size exclusion (FPLC or fast protein liquid chromatography) chromatogram. The blue trace is characteristic of the capsid CP (monitored at 280 nm), whereas the black trace (inset) is characteristic of the ZnPc dye (monitored at 682 nm). Elution volume of the protein cages ~1.3 mL. (c) TEM image. Inset: histogram showing the diameter distribution of capsids filled with Gd-DOTAC10/ZnPc micelles. Scale bar: 50 nm. (Reprinted from *J. Inorg. Biochem.*, 136, Millan, J.G., Brasch, M., Anaya-Plaza, E., de la Escosura, A., Velders, A.H., Reinhoudt, D.N., Torres, T., Koay, M.S., Cornelissen, J.J., Self-assembly triggered by self-assembly: Optically active, paramagnetic micelles encapsulated in protein cage nanoparticles, 140–146. Copyright 2014, with permission from Elseiver.)

and quantum yields, and emission in the therapeutical window (NIR spectral region), all these properties enabling imaging in vivo (Osterloh and Vicente, 2002). Their versatility in cancer imaging and other pathological circumstances was further displayed by their use as radiolabeled imaging probes and in the development of CAs for MRI and PET (Lee et al., 2010; Gros et al., 2011; Shi et al., 2011; Eggenspiller et al., 2013). Currently, the important roles of porphyrin molecules in imaging and PDT (and selective uptake in diseased tissue) and their utility in theranostic applications have been reviewed (Pandey et al., 2005; Lupu et al., 2009; Cheng et al., 2010; Lovell et al., 2010; Ethirajan et al., 2011; McCann et al., 2011; Josefsen and Boyle, 2012; Lovell and Lo, 2012; Poyer et al., 2012; Bozzini et al., 2013). Among different combinations, the inclusions of PSs for PDT and CA for MRI into a single stage would have appreciable advantage for the design of theragnostic tools since both PDT and MRI use nondestructive radiation. The groups of Hoffman and Pandey have synthesized one such solution tumor-avid porphyrins; the gadophrin-2 conjugate has been extensively studied and determined to be necrosis avid (Hofmann et al., 1999). Pandey's group (Roswell Park Cancer Institute, USA) has widely studied multimodal CAs based on PS conjugates (Li et al., 2005; Pandey et al., 2005). The conjugates can be promoted in PDT, as CAs (PET or MRI), and/or in fluorescence imaging allowing tissue imaging (pre-, during, and post-PDT) to determine treatment outcome. Work has been managed to generate a contrast-enhancement agent that can target living tumor cells, particularly those that are strongly undergoing metabolic processes (Ethirajan et al., 2011).

Recent advances in nanotechnologies have allowed us to utilize various nanocrystals (NCs) in biomedical fields such as drug delivery, bioimaging, and therapeutics (Lee et al., 2010; Ke et al., 2011; Liang et al., 2011; Nyström and Wooley, 2011; Yoon et al., 2014). Nowadays, most of the preclinically used magnetic nanoparticles consist of magnetite (Fe_3O_4) and maghemite (Fe_2O_3) nanoparticles and SPIONs that are known as T_2 CAs. Recently, the use of SPIONs includes dendrimer porphyrin (DP) as theranostic agent has been investigated by Yoon and coworkers (2014). They have prepared SPIONs-embedded polystyrene NPs (SPIONs@PS), which were utilized as the sacrificial template for the formation of layer-by-layer (LbL) by alternative deposition of positively charged polyelectrolyte (poly (allylamine hydrochloride); PAH) and photofunctional DP (Figure 11.8). NCs showed strong enough magnetic property (>20 emu g^{-1}) for MRI application with typical superparamagnetic behavior, leading to corresponding T_2 relaxivity coefficient (r_2) value of 93.5 mM^{-1} s^{-1}. Cell viability study upon light irradiation demonstrated that NCs can successfully work in PS formulation for PDT.

Additionally, manganese oxide (MnO) nanoparticles have recently found to be interesting candidates as T_1 CAs. Schladt and coworkers (2010) described the synthesis of highly water-soluble multifunctional MnO NP system carrying protoporphyrin IX as a PS (Figure 11.9). Monodisperse MnO NCs were synthesized by the oleate route and finally functionalized with a dopamine-PEGprotoporphyrin IX (DA-PEG-PP) ligand. Laser light radiation (PDT) (635 nm, incident dose of 72 J cm^{-2}) of Caki-1 cells incubated with protoporphyrin IX-functionalized MnO nanoparticles leads to cell death by apoptosis due to formation of reactive singlet oxygen ($^1O_2$) proposed by photoactivation of protoporphyrin IX and MnO nanoparticles show a strong T_1 contrast enhancement effect for MRI. Therefore, hydrophilic protoporphyrin IX-functionalized MnO nanoparticles demonstrates great potential for application not only as imaging agents for MRI and fluorescence microscopy but also as target systems for PDT.

Another important family of T_1 paramagnetic CAs are Mn complexes (Wang and Westmoreland, 2009). Mn porphyrins have demonstrated great potential for the use of T_1 CAs in tumor imaging due to the good stability, high longitudinal relaxivity, and tumorous "preferential uptake" property (Zhang et al., 2009). Exclusively, a water-soluble metalloporphyrin of Mn(III)-meso-tetrakis(4-sulfonatophenyl) porphyrin (Mn-TPPS4) has been described as a stable and cell-permeable CA with comparable longitudinal (T_1) magnetic resonance relaxivity with that of the commercial MRI CAs Gd-DTPA (Lee et al., 2010; Pan et al., 2011) and promoting to localize in tumors (Fiel et al., 1987; Lyon et al., 1987). Nevertheless, like the other paramagnetic metal complexes, Mn porphyrins suffer from short half-lives in vivo, contributing to poor imaging outcomes (Zong et al., 2005). Therefore, the nanoparticles combining with Mn complexes are acquiring enormous attention. Liang et al. (2014) reported on a versatile theranostic porphyrin dyad nanoparticles (TPD NPs) for the MRI-guided PDT by employing two types of porphyrin derivatives: metal-free porphyrin as a PS for PDT of cancer and Mn-porphyrin as a T_1 CA for MRI. Covalent attachment of porphyrins to TPD NPs prevents premature release during systemic circulation. In addition, TPD NPs (~60 nm) could passively accrue in tumors and be avidly taken up by tumor cells. The PDT and MRI capabilities of TPD NPs can be conveniently modulated by varying the molar ratio of metal-free porphyrin/Mn-porphyrin. At the optimal molar ratio of 40.1%, the total drug loading content is up to 49.8%, 31.3% for metal-free porphyrin, and 18.5% for Mn porphyrin. The laser light ablated the tumor completely within 7 days in the presence of TPD NPs and the tumor growth inhibition was 100%. The relaxivities were determined to be 20.58 s^{-1} mM^{-1} for TPD NPs, about four times as much as that of Mn-porphyrin (5.16 s^{-1} mM^{-1}). After 24 h intravenous injection of TPD NPs, MRI images demonstrated that the complete tumor area remained much brighter than the surrounding healthy tissue, allowing one to guide the laser light to the desired tumor site for photodynamic ablation.

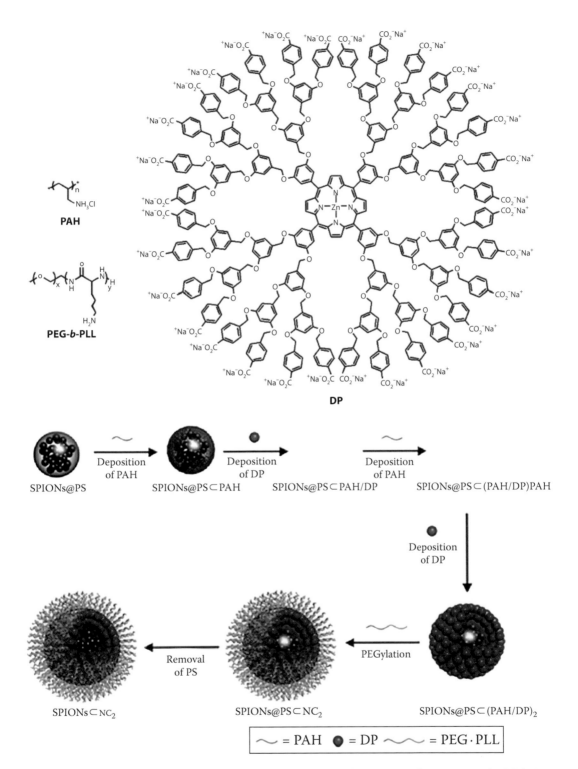

Figure 11.8 Procedures for the fabrication of SPIONs⊂NCn and structures of PAH, DP and PEG-*b*-PLL. (Reprinted with permission from Yoon, H.-J., Lim, T.G., Kim, J.-H., Cho, Y.M., Kim, Y.S., Chung, U.S., Kim, J.H., Choi, B.W., Koh, W.-G., Jang, W.-D., Fabrication of multifunctional layer-by-layer nanocapsules toward the design of theragnostic nanoplatform, *Biomacromolecules*, 15, 1382–1389. Copyright 2014 American Chemical Society.)

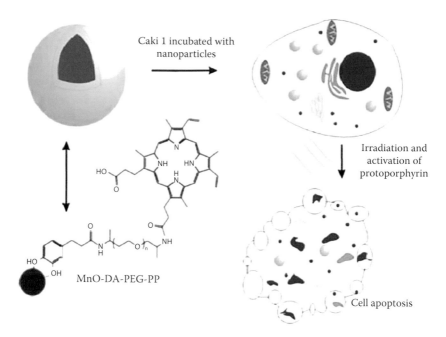

Figure 11.9 MnO nanoparticles functionalized using a multifunctional polymeric ligand through suitable anchor groups and carrying amine moieties. Protoporphyrin is bound to PEG800 shell via an amide bond. The protoporphyrin IX tagged MnO nanoparticles are used as photodynamic therapeutic agents to induce localized and intracellularly induced apoptosis in Caki-1 cells. (From Schladt, T.D., Schneider, K., Shukoor, M.I., Natalio, F., Bauer, H., Tahir, M.N., Weber, S. et al., Highly soluble multifunctional MnO nanoparticles for simultaneous optical and MRI imaging and cancer treatment using photodynamic therapy, *J. Mater. Chem.*, 20, 8297–8304, 2010. Reproduced by permission of The Royal Society of Chemistry.)

However, most of the clinically applied diagnostic and therapeutic drugs are organic or coordination compounds, in which their physiological mechanism has been well understood. Therefore, development of metal coordination or organometallic compounds as theranostic agents that combine both diagnostic and therapeutic functions is more attractive in clinical application. Luo et al. (2014) present a compound has four Gd(III)-DTTA (gadolinium-diethylenetriamine tetraacetic acid) chelate moieties are combined to tetraphenylporphyrin (TPP) through covalent linkages, complex 6 (Figure 11.10). Attachment of four Gd-DTTA groups to a rigid TPP moiety causes a higher relaxivity ($14.1\ mM^{-1}\ s^{-1}$) per Gd(III) than those of MRI CAs ($3.0–6.0\ mM^{-1}\ s^{-1}$) in clinical diagnosis. The four negative charges of complex 6 show excellent water solubility and human serum albumin (HSA) binding character. Also, the signal intensity of T_1-weighted phantom of MRI was significantly enhanced upon binding to HSA (Figure 11.11). Upon binding to HSA, the relaxivity is remarkably increased from 14.1 to $29.2\ mM^{-1}\ s^{-1}$. Due to better water solubility compared with free TPP, the capability of complex 6 to generate singlet oxygen is considerably improved upon irradiation with a far-red light (650 ± 20 nm). The higher far-red excitation (650 nm) and emission (665 nm) ensure complex 6 is applicable to PDT and PDD in deep tissue.

The utilization of porphyrin PSs as theranostic agents also is starting to show extraordinary potential of the capacity of a solitary substance to act as a double imaging and PDT agent and holds important advantages in the recognition and treatment of tumors and other disease models. Moreover, imaging combined with PDT has the potential to provide personalized medicine treatments, which means patient-targeted therapy.

11.3.2.3 PORPHYRAZINES

Pz derivatives exhibit NIR absorption/emission (~700–900 nm; Michel et al., 2001). Some derivatives of Pzs show tumor-specific accumulation and have high quantum yield of singlet oxygen generation. These properties can be candidate Pzs as potential tumor optical imaging and PDT agents in cancer treatment (Hammer et al., 2005; Vesper et al., 2006; Fuchter et al., 2008; Song et al., 2010; Trivedi et al., 2010).

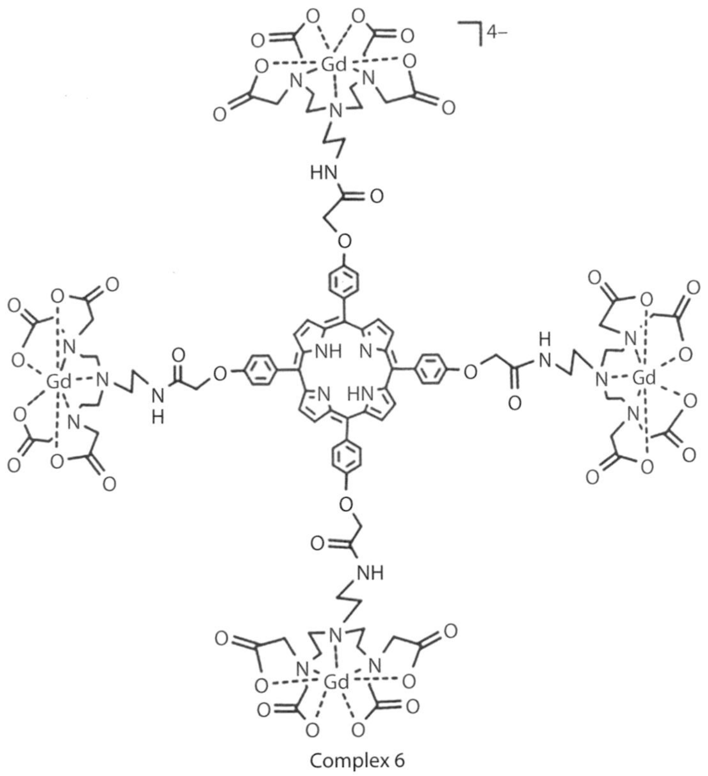

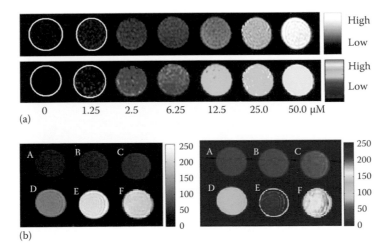

Complex 6

Figure 11.10 Structure of complex 6. (Reprinted with permission from Luo, J., Chen, L.-F., Hu, P., Chen, Z.-N., Tetranuclear gadolinium(III) porphyrin complex as a theranostic agent for multimodal imaging and photodynamic therapy, *Inorg. Chem.*, 53, 4184–4191. Copyright 2014 American Chemical Society.)

Figure 11.11 (a) T_1-weighted phantom MR images for complex 6 with a concentration of 0–50.0 µM. (b) T_1-weighted phantom MR images for complex 6. (A) 100 mM 2-[4-(2-hydroxyethyl)piperazin-1-yl]ethanesulfonic acid (HEPES) buffer solution (pH = 7.2); (B) 100 mM HEPES buffer solution with 0.6 mM HSA; (C) HS; (D) 31.25 µM complex 6 in 100 mM HEPES solution; (E) 31.25 µM complex 6 in 100 mM HEPES solution with 0.6 mM HSA; (F) 31.25 µM complex 6 in HS. (Reprinted with permission from Luo, J., Chen, L.-F., Hu, P., Chen, Z.-N., Tetranuclear gadolinium(III) porphyrin complex as a theranostic agent for multimodal imaging and photodynamic therapy, *Inorg. Chem.*, 53, 4184–4191. Copyright 2014 American Chemical Society.)

MRI is a more effective diagnostic tool in clinical and experimental use to obtain three-dimensional, high-resolution images of deep tissues, but they lack the intense MRI required for use as an effective CA. Coalition of these two types of CA and PDT agent into a single "theranostic" agent (therapeutic/diagnostic) would provide victory against cancer.

A series of multimodal imaging agents were prepared with conjugation of zinc metalated fluorescent Pz derivatives to one, four, or eight paramagnetic Gd(III) complexes as CA in MRI (Song et al., 2010). The structure of these Pz conjugates is presented in Figure 11.12, and ionic relaxivity of these complexes (Zn-Pz-nGd(III) (n = 1, 4, 8)) compared with Gd595 is given in Table 11.3. Among these conjugates, Zn-Pz-8Gd(III)

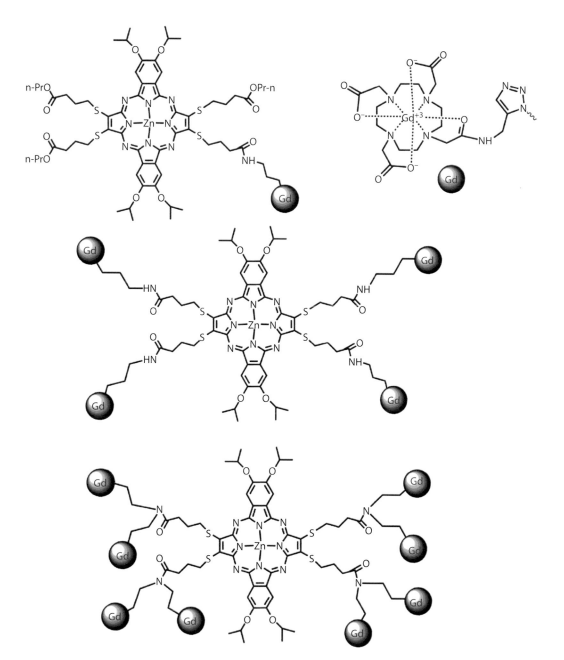

Figure 11.12 Structure of ZnPz-nGd(III) (n = 1, 4, 8). (Adapted from Song, Y. et al., *Bioconjug. Chem.*, 21, 2267–2275, 2010.)

Table 11.3 Molecular and Gd(III) ionic relaxivity of Zn-Pz-nGd(III) (n = 1, 4, 8) complexes in water at 37°C, 60 MHz

Compounds	MW (g/mol)	Gd(III) ionic r_1 (mM^{-1} s^{-1})	Molecular r_1 (mM^{-1} s^{-1})
Gd595	595.7	3.21	3.21
Zn-Pz-1Gd(III)	1985.6	4.20[a]	4.20[a]
Zn-Pz-4Gd(III)	3893.9	10.5	42
Zn-Pz-8Gd(III)	6496.9	12.8	102.4

Source: Song, Y., Zong, H., Trivedi, E.R., Vesper, B.J., Waters, E.A., Barrett, A.G.M., Radosevich, J.A., Hoffman, B.M., and Meade, T.J., Synthesis and characterization of new porphyrazine-Gd(III) conjugates as multimodal MR contrast agents, *Bioconjug. Chem.*, 21, 2267–2275, 2010. Reproduced by permission of The Royal Society of Chemistry.

[a] Measured in DMSO/water, v/v = 1:1.5.

exhibited the highest ionic relaxivity and molecular relaxivity. Unlike current clinical MRI agents, Zn-Pz-1Gd(III) is taken up by cells. This agent demonstrated intracellular fluorescence by confocal microscopy and provided significant contrast enhancement in MR images, as well as marked phototoxicity in assays of cellular viability. The Pz-Gd(III) conjugates exhibited improved ionic and molecular relaxivities relative to well-known single-molecule MRI agents. Furthermore, the photophysical properties that make the Pz class of molecules attractive for biological applications were preserved and the water solubility properties of these compounds were enhanced after addition of the hydrophilic Gd(III) moieties. The results of Pz-based-MRI multimodal agent suggested that Pz agents possess a new potential for use in cancer imaging by both MRI and NIR fluorescence, while acting as a platform for PDT. Thus, multimodal and multifunctional Pzs have the potential to serve as dual MRI-NIR/antitumor therapeutic agents capable of targeting specific tumor types.

11.3.2.4 CHLORINS

Chlorins consisting of three pyrroles and one pyrroline coupled through four ≡CH-linkages exhibit deeper penetration of PDT-induced necrosismas and their absorption wavelength at the "phototherapeutic window" of 600–800 nm. Chlorin-type structures are used as photosensitizing agents in PDT.

Identification of diagnostic materials has been one of the goals of CA research in MRI. Since the ring structure of chlorins is too small to adequately accommodate Gd, Gd-labeled metallochlorins may be unstable as a CA for MRI. One attempt to overcome the stability problem for theranostic applications is to link the most commonly used paramagnetic gadolinium ion to chlorin-based PS, which has the preferential uptake by tumors, and chlorin-based paramagnetic metal chelates and complexes have attracted a lot of interest (Galindev et al., 2009).

The Gd-labeled metallochlorin derivative, Gd-chlorin (PB Chlorin), was synthesized and investigated by using a simple tissue phantom to test its efficacy as an MRI CA (Kim et al., 2006). This study demonstrated the potential activity of Gd-chlorin as not only a MRI CA, but also as a PDT PS by using a simple tissue phantom and conducting a very brief MRI experiment. The structure of PB Chlorin is presented in Figure 11.13.

Among chlorophyll-*a* derivatives, 3-devinyl-3-(1-hexyloxy)ethyl-pyropheophorbide-*a* (HPPH), which is in phase II human clinical trial for PDT, has been studied by using HPPH as a "vehicle" for delivering Gd(III) complexes to tumors as a tumor selective CA for MRI by Pandey et al. (Chen et al., 2002, 2004; Bellnier et al., 2003; Li et al., 2003; Pandey et al., 2006).

They prepared a series of bifunctional agents including two Gd(III) atoms per HPPH molecule that remained tumor-avid and PDT-active and yielded improved MR tumor conspicuity compared to their corresponding mono-Gd(III)-analogs (Li et al., 2005). The structure of these agents is presented in Figure 11.14. Also, different chlorin-based Gd(III) chelates were synthesized by Gavinda et al. (Chen et al., 2002) in order to develop a single bifunctional agent that could be clinically utilized both as a CA for the enhancement of MRI signal and a PS for PDT.

A novel class of polymer-based theranostic agent, namely polymeric micelles of IR825@C18PMH-PEG-Ce6-Gd, including a chlorine derivative, Ce6 as PS for multimodal imaging, and therapy of cancer was prepared by Hua Gong et al. (2014). The structure of this nanomicelles is presented in Figure 11.15. In this system, Ce6 could form a chelate with Gd^{3+} to allow T$_1$-weighted MR imaging. The r$_1$ relaxivity of the

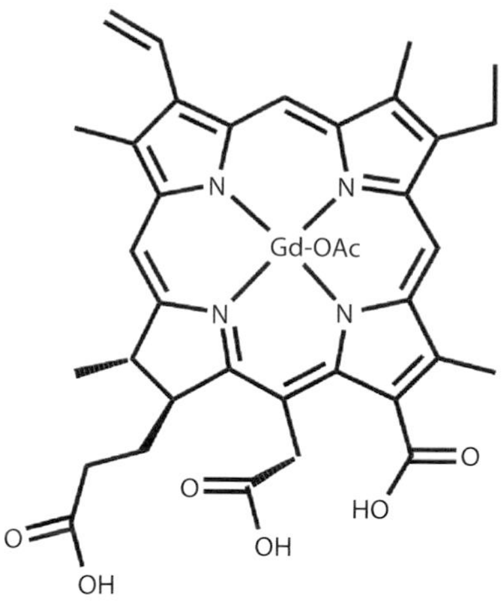

Figure 11.13 Structure of PB-chlorin. (Adapted from Kim, J.-K. et al., *Arch. Pharm. Res.*, 29, 188–190, 2006.)

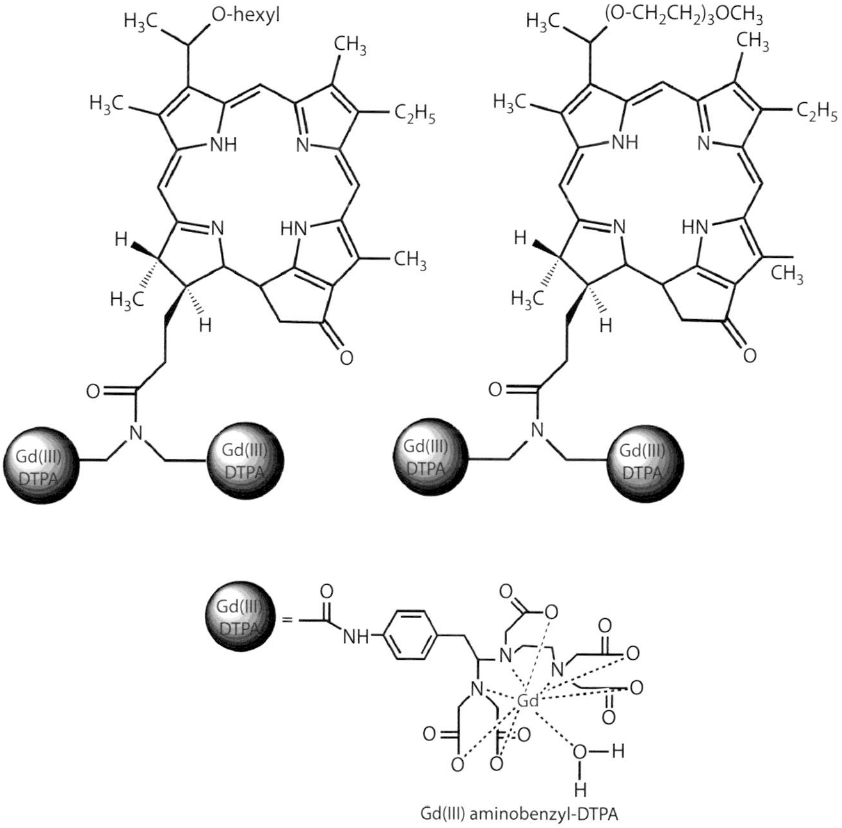

Gd(III) aminobenzyl-DTPA

Figure 11.14 Structure of bifunctional agents including two Gd(III) atoms per HPPH molecule. (Adapted from Li, G. et al., *Bioconjug. Chem.*, 16, 32–42, 2005.)

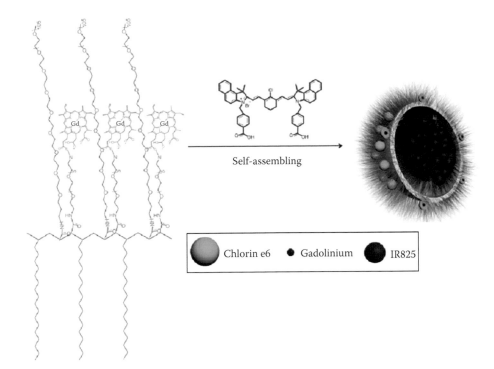

Figure 11.15 Structure of IR825@C18PMH-PEG-Ce6-Gd nanomicelles. Ce6 is anchored on the backbone of C18PMH-PEG polymer via a short PEG linker. Gd^{3+} forms a chelate complex with Ce6. IR825, a water-insoluble NIR dye, is then encapsulated inside the formed nanomicelles. (Reprinted from Gong, H., Dong, Z., Liu, Y., Yin, S., Cheng, L., Xi, W., Xiang, J., Liu, K., Li, Y., Liu, Z.: Engineering of multifunctional nano-micelles for combined photothermal and photodynamic therapy under the guidance of multimodal imaging. *Adv. Funct. Mater.* 2014. 24. 6492–6502. Copyright Wiley-VCH Verlag GmbH & Co. KGaA. Reproduced with permission.)

IR825@ C18PMH-PEG-Ce6-Gd formulation was found to be seven times higher than that of Magnevist, a clinical Gd-based T_1-weighted CA (Figure 11.16). In the animal experiments, combined photodynamic and photothermal therapy was carried out, achieving a remarkable synergist effect in inhibiting tumor growth. The results have demonstrated that the multifunctional nanomicelles may be of great promise in cancer theranostics.

Fluorescence imaging and MRI have different sensitivities, spatial resolutions, and imaging depths. Therefore, various multimodal imaging probes combining different imaging modalities have been developed for a more accurate imaging and diagnosis. For example, nanoparticles combining fluorescence imaging modality and MRI modality can offer the advantages of fluorescence imaging and MRI NaGdF$_4$-based UCNPs have been developed as multimodal imaging probes and the energy conversion process of UCNPs can be exploited for therapeutic applications (Park et al., 2012; Wang et al., 2013). Park et al. reported on dual-mode in vivo tumor imaging and PDT treatment using UCNPs combined with PSs for multimodal imaging (Figure 11.17). Hexagonal phase NaYF$_4$:Yb,Er/NaGdF$_4$ core–shell UCNPs were used for upconversion luminescence imaging and MRI. Owing to the enhanced permeability and retention (EPR) effect, intravenously injected UCNPs were accumulated at the tumors. Ce6 as PS was incorporated in the UCNPs for inducing a therapeutic effect. UCNP–Ce6 nanoparticles were readily accumulated in tumor sites, and tumors could be clearly observed by both upconversion luminescence imaging and MRI (Park et al., 2012). These results demonstrated that UCNP–Ce6 could be used as dual-mode imaging probes and as PDT agents for theranostic.

11.3.2.5 TEXAPHYRINS

Texaphyrins are colored pentaaza Schiff base macrocycles expanded porphyrins. The chemical versatility of this macrocycle makes attractive texaphyrins by offering several sites for chemical modification and functionalization. NIR wavelength absorption properties of metalated texaphyrin derivatives make them ideal

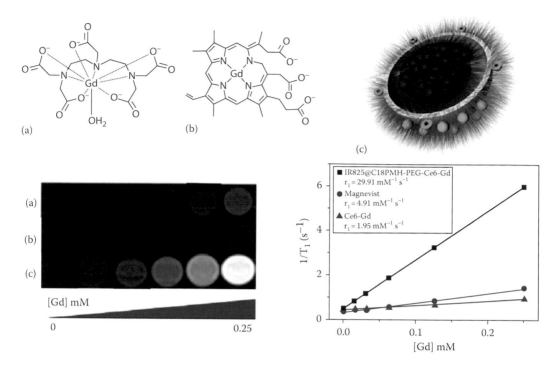

Figure 11.16 T_1-weighted MR images and T_1 relaxation rate of Magnevist (DTPA-Gd) (a), Ce6 chelated with gadolinium (Ce6-Gd) (b) and IR825@C18PMHPEG-Ce6-Gd (c) measured at different gadolinium concentrations. IR825@C18PMH-PEG-Ce6-Gd showed a rather high r_1 relaxivity, which appeared to be ≈7 times higher than that of Magnevist, a clinically used agent. (Reprinted from Gong, H., Dong, Z., Liu, Y., Yin, S., Cheng, L., Xi, W., Xiang, J., Liu, K., Li, Y., Liu, Z.: Engineering of multifunctional nano-micelles for combined photothermal and photodynamic therapy under the guidance of multimodal imaging. *Adv. Funct. Mater.* 2014. 24. 6492–6502. Copyright Wiley-VCH Verlag GmbH & Co. KGaA. Reproduced with permission.)

PDT agents with greater tissue penetration of activating light. Lantanide texaphyrin complexes are experimental drugs that exhibit photoactivated anticancer activity in the clinical trials for the treatment of various cancers, and Gd-texaphyrin derivatives are used as CA for MRI (Sessler et al., 1993; Geraldes et al., 1995; Hussain and Chakravarty, 2012; Preihs et al., 2013). Gd-texaphyrin complex, motexafin gadolinium (MGd), has been studied as a radio- and chemosensitizer for the treatment of Viala cancer (Evens, 2004) and has been evaluated through phase III clinical trials for the treatment of brain metastases of non-small-cell lung cancer (Meyers et al., 2004). The structure of this complex is shown in Figure 11.18. In the first biological experiments, MGd was shown to localize selectively in tumor cells as evidenced from the MRI studies of the highly paramagnetic MGd complex (Viala et al., 1999; Hussain and Chakravarty, 2012). The centrally coordinated paramagnetic metal cation Gd(III) serves to enhance the effective spin–lattice relaxation (T_1). Phase IB and phase II multidose trials of gadolinium texaphyrin as a radiation sensitizer detectable at MRI were studied by Viala et al. and gadolinium texaphyrin followed by whole-brain radiation therapy were administered to patient with brain metastases (Viala et al., 1999). The primary results indicate that gadolinium texaphyrin is tumor selective and that brain metastases can be depicted at MRI long after the administration of gadolinium texaphyrin (Woodburn et al., 1996).

LuTx has the desired characteristic of a PDT agent such as accumulation of abnormal tissue, activation by tissue-penetrating light, and water solubility (Woodburn et al., 1996). In vivo study against SMT-F murine mammary tumors and diet-induced atheromatous plaque in rabbit was carried out by combination of paramagnetic gadolinium texaphyrin (MGd) CA and LuTx as PDT agent for theranostic. This study demonstrated that texaphyrin localizes in cancer and the plaque and PDT with LuTx caused selective photodamage to the diseased tissue (Woodburn et al., 1996). The structure of LuTx (**2**) is given in Figure 11.18.

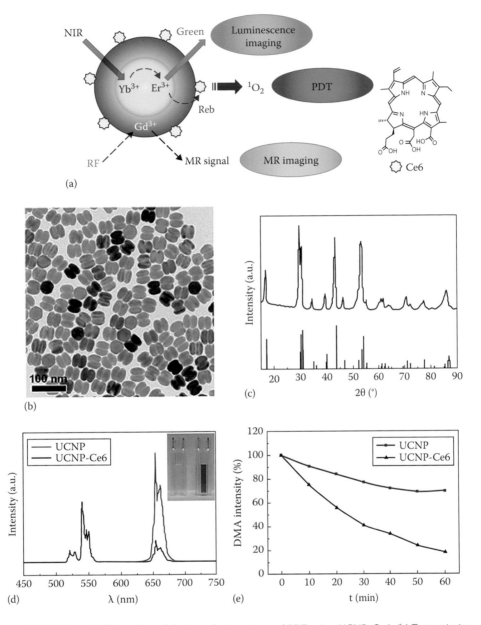

Figure 11.17 (a) Schematic illustration of dual-mode imaging and PDT using UCNP–Ce6. (b) Transmission electron microscopy (TEM) image of core–shell UCNPs. (c) XRD pattern of core–shell UCNPs. Bottom line pattern is that of hexagonal phase NaYF$_4$ (JCPDS 16-0334). (d) Emission spectra of UCNPs and UCNP–Ce6 under 980 nm excitation. Inset is the photograph of UCNPs (colorless) and UCNP–Ce6 solutions (green). (e) Change of DMA fluorescence due to generation of singlet oxygen from UCNPs and UCNP–Ce6 under 980 nm irradiation. (Reprinted from Park, Y.I., Kim, H.M., Kim, J.H., Moon, K.C., Yoo, B., Lee, K.T., Lee, N. et al.: Theranostic probe based on lanthanide-doped nanoparticles for simultaneous in vivo dual-modal imaging and photodynamic therapy. *Adv. Mater.* 2012. 24. 5755–5761. Copyright Wiley-VCH Verlag GmbH & Co. KGaA. Reproduced with permission.)

Typical MRI CAs are comprised of either paramagnetic materials for T_1-weighted scans or superparamagnetic nanoparticles for T_2-weighted scans. Single-mode CAs are effective for accurate imaging of small biological targets. So, dual-mode MRI CA (DMCAs) including both nanoparticles consists of a T_2 active core and a T_1-active material were developed (Choi et al., 2010; Yoo et al., 2012; Preihs et al., 2013). A DMCA system (GdTx-MNP) was prepared with using Gd(III) texaphyrin as the T_1 contrast material by

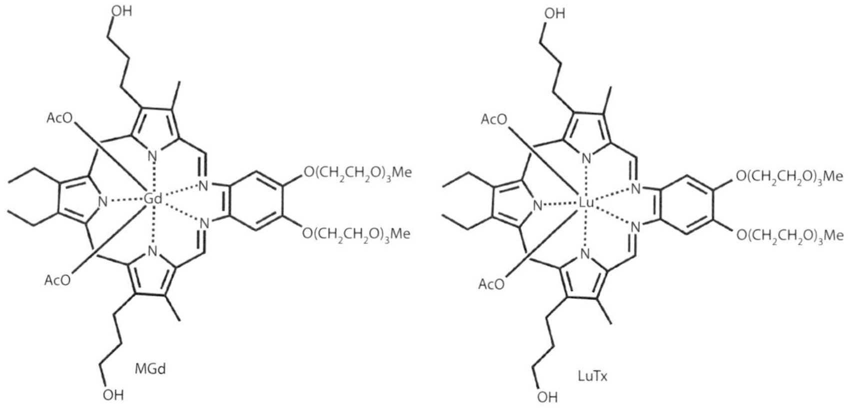

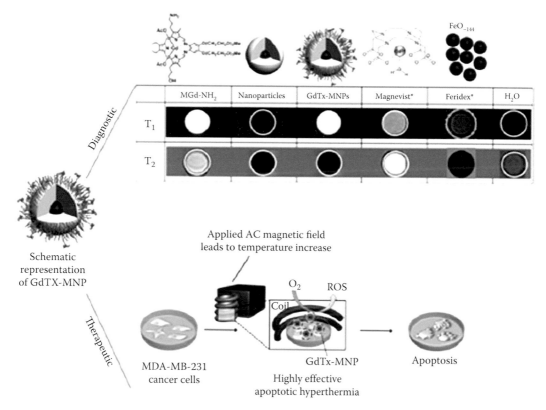

Figure 11.18 Structures of motexafin gadolinium (MGd) and LuTx.

Figure 11.19 DMCA enhancements (T_1 and T_2 modes are shown; note that a bright contrast in the T1 mode and a dark contrast in the T_2 mode are desired in MRI images of tumorous tissues) and anticancer activity that is ascribed to a combination of sensitization (ROS production) and hyperthermia (Yoo et al., 2012). (Reprinted with permission from Preihs, C., Arambula, J.F., Magda, D., Jeong, H., Yoo, D., Cheon, J., Siddik, Z.H., Sessler, J.L., Recent developments in texaphyrin chemistry and drug discovery, *Inorg. Chem.*, 52, 12184–12192. Copyright 2013 American Chemical Society.)

Yoo et al. (2012). In this study, Gd(III) texaphyrin was covalently linked to the surface of magnetic NP constructs consisting of a zinc-doped iron oxide T_2 core. This system was then tested as DMCAs comparing with CAs; Magnevist and Feridex display either only bright T_1 or dark T_2 contrast in a MRI phantom study. GdTx-MNP was found to give rise to intense MRI signals in both T_1 and T_2 modes (Figure 11.19). Additionally, this study demonstrated that the GdTx-MNP construct could effectively sensitize cancer

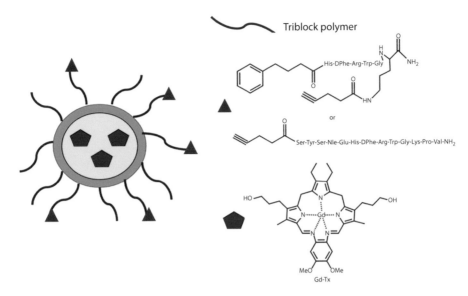

Figure 11.20 Structure of Gd-Tx micelles. (Reprinted with permission from Barkey, N.M., Preihs, C., Cornnell, H.H., Martinez, G., Carie, A., Vagner, J., Xu, L. et al., Development and in vivo quantitative magnetic resonance imaging of polymer micelles targeted to the melanocortin 1 receptor, *J. Med. Chem.*, 56, 6330–6338. Copyright 2013 Americal Chemical Society.)

cells (MDAMB-231, a breast cancer cell line) in vitro and in vivo and apoptosis of the cells was exhibited with ROS producing the texaphyrins, making them highly sensitive to apoptotic magnetic hyperthermia at low temperatures (Yoo et al., 2012).

In another study, Barkey et al. prepared Gd(III) texaphyrin (Gd-Tx) complex encapsulated in an Intezyne's Versatile Encapsulation and Crosslinking Technology (IVECT) micellar system, stabilized through Fe(III) cross-linking and targeted with a specific ligand for the melanocortin 1 receptor (MCI1R) as surface marker in melanoma (Figure 11.20). The comparative MRI experiments indicated that Gd-Tx micelles have an ability to specifically accumulate in MCI1R-expressing tumors in vitro and in vivo more effectively than untargeted and un-cross-linked Gd-Tx micelles. This study concluded that this targeted system is capable of delivering payloads in a tumor-selective fashion (Barkey et al., 2013).

11.4 CONCLUSION AND OUTLOOK

Over the last two decades, the clinical use of PDT has greatly increased. It can be applied either alone or in combination with other therapeutic modalities such as chemotherapy, surgery, radiotherapy, or immunotherapy. Although porphyrins and phthalocyanines share a tetrapyrrolic backbone as PSs, there are literally unlimited variations on substituent components of porphyrins. In addition, by inserting a chelated metal within the porphyrin, even more possibilities exist. PSs have limited applications for detecting deeply seated tumors. Therefore, the recent approaches for developing PS as bifunctional agents provide a unique approach for tumor detection and therapy. The researches have focused on this approach in developing "multifunctional agents" for MRI–PDT and PET–PDT. Advances steadily being made in the design of targeting vehicles used for delivery therapies could lead to the development of "multifunctional theranostics." Different laboratories are investigating the use of activable and nanoparticles approaches to achieve the desired objective of progressing improved target-specific multimodality agents and for developing PDT agents with imaging capability (multifunctional agents) enhanced tumor specificity still being a challenge.

ABBREVIATIONS

ALA	5-Aminolevulinic acid
CAs	Contrast agents
CT	Computed tomography
DA-PEG-PP	Dopamine-PEGprotoporphyrin IX
DMCAs	Dual modal contrast agents
DNP	Dynamic nuclear polarization
DOTA	1,4,7,10-Tetraazacyclododecane-1,4,7,10-tetraacetic acid
DOTAC10	1,4,7,10-Tetraaza-1-(1-carboxymethylundecane)-4,7,10-triacetic acid cyclododecane
DTPA	Diethylene triamine pentaacetic acid
DTTA	Diethylenetriamine tetraacetic acid
EPR	Enhanced permeability and retention
FDA	United States Food and Drug Administration
HpD	Hematoporphyrin derivative
HPPH	3-Devinyl-3-(1-hexyloxy)ethyl-pyropheophorbide-a
HSA	Human serum albumin
HT29	Human colorectal adenocarcinoma cell line
LbL	Layer by layer
LuTx	Lutetium texaphyrin
MCF-7	Human breast adenocarcinoma cell line
MCl1R	Melanocortin 1 receptor
MGd	Motexafin gadolinium
MMP	Matrix metalloproteinases
MNP	Magnetic nanoparticle
Mn-TPPS4	Mn(III)-meso-tetrakis(4-sulfonatophenyl) porphyrin
MRI	Magnetic resonance imaging
MRS	Magnetic resonance spectroscopy
NCs	Nanocrystals
NIR	Near-infrared
NIRF	Near-infrared fluorescence
NMR	Nuclear magnetic resonance
NPs	Nanoparticles
PAH	Poly(allylamine hydrochloride)
PASADENA	Para-hydrogen and synthesis allow dramatically enhanced net alignment
Pc	Phthalocyanine
Pc4	Silicon phthalocyanine [HOSiPcOSi$(CH_3)_2(CH_2)_3$N-$(CH_3)_2$]
PDD	Photodynamic diagnosis
PDT	Photodynamic therapy
PEG	Polyethylene glycol
PET	Positron emission tomography
PLGA	Poly(lactic-*co*-glycolic acid)
PS	Photosensitizers
Pz	Porphyrazine
SEOP	Spin-exchange optical pumping
SPECT	Single photon-emission computed tomography
SPIONs	Superparamagnetic iron oxide nanoparticles
THPP	*Meso*-tetrakis (4-hydroxyphenyl) porphyrin
TPD NPs	Theranostic porphyrin dyad nanoparticles
UCNPs	Upconverting nanoparticles
US	Ultrasound

REFERENCES

Abragam A, Goldman M (1978) Principles of dynamic nuclear polarisation. *Reports on Progress in Physics.* **41**:395.

Agostinis P, Berg K, Cengel KA, Foster TH, Girotti AW, Gollnick SO, Hahn SM et al. (2011) Photodynamic therapy of cancer: An update. *CA: A Cancer Journal for Clinicians.* **61**:250–281.

Ali H, van Lier JE (1999) Metal complexes as photo- and radiosensitizers. *Chemical Reviews* **99**:2379–2450.

Ali H, van Lier JE (2010) 16 Porphyrins and phthalocyanines as photosensitizers and radiosensitizers. In: *Handbook of Porphyrin Science* (Kadish KM, Smith, KM, Guilard R, eds.), pp. 1–119. World Scientific Publishing, Singapore.

Allen M, Bulte JWM, Liepold L, Basu G, Zywicke HA, Frank JA, Young M, Douglas T (2005) Paramagnetic viral nanoparticles as potential high-relaxivity magnetic resonance contrast agents. *Magnetic Resonance in Medicine.* **54**:807–812.

Allison RR, Sibata CH (2010) Oncologic photodynamic therapy photosensitizers: A clinical review. *Photodiagnosis and Photodynamic Therapy.* **7**:61–75.

Anderson EA, Isaacman S, Peabody DS, Wang EY, Canary JW, Kirshenbaum K (2006) Viral nanoparticles donning a paramagnetic coat: Conjugation of MRI contrast agents to the MS2 capsid. *Nano Letters.* **6**:1160–1164.

Aratani N, Osuka A (2010) 1 Synthetic strategies toward multiporphyrinic architectures. In: *Handbook of Porphyrin Science* (Kadish KM, Smith KM, Guilard R, eds.), pp. 1–132. World Scientific Publishing, Singapore.

Ardenkjær-Larsen JH, Fridlund B, Gram A, Hansson G, Hansson L, Lerche MH, Servin R, Thaning M, Golman K (2003) Increase in signal-to-noise ratio of >10,000 times in liquid-state NMR. *Proceedings of the National Academy of Sciences.* **100**:10158–10163.

Aydin Tekdas D, Garifullin R, Senturk B, Zorlu Y, Gundogdu U, Atalar E, Tekinay AB et al. (2014) Design of a Gd-DOTA-phthalocyanine conjugate combining MRI contrast imaging and photosensitization properties as a potential molecular theranostic. *Photochemistry and Photobiology.* **90**:1376–1386.

Balaban TS (2010) 3 Self-assembling porphyrins and chlorins as synthetic mimics of the chlorosomal bacteriochlorophylls. In: *Handbook of Porphyrin Science* (Kadish KM, Smith KM, Guilard R, eds.), pp. 221–306. World Scientific Publishing, Singapore.

Barkey NM, Preihs C, Cornnell HH, Martinez G, Carie A, Vagner J, Xu L et al. (2013) Development and in vivo quantitative magnetic resonance imaging of polymer micelles targeted to the melanocortin 1 receptor. *Journal of Medicinal Chemistry.* **56**:6330–6338.

Bellnier DA, Greco WR, Loewen GM, Nava H, Oseroff AR, Pandey RK, Tsuchida T, Dougherty TJ (2003) Population pharmacokinetics of the photodynamic therapy agent 2-[1-hexyloxyethyl]-2-devinyl pyropheophorbide-a in cancer patients. *Cancer Research.* **63**:1806–1813.

Bentolila LA, Michalet X, Pinaud FF, Tsay JM, Doose S, Li JJ, Sundaresan G, Wu AM, Gambhir SS, Weiss S (2005) Quantum dots for molecular imaging and cancer medicine. *Discovery Medicine.* **5**:213–218.

Bilalis P, Chatzipavlidis A, Tziveleka L-A, Boukos N, Kordas G (2012) Nanodesigned magnetic polymer containers for dual stimuli actuated drug controlled release and magnetic hyperthermia mediation. *Journal of Materials Chemistry.* **22**:13451–13454.

Boesch C (2007) Musculoskeletal spectroscopy. *Journal of Magnetic Resonance Imaging.* **25**:321–338.

Bowers CR, Weitekamp DP (1986) Transformation of symmetrization order to nuclear-spin magnetization by chemical reaction and nuclear magnetic resonance. *Physical Review Letters.* **57**:2645–2648.

Bozzini G, Colin P, Betrouni N, Maurage CA, Leroy X, Simonin S, Martin-Schmitt C, Villers A, Mordon S (2013) Efficiency of 5-ALA mediated photodynamic therapy on hypoxic prostate cancer: A preclinical study on the Dunning R3327-AT2 rat tumor model. *Photodiagnosis and Photodynamic Therapy.* **10**:296–303.

Brasch M, de la Escosura A, Ma Y, Uetrecht C, Heck AJR, Torres T, Cornelissen JJLM (2011) Encapsulation of phthalocyanine supramolecular stacks into virus-like particles. *Journal of the American Chemical Society.* **133**:6878–6881.

Brown SB, Brown EA, Walker I (2004) The present and future role of photodynamic therapy in cancer treatment. *The Lancet Oncology.* **5**:497–508.

Cai W, Shin D-W, Chen K, Gheysens O, Cao Q, Wang SX, Gambhir SS, Chen X (2006) Peptide-labeled near-infrared quantum dots for imaging tumor vasculature in living subjects. *Nano Letters.* **6**:669–676.

Caravan P (2006) Strategies for increasing the sensitivity of gadolinium based MRI contrast agents. *Chemical Society Reviews.* **35**:512–523.

Caravan P, Ellison JJ, McMurry TJ, Lauffer RB (1999) Gadolinium(III) chelates as MRI contrast agents: Structure, dynamics, and applications. *Chemical Reviews.* **99**:2293–2352.

Cassidy PJ, Radda GK (2005) Molecular imaging perspectives. *Journal of the Royal Society Interface.* **2**:133–144.

Chan KW-Y, Wong W-T (2007) Small molecular gadolinium(III) complexes as MRI contrast agents for diagnostic imaging. *Coordination Chemistry Reviews.* **251**:2428–2451.

Chen N, He Y, Su Y, Li X, Huang Q, Wang H, Zhang X, Tai R, Fan C (2012) The cytotoxicity of cadmium-based quantum dots. *Biomaterials.* **33**:1238–1244.

Chen Y, Graham A, Potter W, Morgan J, Vaughan L, Bellnier DA, Henderson BW, Oseroff A, Dougherty TJ, Pandey RK (2002) Bacteriopurpurinimides: Highly stable and potent photosensitizers for photodynamic therapy. *Journal of Medicinal Chemistry.* **45**:255–258.

Chen Y, Sumlin A, Morgan J, Gryshuk A, Oseroff A, Henderson BW, Dougherty TJ, Pandey RK (2004) Synthesis and photosensitizing efficacy of isomerically pure bacteriopurpurinimides. *Journal of Medicinal Chemistry.* **47**:4814–4817.

Cheng S-H, Lee C-H, Chen M-C, Souris JS, Tseng F-G, Yang C-S, Mou C-Y, Chen C-T, Lo L-W (2010) Tri-functionalization of mesoporous silica nanoparticles for comprehensive cancer theranostics—The trio of imaging, targeting and therapy. *Journal of Materials Chemistry.* **20**:6149–6157.

Cherry SR (2004) In vivo molecular and genomic imaging: New challenges for imaging physics. *Physics in Medicine and Biology.* **49**:R13–R48.

Cho MH, Lee EJ, Son M, Lee J-H, Yoo D, Kim J-w, Park SW, Shin J-S, Cheon J (2012) A magnetic switch for the control of cell death signalling in in vitro and in vivo systems. *Nature Materials.* **11**:1038–1043.

Choi J-s, Lee J-H, Shin T-H, Song H-T, Kim EY, Cheon J (2010) Self-confirming "AND" logic nanoparticles for fault-free MRI. *Journal of the American Chemical Society.* **132**:11015–11017.

Danhier F, Ansorena E, Silva JM, Coco R, Le Breton A, Preat V (2012) PLGA-based nanoparticles: An overview of biomedical applications. *Journal of Controlled Release.* **161**:505–522.

Danhier F, Lecouturier N, Vroman B, Jerome C, Marchand-Brynaert J, Feron O, Preat V (2009) Paclitaxel-loaded PEGylated PLGA-based nanoparticles: In vitro and in vivo evaluation. *Journal of Controlled Release.* **133**:11–17.

Das M, Mishra D, Dhak P, Gupta S, Maiti TK, Basak A, Pramanik P (2009) Biofunctionalized, phosphonate-grafted, ultrasmall iron oxide nanoparticles for combined targeted cancer therapy and multimodal imaging. *Small.* **5**:2883–2893.

Datta A, Hooker JM, Botta M, Francis MB, Aime S, Raymond KN (2008) High relaxivity gadolinium hydroxypyridonate-viral capsid conjugates: Nanosized MRI contrast agents. *Journal of the American Chemical Society.* **130**:2546–2552.

De Stefano N, Filippi M, Miller D, Pouwels PJ, Rovira A, Gass A, Enzinger C, Matthews PM, Arnold DL (2007) Guidelines for using proton MR spectroscopy in multicenter clinical MS studies. *Neurology.* **69**:1942–1952.

Di Corato R, Bigall NC, Ragusa A, Dorfs D, Genovese A, Marotta R, Manna L, Pellegrino T (2011) Multifunctional nanobeads based on quantum dots and magnetic nanoparticles: Synthesis and cancer cell targeting and sorting. *ACS Nano.* **5**:1109–1121.

Dumoulin F (2012) Design and conception of photosensitisers. In: *Photosensitizers in Medicine, Environment, and Security* (Nyokong T, Ahsen V, eds.), pp. 1–46. Springer, Amsterdam, the Netherlands.

Eggenspiller A, Michelin C, Desbois N, Richard P, Barbe J-M, Denat F, Licona C et al. (2013) Design of por-phyrin-dota-like scaffolds as all-in-one multimodal heterometallic complexes for medical imaging. *European Journal of Organic Chemistry.* **2013**:6629–6643.

Elsadek B, Kratz F (2012) Impact of albumin on drug delivery—New applications on the horizon. *Journal of Controlled Release.* **157**:4–28.

Ethirajan M, Chen Y, Joshi P, Pandey RK (2011) The role of porphyrin chemistry in tumor imaging and photodynamic therapy. *Chemical Society Reviews.* **40**:340–362.

Evens AM (2004) Motexafin gadolinium: A redox-active tumor selective agent for the treatment of cancer. *Current Opinion in Oncology.* **16**:576–580.

Fei B, Wang H, Meyers JD, Feyes DK, Oleinick NL, Duerk JL (2007) High-field magnetic resonance imaging of the response of human prostate cancer to Pc 4-based photodynamic therapy in an animal model. *Lasers in Surgery and Medicine.* **39**:723–730.

Fiel RJ, Button TM, Gilani S, Mark EH, Musser DA, Henkelman RM, Bronskill MJ, van Heteren JG (1987) Proton relaxation enhancement by manganese(III)TPPS4 in a model tumor system. *Magnetic Resonance Imaging.* **5**:149–156.

Filonenko EV (2015) The history of development of fluorescence diagnosis and photodynamic therapy and their capabilities in oncology. *Russian Journal of General Chemistry.* **85**:211–216.

Frullano L, Meade T (2007) Multimodal MRI contrast agents. *JBIC, Journal of Biological Inorganic Chemistry.* **12**:939–949.

Fuchter MJ, Zhong C, Zong H, Hoffman BM, Barrett AGM (2008) Porphyrazines: Designer macrocycles by peripheral substituent change. *Australian Journal of Chemistry.* **61**:235–255.

Galindev O, Dalantai M, Ahn WS, Shim YK (2009) Gadolinium complexes of chlorin derivatives applicable for MRI contrast agents and PDT. *Journal of Porphyrins and Phthalocyanines.* **13**:823–831.

Garimella PD, Datta A, Romanini DW, Raymond KN, Francis MB (2011) Multivalent high-relaxivity MRI contrast agents using rigid cysteine-reactive gadolinium complexes. *Journal of the American Chemical Society.* **133**:14704–14709.

Geraldes CFGC, Sherry AD, Vallet P, Maton F, Muller RN, Mody TD, Hemmi G, Sessler JL (1995) Nuclear magnetic relaxation dispersion studies of water-soluble gadolinium(iii)-texaphyrin complexes. *Journal of Magnetic Resonance Imaging.* **5**:725–729.

Gong H, Dong Z, Liu Y, Yin S, Cheng L, Xi W, Xiang J, Liu K, Li Y, Liu Z (2014) Engineering of multifunctional nano-micelles for combined photothermal and photodynamic therapy under the guidance of multimodal imaging. *Advanced Functional Materials.* **24**:6492–6502.

Gros CP, Eggenspiller A, Nonat A, Barbe J-M, Denat F (2011) New potential bimodal imaging contrast agents based on DOTA-like and porphyrin macrocycles. *Medicinal Chemistry Communications.* **2**:119–125.

Hammer ND, Lee S, Vesper BJ, Elseth KM, Hoffman BM, Barrett AG, Radosevich JA (2005) Charge dependence of cellular uptake and selective antitumor activity of porphyrazines. *Journal of Medicinal Chemistry.* **48**:8125–8133.

Henderson BW, Dougherty TJ (1992) How does photodynamic therapy work? *Photochemistry and Photobiology.* **55**:145–157.

Hengerer A, Grimm J (2006) Molecular magnetic resonance imaging. *Biomedical Imaging and Intervention Journal.* **2**:e8.

Herschman HR (2003) Molecular imaging: Looking at problems, seeing solutions. *Science.* **302**:605–608.

Hilderbrand SA, Weissleder R (2010) Near-infrared fluorescence: Application to in vivo molecular imaging. *Current Opinion in Chemical Biology.* **14**:71–79.

Hofmann B, Bogdanov A, Jr., Marecos E, Ebert W, Semmler W, Weissleder R (1999) Mechanism of gadophrin-2 accumulation in tumor necrosis. *Journal of Magnetic Resonance Imaging.* **9**:336–341.

Hooker JM, Datta A, Botta M, Raymond KN, Francis MB (2007) Magnetic resonance contrast agents from viral capsid shells: A comparison of exterior and interior cargo strategies. *Nano Letters.* **7**:2207–2210.

Huang H, Delikanli S, Zeng H, Ferkey DM, Pralle A (2010) Remote control of ion channels and neurons through magnetic-field heating of nanoparticles. *Nature Nanotechnology.* **5**:602–606.

Huang P, Lin J, Wang X, Wang Z, Zhang C, He M, Wang K et al. (2012a) Light-triggered theranostics based on photosensitizer-conjugated carbon dots for simultaneous enhanced-fluorescence imaging and photodynamic therapy. *Advanced Materials.* **24**:5104–5110.

Huang Y, He S, Cao W, Cai K, Liang XJ (2012b) Biomedical nanomaterials for imaging-guided cancer therapy. *Nanoscale.* **4**:6135–6149.

Huang Z (2005) A review of progress in clinical photodynamic therapy. *Technology in Cancer Research and Treatment.* **4**:283–293.

Hussain A, Chakravarty A (2012) Photocytotoxic lanthanide complexes. *Journal of Chemical Sciences.* **124**:1327–1342.

Jokerst JV, Lobovkina T, Zare RN, Gambhir SS (2011) Nanoparticle PEGylation for imaging and therapy. *Nanomedicine (London, England).* **6**:715–728.

Josefsen LB, Boyle RW (2008) Photodynamic therapy and the development of metal-based photosensitisers. *Metal-Based Drugs.* **2008**:276109.

Josefsen LB, Boyle RW (2012) Unique diagnostic and therapeutic roles of porphyrins and phthalocyanines in photodynamic therapy, imaging and theranostics. *Theranostics.* **2**:916–966.

Josephs D, Spicer J, O'Doherty M (2009) Molecular imaging in clinical trials. *Targeted Oncology.* **4**:151–168.

Juarranz Á, Jaén P, Sanz-Rodríguez F, Cuevas J, González S (2008) Photodynamic therapy of cancer. Basic principles and applications. *Clinical and Translational Oncology.* **10**:148–154.

Juzeniene A, Peng Q, Moan J (2007) Milestones in the development of photodynamic therapy and fluorescence diagnosis. *Photochemical and Photobiological Sciences* **6**:1234–1245.

Karunakaran SC, Babu PS, Madhuri B, Marydasan B, Paul AK, Nair AS, Rao KS et al. (2013) In vitro demonstration of apoptosis mediated photodynamic activity and NIR nucleus imaging through a novel porphyrin. *ACS Chemical Biology.* **8**:127–132.

Ke H, Wang J, Dai Z, Jin Y, Qu E, Xing Z, Guo C, Yue X, Liu J (2011) Gold-nanoshelled microcapsules: A theranostic agent for ultrasound contrast imaging and photothermal therapy. *Angewandte Chemie International Edition.* **50**:3017–3021.

Kelkar SS, Reineke TM (2011) Theranostics: Combining imaging and therapy. *Bioconjugate Chemistry.* **22**:1879–1903.

Kessel D (1992) Photodynamic therapy and neoplastic disease. *Oncology Research.* **4**:219–225.

Kim J-K, Kim D-M, Kang M-S, Kim H-K, Kim J-S, Yu E-K, Jeong J-H (2006) Gadolinium-chlorin is potentially a new tumor specific MRI contrast agent. *Archives of Pharmacal Research.* **29**:188–190.

Kinsella TJ, Baron ED, Colussi VC, Cooper KD, Hoppel CL, Ingalls ST, Kenney ME et al. (2011) Preliminary clinical and pharmacologic investigation of photodynamic therapy with the silicon phthalocyanine photosensitizer pc 4 for primary or metastatic cutaneous cancers. *Frontiers Oncology.* **1**:14.

Konan YN, Gurny R, Allémann E (2002) State of the art in the delivery of photosensitizers for photodynamic therapy. *Journal of Photochemistry and Photobiology B: Biology.* **66**:89–106.

Krzystek J, Telser J, Pardi LA, Goldberg DP, Hoffman BM, Brunel LC (1999) High-frequency and -field electron paramagnetic resonance of high-spin manganese(III) in porphyrinic complexes. *Inorganic Chemistry.* **38**:6121–6129.

Lee J-H, Jang J-T, Choi J-S, Moon SH, Noh S-H, Kim J-W, Kim J-G, Kim I-S, Park KI, Cheon J (2011) Exchange-coupled magnetic nanoparticles for efficient heat induction. *Nature Nanotechnology.* **6**:418–422.

Lee J-H, Kim ES, Cho MH, Son M, Yeon S-I, Shin J-S, Cheon J (2010c) Artificial control of cell signaling and growth by magnetic nanoparticles. *Angewandte Chemie International Edition.* **49**:5698–5702.

Lee S-M, Song Y, Hong BJ, MacRenaris KW, Mastarone DJ, O'Halloran TV, Meade TJ, Nguyen ST (2010a) Modular polymer-caged nanobins as a theranostic platform with enhanced magnetic resonance relaxivity and pH-responsive drug release. *Angewandte Chemie International Edition.* **49**:9960–9964.

Lee T, Zhang X-a, Dhar S, Faas H, Lippard SJ, Jasanoff A (2010b) In vivo imaging with a cell-permeable porphyrin-based MRI contrast agent. *Chemistry and Biology.* **17**:665–673.

Li G, Graham A, Chen Y, Dobhal MP, Morgan J, Zheng G, Kozyrev A, Oseroff A, Dougherty TJ, Pandey RK (2003) Synthesis, comparative photosensitizing efficacy, human serum albumin (site II) binding ability, and intracellular localization characteristics of novel benzobacteriochlorins derived from vic-dihydroxybacteriochlorins. *Journal of Medicinal Chemistry.* **46**:5349–5359.

Li G, Slansky A, Dobhal MP, Goswami LN, Graham A, Chen Y, Kanter P et al. (2005) Chlorophyll-a analogues conjugated with aminobenzyl-DTPA as potential bifunctional agents for magnetic resonance imaging and photodynamic therapy. *Bioconjugate Chemistry*. **16**:32–42.

Liang X, Li X, Jing L, Yue X, Dai Z (2014) Theranostic porphyrin dyad nanoparticles for magnetic resonance imaging guided photodynamic therapy. *Biomaterials*. **35**:6379–6388.

Liang X, Li X, Yue X, Dai Z (2011) Conjugation of porphyrin to nanohybrid cerasomes for photodynamic diagnosis and therapy of cancer. *Angewandte Chemie International Edition*. **50**:11622–11627.

Liepold L, Anderson S, Willits D, Oltrogge L, Frank JA, Douglas T, Young M (2007) Viral capsids as MRI contrast agents. *Magnetic Resonance in Medicine*. **58**:871–879.

Liepold LO, Abedin MJ, Buckhouse ED, Frank JA, Young MJ, Douglas T (2009) Supramolecular protein cage composite MR contrast agents with extremely efficient relaxivity properties. *Nano Letters*. **9**:4520–4526.

Lim JM, Yoon M-C, Kim KS, Shin J-Y, Kim D (2010) 6 Photophysics and photochemistry of various expanded porphyrins. In: *Handbook of Porphyrin Science* (Kadish KM, Smith KM, Guilard R, eds.), pp. 507–558. World Scientific Publishing, Singapore.

Liu Y, Huang Y, Boamah PO, Zhang Q, Liu Y, Hua M (2014) Synthesis and in vitro evaluation of manganese(II)-porphyrin modified with chitosan oligosaccharides as potential MRI contrast agents. *Chemical Research in Chinese Universities*. **30**:549–555.

Lovell JF, Lo P-C (2012) Porphyrins and phthalocyanines for theranostics. *Theranostics*. **2**:815–816.

Lovell JF, Jin CS, Huynh E, Jin H, Kim C, Rubinstein JL, Chan WCW, Cao W, Wang LV, Zheng G (2011) Porphysome nanovesicles generated by porphyrin bilayers for use as multimodal biophotonic contrast agents. *Nature Materials*. **10**:324–332.

Lovell JF, Liu TW, Chen J, Zheng G (2010) Activatable photosensitizers for imaging and therapy. *Chemical Reviews* **110**:2839–2857.

Lucon J, Qazi S, Uchida M, Bedwell GJ, LaFrance B, Prevelige PE, Douglas T (2012) Use of the interior cavity of the P22 capsid for site-specific initiation of atom-transfer radical polymerization with high-density cargo loading. *Nature Chemistry*. **4**:781–788.

Luo J, Chen L-F, Hu P, Chen Z-N (2014) Tetranuclear gadolinium(III) porphyrin complex as a theranostic agent for multimodal imaging and photodynamic therapy. *Inorganic Chemistry*. **53**:4184–4191.

Luo S, Zhang E, Su Y, Cheng T, Shi C (2011) A review of NIR dyes in cancer targeting and imaging. *Biomaterials*. **32**:7127–7138.

Lupu M, Thomas CD, Maillard P, Loock B, Chauvin B, Aerts I, Croisy A, Belloir E, Volk A, Mispelter J (2009) 23Na MRI longitudinal follow-up of PDT in a xenograft model of human retinoblastoma. *Photodiagnosis and Photodynamic Therapy*. **6**:214–220.

Lyon RC, Faustino PJ, Cohen JS, Katz A, Mornex F, Colcher D, Baglin C, Koenig SH, Hambright P (1987) Tissue distribution and stability of metalloporphyrin MRI contrast agents. *Magnetic Resonance in Medicine*. **4**:24–33.

Mankoff DA, Link JM, Linden HM, Sundararajan L, Krohn KA (2008) Tumor receptor imaging. *Journal of Nuclear Medicine*. **49** (Suppl. 2):149S–163S.

Mathews MS, Chighvinadze D, Gach HM, Uzal FA, Madsen SJ, Hirschberg H (2011) Cerebral edema following photodynamic therapy using endogenous and exogenous photosensitizers in normal brain. *Lasers in Surgery and Medicine*. **43**:892–900.

McCann TE, Kosaka N, Turkbey B, Mitsunaga M, Choyke PL, Kobayashi H (2011) Molecular imaging of tumor invasion and metastases: The role of MRI. *NMR in Biomedicine*. **24**:561–568.

Meikle SR, Kench P, Kassiou M, Banati RB (2005) Small animal SPECT and its place in the matrix of molecular imaging technologies. *Physics in Medicine and Biology*. **50**:R45–R61.

Meyers CA, Smith JA, Bezjak A, Mehta MP, Liebmann J, Illidge T, Kunkler I et al. (2004) Neurocognitive function and progression in patients with brain metastases treated with whole-brain radiation and motexafin gadolinium: Results of a randomized phase III trial. *Journal of Clinical Oncology*. **22**:157–165.

Michalet X, Pinaud FF, Bentolila LA, Tsay JM, Doose S, Li JJ, Sundaresan G, Wu AM, Gambhir SS, Weiss S (2005) Quantum dots for live cells, in vivo imaging, and diagnostics. *Science*. **307**:538–544.

Michel SLJ, Hoffman BM, Baum SM, Barrett AGM (2001) Peripherally functionalized porphyrazines: Novel metallomacrocycles with broad, untapped potential. In: *Progress in Inorganic Chemistry*, Vol. 50 (Karlin KD, ed.), pp. 473–590. John Wiley & Sons, New York.

Millan JG, Brasch M, Anaya-Plaza E, de la Escosura A, Velders AH, Reinhoudt DN, Torres T, Koay MS, Cornelissen JJ (2014) Self-assembly triggered by self-assembly: Optically active, paramagnetic micelles encapsulated in protein cage nanoparticles. *Journal of Inorganic Biochemistry*. **136**:140–146.

Modo MMJ, Bulte JWM, Kim EE (2007) Molecular and cellular MR imaging. *Journal of Nuclear Medicine*. **48**:2087.

Namiki Y, Namiki T, Yoshida H, Ishii Y, Tsubota A, Koido S, Nariai K et al. (2009) A novel magnetic crystal-lipid nanostructure for magnetically guided in vivo gene delivery. *Nature Nanotechnology*. **4**:598–606.

Ng KK, Lovell JF, Zheng G (2011) Lipoprotein-inspired nanoparticles for cancer theranostics. *Accounts of Chemical Research*. **44**:1105–1113.

Norum OJ, Gaustad JV, Angell-Petersen E, Rofstad EK, Peng Q, Giercksky KE, Berg K (2009) Photochemical internalization of bleomycin is superior to photodynamic therapy due to the therapeutic effect in the tumor periphery. *Photochemistry and Photobiology*. **85**:740–749.

Nyström AM, Wooley KL (2011) The importance of chemistry in creating well-defined nanoscopic embedded therapeutics: Devices capable of the dual functions of imaging and therapy. *Accounts of Chemical Research*. **44**:969–978.

O'Connor AE, Gallagher WM, Byrne AT (2009) Porphyrin and nonporphyrin photosensitizers in oncology: Preclinical and clinical advances in photodynamic therapy. *Photochemistry and Photobiology*. **85**:1053–1074.

Osterloh J, Vicente MGH (2002) Mechanisms of porphyrinoid localization in tumors. *Journal of Porphyrins and Phthalocyanines*. **06**:305–324.

Pan D, Caruthers SD, Senpan A, Schmieder AH, Wickline SA, Lanza GM (2011) Revisiting an old friend: Manganese-based MRI contrast agents. *Wiley Interdisciplinary Reviews: Nanomedicine and Nanobiotechnology*. **3**:162–173.

Panchapakesan B, Book-Newell B, Sethu P, Rao M, Irudayaraj J (2011) Gold nanoprobes for theranostics. *Nanomedicine (London, England)*. **6**:1787–1811.

Pandey RK, Goswami LN, Chen Y, Gryshuk A, Missert JR, Oseroff A, Dougherty TJ (2006) Nature: A rich source for developing multifunctional agents. tumor-imaging and photodynamic therapy. *Lasers in Surgery and Medicine*. **38**:445–467.

Pandey SK, Gryshuk AL, Sajjad M, Zheng X, Chen Y, Abouzeid MM, Morgan J et al. (2005) Multimodality agents for tumor imaging (PET, fluorescence) and photodynamic therapy. A possible "see and treat" approach. *Journal of Medicinal Chemistry*. **48**:6286–6295.

Park YI, Kim HM, Kim JH, Moon KC, Yoo B, Lee KT, Lee N et al. (2012) Theranostic probe based on lanthanide-doped nanoparticles for simultaneous in vivo dual-modal imaging and photodynamic therapy. *Advanced Materials*. **24**:5755–5761.

Pass HI (1993) Photodynamic therapy in oncology: Mechanisms and clinical use. *Journal of the National Cancer Institute*. **85**:443–456.

Peng E, Wang F, Xue JM (2015) Nanostructured magnetic nanocomposites as MRI contrast agents. *Journal of Materials Chemistry B*. **3**:2241–2276.

Pernia Leal M, Torti A, Riedinger A, La Fleur R, Petti D, Cingolani R, Bertacco R, Pellegrino T (2012) Controlled release of doxorubicin loaded within magnetic thermo-responsive nanocarriers under magnetic and thermal actuation in a microfluidic channel. *ACS Nano*. **6**:10535–10545.

Pokorski JK, Breitenkamp K, Liepold LO, Qazi S, Finn MG (2011) Functional virus-based polymer–protein nanoparticles by atom transfer radical polymerization. *Journal of the American Chemical Society*. **133**:9242–9245.

Poyer F, Thomas CD, Garcia G, Croisy A, Carrez D, Maillard P, Lupu M, Mispelter J (2012) PDT induced bystander effect on human xenografted colorectal tumors as evidenced by sodium MRI. *Photodiagnosis and Photodynamic Therapy*. **9**:303–309.

Prasuhn Jr DE, Kuzelka J, Strable E, Udit AK, Cho S-H, Lander GC, Quispe JD et al. (2008) Polyvalent display of heme on hepatitis B virus capsid protein through coordination to hexahistidine tags. *Chemistry and Biology*. **15**:513–519.

Prasuhn JDE, Yeh RM, Obenaus A, Manchester M, Finn MG (2007) Viral MRI contrast agents: Coordination of Gd by native virions and attachment of Gd complexes by azide-alkyne cycloaddition. *Chemical Communications*. **12**:1269–1271.

Preihs C, Arambula JF, Magda D, Jeong H, Yoo D, Cheon J, Siddik ZH, Sessler JL (2013) Recent developments in texaphyrin chemistry and drug discovery. *Inorganic Chemistry*. **52**:12184–12192.

Pysz MA, Gambhir SS, Willmann JK (2010) Molecular imaging: Current status and emerging strategies. *Clinical Radiology*. **65**:500–516.

Qiao XF, Zhou JC, Xiao JW, Wang YF, Sun LD, Yan CH (2012) Triple-functional core-shell structured upconversion luminescent nanoparticles covalently grafted with photosensitizer for luminescent, magnetic resonance imaging and photodynamic therapy in vitro. *Nanoscale*. **4**:4611–4623.

Rai P, Mallidi S, Zheng X, Rahmanzadeh R, Mir Y, Elrington S, Khurshid A, Hasan T (2010) Development and applications of photo-triggered theranostic agents. *Advanced Drug Delivery Reviews*. **62**:1094–1124.

Rhee J-K, Baksh M, Nycholat C, Paulson JC, Kitagishi H, Finn MG (2012) Glycan-targeted virus-like nanoparticles for photodynamic therapy. *Biomacromolecules*. **13**:2333–2338.

Sanson C, Diou O, Thévenot J, Ibarboure E, Soum A, Brûlet A, Miraux S et al. (2011) Doxorubicin loaded magnetic polymersomes: Theranostic nanocarriers for MR imaging and magneto-chemotherapy. *ACS Nano*. **5**:1122–1140.

Scherer RL, McIntyre JO, Matrisian LM (2008b) Imaging matrix metalloproteinases in cancer. *Cancer Metastasis Reviews*. **27**:679–690.

Scherer RL, VanSaun MN, McIntyre JO, Matrisian LM (2008a) Optical imaging of matrix metalloproteinase-7 activity in vivo using a proteolytic nanobeacon. *Molecular Imaging*. **7**:118–131.

Schladt TD, Schneider K, Shukoor MI, Natalio F, Bauer H, Tahir MN, Weber S et al. (2010) Highly soluble multifunctional MnO nanoparticles for simultaneous optical and MRI imaging and cancer treatment using photodynamic therapy. *Journal of Materials Chemistry*. **20**:8297–8304.

Sessler JL, Mody TD, Hemmi GW, Lynch V, Young SW, Miller RA (1993) Gadolinium(III) texaphyrin: A novel MRI contrast agent. *Journal of the American Chemical Society*. **115**:10368–10369.

Shi J, Liu TW, Chen J, Green D, Jaffray D, Wilson BC, Wang F, Zheng G (2011) Transforming a targeted porphyrin theranostic agent into a PET imaging probe for cancer. *Theranostics*. **1**:363–370.

Soares DP, Law M (2009) Magnetic resonance spectroscopy of the brain: Review of metabolites and clinical applications. *Clinical Radiology*. **64**:12–21.

Sokolova V, Epple M (2008) Inorganic nanoparticles as carriers of nucleic acids into cells. *Angewandte Chemie International Edition*. **47**:1382–1395.

Son SJ, Reichel J, He B, Schuchman M, Lee SB (2005) Magnetic nanotubes for magnetic-field-assisted bioseparation, biointeraction, and drug delivery. *Journal of the American Chemical Society*. **127**:7316–7317.

Song E-Q, Hu J, Wen C-Y, Tian Z-Q, Yu X, Zhang Z-L, Shi Y-B, Pang D-W (2011) Fluorescent-magnetic-biotargeting multifunctional nanobioprobes for detecting and isolating multiple types of tumor cells. *ACS Nano*. **5**:761–770.

Song Y, Zong H, Trivedi ER, Vesper BJ, Waters EA, Barrett AGM, Radosevich JA, Hoffman BM, Meade TJ (2010) Synthesis and characterization of new porphyrazine-Gd(III) conjugates as multimodal MR contrast agents. *Bioconjugate Chemistry*. **21**:2267–2275.

Sosnovik DE, Weissleder R (2007) Emerging concepts in molecular MRI. *Current Opinion in Biotechnology*. **18**:4–10.

Stephanopoulos N, Carrico ZM, Francis MB (2009) Nanoscale integration of sensitizing chromophores and porphyrins with bacteriophage MS2. *Angewandte Chemie International Edition*. **48**:9498–9502.

Stephanopoulos N, Tong GJ, Hsiao SC, Francis MB (2010) Dual-surface modified virus capsids for targeted delivery of photodynamic agents to cancer cells. *ACS Nano*. **4**:6014–6020.

Tamada T, Ito K, Sone T, Yamamoto A, Yoshida K, Kakuba K, Tanimoto D, Higashi H, Yamashita T (2009) Dynamic contrast-enhanced magnetic resonance imaging of abdominal solid organ and major vessel: Comparison of enhancement effect between Gd-EOB-DTPA and Gd-DTPA. *Journal of Magnetic Resonance Imaging.* **29**:636–640.

Thomas CR, Ferris DP, Lee J-H, Choi E, Cho MH, Kim ES, Stoddart JF, Shin J-S, Cheon J, Zink JI (2010) Noninvasive remote-controlled release of drug molecules in vitro using magnetic actuation of mechanized nanoparticles. *Journal of the American Chemical Society.* **132**:10623–10625.

Triesscheijn M, Baas P, Schellens JH, Stewart FA (2006) Photodynamic therapy in oncology. *The Oncologist.* **11**:1034–1044.

Trivedi ER, Vesper BJ, Weitman H, Ehrenberg B, Barrett AG, Radosevich JA, Hoffman BM (2010) Chiral bis-acetal porphyrazines as near-infrared optical agents for detection and treatment of cancer. *Photochemistry and Photobiology.* **86**:410–417.

Van de Wiele C, Oltenfreiter R (2006) Imaging probes targeting matrix metalloproteinases. *Cancer Biotherapy and Radiopharmaceuticals.* **21**:409–417.

van der Graaf M (2010) In vivo magnetic resonance spectroscopy: Basic methodology and clinical applications. *European Biophysics Journal.* **39**:527–540.

van Geel IP, Oppelaar H, Rijken PF, Bernsen HJ, Hagemeier NE, van der Kogel AJ, Hodgkiss RJ, Stewart FA (1996) Vascular perfusion and hypoxic areas in RIF-1 tumours after photodynamic therapy. *British Journal of Cancer.* **73**:288–293.

Vesper BJ, Lee S, Hammer ND, Elseth KM, Barrett AG, Hoffman BM, Radosevich JA (2006) Developing a structure–function relationship for anionic porphyrazines exhibiting selective anti-tumor activity. *Journal of Photochemistry and Photobiology. B.* **82**:180–186.

Viala J, Vanel D, Meingan P, Lartigau E, Carde P, Renschler M (1999) Phases IB and II multidose trial of gadolinium texaphyrin, a radiation sensitizer detectable at MR imaging: Preliminary results in brain metastases. *Radiology.* **212**:755–759.

Walker TG, Happer W (1997) Spin-exchange optical pumping of noble-gas nuclei. *Reviews of Modern Physics.* **69**:629–642.

Wang C, Cheng L, Liu Y, Wang X, Ma X, Deng Z, Li Y, Liu Z (2013) Imaging-guided pH-sensitive photodynamic therapy using charge reversible upconversion nanoparticles under near-infrared light. *Advanced Functional Materials.* **23**:3077–3086.

Wang L, An Y, Yuan C, Zhang H, Liang C, Ding F, Gao Q, Zhang D (2015) GEM-loaded magnetic albumin nanospheres modified with cetuximab for simultaneous targeting, magnetic resonance imaging, and double-targeted thermochemotherapy of pancreatic cancer cells. *International Journal of Nanomedicine.* **10**:2507–2519.

Wang S, Westmoreland TD (2009) Correlation of relaxivity with coordination number in six-, seven-, and eight-coordinate Mn(II) complexes of pendant-arm cyclen derivatives. *Inorganic Chemistry.* **48**:719–727.

Weissleder R, Mahmood U (2001) Molecular imaging. *Radiology.* **219**:316–333.

Werner EJ, Datta A, Jocher CJ, Raymond KN (2008) High-relaxivity MRI contrast agents: Where coordination chemistry meets medical tmaging. *Angewandte Chemie International Edition.* **47**:8568–8580.

Wester HJ (2007) Nuclear imaging probes: From bench to bedside. *Clinical Cancer Research.* **13**:3470–3481.

Winsborrow BG, Grondey H, Savoie H, Fyfe CA, Dolphin D (1997) Magnetic resonance imaging evaluation of photodynamic therapy-induced hemorrhagic necrosis in the murine M1 tumor model. *Photochemistry and Photobiology.* **66**:847–852.

Woodburn KW, Fan Q, Kessel D, Wright M, Mody TD, Hemmi G, Magda D et al. (1996) Phototherapy of cancer and atheromatous plaque with texaphyrins. *Journal of Clinical Laser Medicine and Surgery.* **14**:343–348.

Xuan SH, Lee SF, Lau JT, Zhu X, Wang YX, Wang F, Lai JM et al. (2012) Photocytotoxicity and magnetic relaxivity responses of dual-porous gamma-Fe_2O_3@meso-SiO_2 microspheres. *ACS Applied Materials and Interfaces.* **4**:2033–2040.

Yan GP, Li Z, Xu W, Zhou CK, Yang L, Zhang Q, Li L et al. (2011) Porphyrin-containing polyaspartamide gadolinium complexes as potential magnetic resonance imaging contrast agents. *International Journal of Pharmaceutics*. **407**:119–125.

Yi X, Wang F, Qin W, Yang X, Yuan J (2014) Near-infrared fluorescent probes in cancer imaging and therapy: An emerging field. *International Journal of Nanomedicine*. **9**:1347–1365.

Yoo D, Jeong H, Preihs C, Choi J-S, Shin T-H, Sessler JL, Cheon J (2012) Double-effector nanoparticles: A synergistic approach to apoptotic hyperthermia. *Angewandte Chemie International Edition*. **51**:12482–12485.

Yoo D, Lee J-H, Shin T-H, Cheon J (2011) Theranostic magnetic nanoparticles. *Accounts of Chemical Research*. **44**:863–874.

Yoon H-J, Lim TG, Kim J-H, Cho YM, Kim YS, Chung US, Kim JH, Choi BW, Koh W-G, Jang W-D (2014) Fabrication of multifunctional layer-by-layer nanocapsules toward the design of theragnostic nanoplatform. *Biomacromolecules*. **15**:1382–1389.

Zeng L, Xiang L, Ren W, Zheng J, Li T, Chen B, Zhang J, Mao C, Li A, Wu A (2013) Multifunctional photosensitizer-conjugated core-shell $Fe_3O_4@NaYF_4$:Yb/Er nanocomplexes and their applications in T_2-weighted magnetic resonance/upconversion luminescence imaging and photodynamic therapy of cancer cells. *RSC Advances*. **3**:13915–13925.

Zhang Z, He R, Yan K, Guo Q-N, Lu Y-G, Wang X-X, Lei H, Li Z-Y (2009) Synthesis and in vitro and in vivo evaluation of manganese(III) porphyrin–dextran as a novel MRI contrast agent. *Bioorganic and Medicinal Chemistry Letters*. **19**:6675–6678.

Zong Y, Wang X, Goodrich KC, Mohs AM, Parker DL, Lu Z-R (2005) Contrast-enhanced MRI with new biodegradable macromolecular Gd(III) complexes in tumor-bearing mice. *Magnetic Resonance in Medicine*. **53**:835–842.

Theranostic applications of photodynamic molecular beacons

WENTAO SONG, YANG ZHOU, AND JONATHAN F. LOVELL

12.1 INTRODUCTION

12.1.1 PHOTODYNAMIC THERAPY

Photodynamic molecular beacons have the capacity for fluorescence imaging, like conventional molecular beacons, but can also be used as activatable probes for photodynamic therapy (PDT). PDT is based on light irradiation of photosensitizers to generate reactive singlet oxygen that destroys target cells and tissues with minimal invasion (Dougherty et al., 1998). Singlet oxygen will cause damage to cellular targets, resulting in apoptosis and necrosis of irradiated cells. At the same time, the vascular network that is carrying oxygen and nutrients to the irradiated area shuts down and furthermore an immune system response is generated against the target cells (Lovell et al., 2010a). There are advantages of PDT as compared with conventional therapies due to the relatively nontoxic nature of the photosensitizer in nonirradiated parts of the body and the selectivity in which light can be applied with spatial control. Repeated doses can be administered to treat the patient without the risk of cumulative toxicity and PDT resistance has not yet been reported. PDT can also lead to rapid healing with excellent cosmetic outcomes for dermatological indications, leaving little or no scarring. Side effects to surrounding healthy tissues and organs can be minimized with proper treatment planning (Wilson and Patterson, 2008). PDT has shown its clinical potential in the past couple of decades. Clinical applications cover a variety of different cancer treatments, including skin, lung, esophagus, bladder, head and neck, brain, ocular melanoma, ovarian, prostate, renal cell, cervix, pancreas, and bone carcinomas. PDT has also been used for the treatment of dysplasias, papillomas, rheumatoid arthritis, actinic keratosis, cosmetic indications, psoriasis, neovascularization in age-associated macular degeneration, endometrial ablation, port wine stains, atherosclerotic plaques, and prophylaxis against arterial restenosis (Sharman et al., 1999; Huang, 2005; Lovell et al., 2010a). Bacterial and fungal infections have been shown to be candidates for PDT treatment for over 30 years (Hamblin and Hasan, 2004). PDT can be used as a stand-alone treatment or combined with other therapeutic modalities such as chemotherapy, surgery, radiotherapy, or immunotherapy.

PDT relies on the combined interaction between a photosensitizer, light, and oxygen in order to generate cytotoxic singlet oxygen. Light, at a specific irradiation wavelength, is absorbed by a photosensitizer in its low energy ground state. The absorbed photons promote the photosensitizer to an excited singlet state. Thermal decay and emission of fluorescence can return the photosensitizer to the ground state. Intersystem crossing occurs for a portion of the photosensitizer population, leading to the formation of a lower energy excited triplet state. Type I and type II processes in PDT are the two mechanisms that generate reactive species from the photosensitizer excited triplet state (Dougherty et al., 1998). In type I processes, electrons get transferred from the photosensitizer to various receptor molecules, and free radical production via the superoxide anion, hydroxyl radical, or hydrogen peroxide (Leanne and Ross, 2008). In type II processes, the excited triplet state photosensitizer interacts with molecular oxygen to produce reactive singlet oxygen. The type II reaction is thought to be more relevant to clinical PDT and singlet oxygen is an effector for destruction of target cells and tissue. Singlet oxygen diffuses only small distances in biological environments, but rapidly reacts with nearby cellular components, including lipids, amino acid residues, and nucleic acids, leading to cell death. Cell death occurs via apoptosis or necrosis, with the mechanism dependent upon factors such as the localization of the photosensitizer within the cell and the amount of singlet oxygen generated (Pervaiz and Olivo, 2006). It has been suggested that photosensitizer localization in the mitochondria or endoplasmic reticulum favors apoptosis whereas photosensitizer localization in the plasma membrane or lysosome favors necrosis (Wilson and Patterson, 2008). Beyond destruction of irradiated cells, PDT also triggers local inflammation and immune responses that can have broader effects against cancers in vivo (Castano et al., 2006).

12.2 TRADITIONAL MOLECULAR BEACONS

Molecular beacons were first described nearly 20 years ago as oligonucleotide probes that increase their fluorescence in response to specific and complementary nucleic acids (Tyagi and Kramer, 1996). Coupled with polymerase chain reaction, molecular beacons provide an innovative method to monitor the presence of small amounts of nucleic acids with excellent specificity. This discovery, demonstrating that a specific and rationally designed nanoscale probe could generate activatable fluorescence, based on recognition of a target molecule has had a profound effect on smart probe design (Lovell and Zheng, 2008). Subsequently, the term molecular beacon has been used to describe other types of optical probes beyond oligonucleotide detection and it is worthwhile noting some common elements of classical molecular beacons.

12.2.1 FLUOROPHORE AND QUENCHER

Common fluorophores that have been used for traditional molecular beacons include 5-(2'-aminoethyl) aminonapthalene-1-sulfonic acid (EDANS), fluorescein (Fam), tetrachloro-6-carboxyfluorescein (Tet), hexachloro-6-carboxy fluorescein (Hex), tetramethylrhodamine (Tamra), and 5-carboxyrhodamine-X (Rox) (Rodríguez-Lázaro et al., 2004). The choice of reporter dye and quencher is flexible and depends on the application. Multicolor molecular beacons with different excitation and different emission wavelengths enable unambiguous multiplexed target detection in a single solution (Tyagi et al., 2000). With appropriate conjugation chemistry, photosensitizers such as phthalocyanines, can readily be used in the fluorophore position to generate photodynamic molecular beacons (Nesterova et al., 2009).

A quenching moiety is responsible for energy capture and transfer from the excited fluorophore when it is in the "off" position (Fabbrizzi et al., 1996). A commonly used quencher is 4-(4-dimethylaminophenylazo) benzoic acid (dabcyl). Dabcyl is a hydrophobic molecule and serves as a universal quencher for numerous fluorophores (Giesendorf et al., 1998). Dabcyl can quench over 95% of the fluorescence of EDANS and fluorescein within molecular beacon constructs (Tyagi et al., 2000). However, quenching efficiency decreases for dyes emitting at longer wavelength. More recently, gold nanoparticles from 1 to 4 nm in diameter have been used as fluorescence quenchers as they have excellent quenching efficiency (Dubertret et al., 2001).

Some quenchers deactivate the fluorophore by forming a ground state complex via contact quenching. Alternatively, Förster resonance energy transfer (FRET) can also be used as another quenching mechanism. FRET occurs between a donor fluorophore and an acceptor chromophore via dipole–dipole interactions (Forster, 1946). The fluorescence of the donor molecular is quenched whereas the emission of the acceptor fluorophore is enhanced only when the molecules come in close proximity (but not necessarily in direct contact). FRET efficiency can be predicted based on the overlap of emission spectrum of the donor and extinction spectrum of the acceptor (Carmel et al., 1973; Matayoshi et al., 1990).

12.2.2 PROBE SEQUENCE

The probe sequence is responsible for generating the unique hairpin-loop structure of classical molecular beacons that leads to proximal positioning of fluorophore and quencher in the "off" position, and increased separation between fluorophore and quencher in the "on" position. In general, the length of the sequence is between 15 and 30 nucleotides and should not form any secondary structure. Target affinity can be improved by increasing the length of the sequence but at the cost of reduced specificity. The beacon should be able to dissociate itself from the target strand at temperatures 7°C–10°C higher than that of the annealing temperature. The percentage of paired guanine and cytosine nucleotides can be used to predict the melting temperature (Goel et al., 2005). Faster hybridization kinetics can be achieved with short-stemmed portions but this will result in lower signal-to-background ratios. Additionally, nucleotide bases themselves can sometimes affect fluorophore brightness and generally exhibit quenching in the order of G > A > C > T (Drake and Tan, 2004).

12.2.3 MOLECULAR BEACONS FOR IMAGING

Molecular beacons have been used for cellular imaging of the temporal and spatial distribution of nucleic acids in living cells (Bratu et al., 2003). Beyond detection of nucleic acids, molecular beacons have shown good potential for imaging cancer and some cellular activities in vivo, via fluorescence emission changes in response to specific molecular targets. Peptide-based beacons have been developed to respond to specific molecular markers of biological pathways and disease progression. Peptide-based molecular beacons usually are activated by irreversible proteolytic cleavage of a fluorophore and quencher system to generate a detectable change in a fluorometric readout. The molecular beacons can be designed by linking a fluorophore and quencher together by a linear peptide substrate that is cleaved by the target protease (Carmel et al., 1973). Generally, the molecular beacon consists of one fluorescence emitter and a fluorescence quencher (Pham et al., 2004; Bullok and Piwnica-Worms, 2005). Following enzymatic cleavage, fluorophore and quencher are free to diffuse away from each other, thereby reducing quenching or energy transfer and increasing the donor fluorescence. Compared to nucleic acid molecular beacons, which physically confine the fluorophore and quencher in contact, peptide beacons usually have greater separation and use of appropriate FRET quenching design is important to ensure a large increase in fluoresce signal occurs following beacon activation. If a FRET donor and acceptor pair are used, both an increase in donor emission and a decrease in the acceptor fluorescence can be used for monitoring proteolytic activity in a ratiometric fashion (Lovell et al., 2011). Many of the first peptide-based molecular beacons were used in the elucidation of enzyme kinetics and enzymatic activity of samples (Carmel et al., 1973). Enzyme activity can be quantified in homogenized cells or tissues overexpressing the target enzyme. High signal amplification is an advantageous property of enzyme-activated beacons, since a single protease can cleave multiple peptide linkers, resulting in the activation of large number of beacons. Various molecular beacon design strategies can be applied to enzyme targets (Weissleder and Ntziachristos, 2003; Lovell et al., 2010a).

Molecular beacons have been used in vivo since at least 1999 and subsequently there has been research interest and research commercialization (in the preclinical market) of this topic based on its broad potential

(Weissleder et al., 1999). Since molecular beacons are capable of imaging specific disease-associated protease activity, they can also monitor the efficacy of protease inhibitor therapy. Image guidance can provide a demarcation between tumor and healthy tissue during surgical procedures (tumor margins). Contribution of multiple different proteases involved in disease progression also can be evaluated (Weissleder et al., 1999; Bremer et al., 2001; Weissleder and Ntziachristos, 2003). The use of near infrared (NIR) fluorophores and concurrent development of NIR imaging systems has been beneficial for in vivo molecular beacon imaging (Weissleder and Ntziachristos, 2003). Detection of increased NIR fluorescence in response to specific disease targets by protease activatable probes is a promising tool for imaging diseases in vivo (Tan et al., 2004; Stefflova et al., 2007b).

12.3 PHOTODYNAMIC MOLECULAR BEACONS

Photodynamic molecular beacons are based on conventional molecular beacon designs but make use of a photosensitizer instead of a standard fluorophore. These can be used for both imaging and therapy since most photosensitizers have near infrared fluorescence properties in addition to singlet oxygen generation capacity. Therefore, they are intrinsically suited for theranostic applications. In a typical photodynamic molecular beacon, the photosensitizer is linked to a quenching molecule, so that it is inactive until the linker is cleaved by a specific enzyme or target (e.g., Figure 12.1).

One important characteristic of photodynamic molecular beacons is that photosensitizer selectivity does not depend solely on photosensitizer targeting and accumulation but also depends on target tissue-specific unquenching of the beacon. Thus, in theory, a higher dose of photodynamic beacon could be administered

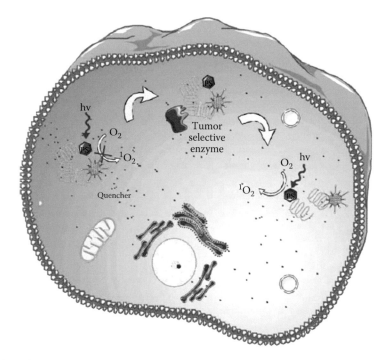

Figure 12.1 Photodynamic therapy molecular beacons. A peptide linker that is a substrate of a cancer-associated enzyme (e.g., a protease) is conjugated to a photosensitizer (PS) and a singlet oxygen ($^1O_2$) quencher. The proximity of the photosensitizer and quencher ensures inhibition of $^1O_2$ generation during irradiation of normal cells. In the presence of an enzyme, the substrate sequence is cleaved and the photosensitizer and quencher are separated, thereby enabling photoactivation of the PS. hv indicates light; O_2, molecular oxygen. (From Agostinis, P. et al.: Photodynamic therapy of cancer: An update. *Cancer J. Clin.* 2011. 61. 250–281. Copyright Wiley-VCH Verlag GmbH & Co. Reproduced with permission.)

and the tissues that do not express the activating stimulus (e.g., possibly normal skin and adjacent healthy tissue) would be less impacted by the treatment irradiation or by sunlight exposure. Since PDT is already a highly selective treatment modality due to the spatially controlled delivery of the irradiation light, the addition of a molecular activation step would add more complexity to the treatment, but also add another safeguard for patient safety.

Based on their potential for theranostics, numerous photodynamic molecular beacons have been described, in many different forms (Chen et al., 2004; Stefflova et al., 2006a,b; Chen et al., 2007, 2008, 2009; Zheng et al., 2007; Lovell et al., 2010a). In one example, asymmetric photodynamic hairpin beacons were developed to balance high quenching efficiency with two step activation (cleavage and dissociation) to enhance tumor cell uptake (Chen et al., 2009). In this report, the authors described the synthesis and characterization of an MMP7-triggered photodynamic molecular beacon using pyropheophorbide-a as the photosensitizer, another molecule as a dual fluorescence and singlet oxygen quencher, and a short peptide sequence as the MMP7 cleavable linker.

The design of photodynamic molecular beacons is in large part similar to that of conventional molecular beacons. The photosensitizer is silenced by a quenching mechanism, with respect to both photosensitizer fluorescence and photosensitizer singlet oxygen generation, until the beacon is activated by a molecular stimulus. Fluorescence and PDT activity is restored upon beacon activation (Zheng et al., 2007). FRET theory can be used to select an appropriate quencher for the PS (Lovell et al., 2009). Other unique quenchers can be used, such as carotenoids, which are able to directly scavenge photosensitizer-generated singlet oxygen, in addition to deactivating the excited state photosensitizer (Chen et al., 2007). Although there are many classes of photosensitizer molecules, porphyrins and related compounds are frequently used for photodynamic molecular beacons. Porphyrins can be chemically conjugated with relative ease and have been used for numerous phototherapeutic and theranostic applications such as PDT, imaging, and other applications such as photothermal therapy, light-triggered drug release, and higher order multimodal imaging (Zhang and Lovell, 2012; Jin et al., 2013; Huang et al., 2015; Rieffel et al., 2015). Photosensitizers that have optical absorption between 650 and 900 nm range are usually selected due to superior tissue penetration of light and lower background fluorescence due to the intrinsic optical properties of tissue (Stefflova et al., 2007a).

Tumor-specific enzymes can act as the activator for photodynamic beacons if they are constructed with an appropriate linker sequence. This will result in the cleavage of the linker by enzymatic cleavage in the specific diseased cells and tissue, restoring singlet oxygen generation and fluorescence. This approach has been used to image specific proteolytic activation of photodynamic molecular beacons in breast cancer vertebral metastases (Liu et al., 2011). Since vertebral metastases are a common occurrence in breast cancer patients, such an approach could eventually allow clinicians to first identify and locate the sites of metastases and then insert a fiber optic laser fiber to treat them. Matrix metalloproteinase (MMPs), proteases overexpressed in the disease, were able to activate the beacon. Therapy and imaging has been carried out by a cancer-specific beacon with a built-in apoptosis sensor (Stefflova et al., 2006a). The caspase-3 cleavable peptide sequence (KGDEVDGSGK) served as a linker, and pyropheophorbide-a served as a fluorescent photosensitizer, BHQ-3 was the quencher, and folic acid served as a targeting moiety. The construct preferentially accumulated in cells that overexpressed cell surface folate receptors demonstrating the efficacy of the targeting moiety. Singlet oxygen was generated following cell uptake, leading to cell death, which in turn increased the expression of caspase-3. Capase-3 resulted in beacon cleavage, which could be used to identify dying cells via restoration of fluorescence emission. A related approach used 5-carboxy-X-rhodamine (Rox) as a donor and pyro as an acceptor with a caspase-3-specific peptide sequence. This design was more effectively to be able to induce and detect apoptosis, since the photosensitizer was not quenched prior to activation (Lovell et al., 2011). Such photodynamic molecular beacon designs offer new potential strategies to better guide treatment by enabling direct molecular feedback of cell death during treatment.

Other approaches like the combination of photosensitizers with single-walled carbon nanotubes as quenchers have been reported (Zhu et al., 2008). Single-walled carbon nanotubes have been used as efficient fluorescence quenchers and intracellular delivery vehicles (Kam et al., 2006; Zhu et al., 2010). The control of fluorescence and light-activated singlet oxygen was achieved by attachment of the photosensitizer chlorin e6 to one end of an aptamer, which like other single-stranded nucleic acids, can be readily adsorbed to single-walled carbon nanotubes. Chlorin e6 was released from the nanotubes upon the aptamer binding to its target, thereby leading to unquenching of fluorescence and singlet oxygen generation. The development of photodynamic molecular beacons is limitless and light-activated control is not the only strategy. Lanthanum fluoride nanoparticles covalently linked to photosensitizer have been introduced as an x-ray-activated system and capable of yielding singlet oxygen as well. Such a design offers new opportunities for photodynamic beacons in deep human tissue (Liu et al., 2008).

Zheng et al. (2007) was pioneering in using traditional molecular beacon concepts with a photosensitizer to produce photodynamic molecular beacons. These molecules exhibited quenching that suppressed their production of $^1O_2$ in their latent state. They could be activated by interaction with a tumor-specific molecular marker, in this case the matrix metalloproteinase MMP-7. The clinical implementation of strategies such as these has the potential to improve the activity of the photosensitizer at the site of the tumor. An essential component of any targeting strategy is the ability to verify the targeting of the drug to the desired target and to separate the effects of targeting and beacon activation. The distribution and activation of the photosensitizer can be determined optically using fluorescence imaging. Porphyrins can also be stably labeled with radioisotopes to image the localization and not the activation of the beacon using PET or SPECT techniques (Liu et al., 2012; Lee et al., 2014; Zhang et al., 2014).

The diagnosis and treatment of epithelial cancer using a peptide photodynamic molecular beacon has been reported (Lo et al., 2008). Fibroblast activation protein is a cell surface serine protease in cancer-related fibroblasts of human epithelial carcinomas. The fluorescence and singlet oxygen generation was restored when the peptide loop specific to the protease was cleaved. Therapeutic efficacy was demonstrated in cells overexpressing the enzyme. Therefore, numerous proteases have been demonstrated to be suitable activators of photodynamic molecular beacons.

Taking advantage of their strong absorption in the near-infrared region, gold nanorods have proven to be an efficient material for photothermal therapy (PTT) and are also efficient photosensitizer quenchers. In order to manipulate the quenching and recovery of photosensitizer fluorescence, a photosensitizer-conjugated beacon was designed, which was assembled onto gold nanorods, thus achieving controlled singlet oxygen generation for PDT (Wang et al., 2012). The strategy of utilizing selective activatable photosensitizers combined with the synergistic effect of PTT and PDT could be a potent therapeutic regimen against cancer cells than nonspecific methods using either PTT or PDT alone (Figure 12.2).

Traditional molecular beacon architecture has been used in activatable photosensitizers, as shown in Figure 12.3. A pyropheophorbide-a photosensitizer was held in place next to a carotenoid quencher by a 6-base stem with a loop portion specific for the cRaf-1 oncogene (Chen et al., 2008). This photodynamic molecular beacon used a modified 2′-O-methyl backbone to avoid nuclease degradation. Upon incubation with cRaf-1 expressing cells, the photodynamic molecular beacon was taken up into the cells which were dependent on the presence of the hydrophobic pyropheophorbide-a photosensitizer. Once in the cell, the photodynamic molecular beacon became activated. However, a photodynamic molecular beacon with a scrambled sequence showed much less activation, implying specific beacon opening by cRAF-1 mRNA. PDT was also performed and showed that the photodynamic molecular beacon was capable of destroying the target cells. Another photodynamic molecular beacon was developed that relied on self-quenching, rather than a dark quencher (Nesterova et al., 2009). To achieve quenching, the beacon held two molecules of a zinc phthalocyanine photosensitizer, conjugated to the 5′ and 3′ termini of the beacon together via a 5-base stem. This construct demonstrated good quenching and activation, with the target inducing a 45-fold increase in photodynamic molecular beacon fluorescence.

Singlet oxygen modulation in response to nucleic acid target binding has been demonstrated using other types of DNA-based activatable photosensitizers (Cló et al., 2006). Pyropheophorbide and black hole quencher were conjugated on the two ends of an oligonucleotide strands and acted as a fluorescent and photosensitizing reporter and a quencher, respectively. The fluorescence emission and singlet oxygen production was quenched due to the short distance in between hybridized sequences. The fluorescence was restored more than 85% when there was an excess complementary sequence present in the solution after hybridization to displace binding next to the quencher. Other approaches have shown that the use of multiple quenching moieties can induce highly effective beacon quenching (Lovell et al., 2010c). Interestingly, the large number

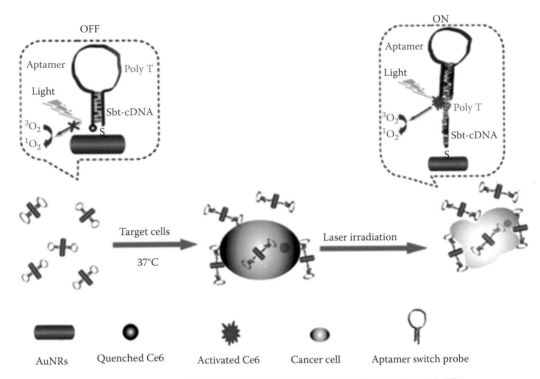

Sequence: 5′–SH–CTA ACC GTT TTT TTT TTT TTT TTT TTT TTT TTT TTT TTT TAT CTA
ACT GCT GCC CCG CCG GGA AAA TAC TGT ACG GTT AGA–Ce6–3′

Figure 12.2 Schematic of photosensitizer—gold nanorods for PTT and PDT. (Reprinted with permission from Wang, P. et al., Assembly of aptamer switch probes and photosensitizer on gold nanorods for targeted photothermal and photodynamic cancer therapy, *ACS Nano*, 6, 5070–5077. Copyright 2012 American Chemical Society.)

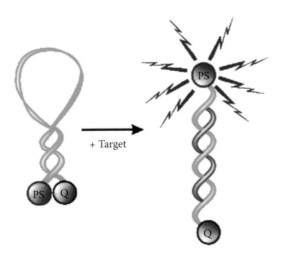

Figure 12.3 A simple nucleic acid-based photodynamic molecular beacon. A complementary stem portion maintains the photosensitizer (red) and quencher (blue) close together until a nucleic acid target (orange) binds to the loop portion of the beacon. Upon target hybridization, quenching efficiency decreases and singlet oxygen production increases. (Reprinted with permission from Lovell, J.F. et al., Activatable photosensitizers for imaging and therapy, *Chem. Rev.*, 110, 2839–2857. Copyright 2010a American Chemical Society.)

of quenchers increased the hydrophobicity of the beacon, enabling insertion of the beacon into lipophilic nanoparticles and physical responses, in the form of induced nanoparticle aggregation, to beacon target recognition (Lovell et al., 2010b). Some photodynamic beacons themselves have been developed that can be activated by other beacons (Lou and Lovell, 2014).

Other stimuli can be used to modulate photodynamic molecular beacons, such as pH. The pH-sensitive DNA i-motif was used to control photosensitized singlet oxygen generation (Tørring et al., 2010). The absence of acidic condition will keep the photosensitizer and quencher together in an i-motif quadruplex. Quenching effects prevent the formation of the triplet state photosensitizer and subsequent generation of singlet oxygen. Singlet oxygen production increased following separation between photosensitizer and quencher induced by i-motif quadruplex when solution pH increased beyond 5. This approach presents the modulation of photodynamic activity in response to changes in the chemical environment (pH).

12.4 CONCLUSION AND OUTLOOK

Photodynamic molecular beacons bridge the research fields of PDT and molecular recognition. So far, proof of principle has been established that numerous stimuli can be used for activation and restoration of fluorescence and singlet oxygen generation. These include activation by nucleic acid sequences and enzymatic activity found in diseases cells and tissues. Photodynamic molecular beacons add a layer of complexity beyond conventional photosensitizers and therefore the correct clinical indications must be identified in which photodynamic molecular beacons offer a compelling treatment approach. Further translational studies are required to realize the theranostic benefit photodynamic molecular beacons can offer.

REFERENCES

Agostinis P et al. (2011) Photodynamic therapy of cancer: An update. *A Cancer Journal for Clinicians* **61**:250–281.

Bratu DP et al. (2003) Visualizing the distribution and transport of mRNAs in living cells. *Proceedings of the National Academy of Sciences* **100**:13308–13313.

Bremer C, Tung C-H, Weissleder R (2001) In vivo molecular target assessment of matrix metalloproteinase inhibition. *Nature Medicine* **7**:743–748.

Bullok K, Piwnica-Worms D (2005) Synthesis and characterization of a small, membrane-permeant, caspase-activatable far-red fluorescent peptide for imaging apoptosis. *Journal of Medicinal Chemistry* **48**:5404–5407.

Carmel A, Zur M, Yaron A, Katchalski E (1973) Use of substrates with fluorescent donor and acceptor chromophores for the kinetic assay of hydrolases. *FEBS Letters* **30**:11–14.

Castano AP, Mroz P, Hamblin MR (2006) Photodynamic therapy and anti-tumour immunity. *Nature Reviews Cancer* **6**:535–545.

Chen J et al. (2004) Protease-triggered photosensitizing beacon based on singlet oxygen quenching and activation. *Journal of the American Chemical Society* **126**:11450–11451.

Chen J et al. (2007) Using the singlet oxygen scavenging property of carotenoid in photodynamic molecular beacons to minimize photodamage to non-targeted cells. *Photochemical and Photobiological Sciences* **6**:1311–1317.

Chen J et al. (2008) A tumor mRNA-triggered photodynamic molecular beacon based on oligonucleotide hairpin control of singlet oxygen production. *Photochemical and Photobiological Sciences* **7**:775–781.

Chen J et al. (2009) "Zipper" molecular beacons: A generalized strategy to optimize the performance of activatable protease probes. *Bioconjugate Chemistry* **20**:1836–1842.

Cló E et al. (2006) DNA-programmed control of photosensitized singlet oxygen production. *Journal of the American Chemical Society* **128**:4200–4201.

Dougherty TJ et al. (1998) Photodynamic therapy. *Journal of the National Cancer Institute* **90**:889–905.

Drake TJ, Tan W (2004) Molecular beacon DNA probes and their bioanalytical applications. *Applied Spectroscopy* **58**:269A–280A.

Dubertret B, Calame M, Libchaber AJ (2001) Single-mismatch detection using gold-quenched fluorescent oligonucleotides. *Nature Biotechnology* **19**:365–370.

Fabbrizzi L et al. (1996) Sensing of transition metals through fluorescence quenching or enhancement. *A Review Analyst* **121**:1763–1768.

Forster T (1946) Energiewanderung und fluoreszenz. *Naturwissenschaften* **33**:166–175.

Giesendorf BA et al. (1998) Molecular beacons: A new approach for semiautomated mutation analysis. *Clinical Chemistry* **44**:482–486.

Goel G et al. (2005) Molecular beacon: A multitask probe. *Journal of Applied Microbiology* **99**:435–442.

Hamblin MR, Hasan T (2004) Photodynamic therapy: A new antimicrobial approach to infectious disease? *Photochemical and Photobiological Sciences* **3**:436–450.

Huang H, Song W, Rieffel J, Lovell JF (2015) Emerging applications of porphyrins in photomedicine. *Frontiers in Physics* **3**:23.

Huang Z (2005) A review of progress in clinical photodynamic therapy. *Technology in Cancer Research and Treatment* **4**:283–293.

Jin CS, Lovell JF, Chen J, Zheng G (2013) Ablation of hypoxic tumors with dose-equivalent photothermal, but not photodynamic, therapy using a nanostructured porphyrin assembly. *ACS Nano* **7**:2541–2550.

Kam NWS, Liu Z, Dai H (2006) Carbon nanotubes as intracellular transporters for proteins and DNA: An investigation of the uptake mechanism and pathway. *Angewandte Chemie* **118**:591–595.

Leanne BJ, Ross WB (2008) Photodynamic therapy and the development of metal-based photosensitisers. *Metal-Based Drugs* **2008**:276109.

Lee J-H et al. (2014) 99mTc-labeled porphyrin-lipid nanovesicles. *Journal of Liposome Research* **25**:1–6.

Liu TW et al. (2011) Imaging of specific activation of photodynamic molecular beacons in breast cancer vertebral metastases. *Bioconjugate Chemistry* **22**:1021–1030.

Liu TW et al. (2012) Intrinsically copper-64-labeled organic nanoparticles as radiotracers. *Angewandte Chemie International Edition* **51**:13128–13131.

Liu Y, Chen W, Wang S, Joly AG (2008) Investigation of water-soluble x-ray luminescence nanoparticles for photodynamic activation. *Applied Physics Letters* **92**:043901.

Lo P-C et al. (2008) Photodynamic molecular beacon triggered by fibroblast activation protein on cancer-associated fibroblasts for diagnosis and treatment of epithelial cancers. *Journal of Medicinal Chemistry* **52**:358–368.

Lou K, Lovell JF (2014) A quenched binuclear ruthenium (II) dimer activated by another photosensitizer. *Chemical Communications* **50**:3231–3233.

Lovell JF, Jin H, Ng KK, Zheng G (2010b) Programmed nanoparticle aggregation using molecular beacons. *Angewandte Chemie International Edition* **49**:7917–7919.

Lovell JF, Liu TW, Chen J, Zheng G (2010a) Activatable photosensitizers for imaging and therapy. *Chemical Reviews* **110**:2839–2857.

Lovell JF, Zheng G (2008) Activatable smart probes for molecular optical imaging and therapy. *Journal of Innovative Optical Health Sciences* **1**:45–61.

Lovell JF et al. (2009) FRET quenching of photosensitizer singlet oxygen generation. *The Journal of Physical Chemistry B* **113**:3203–3211.

Lovell JF et al. (2010c) Facile synthesis of advanced photodynamic molecular beacon architectures. *Bioconjugate Chemistry* **21**:1023–1025.

Lovell JF et al. (2011) Porphyrin FRET acceptors for apoptosis induction and monitoring. *Journal of the American Chemical Society* **133**:18580–18582.

Matayoshi ED, Wang GT, Krafft GA, Erickson J (1990) Novel fluorogenic substrates for assaying retroviral proteases by resonance energy transfer. *Science* **247**:954–958.

Nesterova IV et al. (2009) Phthalocyanine dimerization-based molecular beacons using near-IR fluorescence. *Journal of the American Chemical Society* **131**:2432–2433.

Pervaiz S, Olivo M (2006) Art and science of photodynamic therapy. *Clinical and Experimental Pharmacology and Physiology* **33**:551–556.

Pham W, Choi Y, Weissleder R, Tung C-H (2004) Developing a peptide-based near-infrared molecular probe for protease sensing. *Bioconjugate Chemistry* **15**:1403–1407.

Rieffel J et al. (2015) Hexamodal imaging with porphyrin-phospholipid-coated upconversion nanoparticles. *Advanced Materials* **27**:1785–1790.

Rodríguez-Lázaro D, D'agostino M, Pla M, Cook N (2004) Construction strategy for an internal amplification control for real-time diagnostic assays using nucleic acid sequence-based amplification: Development and clinical application. *Journal of Clinical Microbiology* **42**:5832–5836.

Sharman WM, Allen CM, Van Lier JE (1999) Photodynamic therapeutics: Basic principles and clinical applications. *Drug Discovery Today* **4**:507–517.

Stefflova K, Chen J, Li H, Zheng G (2006a) Targeted photodynamic therapy agent with a built-in apoptosis sensor for in vivo near-infrared imaging of tumor apoptosis triggered by its photosensitization in situ. *Molecular Imaging* **5**:520.

Stefflova K, Chen J, Zheng G (2007a) Killer beacons for combined cancer imaging and therapy. *Current Medicinal Chemistry* **14**:2110–2125.

Stefflova K, Chen J, Zheng G (2007b) Using molecular beacons for cancer imaging and treatment. *Front Bioscience* **12**:4709–4721.

Stefflova K et al. (2006b) Photodynamic therapy agent with a built-in apoptosis sensor for evaluating its own therapeutic outcome in situ. *Journal of Medicinal Chemistry* **49**:3850–3856.

Tan W, Wang K, Drake TJ (2004) Molecular beacons. *Current Opinion in Chemical Biology* **8**:547–553.

Tørring T et al. (2010) Reversible pH-regulated control of photosensitized singlet oxygen production using a DNA i-Motif. *Angewandte Chemie* **122**:8095–8097.

Tyagi S, Kramer FR (1996) Molecular beacons: Probes that fluoresce upon hybridization. *Nature Biotechnology* **14**:303–308.

Tyagi S, Marras SA, Kramer FR (2000) Wavelength-shifting molecular beacons. *Nature Biotechnology* **18**:1191–1196.

Wang J et al. (2012) Assembly of aptamer switch probes and photosensitizer on gold nanorods for targeted photothermal and photodynamic cancer therapy. *ACS Nano* **6**:5070–5077.

Weissleder R, Ntziachristos V (2003) Shedding light onto live molecular targets. *Nature Medicine* **9**:123–128.

Weissleder R, Tung C-H, Mahmood U, Bogdanov A (1999) In vivo imaging of tumors with protease-activated near-infrared fluorescent probes. *Nature Biotechnology* **17**:375–378.

Wilson BC, Patterson MS (2008) The physics, biophysics and technology of photodynamic therapy. *Physics in Medicine and Biology* **53**:R61.

Zhang Y, Lovell JF (2012) Porphyrins as theranostic agents from prehistoric to modern times. *Theranostics* **2**:905.

Zhang Y et al. (2014) Non-invasive multimodal functional imaging of the intestine with frozen micellar naphthalocyanines. *Nature Nanotechnology* **9**:631–638.

Zheng G et al. (2007) Photodynamic molecular beacon as an activatable photosensitizer based on protease-controlled singlet oxygen quenching and activation. *Proceedings of the National Academy of Sciences* **104**:8989–8994.

Zhu Z et al. (2008) Regulation of singlet oxygen generation using single-walled carbon nanotubes. *Journal of the American Chemical Society* **130**:10856–10857.

Zhu Z et al. (2010) Single-walled carbon nanotube as an effective quencher. *Analytical and Bioanalytical Chemistry* **396**:73–83.

Tumor-specific imaging and photodynamic therapy targeting the urokinase receptor

ZAFAR IQBAL, LONGGUANG JIANG, ZHUO CHEN, CAI YUAN,
RUI LI, KE ZHENG, XIAOLEI ZHOU, JINCAN CHEN, PING HU,
AND MINGDONG HUANG

ABBREVIATIONS

ATF	Amino-terminal fragment, residue 1–143 of uPA
ECM	Extracellular matrix
MMP	Matrix metalloproteinase
MRI	Magnetic resonance imaging
PAI-1	Plasminogen activator inhibitor 1
PET	Positron emission therapy
SMB	Somatomedin B domain of vitronectin
suPAR	Soluble uPAR
uPA	Urokinase-type plasminogen activator
uPAR	uPA receptor

13.1 UROKINASE/UROKINASE RECEPTOR SYSTEM IN FIBRINOLYSIS AND CANCER

Plasminogen is a major plasma protein (Table 13.1) synthesized by the liver that circulates in blood at a high concentration (1500 nM). Plasminogen is an inactive serine protease or zymogen. The activated form of plasminogen, or plasmin, is the only enzyme responsible for the degradation of the major component of a blood clot, fibrin. A feature of plasmin is that it has relatively low specificity toward its substrates compared

Table 13.1 uPA/uPAR is a critical component of the fibrinolytic system

Property	Plasminogen	t-PA	u-PA	α$_2$-Plasmin inhibitor	PAI-1	PAI-2	uPAR
MW/No. of residue	92 kDa/791	72 kDa/527	54 kDa/411	70 kDa/452	52 kDa/402	47 kDa/393	55 kDa/313
Sources	Liver	Endothelium	Endothelium/ Liver	Kidney/Liver	Endothelium, monocytes, fat tissue, liver	Placenta, Endothelium	Endothelium/ Monocytes/ Neutrophils
Conc. (nM)	1500	0.075	0.150	900	0.1–0.4	ND	0.04
Plasma half lives	48 h	5 min	8 min				

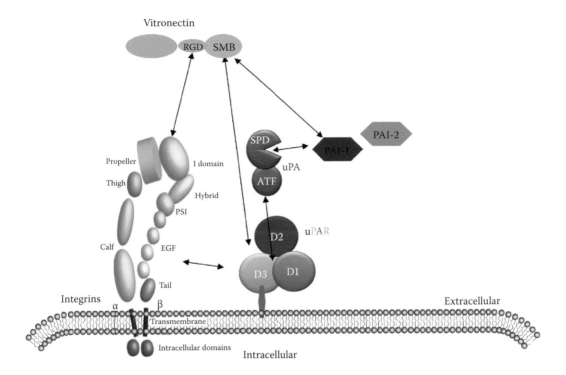

Figure 13.1 Schematic representation of the uPA/uPAR system. uPAR has three domains (D1–D3) and is anchored to the membrane surface through a GPI anchor. uPAR binds to the amino-terminal fragment (ATF, blue) of uPA. The serine protease domain (SPD) of uPA is inhibited by either PAI-1 or PAI-2. Vitronectin, found in blood and extracellular matrix, can bind to either PAI-1 or uPAR through its Somatomedin B (SMB) domain. Integrins can interact with uPAR at either residue 130–139 [4] or residues 240–248 [5].

to typical proteases. Thus, plasmin was shown to be capable of degrading a number of extracellular matrices, for example, fibrin, fibronectin, laminin, and collagen type VI. Plasmin also activates certain other proteases, for example, matrix metalloproteases, collagenases, and stromolysin-1 [1].

Plasminogen is activated by two primary plasminogen activators (PA): the human tissue-type plasminogen activator (tPA) and urokinase-type plasminogen activator (uPA) (both are also serine proteases). Both PAs are inhibited by two plasminogen activator inhibitors: plasminogen activator inhibitor-1 (PAI-1) and plasminogen activator inhibitor-2 (PAI-2) (Figure 13.1; Table 13.1) [2]. PAI-1 appears to be more important than PAI-2 because PAI-2 is found only in the placenta and in the intracellular space and its (patho) physiological role has not yet been fully established.

tPA itself has high intrinsic proteolytic activity without being activated. However, it is also regulated through its high specificity toward the blood clot (fibrin). Thus, recombinant tPA is used as an FDA-approved fibrinolytic drug for myocardial infarction and ischemic stroke. On the other hand, uPA regulation involves zymogen activation, PAI-1 inhibition, and binding to its cellular receptor, uPAR. uPAR is generally regarded as a cellular receptor for proteases because it colocalizes with uPA, and thus plasmin activity, in plasma and the pericellular space.

uPA, uPAR, and two plasminogen activator inhibitors are together termed the "uPA/uPAR system." uPAR has a low expression level in most quiescent cells but is greatly upregulated in activated immune cells (monocytes, neutrophils) and in tumor cells. A common hypothesis of the connection between uPAR and tumor metastasis is that the tumor hijacks the uPA/uPAR system to concentrate the plasmin-mediated proteolytic activity into the pericellular region so that the tumor is able to degrade the extracellular matrix (ECM) and thus migrate or metastasize from its original location [3].

13.1.1 UROKINASE-TYPE PLASMINOGEN ACTIVATOR

The urokinase-type plasminogen activator (uPA) is synthesized as a 411 residue, single-chain glycoprotein that contains 24 cysteine residues that form 12 disulfide bonds. The single-chain uPA (scuPA) possesses only a low amidolytic activity but can be activated by, for example, plasmin, into a two-chain form (tcuPA), which is highly active in converting plasminogen into plasmin. The scuPA is composed of an amino-terminal fragment (ATF, amino acid residues 1–135) [6], which contains six disulfide bonds, and is responsible for the high-affinity binding to its cellular receptor (uPAR), and a carboxyl-terminal serine protease domain (SPD, residues 159–411) [7] that contains 5 disulfide bonds together with the catalytic proteolytic site. The ATF includes an amino-terminal epidermal growth factor-like domain (GFD, residues 1–46) and a kringle domain (residues 56–135) [8,9]. The GFD domain is responsible for concentrating uPA on the cell surface by binding to uPAR. This interaction is specific since other homologous growth factors do not show appreciable binding affinity for the uPAR. The kringle domain is required to stabilize the binding between uPA and uPAR [10,11].

Physiologically, uPA also affects the processes of cell adhesion, cell migration, and tissue remodeling. Abnormal uPA expression is associated with a number of clinical conditions, including postinfarction cardiac rupture [12], aortic aneurisms [13], arthritis [14], multiple sclerosis [15], and the metastasis process in cancer [16,17]. uPA and PAI-1 are recommended by United States and Europe as level-1 markers for breast cancer diagnosis and their levels in breast cancer have been shown to be inversely proportional to cancer patient survival time [18].

13.1.2 uPA RECEPTOR

Urokinase plasminogen activator receptor (uPAR, or CD87) is a membrane glycoprotein containing three cysteine-rich Ly6/uPAR domains (about 55–60 kDa) and is attached to the plasma membrane (via its carboxy-terminus) through a glycosyl phosphatidyl inositol (GPI) anchor [19]. Besides uPA, uPAR interacts with an array of extracellular proteins, including vitronectin, integrins, G-protein-coupled receptors, and others [19] (Figure 13.1). These interactions are important for uPAR to its extracellular signal to the uPAR intracellular domain [20].

Once formed, uPA/uPAR complex at the surface is inhibited by PAI-1 and the ternary complex is recognized by the low-density lipoprotein receptor LRP-1 (LDL receptor-related protein-1) or vLDLR [21,22] and is internalized. Once it has entered the cells, the uPA/PAI-1 complex is degraded in the lysosomes, whereas uPAR is relocated back to the cell surface [23].

The receptor binding of uPA is mediated by the amino-terminal fragment (ATF) of uPA, and has a high dissociation constant (K_d = 0.28 nM) and a slow off rate [24,25], whereas the catalytic carboxyl-terminal domain of uPA does not have a direct interaction with the receptor or proteolytic activity [26]. The binding affinity of ATF to uPAR is indistinguishable from that of the full-length uPA.

Crystal structural studies of uPAR [11,27–29] have revealed uPAR adopts a compact shape with its three globular domains (D1-D3) arranged in a triangular pattern, forming a central cavity that recognizes ATF (Figure 13.2) or an antagonist peptides. The other ligand, the somatomedin B domain (SMB; residues 1–44) of vitronectin [29] (Figure 13.1), binds at the outer side on the interface between D1 and D2 domains (Figure 13.2). More specifically, uPAR binds to the ATF Ω-loop (residues 22–28) consisting of two antiparallel β-strands with the K23, Y24, and F25 being the key amino acid residues [11]. Computational modeling of uPAR also confirmed that the Ω-loop of ATF is the key region for the binding of ATF to uPAR [30,31]. Small angle x-ray scattering (SAXS) showed that uPAR can be much more flexible in solution than observed in crystal structure [32].

13.1.3 uPAR IN TUMOR METASTASIS

Tumor metastasis is a process by which cancerous cells spread to distant tissues through blood or lymphatic circulation. The detached cells from the primary tumor migrate to a different location and grow into new colonies of cells, ultimately ending into new tumors. The original source may be a primary lesion or circulating tumor cells that have detached from another metastatic tumor [33]. The metastatic process involves multiple stages starting from the detachment of cells from the parent primary tumor, followed by invasion

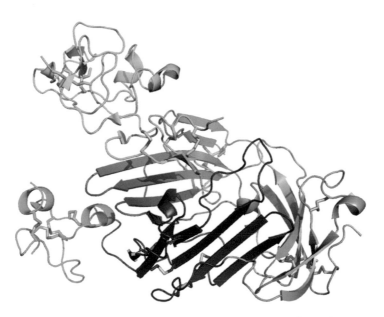

Figure 13.2 The structure of suPAR:ATF:SMB complex. D1 (orange), D2 (purple), and D3 (green) of suPAR form a hydrophobic cavity to recognize ATF (cyan). SMB binds at the outer side on the interface between D1 and D2 domains. Disulfide bonds are shown as sticks.

of these cells into the surrounding tissues and blood vessels. Later on, systemic dissemination of these cells to a distant organ followed by a cell adhesion and extravasation process, to form the metastatic tumor. The formation of a new vascular system is then initiated to sustain the newly formed colony of cells [34]. Each of the steps involved in the progression of a metastatic lesion is governed by complex gene alterations and encoded products [35].

The uPA/uPAR system plays a critical role in tumor invasion, metastasis [36,37], and angiogenesis [38]. uPAR takes part in many steps of metastatic processes in association with other proteins like uPA, vitronectin (VN), and integrins. The participation of uPAR in metastasis is shown by a number of observations: (1) The uPAR level is overexpressed [39,40] in tumor cells (100–500 fold higher than that in normal cells) and is always found on the extracellular surface of invading cells [41,42]. Elevated levels of soluble uPAR in plasma or tumor tissue lysates are usually associated with poor patient prognosis and survival [43,44]. uPAR mRNA is overexpressed in isolated bone marrow and peripheral blood cells from gastric cancer patients [45]. (2) Disruption of the uPA/uPAR interaction leads to the suppression of various cancer types [46]. (3) Knockdown of uPAR inhibits angiogenesis, thereby improving the survival rate of animals in in vivo experiments [47–51]. Downregulation of uPAR by antisense mRNA also led to the suppression of metastasis of tumors in animal models in vivo [52–54]. These and other findings have led to the widely held proposition that uPA/uPAR system could serve as a good potential target for the detection of cancer and as a treatment to retard tumor growth and metastasis.

The role of uPAR in the migration and proliferation of tumor is also likely independent of its function as a proteolysis receptor [55,56]. A direct interaction between uPAR and integrin seems necessary for the movement of the tumor cells from one part of the body to the other. For example, the interaction of uPAR with β1/β3 integrins is responsible for the amoeboid and mesenchymal invasion of prostate cancer cells [57]. It has been found that β-catenin is involved in uPA/uPAR gene expression in association with NF-kB transcription factor [58].

Many biomarkers can be utilized as oncogenic targets for drug delivery, imaging, and therapy. It should be noted that not every biomarker can be utilized as an oncotarget for imaging and therapy. Only those protein molecules which are homogenously expressed in the cancerous cells at a level at least 10-fold in excess of that found in normal cells can be exploited as biomarkers for oncotargeted imaging and therapy [59]. The presence of high levels of uPAR in the hypoxic regions of solid tumors, invasive borders [60], and in the tumor-associated stromal cells [61–63] suggests it could be a highly selective and specific target for imaging.

13.1.4 INHIBITORS OF uPAR AND BIOIMAGING

The upregulated expression of uPAR in neoplastic cells is recognized as a poor prognostic marker for patients with various cancers [43]. Inhibition of the binding between uPAR and its ligands has been proposed to limit the establishment of tumor micrometastasis or even primary tumors [55,64]. Over the years, a number of uPAR antagonists have been developed, including organic molecules [46,65,66], peptides, proteins, or monoclonal antibodies [67]. uPAR inhibitors have been successfully used for targeted imaging of uPAR using positron emission therapy (PET), magnetic resonance imaging (MRI), and single photon emission computer tomography (SPECT) [68]. Of these inhibitors, only the protein or peptide-based inhibitors were shown to exhibit the utility for imaging by targeting uPAR-expressing tumors, and these will be discussed here in detail.

Peptidic and antibody inhibitors of uPAR have been exploited as imaging probes by appropriate modification using various imaging techniques. For example, an alkylated peptide consisting of 11 amino acid residues (VSNKYFSNIHW) was encapsulated in the outer layer of liposomal nanoparticles. The nanoparticle conjugated peptide was specifically taken up in high concentration by uPAR-positive human prostate cancer cells (DU145), as compared to receptor-negative HEK293 cells [69] when visualized by fluorescence microscopy after 2 h of incubation in vitro. A dimeric linear peptide antagonist AE120 was labeled with ^{111}In bound at the DOTA located at the C-terminal of the peptide. The complex was assessed by SPECT in tumor-bearing mice 4 h after injection [70]. A monomer form of AE120 agonist (AE105) with high binding affinity with human uPAR ($K_d \sim 0.4$ nM) [71] was conjugated with a metal chelator (DOTA) to from DOTA:AE105 complex. This complex was further labeled with radioisotopes of [64]Cu [72,73], [177]Lu [74–77], and [68]Ga [75–77] for micro-PET imaging of human uPAR-positive and negative tumor cell lines in vivo. The [64]Cu:DOTA:AE105 complex showed high tumor specificity toward uPAR-positive U87MG human glioblastoma cells xenografted in a mouse model, as compared to the uPAR-negative human breast cancer MDA-MB-435 [72]. Similar results were reported for three different tumor xenografts indicating the higher accumulation of the complex in uPAR positive implants [73]. Comparing the ^{64}Cu with the ^{68}Ga complex, it has been deduced that the latter can reduce the nonspecific uptake of complex in tissues like liver accompanied by reduced tumor uptake. However, overall results revealed 5-fold increase of the ^{68}Ga conjugate in tumor-to-liver ratio and 1.4-fold reduction in absolute tumor accumulation. Moreover, higher muscle uptake for ^{68}Ga containing complexes was also observed, leading to poor PET images. Therefore, going back to Cu, the chelator was replaced to form Cu:[CB:TE2A]:AE105 and Cu:[CB:TE2A-PA]:AE105 conjugates. Although the complex Cu:[CB:TE2A-PA]:AE105 exhibited improved tumor uptake and higher tumor-to-liver ratios 1 h after injection, a significant increase in tumor uptake for [64]Cu:DOTA:AE105 was observed in same cell line (U87MG) 22 h postinjection [76]. The authors concluded that [64]Cu:DOTA:AE105 complex seems to be a preferable imaging probe for PET applications. The [64]Cu:DOTA complex was comparatively unstable and the prolonged circulation time of this complex in blood may lead to the leakage of Cu from the complex. In an alternative approach to avoid the use of metal, the peptide was conjugated with the AlF complex of NOTA to form the ^{19}F complex (^{19}F-AlF:NOTA:AE105) for PET imaging of uPAR-positive prostate cancer cells, PC-3 [77]. Using a PC-3 transplanted mouse model, the optimal tumor-to-background contrast was achieved in 1 h in addition to high tumor specificity and uptake, as compared to the metalized complexes. Considering the fact that both studies utilized different cell lines, a comparison was drawn on the basis of previously described technique which involves correlation between uPAR expression and uptake of the drug by tumor cells [76].

Antibodies that interact with uPAR may control the uPA/uPAR system-mediated signaling processes involved in the invasion and metastasis of tumors. Human recombinant antibodies that compete against uPA and β1 integrins for uPAR binding have been identified using a human Fab library and phage display technology. Two of these human Fabs (2G10 and 2E9) were found to be uPAR antagonistic antibodies, preventing the association of uPA with uPAR whereas 3C6 was hindering the binding of β1 integrin with uPAR. The results showed that these competitive antibodies disrupt the cell signaling and invasion processes initiated by uPA/uPAR system in H1299 lung cancer cell line in vitro [78]. 3C6 and 2G10 were also employed as imaging probes for the detection of uPAR in breast cancer xenografts visualized by SPECT in vivo [79].

13.2 ATF-BASED PHOTOSENSITIZERS FOR PHOTODYNAMIC THERAPY AND IMAGING

ATF is the main fragment responsible for binding to uPAR and has been used in both imaging and photodynamic therapy (PDT) by targeting uPAR.

A fluorescent dye Cy5.5 that was conjugated with ATF to form an uPAR targeted multimodality imaging probe was developed by Yang et al. The Cy5.5-ATF complex was conjugated with iron oxide nanoparticles and was employed for imaging of uPAR-overexpressing tumors [80] such as breast [81] and pancreatic cells [82] visualized by MRI or near infrared (NIR) fluorescence microscopy, in a tumor-implanted nude mouse model. ATF has been utilized in the uPAR-targeting drug delivery of noscapine, a naturally occurring antitumor alkaloid, in uPAR-overexpressed tumors [83]. Noscapine was adsorbed on the surface of polymer-coated iron oxide nanoparticles. The drug was delivered to the prostate cancer cells (PC3) in vitro through guided delivery of ATF. For optical visualization, the ATF was conjugated with fluorescent dye Cy5.5. The cell line was incubated with the noscapine-loaded nanoparticles and showed high drug uptake mediated by the uPAR as indicated by MRI and by NIR optical methods. In addition, the uPAR-targeting nanoparticle drug showed 6-fold higher cytotoxicity against the cell line as compared to the drug alone [83]. The use of magnetic iron oxide nanoparticles (IONPs) in drug delivery and MRI imaging is well documented. The uPAR-oriented multifunctional theranostic agents comprising of nanoparticles, ATF, and chemotherapeutics have been designed for drug delivery and imaging. A chemotherapeutic agent, gemcitabine (Gem), conjugated with IONPs via a tetrapeptide (GFLG) linker was linked with ATF to target the uPAR in pancreatic cancer and tumor stromal cells [84]. The multifunctional probe, ATF:IONP:Gem, was able to enter cells by receptor-mediated endocytosis, was released intracellularly, and allowed the visualization of drug accumulations in cancer through MRI. Systemic delivery of the ATF:IONP:Gem inhibited tumor growth in an orthotopic human pancreatic cancer xenograft model. The targeted delivery of the ATF:IONP:Gem and the presence of drug-resistant residual tumors was detected noninvasively by MRI using both T2-weighted and T1-weighted ultrashort echo time imaging [84]. In another study, a fluorescent drug doxorubicin (Dox) combined with the ATF:IONPs was used for specific delivery and imaging against breast cancer cell line in vitro. The nanoparticle encapsulated drug was fairly stable at pH 7.4, but could be released from the nanoparticles at pH 4.0–5.0 within 2 h. ATF:IONP-bound doxorubicin (Dox) was accumulated in breast cancer cell lines in higher concentration than the equivalent dose of free Dox and produced a stronger inhibitory effect on tumor cell growth, making it feasible to monitor drug delivery using MRI [85]. Dox is a highly efficient chemotherapy agent that can cause cardiotoxicity, limiting its clinical application. Recently, Dox-associated cardiotoxicity was minimized by embedding Dox inside recombinant human serum albumin (HSA) fused with ATF (ATF-HSA). HSA functions physiologically as a fatty acid carrier in blood flow and can also bind exogenous drugs in the circulation. The in vivo administration of ATF-HSA:DOX complex to hepatoma H22 tumor bearing mice showed high specificity and good antitumor efficacy of the complex as compared to free Dox, and at the same time, lower cardiotoxicity [86]. Lanthanide-doped upconversion nanoparticles (UCNPs) were conjugated with ATF and exhibited specific recognition of cancer cells overexpressing uPAR [87,88]. A uPAR targeted imaging probe was developed by the conjugation of NIR-830 dye with ATF and IONPs and was specifically targeted to orthotopic mouse models with mammary tumors after systemic delivery. FMT enabled the detection of both locally recurrent tumor and lung metastasis in the mammary tumor model 72 h after systemic administration of the uPAR-targeted NIR-830-labeled ATF imaging probes [89].

Precise localization of tumor margins is a key prognostic factor for the survival of cancer patients with resectable tumors [90]. The patients with smeared and undefinable tumor margins require additional surgery or postoperative radio- or chemotherapy [91,92]. Therefore, a reliable optical probe is likely to be useful in real-time detection of tumor margins during the surgical resection process. Five different optical imaging probes have been designed and evaluated taking advantage of two different tumor cell receptors, that is, uPAR and Epidermal Growth Factor receptor (EGFR). Recombinant ATF or anti-EGFR single-chain antibodies

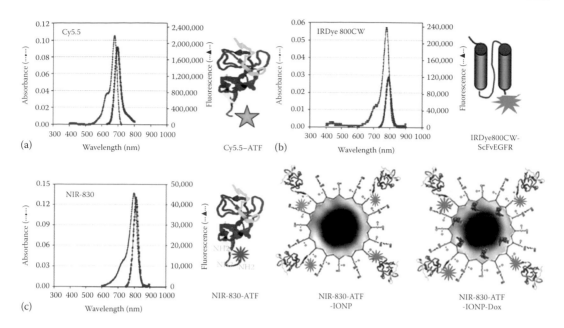

Figure 13.3 Schematic of optical imaging probes labeled with different NIR dyes. (a) Cy5.5-recombinant ATF imaging probe has an excitation wavelength of 680 nm and an emission wavelength of 694 nm. (b) IRDye800CW labeled single chain antibody (ScFvEGFR) imaging probe has an excitation wavelength of 780 nm and emission wavelength of 790 nm. (c) Three NIR-830 dye-labeled optical imaging probes were produced, including NIR-830:ATF peptide probe, NIR-830:ATF:IONP nanoparticle probe, and NIR-830:ATF-theranostic IONP carrying Dox. NIR-830 dye-labeled probes have an excitation wavelength of 800 nm and emission wavelength of 825 nm. (Adapted from Yang, L.L. et al., *Theranostics*, 4, 106, 2014. With permission.)

(scFv) were labeled with NIR dyes followed by coupling with IONPs to form either peptide imaging probes or peptide-conjugated nanoparticle imaging probes (Figure 13.3). In vivo imaging of the probes after systemic delivery, in mice bearing syngeneic mouse mammary tumors or human orthotopic breast or pancreatic cancers, showed the specific accumulation of these probes in the tumor and stromal margins. Histological analysis of the tumor tissues revealed that the uPAR-targeted nanoparticles were present in the tumor edge and stromal cells immediately adjacent to the tumor border. Furthermore, residual tumor detection was possible by optical imaging, followed by resection [93].

PDT is now emerging as a minimally invasive oncologic [94,95] as well as nononcologic [96,97] therapeutic modality. The therapeutic function of PDT requires the presence of photosensitizers (PSs), molecular oxygen, and visible light in the pathological tissues. Upon light illumination the PS is activated and transfers light energy to the surrounding molecular oxygen, and ultimately generates cytotoxic reactive oxygen species (ROS) that consequently lead to cell death and tissue destruction. A number of PSs have been approved for oncological and nononcological clinical applications, with Photofrin being the pioneer [98]. Dark toxicity and lack of tumor specificity are among the major shortcomings in currently employed PS [99,100]. Different strategies have been adopted to overcome these problems leading to the evolution of second- and third-generation PS. Among various other approaches [101–103], the bioconjugation of PS to the tumor-specific carrier molecules, such as antibodies, synthetic peptides, or recombinant proteins (e.g., epidermal growth factors, EGF) [104,105], is now an extensive area of research. Considering the prime role of the uPA/uPAR system and its components in tumor formation and metastasis, a new generation of PS aimed at receptor-mediated targeting is currently being explored. As examples, poly-lysine conjugated with PSs (chlorin-e6, Ce6 [106] or pheophorbide a, PFA [107]) via peptide linker to form a polymeric photosensitizer prodrug was reported to be specific to tumors expressing uPA. The PSs on the polylysine interact with each other and do not have photosensitizing activity due to quenching. The linkers in these conjugates have sequences corresponding to the uPA cleavage site. As mentioned earlier, uPA is typically found at high concentration in breast tumor tissues and can mediate proteolytic cleavage of these peptide linkers, releasing PSs and leading to the restoration of photosensitizing activity [107–109] with tumor specificity. Similarly, protease-sensitive PSs such as PHA [110,111] and Ce6 [112] that are activatable through enzymatic cleavage by MMP-2 [111] or MMP-7 [110] or Cathepsin B [112] have also been reported.

In these cases, PS molecules are typically noncytotoxic due to intramolecular fluorescence quenching. Followed by receptor-mediated tumor accumulation, the photosensitizer can be activated by cleavage by various stimuli, for example, tissue environment or enzymes [98].

Phthalocyanines (Pcs) are a versatile class of macrocyclic compounds that possess great potential for imaging and PDT applications, owing to their improved photophysical and photochemical properties over the classical porphyrin photosensitizers [113,114]. uPAR-targeted tumor accumulation of mono-substituted β-carboxy phthalocyanine zinc (CPZ) was achieved by conjugating the CPZ with ATF. ATF was covalently linked to the CPZ through a linker allowing the amide bond formation between the two compounds. The formed ATF:CPZ complex was analyzed and showed promising in vitro photodynamic efficacy against uPAR-overexpressing cell lines. The photosensitizer was preferentially accumulated in the tumor region in H22 tumor-bearing mice showing its potential for tumor imaging [115].

Human serum albumin (HSA) is a plasma protein with long half-life of 19 days. Besides modulating the osmotic pressure and regulating the fluid distribution in the body compartments, HSA possesses an extraordinary ligand-binding capacity. HSA plays a vital role in the transportation and metabolism of fatty acids, thyroxine, heme, and bilirubin. In addition, HSA is capable of tightly binding to many drugs such as aspirin, carboplatin, and cisplatin with up to nanomolar dissociation constants. The long plasma half-life and its binding affinity with numerous ligands have introduced HSA as a promising candidate in drug delivery of therapeutic peptides, proteins, and other drug molecules [116]. Keeping in view the versatility of HSA in drug delivery, a doxorubicin derivative (INNO-206) that covalently interacted with endogenous albumin showed higher antitumor activity compared to the free doxorubicin derivative in tumor-bearing models. However, it should be noted that HSA itself does not have any highly specific receptor on the tumor cell surface; therefore, it is preferable to be anchored to a tumor-specific molecule to achieve tumor targeting capability. In that context, a recombinant HSA was fused with ATF through its N-terminus for targeting the uPAR on tumors. The ATF-HSA was further loaded with the mono-substituted β-carboxy phthalocyanine zinc (CPZ) onto HSA drug binding sites to form a noncovalent drug–protein complex (1:1) abbreviated as ATF-HSA:CPZ (Figure 13.4). The complex was water soluble, in contrast to the insolubility of CPZ, and was highly stable in aqueous solution. Such formulation of the loading of CPZ inside ATF-HSA did not perturb the receptor-binding capability of ATF by the typically hydrophobic PS CPZ. In vitro ATF-HSA:CPZ showed tumor specificity toward the uPAR-overexpressing tumor cells. In vivo experiments of ATF-HSA:CPZ showed its great potential in tumor imaging by fluorescence molecular tomography and potent antitumor properties in tumor-bearing mouse models with a low dose of 0.080 μmol/kg, or 0.050 mg CPZ/kg of mouse body weight. The study demonstrated that ATF:HSA complex was a promising drug carrier agent with therapeutic potential in both imaging and clinical PDT [117].

Murine uPAR binds to murine ATF 400-fold stronger than to human ATF; therefore, murine ATF is expected to be a much better targeting agent in murine tumor models, and a murine version of this drug carrier was designed and synthesized. The new mATF–HSA complex was loaded with the CPZ to form the ultimate molecular complex mATF–HSA:CPZ. This complex showed good affinity with the murine uPAR in vitro, which proved that the mATF in the mATF–HSA:CPZ construct possessed receptor-binding capability. In fact, mATF–HSA:CPZ showed an improved tumor targeting specificity by FMT imaging and an enhanced PDT efficacy compared to its human counterpart (hATF–HSA:CPZ) in murine H22 tumor-bearing mice, using a dose of 0.080 μmol/kg, or 0.050 mg CPZ/kg of mouse body weight. Therefore, mATF–HSA is a promising drug carrier toward murine-uPAR overexpressing tumors and could be a useful tool to study murine tumor models [118].

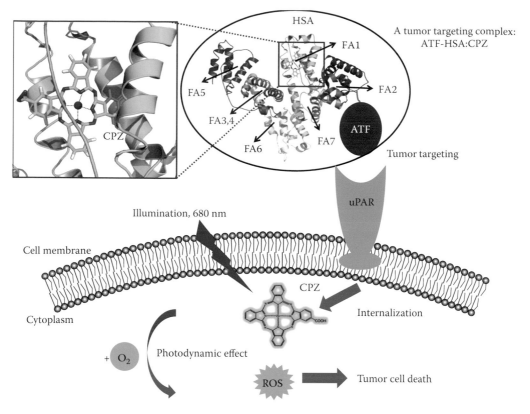

Figure 13.4 A bifunctional recombinant protein ATF:HSA can target tumors through the urokinase receptor (uPAR) that is overexpressed on the tumor cell surfaces. HSA has multiple ligand binding sites (the fatty acid binding sites of HSA are labeled, FA1–FA7). In this study, ATF:HSA was loaded with a large hydrophobic photo-sensitizer, mono-substituted β-carboxy phthalocyanine zinc (ZnPc-COOH, abbreviated as CPZ), which bound at the FA1 site (inset). The ATF:HSA:CPZ displays cytotoxicity toward uPAR-expressing tumor cells upon light illumination.

13.3 SUMMARY

The past years have seen many successful imaging studies utilizing the uPA/uPAR system using reporter molecules based on peptides, antibody, and recombinant proteins. In fact, PET probes based on a uPAR inhibitory peptide (AE105) have entered clinical trials for the diagnosis of aggressive cancers (http://clinicaltrials.gov/). It appears uPA/uPAR system remains promising for the further imaging application.

A fragment of uPA, ATF, has been used extensively in recent years to target uPAR. Recombinant ATF was modified for conjugation to many different type of carriers, for example, nanoparticles, photosensitizers, HSA, or drugs (doxorubicin). Interestingly, such modifications seem to not reduce the capability of ATF to recognize uPAR on the tumor surface. Thus, recombinant ATF has emerged as a versatile targeting agent for uPAR. Small organic molecule inhibitors of uPAR are currently undergoing active development. Although the specificity of these small molecule uPAR inhibitors remains to be demonstrated, in common with many other small molecule drugs, this development is an important direction based on the advantage of good druggability of small molecules and the specific tumor targeting of uPAR inhibitory peptides.

REFERENCES

1. Ngo, J.C. et al., Structural basis for therapeutic intervention of uPA/uPAR system. *Curr Drug Targets*, 2011. **12**: 1729–1743.

2. Dupont, D.M. et al., Biochemical properties of plasminogen activator inhibitor-1. *Front Biosci*, 2009. **14**: 1337–1361.

3. Dano, K. et al., Plasminogen activators, tissue degradation, and cancer. *Adv Cancer Res*, 1985. **44**(2): 139–266.

4. Degryse, B. et al., Domain 2 of the urokinase receptor contains an integrin-interacting epitope with intrinsic signaling activity: Generation of a new integrin inhibitor. *J Biol Chem*, 2005. **280**(26): 24792–24803.

5. Chaurasia, P. et al., A region in urokinase plasminogen receptor domain III controlling a functional association with alpha5beta1 integrin and tumor growth. *J Biol Chem*, 2006. **281**(21): 14852–14863.

6. Stoppelli, M.P. et al., Differentiation-enhanced binding of the amino-terminal fragment of human urokinase plasminogen activator to a specific receptor on U937 monocytes. *Proc Natl Acad Sci USA*, 1985. **82**(15): 4939–4943.

7. Schweinitz, A. et al., Design of novel and selective inhibitors of urokinase-type plasminogen activator with improved pharmacokinetic properties for use as antimetastatic agents. *J Biol Chem*, 2004. **279**(32): s33613–33622.

8. Cooke, R.M. et al., The solution structure of human epidermal growth factor. *Nature*, 1987. **327**(6120): 339–341.

9. Rabbani, S.A. et al., Structural requirements for the growth factor activity of the amino-terminal domain of urokinase. *J Biol Chem*, 1992. **267**(20): 14151–14156.

10. Bdeir, K. et al., The kringle stabilizes urokinase binding to the urokinase receptor. *Blood*, 2003. **102**(10): 3600–3608.

11. Huai, Q. et al., Structure of human urokinase plasminogen activator in complex with its receptor. *Science*, 2006. **311**(5761): 656–659.

12. Heymans, S. et al., Inhibition of plasminogen activators or matrix metalloproteinases prevents cardiac rupture but impairs therapeutic angiogenesis and causes cardiac failure. *Nat Med*, 1999. **5**(10): 1135–1142.

13. Jean-Claude, J. et al., Possible key role for plasmin in the pathogenesis of abdominal aortic aneurysms. *Surgery*, 1994. **116**(2): 472–478.

14. Busso, N. et al., Exacerbation of antigen-induced arthritis in urokinase-deficient mice. *J Clin Invest*, 1998. **102**(1): 41–50.

15. Gveric, D. et al., Plasminogen activators in multiple sclerosis lesions: Implications for the inflammatory response and axonal damage. *Brain*, 2001. **124**(Pt 10): 1978–1988.

16. Almholt, K. et al., Reduced metastasis of transgenic mammary cancer in urokinase-deficient mice. *Int J Cancer*, 2005. **113**(4): 525–532.

17. Andreasen, P.A. et al., The urokinase-type plasminogen activator system in cancer metastasis: A review. *Int J Cancer*, 1997. **72**(1): 1–22.

18. Schmitt, M. et al., Cancer therapy trials employing level-of-evidence-1 disease forecast cancer biomarkers uPA and its inhibitor PAI-1. *Expert Review of Molecular Diagnostics*, 2011. **11**(6): 617–634.

19. Ploug, M., Structure–function relationships in the interaction between the urokinase-type plasminogen activator and its receptor. *Curr Pharm Des*, 2003. **9**(19): 1499–1528.

20. Smith, H.W. and C.J. Marshall, Regulation of cell signalling by uPAR. *Nat Rev Mol Cell Biol*, 2010. **11**(1): 23–36.

21. Binder, B.R. et al., uPAR-uPA-PAI-1 interactions and signaling: A vascular biologist's view. *Thromb Haemost*, 2007. **97**(3): 336–342.

22. Herz, J. et al., LDL receptor-related protein internalizes and degrades uPA-PAI-1 complexes and is essential for embryo implantation. *Cell*, 1992. **71**(3): 411–421.

23. Nykjaer, A. et al., Recycling of the urokinase receptor upon internalization of the uPA: Serpin complexes. *Embo J*, 1997. **16**(10): 2610–2620.

24. Ploug, M. et al., Photoaffinity labeling of the human receptor for urokinase-type plasminogen activator using a decapeptide antagonist. Evidence for a composite ligand-binding site and a short interdomain separation. *Biochemistry*, 1998. **37**(11): 3612–3622.

25. Roldan, A.L. et al., Cloning and expression of the receptor for human urokinase plasminogen activator, a central molecule in cell surface, plasmin dependent proteolysis. *Embo J*, 1990. **9**(2): 467–474.

26. Plesner, T. et al., Structure, function and expression on blood and bone marrow cells of the urokinase-type plasminogen activator receptor, uPAR. *Stem Cells*, 1997. **15**(6): 398–408.

27. Llinas, P. et al., Crystal structure of the human urokinase plasminogen activator receptor bound to an antagonist peptide. *Embo J*, 2005. **24**(9): 1655–1663.

28. Barinka, C. et al., Structural basis of interaction between urokinase-type plasminogen activator and its receptor. *J Mol Biol*, 2006. **363**(2): 482–495.

29. Huai, Q. et al., Crystal structures of two human vitronectin, urokinase and urokinase receptor complexes. *Nat Struct Mol Biol*, 2008. **15**(4): 422–423.

30. Kasumi, T. et al., The effects of vitronectin on specific interactions between urokinase-type plasminogen activator and its receptor: Ab initio molecular orbital calculations. *Mol Simul*, 2013. **39**(10): 769–779.

31. Tsuji, S. et al., The effects of amino-acid mutations on specific interactions between urokinase-type plasminogen activator and its receptor: Ab initio molecular orbital calculations. *J Mol Graph Model*, 2011. **29**(8): 975–984.

32. Mertens, H.D. et al., A flexible multidomain structure drives the function of the urokinase-type plasminogen activator receptor (uPAR). *J Biol Chem*, 2012. **287**(41): 34304–34315.

33. Norton, L. and J. Massagué, Is cancer a disease of self-seeding? *Nat Med*, 2006. **12**(8): 875–878.

34. Billottet, C. et al., Rapid tumor development and potent vascularization are independent events in carcinoma producing FGF-1 or FGF-2. *Oncogene*, 2002. **21**(53): 8128–8139.

35. Gontero, P. et al., Metastasis markers in bladder cancer: A review of the literature and clinical considerations. *Eur Urol*, 2004. **46**(3): 296–311.

36. Lakka, S.S. et al., Adenovirus-mediated antisense urokinase-type plasminogen activator receptor gene transfer reduces tumor cell invasion and metastasis in non-small cell lung cancer cell lines. *Clin Cancer Res*, 2001. **7**(4): 1087–1093.

37. Holst-Hansen, C. et al., Urokinase-type plasminogen activation in three human breast cancer cell lines correlates with their in vitro invasiveness. *Clin Exp Metastasis*, 1996. **14**(3): 297–307.

38. Schnaper, H.W. et al., Plasminogen activators augment endothelial cell organization in vitro by two distinct pathways. *J Cell Physiol*, 1995. **165**(1): 107–118.

39. Duffy, M.J., The urokinase plasminogen activator system: Role in malignancy. *Curr Pharm Des*, 2004. **10**(1): 39–49.

40. Choong, P.F. and A.P. Nadesapillai, Urokinase plasminogen activator system: A multifunctional role in tumor progression and metastasis. *Clin Orthop Relat Res*, 2003(415 Suppl.): S46–S58.

41. Sidenius, N. and F. Blasi, The urokinase plasminogen activator system in cancer: Recent advances and implication for prognosis and therapy. *Cancer Metastasis Rev*, 2003. **22**(2–3): 205–222.

42. Waltz, D.A. et al., Plasmin and plasminogen activator inhibitor type 1 promote cellular motility by regulating the interaction between the urokinase receptor and vitronectin. *J Clin Invest*, 1997. **100**(1): 58–67.

43. Stephens, R.W. et al., Plasma urokinase receptor levels in patients with colorectal cancer: Relationship to prognosis. *J Natl Cancer Inst*, 1999. **91**(10): 869–874.

44. Foekens, J.A. et al., The urokinase system of plasminogen activation and prognosis in 2780 breast cancer patients. *Cancer Res*, 2000. **60**(3): 636–643.

45. Kita, Y. et al., Expression of uPAR mRNA in peripheral blood is a favourite marker for metastasis in gastric cancer cases. *Br J Cancer*, 2009. **100**(1): 153–159.

46. Tyndall, J.D. et al., Peptides and small molecules targeting the plasminogen activation system: Towards prophylactic anti-metastasis drugs for breast cancer. *Recent Pat Anticancer Drug Discov*, 2008. **3**(1): 1–13.

47. Nalla, A.K. et al., Suppression of uPAR retards radiation-induced invasion and migration mediated by integrin beta1/FAK signaling in medulloblastoma. *PLoS One*, 2010. **5**(9): e13006.

48. Kenny, H.A. et al., Targeting the urokinase plasminogen activator receptor inhibits ovarian cancer metastasis. *Clin Cancer Res*, 2011. **17**(3): 459–471.

49. Mazar, A.P., Urokinase plasminogen activator receptor choreographs multiple ligand interactions: Implications for tumor progression and therapy. *Clin Cancer Res*, 2008. **14**(18): 5649–5655.

50. Zhang, J. et al., Activation of urokinase plasminogen activator and its receptor axis is essential for macrophage infiltration in a prostate cancer mouse model. *Neoplasia*, 2011. **13**(1): 23–30.

51. Gondi, C.S. et al., Down-regulation of uPAR and uPA activates caspase-mediated apoptosis and inhibits the PI3K/AKT pathway. *Int J Oncol*, 2007. **31**(1): 19–27.

52. Dass, C.R. et al., Downregulation of uPAR confirms link in growth and metastasis of osteosarcoma. *Clin Exp Metastasis*, 2005. **22**(8): 643–652.

53. Zhang, Y.Y. et al., Metastasis-associated factors facilitating the progression of colorectal cancer. *Asian Pac J Cancer Prev*, 2012. **13**(6): 2437–2444.

54. Rao, J.S. et al., Inhibition of invasion, angiogenesis, tumor growth, and metastasis by adenovirus-mediated transfer of antisense uPAR and MMP-9 in non-small cell lung cancer cells. *Mol Cancer Ther*, 2005. **4**(9): 1399–1408.

55. Blasi, F. and P. Carmeliet, uPAR: A versatile signalling orchestrator. *Nat Rev Mol Cell Biol*, 2002. **3**(12): 932–943.

56. Asuthkar, S. et al., Urokinase-type plasminogen activator receptor (uPAR)-mediated regulation of WNT/ß-catenin signaling is enhanced in irradiated medulloblastoma cells. *J Biol Chem*, 2012. **287**(24): 20576–20589.

57. Margheri, F. et al., The receptor for urokinase-plasminogen activator (uPAR) controls plasticity of cancer cell movement in mesenchymal and amoeboid migration style. *Oncotarget*, 2014. **5**(6): 1538.

58. Moreau, M. et al., ß-Catenin and NF-?B cooperate to regulate the uPA/uPAR system in cancer cells. *Int J Cancer*, 2011. **128**(6): 1280–1292.

59. van Oosten, M. et al., Selecting potential targetable biomarkers for imaging purposes in colorectal cancer using TArget Selection Criteria (TASC): A novel target identification tool. *Trans Oncol*, 2011. **4**(2): 71–82.

60. Krishnamachary, B. et al., Regulation of colon carcinoma cell invasion by hypoxia-inducible factor 1. *Cancer Res*, 2003. **63**(5): 1138–1143.

61. Boonstra, M.C. et al., Expression of uPAR in tumor-associated stromal cells is associated with colorectal cancer patient prognosis: A TMA study. *BMC Cancer*, 2014. **14**(1): 269.

62. Illemann, M. et al., Urokinase-type plasminogen activator receptor (uPAR) on tumor-associated macrophages is a marker of poor prognosis in colorectal cancer. *Cancer Med*, 2014. **3**(4): 855–864.

63. Hildenbrand, R. and A. Schaaf, The urokinase-system in tumor tissue stroma of the breast and breast cancer cell invasion. *Int J Oncol*, 2009. **34**(1): 15–23.

64. Ignar, D.M. et al., Inhibition of establishment of primary and micrometastatic tumors by a urokinase plasminogen activator receptor antagonist. *Clin Exp Metastasis*, 1998. **16**(1): 9–20.

65. Khanna, M. et al., Targeting multiple conformations leads to small molecule inhibitors of the upar.upa protein–protein interaction that block cancer cell invasion. *ACS Chem Biol*, 2011. **6**: 1232–1243.

66. Liu, D. et al., A new class of orthosteric uPAR. uPA small-molecule antagonists are allosteric inhibitors of the uPAR. Vitronectin interaction. *ACS Chem Biol*, 2015. **10**(6): 1521–1534.

67. Jacobsen, B. et al., Structure and inhibition of the urokinase-type plasminogen activator receptor, The Cancer Degradome, 2008, Springer, New York, pp. 699–719.

68. Persson, M. and A. Kjaer, Urokinase-type plasminogen activator receptor (uPAR) as a promising new imaging target: Potential clinical applications. *Clin Physiol Funct Imaging*, 2013. **33**(5): 329–337.

69. Wang, M. et al., Targeting the urokinase plasminogen activator receptor with synthetic self-assembly nanoparticles. *Bioconjug Chem*, 2009. **20**(1): 32–40.

70. Liu, D. et al., Synthesis and characterization of an (111)In-labeled peptide for the in vivo localization of human cancers expressing the urokinase-type plasminogen activator receptor (uPAR). *Bioconjug Chem*, 2009. **20**(5): 888–894.

71. Ploug, M. et al., Peptide-derived antagonists of the urokinase receptor. Affinity maturation by combinatorial chemistry, identification of functional epitopes, and inhibitory effect on cancer cell intravasation. *Biochemistry*, 2001. **40**(40): 12157–12168.

72. Li, Z.B. et al., Imaging of urokinase-type plasminogen activator receptor expression using a 64Cu-labeled linear peptide antagonist by microPET. *Clin Cancer Res*, 2008. **14**(15): 4758–4766.

73. Persson, M. et al., Quantitative PET of human urokinase-type plasminogen activator receptor with 64Cu-DOTA-AE105: Implications for visualizing cancer invasion. *J Nucl Med*, 2012. **53**(1): 138–145.

74. Persson, M. et al., New peptide receptor radionuclide therapy of invasive cancer cells in vivo studies using ^{177}Lu-DOTA-AE105 targeting uPAR in human colorectal cancer xenografts, *Nucl Med Biol*, 2012. **39**(7): 962–969.

75. Persson, M. et al, ^{68}Ga-labeling and in vivo evaluation of a uPAR binding DOTA-and NODAGA-conjugated peptide for PET imaging of invasive cancer. *Nucl Med Biol*, 2012. **394**: 560–569.

76. Persson, M. et al., Improved PET imaging of uPAR expression using new 64Cu-labeled cross-bridged peptide ligands: comparative in vitro and in vivo studies. *Theranostics*, 2013. 3(9): 618–632.

77. Persson, M. et al., First (18)F-labeled ligand for PET imaging of uPAR: In vivo studies in human prostate cancer xenografts. *Nucl Med Biol*, 2013. **40**(5): 618–624.

78. Duriseti, S. et al., Antagonistic anti-urokinase plasminogen activator receptor (uPAR) antibodies significantly inhibit uPAR-mediated cellular signaling and migration. *J Biol Chem*, 2010. **285**(35): 26878–26888.

79. LeBeau, A.M. et al., Imaging the urokinase plasminongen activator receptor in preclinical breast cancer models of acquired drug resistance. *Theranostics*, 2014. **4**(3): 267–279.

80. Leung, K., Cy5.5-Amino-terminal fragment of urokinase-type plasminogen activator conjugated to magnetic iron oxide nanoparticles, in *Molecular Imaging and Contrast Agent Database (MICAD)*, 2004. Bethesda, MD: National Center for Biotechnology Information (US). Available from http://www.ncbi.nlm.nih.gov/books/NBK23353/.

81. Yang, L. et al., Receptor-targeted nanoparticles for in vivo imaging of breast cancer. *Clin Cancer Res*, 2009. **15**(14): 4722–4732.

82. Yang, L. et al., Molecular imaging of pancreatic cancer in an animal model using targeted multifunctional nanoparticles. *Gastroenterology*, 2009. **136**(5): 1514–1525.e2.

83. Abdalla, M.O. et al., Enhanced noscapine delivery using uPAR-targeted optical-MR imaging trackable nanoparticles for prostate cancer therapy. *J Control Release*, 2011. **149**(3): 314–322.

84. Lee, G.Y. et al., Theranostic nanoparticles with controlled release of gemcitabine for targeted therapy and MRI of pancreatic cancer. *ACS Nano*, 2013. **7**(3): 2078–2089.

85. Yang, L. et al., Development of receptor targeted magnetic iron oxide nanoparticles for efficient drug delivery and tumor imaging. *J Biomed Nanotechnol*, 2008. **4**(4): 439–449.

86. Zheng, K. et al., Dual actions of albumin packaging and tumor targeting enhance the antitumor efficacy and reduce the cardiotoxicity of doxorubicin in vivo. *Int J Nanomed*, 2015. **10**: 5327–5342.

87. Ai, Y. et al., Lanthanide-doped $NaScF_4$ nanoprobes: Crystal structure, optical spectroscopy and bio-detection. *Nanoscale*, 2013. **5**(14): 6430–6438.

88. Chen, Z. et al., Lanthanide-doped luminescent nano-bioprobes for the detection of tumor markers. *Nanoscale*, 2015. **7**(10): 4274–4290.

89. Tan, Y. et al., DOT corrected fluorescence molecular tomography using targeted contrast agents for small animal tumor imaging. *J X Ray Sci Technol*, 2013. **21**(1): 43–52.

90. Kimbrough, C.W. et al., Tumor-positive resection margins reflect an aggressive tumor biology in pancreatic cancer. *J Surg Oncol*, 2013. **107**(6): 602–607.

91. Konstantinidis, I.T. et al., Pancreatic ductal adenocarcinoma: Is there a survival difference for R1 resections versus locally advanced unresectable tumors? What is a "true" R0 resection? *Ann Surg*, 2013. **257**(4): 731–736.

92. Jung, W. et al., Factors associated with re-excision after breast-conserving surgery for early-stage breast cancer. *J Breast Cancer*, 2012. **15**(4): 412–419.

93. Yang, L.L. et al., uPAR-targeted optical imaging contrasts as theranostic agents for tumor margin detection. *Theranostics*, 2014. **4**(1): 106–118.

94. Castano, A.P. et al., Photodynamic therapy and anti-tumour immunity. *Nat Rev Cancer*, 2006. **6**(7): 535–545.

95. Schuitmaker, J. et al., Photodynamic therapy: A promising new modality for the treatment of cancer. *J Photochem Photobiol B Biol*, 1996. **34**(1): 3–12.

96. Erikitola, O. et al., Photodynamic therapy for central serous chorioretinopathy. *Eye*, 2014. **28**: 944–957.

97. Mitra, A. and G. Stables, Topical photodynamic therapy for non-cancerous skin conditions. *Photodiagnosis Photodyn Ther*, 2006. **3**(2): 116–127.

98. Lovell, J.F. et al., Activatable photosensitizers for imaging and therapy. *Chem Rev*, 2010. **110**(5): 2839–2857.

99. Paszko, E. et al., Nanodrug applications in photodynamic therapy. *Photodiagnosis Photodyn Ther*, 2011. **8**(1): 14–29.

100. Celli, J.P. et al., Imaging and photodynamic therapy: Mechanisms, monitoring, and optimization. *Chem Rev*, 2010. **110**(5): 2795–2838.

101. Weijer, R. et al., Enhancing photodynamic therapy of refractory solid cancers: Combining second-generation photosensitizers with multi-targeted liposomal delivery. *J Photochem Photobiol C Photochem Rev*, 2015. **23**: 103–131.

102. Lammers, T. et al., Drug targeting to tumors: Principles, pitfalls and (pre-) clinical progress. *J Control Rel*, 2012. **161**(2): 175–187.

103. Danhier, F. et al., To exploit the tumor microenvironment: Passive and active tumor targeting of nanocarriers for anti-cancer drug delivery. *J Control Rel*, 2010. **148**(2): 135–146.

104. Taquet, J.-P. et al., Phthalocyanines covalently bound to biomolecules for a targeted photodynamic therapy. *Curr Med Chem*, 2007. **14**(15): 1673–1687.

105. Pereira, P.M. et al., Antibodies armed with photosensitizers: From chemical synthesis to photobiological applications. *Org Biomolecular Chem*, 2015. **13**(9): 2518–2529.

106. Choi, Y. et al., Protease-mediated phototoxicity of a polylysine–chlorine6 conjugate. *Chem Med Chem*, 2006. **1**(7): 698–701.

107. Gabriel, D. et al., Urokinase-plasminogen-activator sensitive polymeric photosensitizer prodrugs: Design, synthesis and in vitro evaluation. *J Drug Deliv Sci Technol*, 2009. **19**(1): 15–24.

108. Zuluaga, M.F. et al., Enhanced prostate cancer targeting by modified protease sensitive photosensitizer prodrugs. *Mol Pharm*, 2012. **9**(6): 1570–1579.

109. Zuluaga, M.-F. et al., Selective photodetection and photodynamic therapy for prostate cancer through targeting of proteolytic activity. *Mol Cancer Ther*, 2013. **12**(3): 306–313.

110. Zheng, G. et al., Photodynamic molecular beacon as an activatable photosensitizer based on protease-controlled singlet oxygen quenching and activation. *Proc Natl Acad Sci*, 2007. **104**(21): 8989–8994.

111. Jang, B. and Y. Choi, Photosensitizer-conjugated gold nanorods for enzyme-activatable fluorescence imaging and photodynamic therapy. *Theranostics*, 2012. **2**(2): 190.

112. Soo-Min Shon, Y.C. et al., Photodynamic therapy using a protease-mediated theranostic agent reduces cathepsin-b activity in mouse atheromata in vivo. *Arterioscler Thromb Vasc Biol*, 2013. **33**(6): 1360–1365.

113. Tedesco, A.C. et al., Synthesis, photophysical and photochemical aspects of phthalocyanines for photo-dynamic therapy. *Curr Org Chem*, 2003. **7**(2): 187–196.
114. Nyokong, T., Desired properties of new phthalocyanines for photodynamic therapy. *Pure Appl Chem*, 2011. **83**(9): 1763–1779.
115. Chen, Z. et al., Zinc phthalocyanine conjugated with the amino-terminal fragment of urokinase for tumor-targeting photodynamic therapy. *Acta Biomatererialia*, 2014. **10**(10): 4257–4268.
116. Elsadek, B. and F. Kratz, Impact of albumin on drug delivery-New applications on the horizon. *J Control Rel*, 2012. **157**(1): 4–28.
117. Li, R. et al., A novel tumor targeting drug carrier for optical imaging and therapy. *Theranostics*, 2014. **4**(6): 642–659.
118. Zhou, X. et al., A drug carrier targeting murine uPAR for photodynamic therapy and tumor imaging. *Acta Biomater*, 2015. **23**: 116–126.

SMALL ANIMAL IMAGING

Vascular imaging in photodynamic therapy

BIN CHEN

14.1 INTRODUCTION

Photodynamic therapy (PDT) is a treatment modality that combines a light-activatable drug (photosensitizer), activated by light typically in the red or near infrared (NIR) range and ambient oxygen (Agostinis et al., 2011). In the presence of oxygen, photosensitizers are activated by light, which results in the generation of reactive oxygen species (ROS) and consequent biological effects via ROS-mediated oxidative stress. With a sufficient amount of photosensitizer, light and oxygen, PDT is able to induce a rapid and efficient cell death, particularly apoptosis, in a variety of cell lines. Because of its effectiveness in inducing cell death, PDT has been approved for the treatment of different types of cancers, precancers, and noncancer diseases (e.g., age-related macular degeneration [AMD], port-wine stain [PWS] birthmarks) where cell proliferation is abnormally activated (Agostinis et al., 2011).

Although PDT may induce direct toxicity to tumor cells and activate antitumor immunity, the vascular effect has been shown as a major contributing factor to the overall antitumor effect of PDT with most, if not all, current photosensitizers (Chen et al., 2006a). PDT vascular effect can be greatly enhanced by using a short drug-light interval (the time between systemic photosensitizer injection and light illumination) when the photosensitizer is predominantly localized in the vasculature. This vascular-targeted PDT protocol has been successfully used in the clinic for the treatment of AMD with the photosensitizer verteporfin (Brown and Mellish, 2001) and is under clinical trial for prostate cancer treatment with the photosensitizer called Tookad (Azzouzi et al., 2015).

As a means of visualizing internal or small structures and dynamic physiological functions that are otherwise invisible to unaided eyes, imaging, particularly noninvasive imaging, is being increasingly used in experimental biomedical research to unravel biological mechanisms and evaluate perturbations to biological systems. Various imaging methods have also been used to study PDT vascular effect. As a matter of fact, much of what we now know about PDT vascular effects is derived from such imaging studies. In this chapter, current understanding of PDT-induced vascular effect together with major imaging modalities that have been used to obtain such knowledge is reviewed with the goal to illustrate that imaging has become an indispensable tool in the study of PDT vascular effects.

14.2 TUMOR VASCULATURE AS A CANCER THERAPEUTIC TARGET

It has long been recognized that tumor tissues depend on the vasculature for substance exchange (delivery of oxygen and nutrients and removal of metabolic wastes) and the supply of blood and cells (Folkman, 2006). In order to keep up with tumor growth and progression, tumors need to continuously develop new vasculature through multiple mechanisms including angiogenesis (generating new blood vessels from existing ones), vasculogenesis (generating new blood vessels from new vascular progenitor cells), and vascular mimicry (formation of new vessels composed of tumor cells) (Carmeliet and Jain, 2011). Compared with normal vasculature, tumor vasculature exhibits significant abnormalities in blood vessel architecture (e.g., tortuosity, dilatation, irregular branching, lack of pericyte, and basement membrane coverage) and function (e.g., stagnant blood flow, increased vascular permeability) (Baluk et al., 2005). Many angiogenic signaling molecules that cause abnormal tumor vasculature have been identified, among which vascular endothelial growth factor (VEGF) is the most well studied and so far the most potent one (Jain, 2014). Drugs targeting VEGF and inhibiting its signaling have been approved for the treatment of various cancers. In addition to inhibiting angiogenesis by targeting VEGF signaling, eradication of existing tumor blood vessels by vascular-disrupting agents is also being actively explored (Mita et al., 2013). However, despite such successes, current vascular-targeted therapy has not fulfilled the expectation, which raises the debate on what is the best way to exploit vasculature to control tumors (Jain, 2014; Rivera and Bergers, 2015). Nevertheless, obvious survival benefits seen in some patients treated with existing drugs as well as promising results reported in many new studies clearly demonstrate that tumor vasculature is a legitimate cancer treatment target.

14.3 PDT: ESSENTIALLY A VASCULAR-DISRUPTING MODALITY

14.3.1 EARLY STUDIES OF PDT VASCULAR EFFECT

It has long been observed that grazing animals ingesting photosensitizing plants and mammals and those that had been photosensitized by porphyrins develop symptoms such as erythema, edema, and hemorrhage (Spikes, 1975). These symptoms are vascular in nature and are indications of photosensitization-induced vascular damage. The first experimental evidence demonstrating that photosensitization causes direct damages to vascular components is probably the study in 1908 by Hausmann, who reported that rabbit erythrocytes were lysed in the presence of hematoporphyrin or chlorophyll with light illumination (Spikes, 1975). Studies in the 1920s further showed that photosensitization with porphyrins inactivated serum proteins, including albumin, globulins, and fibrinogen, by oxidizing amino acids. In the first PubMed-retrieved experimental study involving photosensitization-induced vascular effect, Castellani et al. reported in 1963 that photosensitization with hematoporphyrin caused blood flow arrest and hemolysis in blood vessels in the rat mesentery (Castellani et al., 1963; Spikes, 1975). These early observations provided important evidence of PDT-induced vascular effects and stimulated systematic research on this topic using more advanced experimental techniques.

14.3.2 Use of imaging methods to study PDT vascular response

One technique that is often used to study PDT vascular response is the use of imaging methods. Different from other techniques, imaging is able to provide both structural and functional information about cells and tissues that are inaccessible or invisible to unaided human eyes. With the aid of imaging, we are able to visualize tissue structural abnormalities and functional changes, which enables disease diagnosis and therapeutic response monitoring. Because therapeutic responses (such as PDT vascular response) are dynamic and include systemic reactions from a biological system to a therapeutic perturbation, it is necessary to combine static snapshot imaging methods with dynamic imaging techniques in order to obtain a comprehensive view of a treatment effect. Imaging modalities that have been used for studying PDT vascular response include static ex vivo imaging systems that are able to reveal structural details at high resolutions, and live imaging systems that are capable of providing longitudinal information in live cells and animals (Figure 14.1). Use of these different imaging modalities at whole body, tissue, cellular, and subcellular levels has revealed a plethora of information about vascular structural and functional alterations caused by PDT with different photosensitizers.

14.3.3 PDT vascular response: Perspectives from different imaging modalities

14.3.3.1 EX VIVO IMAGING BY LIGHT, FLUORESCENCE, AND ELECTRON MICROSCOPY

Various ex vivo microscopic imaging methods including light, fluorescence, and electron microscopy have been used to examine vascular structural changes after PDT at tissue, cell, and subcellular levels. Staining tissue samples with hematoxylin and eosin (H&E) and examining H&E staining sections under a light microscope is the simplest and most common imaging method to observe the effects of PDT on vasculature. Use of this simple imaging method led to the finding that PDT with hematoporphyrin derivatives (HpD) caused blood vessel dilation, vessel congestion with red blood cells, and endothelial cell pyknosis (Zhou et al., 1985; Berenbaum et al., 1986). More importantly, endothelial cell damage was observed while surrounding cells still appeared normal, suggesting that endothelial cells are primary targets of HpD-PDT. Similar findings have been reported in PDT studies using other photosensitizers such as Photofrin (Engbrecht et al., 1999), hypericin (Chen et al., 2002), Tookad (Madar-Balakirski et al., 2010) and verteporfin (Chen et al., 2003).

To further determine the effects of PDT on endothelial cells as well as on vascular supporting cells (pericytes, smooth muscle cells) and structural components (basement membrane), tissue sections can be stained with fluorescence-labeled antibodies and examined with a conventional wide-field fluorescence microscope or confocal fluorescence microscope with increased optical resolution due to the elimination of out-of-focus light. PDT with Photofrin induced a rapid loss of staining for endothelial cell marker CD31, and an increase in apoptotic staining in cells surrounding blood vessels, indicating a direct PDT damage to endothelial cells (Engbrecht et al., 1999). Photofrin was found associated with collagen in tumor blood vessel basement membrane, and Photofrin-PDT caused more vascular congestion and ischemia in tumors with higher collagen content, which suggests that basement membrane is involved in PDT-induced vascular effect (Maas et al., 2012). Immunohistochemical staining of lipid peroxidation, an indicator of ROS production, showed its main localization in tumor blood vessels in tumors treated with Tookad–PDT (Gross et al., 2003). For the photosensitizer verteporfin, light treatment caused an immediate surge in the ROS production (Li et al., 2013) and calcium release (Granville et al., 2001), which resulted in rapid damage to microtubules, cell contraction

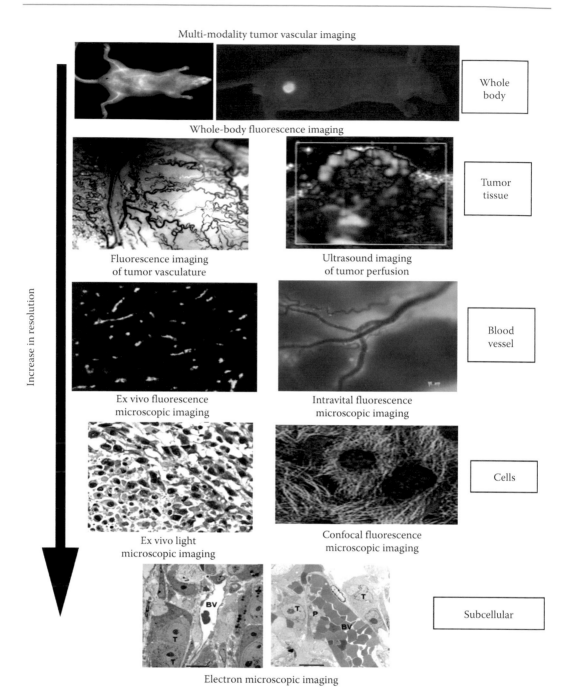

Figure 14.1 Multimodality imaging of PDT vascular effect. Various in vivo and ex vivo imaging modalities ranging from the whole body down to the subcellular level have been integrated to study PDT vascular effect.

(Chen et al., 2006b), and induction of apoptosis (Granville et al., 1999) in endothelial cells. Endothelial cell apoptosis (by TUNEL assay) and proliferation (Ki-67 positive) were examined by immunohistochemistry in choroidal neovascular membranes from AMD patients at different times after verteporfin-PDT (Petermeier et al., 2006) to determine the correlation between endothelial cell death/proliferation and disease recurrence. Increased endothelial cell apoptosis together with reduced cell proliferation was observed at 3 days after PDT, whereas increase in vascularization (CD34 and CD105 positive) and endothelial cell proliferation was commonly found at time points of more than 1 month after treatment when disease recurrence started to happen. All these studies point to the conclusion that PDT with photosensitizers such as Photofrin, Tookad, and verteporfin initiates photochemical reactions at vascular targets such as endothelial cells and basement membranes, which triggers the PDT vascular effect.

Effects of PDT on vascular ultrastructure have been studied with electron microscopy to confirm that the vasculature is a sensitive target of PDT. PDT with hematoporphyrin caused significant endothelial cell damage and blood cell aggregation even before damage to surrounding tumor cells was observed (Reed et al., 1989), suggesting a pivotal role of vascular damage in the overall PDT effect. Examination of mouse tumors by both light and electron microscopy at time points ranging from 0.5 to 24 h after PDT using three photosensitizers, including hematoporphyrin derivative, chlorin and phthalocyanine concluded that tumor destruction by PDT with all three photosensitizers was due to tumor vascular damage rather than direct toxicity to tumor cells (Nelson et al., 1988). Furthermore, the study found that damage to the subendothelial zone of blood vessel wall, an area rich in collagen fibers and other connective tissue elements, was an early observation of PDT-induced vascular effect. Effects of verteporfin-PDT on vasculature have been studied with electron microcopy in AMD patients. Choroidal neovascular membrane surgically removed from a patient at 3 days after PDT with verteporfin showed vessel occlusion by thrombus formation (Moshfeghi et al., 2003). Endothelial cell and pericyte degeneration, thrombus formation, and inflammatory cell infiltration were also reported in a patient at about 1 month after PDT (Ghazi et al., 2001). However, almost no thrombus formation was found at time points of more than 1 month after PDT when the patients' vision started to deteriorate, although evidence of vascular damage (e.g., extravasated erythrocytes and fibrin) still existed, which suggests that sustained verteporfin-PDT outcome depends on complete and permanent vascular occlusion (Moshfeghi et al., 2003). Using electron microscopy, we found that PDT with verteporfin caused rapid mitochondrial swelling and degeneration in endothelial cells both in vitro and in an animal tumor model (Figure 14.2). Clearly, electron microscopic studies not only support the notion that vascular damage is a predominant effect of PDT but also provide important insights into the subcellular target of PDT.

14.3.3.2 IN VIVO OPTICAL IMAGING

Since nothing is more convincing than visualizing therapy-induced tissue structural and functional alterations in living systems and in real time, in vivo imaging has been extensively used for evaluating PDT vascular effects. With its cost-effectiveness, easiness to operate, and high spatial resolution, in vivo optical imaging is certainly the most commonly used in vivo imaging modality in PDT studies. The availability of versatile fluorescence probes, bioluminescent reporters, and the fact that almost all photosensitizers are fluorescent enable the use of multispectral and tomographic fluorescence/bioluminescence imaging to interrogate photosensitizer tissue distribution and PDT effects. In addition to microscopic imaging, the commercial availability of in vivo optical imaging systems greatly promotes macroscopic optical imaging in live animals.

Macroscopic optical imaging of PDT vascular effect typically involves the injection of a fluorescence dye and the capture of fluorescence images as a function of time after injection to visualize blood vessel morphology and probe vascular functions such as blood vessel patency and vascular permeability. Cells can be transfected with fluorescence protein or luciferase genes, which enables the use of noninvasive fluorescence/bioluminescence imaging to report cell viability based on the assumption that dead cells will not be able to emit fluorescence/bioluminescence signal.

Fluorescence angiography using sodium fluorescein or other fluorescent dyes is commonly used for examining vascular structure and function in patients and animals. Due to its high hydrophilicity, sodium fluorescein has no cellular uptake. Following intravenous injection, it is immediately distributed throughout the vascular system and rapidly eliminated through the kidneys. Its bright green fluorescence highlights the pattern of vasculature and alterations in fluorescence intensity are indicative of changes in vascular structure and function. Particularly, hyperfluorescence often suggests leaky blood vessels or high vessel density, whereas hypofluorescence generally indicates perfusion arrest or bleeding. As a common method for examining the retina and choroid vasculature, fluorescein angiography is routinely used in assessing the effectiveness of verteporfin-PDT to occlude choroidal neovasculature in AMD patients (Moshfeghi et al., 2003; Schmidt-Erfurth et al., 2005). It has also been used to evaluate PDT-induced vascular disruption in animal tumor

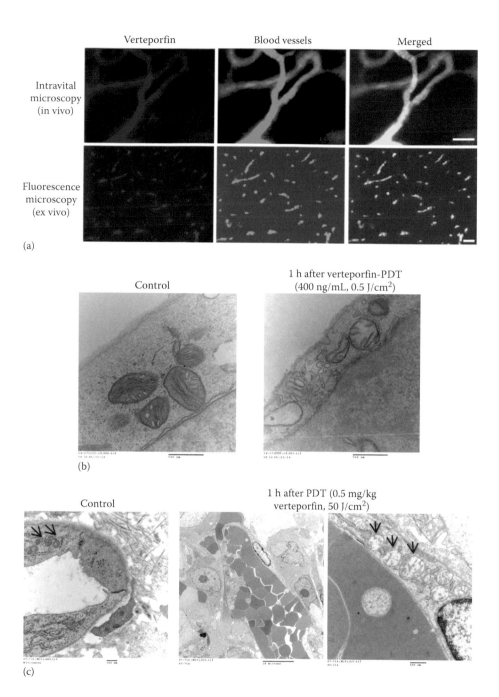

Figure 14.2 (a) Both in vivo and ex vivo fluorescence microscopic imaging demonstrate that verteporfin (0.25 mg/kg) was predominately localized within tumor blood vessels at 15 min after intravenous injection in the orthotopic MatLyLu (MLL) prostate tumor. Tumor blood vessels were visualized by injecting perfusion marker 2000 kDa FITC-dextran. Bars, 100 um. (b) Electron microscopic images of SVEC mouse endothelial cells showing mitochondrial swelling after verteporfin-PDT. (c) Electron microscopic images of PC-3 prostate tumors showing blood vessel congestion and damage to mitochondria (indicated by arrows) after verteporfin-PDT (0.5 mg/kg, 50 J/cm²).

models (Bellnier et al., 1995; Chen et al., 2002). In addition to fluorescein, other fluorescence dyes including indocyanine green (Schmidt-Erfurth et al., 2005), fluorescence dye-labeled albumin (Chen et al., 2008), and high molecular-weight dextran (Madar-Balakirski et al., 2010) have also been used as angiographic tracer molecules. All these studies demonstrate that vascular permeability increase, as indicated by the increase in fluorescence dye exudation in PDT-treated area, was observed within hours after PDT. Occlusion of blood vessels shown by significant decrease in fluorescence occurred at later times (about 24 h). In AMD patients treated with verteporfin-PDT, angiographic fluorescence increase in PDT-treated area, which often occurred within 3 months after PDT, was associated with increased perfusion in the choroidal neovasculature and the worsening of disease (Michels and Schmidt-Erfurth, 2003; Moshfeghi et al., 2003).

Macroscopic in vivo fluorescence/bioluminescence imaging of tumors that have been transfected with fluorescent proteins or luciferase genes represents a convenient and noninvasive imaging method for evaluating tumor cell survival after PDT. We monitored the fluorescence of green fluorescent protein (GFP) in GFP-transfected tumors as a function of time after verteporfin-PDT and observed a dose-dependent inhibition of GFP fluorescence in PDT-treated tumors (Chen et al., 2008). Moreover, we found that tumor regrowth tended to occur at the tumor periphery, which was confirmed by histological examination. Macroscopic fluorescence imaging has also been used to track tumor cell survival in GFP tumors treated with a vascular-targeted PDT using BF2-chelated tetraaryl-azadipyrromethene (ADMP) photosensitizer ADPM06 (Byrne et al., 2009). No recurrence of GFP fluorescence was observed for up to 8 weeks after PDT, suggesting the cure of PDT-treated tumors. With the advantage that no excitation light is needed, in vivo bioluminescence imaging has been used to follow tumor cell survival noninvasively after PDT in luciferase-transfected tumors (Moriyama et al., 2004; Rollakanti et al., 2015). In addition to functioning as a marker for tumor cell survival, GFP fluorescence/bioluminescence can also serve as a gene expression reporter. In this case, GFP or luciferase gene needs to be inserted in a DNA region under the control of an appropriate gene promoter. Activation of gene expression will produce GFP or luciferase, which can be monitored in real time by fluorescence or bioluminescence imaging in live animals. Using tumors expressed with fluorescence or bioluminescence gene expression reporters, PDT has been shown to activate the expression of cell stress genes such as hypoxia-inducible factor (HIF) 1α (Moriyama et al., 2004) and heat shock protein (HSP) 70 (Mitra et al., 2011). It should be pointed out that fluorescent proteins and luciferase are all foreign proteins and therefore immunogenic (Castano et al., 2006). Its immunogenicity may interfere with its application in immunocompetent animals.

To understand the effect of PDT on vascular structure and function at cellular level in live animals, in vivo (intravital) microscopic imaging is needed. As a powerful tool for revealing biomolecular interactions, cellular structures, and dynamic tissue functions in real time at a high resolution, intravital microscopy has been used to study photosensitizer tissue distribution and vascular effect of PDT with a variety of photosensitizing agents including Photofrin (Fingar et al., 1992), verteporfin (Fingar et al., 1999; He et al., 2008; Debefve et al., 2011), MV6401 (Dolmans et al., 2002), aminolevulinic acid (Middelburg et al., 2013), and Tookad (Madar-Balakirski et al., 2010). To facilitate optical imaging, tumors need to be implanted in an external tissue with a shallow depth such as the mouse ear (Madar-Balakirski et al., 2010) or in a window chamber (Dolmans et al., 2002) to enable longitudinal microscopic imaging. Internal tumors need to be surgically exposed for intravital imaging (Fingar et al., 1999; He et al., 2008). As in fluorescence angiography, intravital microscopy also requires the intravenous injection of fluorescent dyes to highlight blood vessels and probe vascular functions. To measure blood cell velocity and determine cell adhesion, blood cells are often labeled with a fluorescent dye and injected back into the vascular system of animals (He et al., 2008; Madar-Balakirski et al., 2010; Debefve et al., 2011).

Intravital microscopy of the rat cremaster muscle showed that Photofrin-PDT caused vessel constriction and increase in vessel permeability and leukocyte adhesion (Fingar et al., 1992). The cyclooxygenase inhibitor indomethacin was able to inhibit vessel constriction and vascular permeability increase, indicating the involvement of vasoactive metabolites of cyclooxygenase (thromboxane, prostacyclin). An increase in vascular permeability, thrombus formation, and blood flow reduction was observed in animals treated with verteporfin-PDT in a dose- and time-dependent manner (Fingar et al., 1999; He et al., 2008; Debefve et al., 2010). Notably, blood vessels with lower flow rates were more sensitive to verteporfin-PDT-induced vascular shutdown than vessels with a higher flow rate. In agreement with light and electron microscopic studies, intravital fluorescence microscopic imaging demonstrated in live animals that verteporfin-PDT decreased endothelial cell viability and caused platelet aggregation (Khurana et al., 2008). Rapid shutdown of tumor vascular perfusion by thrombus formation was also found after PDT with Tookad and MV6401, which was also confirmed by histological assessment (Dolmans et al., 2002; Madar-Balakirski et al., 2010). All these optical imaging studies point to the conclusion that PDT is essentially a vascular disrupting therapy.

14.3.3.3 ULTRASOUND IMAGING

Ultrasound imaging utilizes high frequency sound echos (typically more than 20 kHz) to probe tissue structure and function. Compared with optical light, ultrasonic waves have much deeper penetration and less scattering in tissues, enabling visualization of tissues at depths beyond the limit of optical imaging. Because of the high echogenicity of air, ultrasound imaging contrast can be greatly increased by contrast agents, which are typically emulsions of gas–liquid particles composed of a gaseous core surrounded by a phospholipid shell (Kircher and Willmann, 2012). As a sensitive and noninvasive imaging modality, ultrasound imaging reveals tissue structural details based on the difference in echogenicity and enables the detection of vascular functional change based on the frequency shift in the reflected echo (Doppler effect) when emitted sonic wave encounters moving objects such as circulating blood cells.

Power Doppler ultrasonography has been successfully used for examining the effects of PDT on tumor vascular function (Yu et al., 2005; Ohlerth et al., 2006). Different from color Doppler ultrasonography which uses the frequency shift of reflected echo to estimate the velocity and direction of moving blood cells, power Doppler ultrasonography shows changes in the amplitude of reflected signal to indicate the total number of moving blood cells (perfusion). Power Doppler ultrasonography has been shown to be more sensitive than color Doppler ultrasonography for vascular imaging of small blood vessels and at low blood flow rate, which are often found in tumor tissues. Thus, it is commonly used for tumor diagnosis and assessing the effect of anticancer treatments on tumor vasculature. Power Doppler ultrasonography demonstrates that PDT with Photofrin induced significant reduction in tumor perfusion as early as 15 min after PDT and tumor perfusion continued to decline for at least 6.5 h following treatment in an animal tumor model (Yu et al., 2005). PDT with another photosensitizer, Foscan, almost completely inhibited tumor perfusion at 5 min after treatment, which did not recover for up to 24 h (Ohlerth et al., 2006). These results are in agreement with optical imaging finding and histological assessment, indicating a strong vascular effect induced by PDT.

14.3.3.4 PHOTOACOUSTIC/OPTOACOUSTIC IMAGING

Photoacoustic imaging is an emerging hybrid imaging modality that combines the high spatial resolution of optical imaging with the deep tissue penetration of ultrasound imaging (Taruttis et al., 2015). Typically the tissue is illuminated with a short pulse of laser light, which is absorbed by the endogenous and exogenous photoacoustic contrast agents and causes these agents to undergo thermoelastic expansion and release acoustic pressure waves. Detection of this acoustic signal by ultrasound transducers is used to reconstruct images based on tissue optical absorption. Because the absorption of contrast agents is both wavelength- and concentration-dependent, dynamic multispectral photoacoustic imaging is able to extract important tissue structural and functional information noninvasively by interrogating the absorption property of a variety of endogenous (hemoglobin, deoxyhemoglobin, and melanin) and exogenous (indocyanine green, methylene blue) contrast agents in tissues.

Although there is little study of using photoacoustic imaging to assess PDT vascular effect, there are reports showing that photoacoustic imaging can be used to determine photosensitizer tissue distribution (Hirao et al., 2010) and some photosensitizers with strong photoacoustic property can even function as photoacoustic contrast agents (Ho et al., 2014). Among several common photosensitizers examined, zinc phthalocyanine (ZnPc) was found to have the highest photoacoustic property, followed in order by protoporphyrin IX (PpIX), chlorin e6 (Ce6), and methylene blue (MB) (Ho et al., 2014). With recent availability of commercial photoacoustic scanners, it is expected to see studies of using this emerging imaging technology to characterize PDT vascular effect.

14.3.3.5 COMPUTED TOMOGRAPHY IMAGING

Computed tomography (CT) imaging uses x-ray to generate tissue images from different angles and relies on digital processing to combine all digital images to reconstruct cross-sectional (tomographic) tissue images in three dimensions (Kircher and Willmann, 2012). CT imaging is fast, readily available, and therefore widely used in clinic for anatomic imaging. However, its sensitivity for imaging the soft tissue is relatively low because CT imaging contrast is solely dependent on mass attenuation to x-ray and the difference between soft tissues in x-ray attenuation is often not that great. This limitation can be somewhat corrected by using CT contrast agents with enhanced x-ray absorption. Small iodinated molecules are commonly used as CT contrast agents. The fast pharmacokinetics of these highly hydrophilic iodinated agents enables using dynamic CT imaging to assess tissue perfusion and viability. Compared with surrounding tissues, changes in the enhancement of contrast-enhanced CT images suggest alterations in tissue blood perfusion and lack of enhancement typically indicates tissue necrosis.

CT imaging is an anatomic imaging modality good for revealing tissue morphology and structure that has been used for assessing changes in tumor size after PDT in lung (Kato et al., 2003) and esophageal (Tan et al., 1999) cancers. More recent studies suggest that contrast-enhanced dynamic CT imaging provides a noninvasive approach for evaluating photosensitizer tissue uptake and PDT-induced tissue necrosis, and can serve as a surrogate for predicating PDT treatment response. Vascular-targeted PDT with the photosensitizer Tookad induced a well-demarcated area of tumor necrosis shown by CT imaging with an iodinated contrast agent in a spontaneous dog prostate tumor (Huang et al., 2005). Dynamic CT imaging using an iodine-based contrast agent iohexol showed enhanced blood flow, visualized blood volume, and vascular permeability surface area in the rim of tumors implanted in the pancreas of rabbits, compared with surrounding normal pancreatic tissues (Elliott et al., 2015). In contrast, these vascular parameters were reduced in the tumor core. Importantly, photosensitizer verteporfin fluorescence at 1 h after intravenous injection was highly correlated with these vascular parameters, suggesting that contrast-enhanced CT imaging would be predicative of verteporfin uptake. In a pilot study involving 15 pancreatic cancer patients treated with verteporfin-PDT, venous-phase blood contrast enhancement obtained by taking CT scans before and after contrast injection exhibited significant correlation with tumor necrotic volume determined by post-PDT CT scans (Jermyn et al., 2014). A possible explanation for such a correlation between CT image enhancement and PDT outcomes could be that greater contrast enhancement indicates better blood perfusion/tissue oxygenation and photosensitizer distribution, which results in more effective photochemical reactions and better PDT treatment outcome.

14.3.3.6 MAGNETIC RESONANCE IMAGING

Magnetic resonance imaging (MRI) utilizes radiofrequency pulses to manipulate the motion of polar molecules in a magnetic field to generate image contrast (Gallagher, 2010). Because water is the most abundant polar molecule in the human body, MRI is sensitive for detecting the spatial distribution and diffusion of water molecules in different tissues. As most soft tissues like brain and internal organs have a high water content, MRI is often used for imaging the structure and function of these soft tissues.

Different MRI imaging techniques without contrast agent have been widely used in both preclinical and clinical studies for assessing PDT-induced tumor necrosis. Due to the difference in the content of water molecules, as well as other polar biomolecules between normal and necrotic areas, MRI without contrast agent has been shown to be sensitive for noninvasive imaging of tissue necrosis after PDT (Dodd et al., 1989). Vascular-targeted PDT with the photosensitizer Tookad effectively induced tumor necrosis in a mouse prostate tumor model, as indicated by T2-weighted MRI imaging (Koudinova et al., 2003). Diffusion-weighted magnetic resonance imaging (DW-MRI) indicated that Tookad–PDT induced a unique biphasic change in the apparent diffusion coefficient (ADC) within 24 h after PDT, that is, an initial decrease followed by later increase in ADC (Plaks et al., 2004). Although the mechanism for causing this initial decrease in ADC was not clear, it appeared to correlate with subsequent tumor necrosis, suggesting a predicative value as an early therapeutic response marker.

With the ability to image vascular structure and function noninvasively in real time, dynamic contrast-enhanced magnetic resonance imaging (DCE-MRI) is often used to evaluate the effects of PDT on tumor vasculature and predicate tumor response to PDT, particularly vascular-targeted PDT. DCE-MRI typically uses paramagnetic gadolinium ions or gadolinium-labeled contrast agents injected intravenously to interrogate vascular structure and function as they circulate in the blood and diffuse across the blood vessel wall into the tissue interstitial area (O'Connor et al., 2007). This is because gadolinium ions increase T1-weighted MRI signal intensity by interacting with water molecules in tissues, and such signal enhancement is dependent on factors such as the amount of gadolinium in the tissue, blood perfusion, and vascular permeability. Thus, by tracking T1-weighted signal enhancement after intravenous bolus injection of a contrast agent, DCE-MRI is able to reveal important information about tissue vascular structure (density, morphology) and function (blood flow, vascular permeability).

Imaged by DCE-MRI using contrast agent gadolinium diethylenetriamine pentaacetate (Gd-DTPA), PDT with a vascular-targeted photosensitizer bacteriochlorophyll-serine significantly reduced T1-weighted gradient echo signal in a mouse tumor model as early as 1 h after treatment and there was no recovery of signal by 24 h post-PDT, indicating an early onset and sustained inhibition of vascular perfusion by PDT (Zilberstein et al., 2001). Similar PDT-induced vascular damage has also been reported with other photosensitizers such as BF2-chelated tetraaryl-azadipyrromethene ADPM06 (Byrne et al., 2009) and verteporfin (Samkoe et al., 2010). DCE-MRI using high molecular weight contrast agents has been used to evaluate the effect of PDT on vascular permeability to macromolecules (Seshadri et al., 2005). Different from Gd-DTPA, which has a molecular weight of less than 1000 Da, macromolecular MRI contrast agent methoxy-PEG succinyl-poly-L-lysine-Gd-DTPA (MacroGd) has an average molecular weight of 530 kDa. MacroGd-MRI showed that PDT, with the photosensitizer 2-[1-hexyloxyethyl]-2-devinyl pyropheophorbide-a (HPPH), significantly increased tumor vascular permeability, resulting in an enhancement of T1-weighted signal, in a mouse tumor model, particularly at lower PDT doses. Although an increase in vascular permeability does not appear to predicate long-term tumor response to PDT, this PDT-induced vascular effect has been explored to enhance drug delivery to tumors (Snyder et al., 2003).

DCE-MRI has important role in predicting photosensitizer tumor uptake and tumor response to vascular-targeted PDT. Using Gd-DTPA as contrast agent, T1-weighted gadolinium signal enhancement provides a noninvasive method for estimating overall tumor perfusion. Because photosensitizer uptake in the tumor depends on functional vasculature, it is not surprising to see that tumor uptake of the photosensitizer verteporfin was positively correlated with T1-weighted MRI signal enhancement in tumor models, suggesting a potential application of DCE-MRI for predicting verteporfin tumor uptake (Samkoe et al., 2013). Because tumor cell survival depends on functional vasculature, a sustained lack of T1-weighted gadolinium signal indicates tissue necrosis. Indeed, Gd-DTPA-based DCE-MRI at 7 days after vascular-targeted PDT with bacteriopheophorbide photosensitizers in prostate cancer patients showed that lack of T1-weighted signal enhancement was positively associated with tumor tissue necrosis assessed at 6 months after PDT, suggesting a prognostic value for predicating PDT treatment outcome (Barrett et al., 2014; Moore et al., 2015).

MRI can also reveal tissue oxygenation status. This MRI technique, termed blood oxygenation level-dependent (BOLD) contrast MRI, is based on the paramagnetic property of deoxyhemoglobin (Gross et al., 2003). Oxygen consumption by photochemical reaction during PDT as well as the deficiency in oxygen delivery due to PDT-induced vascular damage may significantly increase deoxyhemoglobin level, which can be detected by MRI using T2-weighted spin echo sequence. BOLD-MRI is very sensitive to light illumination during PDT and has been proposed to be used to monitor tissue response during PDT in real time (Gross et al., 2003; Tempel-Brami et al., 2007). However, its application in predicting long-term treatment outcome remains to be determined.

14.3.3.7 POSITRON EMISSION TOMOGRAPHY IMAGING

Positron emission tomography (PET) imaging uses imaging probes labeled with positron emitting radio-isotopes such as ^{18}F, ^{11}C, ^{15}O. After a positron is emitted, it annihilates with a nearby electron and generates 2 annihilation photons (each with an energy of 511 keV) traveling in opposite directions. PET imaging has been widely used for cancer detection, monitoring tumor response, and evaluating prognosis (Farwell et al., 2014). The most commonly used radiotracer for PET imaging is 2-deoxy-2-(^{18}F)fluoro-D-glucose (^{18}FDG). As an analog of the cell energy source glucose, ^{18}FDG is rapidly up taken by tumor cells through glucose transporters because tumor cells often exhibit a high rate of glycolysis and increased expression of glucose transporters. Once inside the cell, [18]FDG is phosphorylated by hexokinase to form ^{18}F-deoxyglucose-6-phosphate ([18]FDG-6P). Because it lacks a hydroxyl group at the 2 position, it cannot be metabolized by enzymes farther down the glycolytic pathway, resulting in being trapped within cells (Farwell et al., 2014). Thus, [18]FDG-PET imaging is essentially a noninvasive imaging modality for tumor cell metabolism, a surrogate for tumor cell survival and progression.

PET imaging has been evaluated for assessing and predicting tumor response to PDT. Although reduced [18]FDG tumor uptake was an early observation after PDT with different photosensitizers, tumor [18]FDG uptake kinetics showed significant differences between PDT with a vascular-targeted photosensitizer versus PDT with a tumor cell-targeted photosensitizer (Berard et al., 2006; Boubacar et al., 2015). PDT with a tumor cell-targeted photosensitizer zinc phthalocyanine disulfonate (ZnPcS2) almost completely inhibited [18]FDG tumor uptake during light treatment, suggesting a fast and direct inhibition of glucose uptake in tumor cells, whereas PDT with a vascular-targeted photosensitizer, aluminum phthalocyanine tetrasulfonate (AlPcS4), only partially inhibited tumor [18]FDG uptake during PDT. Tumors showed a robust rebound of [18]FDG uptake shortly after PDT with tumor cell-targeted photosensitizer ZnPcS2. In contrast, recovery of [18]FDG uptake was much less in tumors treated with PDT using vascular-targeted photosensitizer AlPcS4, possibly due to reduced [18]FDG tumor delivery as a result of PDT-induced vascular damage. Although more studies are needed, these results suggest that [18]FDG-PET imaging may be used to determine the therapeutic mechanism of PDT with different photosensitizers.

The potential of using [18]FDG-PET imaging to predict PDT treatment outcome has also been explored. In a study involving four different sulfonated phthalocyanine photosensitizers, it was found that a fast drop in the rate of [18]FDG tumor uptake during PDT, followed by a strong rebound after PDT was indicative of long-term tumor control (Cauchon et al., 2012). This finding appears to indicate that maintaining tissue oxygen by preserving vascular function during PDT is important for sustained tumor response after PDT with tumor cell-targeted photosensitizers.

PET imaging is also useful for monitoring treatment response of vascular-targeted PDT. Vascular-targeted PDT with a nonporphyrin photosensitizer BF2-chelated tetraaryl-azadipyrromethene ADPM06 caused a significant decrease in tumor [18]FDG uptake, which was detected immediately after treatment and maintained for at least 4 h (Byrne et al., 2009). To determine the effect of ADPM06-PDT on tumor cell proliferation, tumors were imaged using ^{18}F-labeled 3'-deoxy-3'-fluorothymidine (^{18}F-FLT) radiotracer (O'Connor et al., 2012). Because ^{18}F-FLT will be preferentially incorporated into the DNA of proliferating cells through DNA replication, ^{18}F-FLT-PET imaging allows direct visualization of proliferating cells. ^{18}F-FLT-PET imaging indicates that ADPM06-PDT resulted in significant reduction in ^{18}F-FLT tumor uptake at 4 h after treatment, which did not recover for at least 24 h. Although these PET imaging studies demonstrate that vascular-targeted PDT damages tumor perfusion and inhibits tumor cell proliferation, it remains to be determined whether it can be used to predict long-term treatment outcome after vascular-targeted PDT.

14.4 CURRENT UNDERSTANDING OF PDT VASCULAR EFFECT

Through all of the earlier imaging studies conducted at the whole body, tissue, cellular, and subcellular level, it is now clear that the vascular effect is a predominant therapeutic mechanism of PDT with nearly all current photosensitizers. This effect appears to originate from an association between photosensitizer molecules and vascular targets in endothelial cells or vascular supporting structures. Although the exact molecular target of PDT remains elusive and may be different depending on photosensitizers, molecules in the mitochondria, endoplasmic reticulum, and basement membrane are possible candidates. Because these vascular targets are in close proximity to the source of oxygen and photosensitizer molecules in the blood, photochemical reactions at these sites are expected to be efficient upon light illumination. PDT-induced oxidative damage to endothelial cells and vascular supporting structures result in the loss of vascular barrier function, causing vascular permeability increase. This vascular dysfunction, together with the release of factors from injured endothelial cells (such as Von Willebrand factor), activates the blood coagulation cascade and causes thrombus formation, which leads to blood flow arrest. Photosensitization of circulating blood cells, particularly platelets and leukocytes when they pass through the light treatment field exacerbates vascular functional disruption by promoting platelet aggregation, leukocyte adhesion, and vessel constriction via releasing vaso-active substances. Reduced blood flow further aggravates PDT-induced damage to the circulating blood cells due to increased exposure to light illumination due to their longer dwell time, which stimulates more thrombus formation and vessel constriction. The interplay of these vascular events may eventually occlude blood vessels and completely shut down vascular function, resulting in tissue hypoxia, ischemia, and ultimate cell death. All these vascular events and their consequent effects on tumor cell death and survival have been captured with various imaging modalities.

14.5 CONCLUSIONS AND FUTURE DIRECTIONS

Intensive research over the past 50 years has generated a tremendous amount of knowledge about the effects and mechanism of PDT, which has led to a successful transition of PDT from the bench to the bedside. As an indispensable tool for biomedical research, imaging with different modalities at levels ranging from the whole body down to the ultrastructural level has been used extensively in PDT studies. Through these multimodality imaging studies, we have come to the conclusion that the vascular effect makes a considerable contribution to the overall PDT outcome. For photosensitizers like Tookad, PDT effect is solely dependent on its vascular effect. PDT using a vascular-targeted protocol, as in the case of verteporfin, has been used in the clinic, and vascular-targeted PDT with Tookad is showing promise in multicenter clinical trials for prostate cancer.

Despite such successes, there are some fundamental issues that remain to be addressed in order to fulfill the potential of PDT. First, although we are able to repeatedly visualize the PDT vascular effect using various imaging modalities, we still do not know the molecular target of PDT. Second, we do not understand why some blood vessels, particularly peripheral tumor blood vessels, are not fully occluded after PDT despite the presence of photo-oxidative damage. In other words, how can we increase the consistence of vascular shutdown of all blood vessels in the treated area? Finally, how to address the resumption of vascular function after PDT, which has been observed in both AMD and cancer patients treated with PDT and results in disease recurrence? Is this an issue of recanalization, angiogenesis, or vasculogenesis? To solve these problems, we need to return to the bench to carry out more hypothesis-driven mechanistic studies and translate basic research findings into clinical therapeutic approaches. It is expected that imaging will continue to play a critical role in this translational PDT research.

ACKNOWLEDGMENTS

I thank my mentors Dr. Peter de Witte and Dr. Brian Pogue for guidance, previous and current lab members for research contribution, and funding agencies (ACS, DoD, NIH) for support. I apologize for not being able to cite all important PDT imaging studies.

REFERENCES

Agostinis P, Berg K, Cengel KA, Foster TH, Girotti AW, Gollnick SO, Hahn SM et al. (2011) Photodynamic therapy of cancer: An update. *CA Cancer J Clin* **61**:250–281.

Azzouzi AR, Barret E, Bennet J, Moore C, Taneja S, Muir G, Villers A et al. (2015) TOOKAD((R)) Soluble focal therapy: Pooled analysis of three phase II studies assessing the minimally invasive ablation of localized prostate cancer. *World J Urol* **33**:945–953.

Baluk P, Hashizume H, McDonald DM (2005) Cellular abnormalities of blood vessels as targets in cancer. *Curr Opin Genet Dev* **15**:102–111.

Barrett T, Davidson SR, Wilson BC, Weersink RA, Trachtenberg J, Haider MA (2014) Dynamic contrast enhanced MRI as a predictor of vascular-targeted photodynamic focal ablation therapy outcome in prostate cancer post-failed external beam radiation therapy. *Can Urol Assoc J* **8**:E708–E714.

Bellnier DA, Potter WR, Vaughan LA, Sitnik TM, Parsons JC, Greco WR, Whitaker J, Johnson P, Henderson BW (1995) The validation of a new vascular damage assay for photodynamic therapy agents. *Photochem Photobiol* **62**:896–905.

Berard V, Rousseau JA, Cadorette J, Hubert L, Bentourkia M, van Lier JE, Lecomte R (2006) Dynamic imaging of transient metabolic processes by small-animal PET for the evaluation of photosensitizers in photodynamic therapy of cancer. *J Nucl Med* **47**:1119–1126.

Berenbaum MC, Hall GW, Hoyes AD (1986) Cerebral photosensitisation by haematoporphyrin derivative. Evidence for an endothelial site of action. *Br J Cancer* **53**:81–89.

Boubacar P, Sarrhini O, Lecomte R, van Lier JE, Bentourkia M (2015) A real-time follow-up of photodynamic therapy during PET imaging. *Photodiagnosis Photodyn Ther* **12**:428–435.

Brown SB, Mellish KJ (2001) Verteporfin: A milestone in opthalmology and photodynamic therapy. *Expert Opin Pharmacother* **2**:351–361.

Byrne AT, O'Connor AE, Hall M, Murtagh J, O'Neill K, Curran KM, Mongrain K et al. (2009) Vascular-targeted photodynamic therapy with BF2-chelated Tetraaryl-Azadipyrromethene agents: A multimodality molecular imaging approach to therapeutic assessment. *Br J Cancer* **101**:1565–1573.

Carmeliet P, Jain RK (2011) Molecular mechanisms and clinical applications of angiogenesis. *Nature* **473**:298–307.

Castano AP, Liu Q, Hamblin MR (2006) A green fluorescent protein-expressing murine tumour but not its wild-type counterpart is cured by photodynamic therapy. *Br J Cancer* **94**:391–397.

Castellani A, Pace GP, Concioli M (1963) Photodynamic effect of haematoporphyrin on blood microcirculation. *J Pathol Bacteriol* **86**:99–102.

Cauchon N, Turcotte E, Lecomte R, Hassessian HM, Lier JE (2012) Predicting efficacy of photodynamic therapy by real-time FDG-PET in a mouse tumour model. *Photochem Photobiol Sci* **11**:364–370.

Chen B, Crane C, He C, Gondek D, Agharkar P, Savellano MD, Hoopes PJ, Pogue BW (2008) Disparity between prostate tumor interior versus peripheral vasculature in response to verteporfin-mediated vascular-targeting therapy. *Int J Cancer* **123**:695–701.

Chen B, Pogue BW, Goodwin IA, O'Hara JA, Wilmot CM, Hutchins JE, Hoopes PJ, Hasan T (2003) Blood flow dynamics after photodynamic therapy with verteporfin in the RIF-1 tumor. *Radiat Res* **160**:452–459.

Chen B, Pogue BW, Hoopes PJ, Hasan T (2006a) Vascular and cellular targeting for photodynamic therapy. *Crit Rev Eukaryot Gene Expr* **16**:279–305.

Chen B, Pogue BW, Luna JM, Hardman RL, Hoopes PJ, Hasan T (2006b) Tumor vascular permeabilization by vascular-targeting photosensitization: Effects, mechanism, and therapeutic implications. *Clin Cancer Res* **12**:917–923.

Chen B, Roskams T, de Witte PA (2002) Antivascular tumor eradication by hypericin-mediated photodynamic therapy. *Photochem Photobiol* **76**:509–513.

Debefve E, Cheng C, Schaefer SC, Yan H, Ballini JP, van den Bergh H, Lehr HA, Ruffieux C, Ris HB, Krueger T (2010) Photodynamic therapy induces selective extravasation of macromolecules: Insights using intravital microscopy. *J Photochem Photobiol B* **98**:69–76.

Debefve E, Mithieux F, Perentes JY, Wang Y, Cheng C, Schaefer SC, Ruffieux C et al. (2011) Leukocyte-endothelial cell interaction is necessary for photodynamic therapy induced vascular permeabilization. *Lasers Surg Med* **43**:696–704.

Dodd NJ, Moore JV, Poppitt DG, Wood B (1989) In vivo magnetic resonance imaging of the effects of photodynamic therapy. *Br J Cancer* **60**:164–167.

Dolmans DE, Kadambi A, Hill JS, Waters CA, Robinson BC, Walker JP, Fukumura D, Jain RK (2002) Vascular accumulation of a novel photosensitizer, MV6401, causes selective thrombosis in tumor vessels after photodynamic therapy. *Cancer Res* **62**:2151–2156.

Elliott JT, Samkoe KS, Gunn JR, Stewart EE, Gardner TB, Tichauer KM, Lee TY et al. (2015) Perfusion CT estimates photosensitizer uptake and biodistribution in a rabbit orthotopic pancreatic cancer model: A pilot study. *Acad Radiol* **22**:572–579.

Engbrecht BW, Menon C, Kachur AV, Hahn SM, Fraker DL (1999) Photofrin-mediated photodynamic therapy induces vascular occlusion and apoptosis in a human sarcoma xenograft model. *Cancer Res* **59**:4334–4342.

Farwell MD, Pryma DA, Mankoff DA (2014) PET/CT imaging in cancer: Current applications and future directions. *Cancer* **120**:3433–3445.

Fingar VH, Kik PK, Haydon PS, Cerrito PB, Tseng M, Abang E, Wieman TJ (1999) Analysis of acute vascular damage after photodynamic therapy using benzoporphyrin derivative (BPD). *Br J Cancer* **79**:1702–1708.

Fingar VH, Wieman TJ, Wiehle SA, Cerrito PB (1992) The role of microvascular damage in photodynamic therapy: The effect of treatment on vessel constriction, permeability, and leukocyte adhesion. *Cancer Res* **52**:4914–4921.

Folkman J (2006) Angiogenesis. *Annu Rev Med* **57**:1–18.

Gallagher FA (2010) An introduction to functional and molecular imaging with MRI. *Clin Radiol* **65**:557–566.

Ghazi NG, Jabbour NM, De La Cruz ZC, Green WR (2001) Clinicopathologic studies of age-related macular degeneration with classic subfoveal choroidal neovascularization treated with photodynamic therapy. *Retina* **21**:478–486.

Granville DJ, Ruehlmann DO, Choy JC, Cassidy BA, Hunt DW, van Breemen C, McManus BM (2001) Bcl-2 increases emptying of endoplasmic reticulum Ca2+ stores during photodynamic therapy-induced apoptosis. *Cell Calcium* **30**:343–350.

Granville DJ, Shaw JR, Leong S, Carthy CM, Margaron P, Hunt DW, McManus BM (1999) Release of cytochrome *c*, Bax migration, Bid cleavage, and activation of caspases 2, 3, 6, 7, 8, and 9 during endothelial cell apoptosis. *Am J Pathol* **155**:1021–1025.

Gross S, Gilead A, Scherz A, Neeman M, Salomon Y (2003) Monitoring photodynamic therapy of solid tumors online by BOLD-contrast MRI. *Nat Med* **9**:1327–1331.

He C, Agharkar P, Chen B (2008) Intravital microscopic analysis of vascular perfusion and macromolecule extravasation after photodynamic vascular targeting therapy. *Pharm Res* **25**:1873–1880.

Hirao A, Sato S, Saitoh D, Shinomiya N, Ashida H, Obara M (2010) In vivo photoacoustic monitoring of photosensitizer distribution in burned skin for antibacterial photodynamic therapy. *Photochem Photobiol* **86**:426–430.

Ho CJ, Balasundaram G, Driessen W, McLaren R, Wong CL, Dinish US, Attia AB, Ntziachristos V, Olivo M (2014) Multifunctional photosensitizer-based contrast agents for photoacoustic imaging. *Sci Rep* **4**:5342.

Huang Z, Chen Q, Luck D, Beckers J, Wilson BC, Trncic N, Larue SM, Blanc D, Hetzel FW (2005) Studies of a vascular-acting photosensitizer, Pd-bacteriopheophorbide (Tookad), in normal canine prostate and spontaneous canine prostate cancer. *Lasers Surg Med* **36**:390–397.

Jain RK (2014) Antiangiogenesis strategies revisited: From starving tumors to alleviating hypoxia. *Cancer Cell* **26**:605–622.

Jermyn M, Davis SC, Dehghani H, Huggett MT, Hasan T, Pereira SP, Bown SG, Pogue BW (2014) CT contrast predicts pancreatic cancer treatment response to verteporfin-based photodynamic therapy. *Phys Med Biol* **59**:1911–1921.

Kato H, Furukawa K, Sato M, Okunaka T, Kusunoki Y, Kawahara M, Fukuoka M et al. (2003) Phase II clinical study of photodynamic therapy using mono-L-aspartyl chlorin e6 and diode laser for early superficial squamous cell carcinoma of the lung. *Lung Cancer* **42**:103–111.

Khurana M, Moriyama EH, Mariampillai A, Wilson BC (2008) Intravital high-resolution optical imaging of individual vessel response to photodynamic treatment. *J Biomed Opt* **13**:040502.

Kircher MF, Willmann JK (2012) Molecular body imaging: MR imaging, CT, and US. Part I. Principles. *Radiology* **263**:633–643.

Koudinova NV, Pinthus JH, Brandis A, Brenner O, Bendel P, Ramon J, Eshhar Z, Scherz A, Salomon Y (2003) Photodynamic therapy with Pd-Bacteriopheophorbide (TOOKAD): Successful in vivo treatment of human prostatic small cell carcinoma xenografts. *Int J Cancer* **104**:782–789.

Li Z, Agharkar P, Chen B (2013) Therapeutic enhancement of vascular-targeted photodynamic therapy by inhibiting proteasomal function. *Cancer Lett* **339**:128–134.

Maas AL, Carter SL, Wileyto EP, Miller J, Yuan M, Yu G, Durham AC, Busch TM (2012) Tumor vascular microenvironment determines responsiveness to photodynamic therapy. *Cancer Res* **72**:2079–2088.

Madar-Balakirski N, Tempel-Brami C, Kalchenko V, Brenner O, Varon D, Scherz A, Salomon Y (2010) Permanent occlusion of feeding arteries and draining veins in solid mouse tumors by vascular targeted photodynamic therapy (VTP) with Tookad. *PLoS One* **5**:e10282.

Michels S, Schmidt-Erfurth U (2003) Sequence of early vascular events after photodynamic therapy. *Invest Ophthalmol Vis Sci* **44**:2147–2154.

Middelburg TA, de Bruijn HS, Tettero L, van der Ploeg van den Heuvel A, Neumann HA, de Haas ER, Robinson DJ (2013) Topical hexylaminolevulinate and aminolevulinic acid photodynamic therapy: Complete arteriole vasoconstriction occurs frequently and depends on protoporphyrin IX concentration in vessel wall. *J Photochem Photobiol B* **126**:26–32.

Mita MM, Sargsyan L, Mita AC, Spear M (2013) Vascular-disrupting agents in oncology. *Expert Opin Investig Drugs* **22**:317–328.

Mitra S, Giesselman BR, De Jesus-Andino FJ, Foster TH (2011) Tumor response to mTHPC-mediated photodynamic therapy exhibits strong correlation with extracellular release of HSP70. *Lasers Surg Med* **43**:632–643.

Moore CM, Azzouzi AR, Barret E, Villers A, Muir GH, Barber NJ, Bott S et al. (2015) Determination of optimal drug dose and light dose index to achieve minimally invasive focal ablation of localised prostate cancer using WST11-vascular-targeted photodynamic (VTP) therapy. *BJU Int* **116**:888–896.

Moriyama EH, Bisland SK, Lilge L, Wilson BC (2004) Bioluminescence imaging of the response of rat gliosarcoma to ALA-PpIX-mediated photodynamic therapy. *Photochem Photobiol* **80**:242–249.

Moshfeghi DM, Kaiser PK, Grossniklaus HE, Sternberg P, Jr., Sears JE, Johnson MW, Ratliff N, Branco A, Blumenkranz MS, Lewis H (2003) Clinicopathologic study after submacular removal of choroidal neovascular membranes treated with verteporfin ocular photodynamic therapy. *Am J Ophthalmol* **135**:343–350.

Nelson JS, Liaw LH, Orenstein A, Roberts WG, Berns MW (1988) Mechanism of tumor destruction following photodynamic therapy with hematoporphyrin derivative, chlorin, and phthalocyanine. *J Natl Cancer Inst* **80**:1599–1605.

O'Connor AE, Mc Gee MM, Likar Y, Ponomarev V, Callanan JJ, O'Shea D F, Byrne AT, Gallagher WM (2012) Mechanism of cell death mediated by a BF2-chelated tetraaryl-azadipyrromethene photodynamic therapeutic: Dissection of the apoptotic pathway in vitro and in vivo. *Int J Cancer* **130**:705–715.

O'Connor JP, Jackson A, Parker GJ, Jayson GC (2007) DCE-MRI biomarkers in the clinical evaluation of antiangiogenic and vascular disrupting agents. *Br J Cancer* **96**:189–195.

Ohlerth S, Laluhova D, Buchholz J, Roos M, Walt H, Kaser-Hotz B (2006) Changes in vascularity and blood volume as a result of photodynamic therapy can be assessed with power Doppler ultrasonography. *Lasers Surg Med* **38**:229–234.

Petermeier K, Tatar O, Inhoffen W, Volker M, Lafaut BA, Henke-Fahle S, Gelisken F et al. (2006) Verteporfin photodynamic therapy induced apoptosis in choroidal neovascular membranes. *Br J Ophthalmol* **90**:1034–1039.

Plaks V, Koudinova N, Nevo U, Pinthus JH, Kanety H, Eshhar Z, Ramon J, Scherz A, Neeman M, Salomon Y (2004) Photodynamic therapy of established prostatic adenocarcinoma with TOOKAD: A biphasic apparent diffusion coefficient change as potential early MRI response marker. *Neoplasia* **6**:224–233.

Reed MW, Wieman TJ, Schuschke DA, Tseng MT, Miller FN (1989) A comparison of the effects of photodynamic therapy on normal and tumor blood vessels in the rat microcirculation. *Radiat Res* **119**:542–552.

Rivera LB, Bergers G (2015) CANCER. Tumor angiogenesis, from foe to friend. *Science* **349**:694–695.

Rollakanti KR, Anand S, Maytin EV (2015) Vitamin D enhances the efficacy of photodynamic therapy in a murine model of breast cancer. *Cancer Med* **4**:633–642.

Samkoe KS, Bryant A, Gunn JR, Pereira SP, Hasan T, Pogue BW (2013) Contrast enhanced-magnetic resonance imaging as a surrogate to map verteporfin delivery in photodynamic therapy. *J Biomed Opt* **18**:120504.

Samkoe KS, Chen A, Rizvi I, O'Hara JA, Hoopes PJ, Pereira SP, Hasan T, Pogue BW (2010) Imaging tumor variation in response to photodynamic therapy in pancreatic cancer xenograft models. *Int J Radiat Oncol Biol Phys* **76**:251–259.

Schmidt-Erfurth U, Niemeyer M, Geitzenauer W, Michels S (2005) Time course and morphology of vascular effects associated with photodynamic therapy. *Ophthalmology* **112**:2061–2069.

Seshadri M, Spernyak JA, Mazurchuk R, Camacho SH, Oseroff AR, Cheney RT, Bellnier DA (2005) Tumor vascular response to photodynamic therapy and the antivascular agent 5,6-dimethylxanthenone-4-acetic acid: Implications for combination therapy. *Clin Cancer Res* **11**:4241–4250.

Snyder JW, Greco WR, Bellnier DA, Vaughan L, Henderson BW (2003) Photodynamic therapy: A means to enhanced drug delivery to tumors. *Cancer Res* **63**:8126–8131.

Spikes JD (1975) Porphyrins and related compounds as photodynamic sensitizers. *Ann N Y Acad Sci* **244**:496–508.

Tan WC, Fulljames C, Stone N, Dix AJ, Shepherd N, Roberts DJ, Brown SB, Krasner N, Barr H (1999) Photodynamic therapy using 5-aminolaevulinic acid for oesophageal adenocarcinoma associated with Barrett's metaplasia. *J Photochem Photobiol B* **53**:75–80.

Taruttis A, van Dam GM, Ntziachristos V (2015) Mesoscopic and macroscopic optoacoustic imaging of cancer. *Cancer Res* **75**:1548–1559.

Tempel-Brami C, Pinkas I, Scherz A, Salomon Y (2007) Detection of light images by simple tissues as visualized by photosensitized magnetic resonance imaging. *PLoS One* **2**:e1191.

Yu G, Durduran T, Zhou C, Wang HW, Putt ME, Saunders HM, Sehgal CM, Glatstein E, Yodh AG, Busch TM (2005) Noninvasive monitoring of murine tumor blood flow during and after photodynamic therapy provides early assessment of therapeutic efficacy. *Clin Cancer Res* **11**:3543–3552.

Zhou CN, Yang WZ, Ding ZX, Wang YX, Shen H, Fan XJ, Ha XW (1985) The biological effects of photodynamic therapy on normal skin in mice–I. A light microscopic study. *Adv Exp Med Biol* **193**:105–109.

Zilberstein J, Schreiber S, Bloemers MC, Bendel P, Neeman M, Schechtman E, Kohen F, Scherz A, Salomon Y (2001) Antivascular treatment of solid melanoma tumors with bacteriochlorophyll-serine-based photodynamic therapy. *Photochem Photobiol* **73**:257–266.

Photosensitizer activity imaging on the microscopic scale

STEFFEN HACKBARTH

15.1 INTRODUCTION

In photobiology, a photosensitizer (PS) is a light-absorbing molecule that mediates a reaction in a cell, tissue, or whole organism in response to light, without undergoing any permanent change itself. Since the PS is normally not consumed during this photodynamic reaction, it can mediate many reaction cycles that can increase the damage to a substrate (the final target of the process). Different types of photosensitization have been distinguished in the literature based on the intramolecular interaction of the PS after being excited. The so-called type II photochemical pathway stands for a direct energy transfer from the PS triplet state to molecular oxygen, forming singlet oxygen ($^1O_2$), the lowest electronically excited state of oxygen. Besides this pathway, electron-transfer reactions there might occur in the substrate or oxygen, followed by chemical reactions of the radicals that are produced. Today there is common agreement (Baier et al. 2005; Snyder et al. 2005;

Redmond and Kochevar 2006; Juzeniene et al. 2007; Jiménez-Banzo et al. 2008b; Cavalcante et al. 2009; Price et al. 2009; Hackbarth et al. 2010; Wang et al. 2010; Jarvi et al. 2011, 2012; Kanofsky 2011; Shen et al. 2011) that $^1O_2$ is the key agent in photosensitization in biological environments. The term "PS activity," as used in this chapter, points toward the amount of $^1O_2$ generated as well as its reactions with the biological environment.

In principle, there are several options to detect $^1O_2$. Indirect methods are based on reactions of $^1O_2$ with sensor molecules, simple quenchers such as diisobenzofuran (DBPF) (Spiller et al. 1997), switchable linked photoinduced electron transfer (PET) pairs like singlet oxygen sensor green (SOSG) (Flors et al. 2006; Krumova and Cosa 2013), or spin traps like tetramethylpiperidine (Han et al. 2011). Another option is given by the tiny but characteristic phosphorescence of $^1O_2$ around 1270 nm (Schlothauer et al. 2009). This luminescence detection is the only direct method to observe $^1O_2$ (Li et al. 2013). Finally, the PS fluorescence together with the singlet and triplet kinetics of the PS can be used as a measure for PS activity under some circumstances. Since this chapter mainly focusses on the detection of $^1O_2$ itself, this PS-oriented method will only be included, when the detection limits of the other methods are discussed (Section 15.4.5).

However, not all of the mentioned methods are good for imaging at the cellular level. First of all, we disqualify those methods that (1) do not allow time-resolved detection and (2) require volumes to be probed that are far greater than cells. This applies to spin traps quantified by ESR (White et al. 2010) or methods that observe the absorption of adducts or products of a chemical reaction with $^1O_2$. Only emission-based methods do not suffer from this limitation. This means just two different detection methods really have to be taken into account: PET sensors and $^1O_2$ luminescence.

Besides the ability to detect $^1O_2$, these two methods have little in common, PET sensors being an indirect sensor activated by a chemical reaction and $^1O_2$ luminescence detection being a direct measurement of the characteristic emission around 1270 nm and the sole detection method allowing a time resolution in the ns scale (Jiménez-Banzo et al. 2008a; Schlothauer et al. 2009; Hackbarth et al. 2012). For both methods in cells, strong limitations apply due to the nature of $^1O_2$ and due to the detection methods themselves.

However, once the microscopic images of singlet oxygen luminescence and SOSG fluorescence were published (Figure 15.1; Zebger et al. 2004; Shen et al. 2011), a new chapter of $^1O_2$ detection on the microscopic scale was opened and high expectations have been raised. Now it is time to discuss what is or what may be possible by imaging and where are the limits.

Figure 15.1 shows the first published attempt to image single cells directly by the detection of the $^1O_2$ luminescence as well as the first report of $^1O_2$ detection based on fluorogenic probes. The latter report was limited to the detection of $^1O_2$ that had left the cell after being generated in the outer cell membrane. Fluorogenic markers are cell impermeable under normal conditions (Shen et al. 2011). However, following special protocols, they can be incorporated into mammalian cells (Gollmer et al. 2011; Pedersen et al. 2014) as found out later.

Besides these two obviously imaging-related methods, time-resolved $^1O_2$ luminescence detection in cell suspensions will be discussed. In heterogeneous environment, the kinetics of $^1O_2$ are much more complicated than they are in solution. In many cases, the local environment is encoded in the luminescence kinetics. Analysis thereof may reveal details on the PS localization even far below microscopic resolution (more on that later), especially if combined with other time-resolved imaging methods that focus on the PS itself (Jiménez-Banzo et al. 2008b ; Hackbarth et al. 2013a).

Even though being very distinct, all the methods trying to observe $^1O_2$ in biological material have to deal with similar issues, which will be discussed as follows:

1. Diffusion of $^1O_2$: It is a small molecule and thus quite mobile, but it decays very fast in cells.
2. Interactions of $^1O_2$ with cellular components: The short lifetime of $^1O_2$ in cells is caused mainly by chemical reactions that will alter the local environment.
3. Sensitivity: $^1O_2$ has a really weak emission and sensors used for detecting fluorescence suffer from insufficient dynamic range

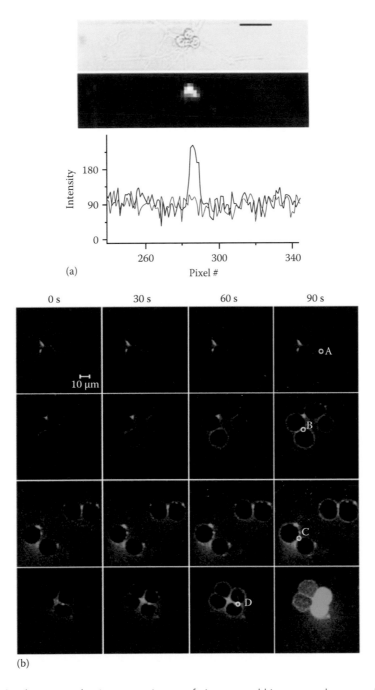

(a)

(b)

Figure 15.1 (a) Singlet oxygen luminescence image of air-saturated hippocampal nerve cells of a rat incubated with tetrakis-methyl-pyridyl-porphyrin (TMPyP). The bright field, the image at 1270 nm, and the light intensity at 1270 nm across selected lines of the latter one are also shown. (b) CNE2 cells incubated with (from top to bottom) 0, 1, 2, and 4 µM Protoporphyrin IX. SOSG is only in the medium, so just the $^1O_2$ leaving the cells can be detected after continuous illumination with 633 nm. ([a]: Reprinted from Zebger, I. et al., *Photochem. Photobiol.*, 79, 319, 2011; [b]: Reprinted from Shen, Y. et al., *Laser Phys. Lett.*, 8, 232, 2011.)

15.2 HOW THE DIFFUSION OF $^1O_2$ AFFECTS ITS DETECTION

Being very heterogeneous, cells have areas with very different properties and morphologies right next to each other. Parameters like the local polarity may change completely within a few nm. The same goes for the solubility of oxygen, pH value, viscosity, and other parameters that may have influence on quantitative imaging.

After generation, $^1O_2$ will diffuse depending on the local environment. In water, the diffusion constant is uniformly reported to be $2 \cdot 10^{-5}$ cm^2 s^{-1} (St-Denis and Fell 1971; Jamnongwong et al. 2010). For lipid layers, values around $1 \cdot 10^{-5}$ cm^2 s^{-1} were reported (Baier et al. 2005). For other cell compartments, there is agreement that the values are at least significantly lower than the one in water (Dutta and Popel 1995; Sidell 1998).

As long as the areas differing in their properties are either small or big compared to the diffusion length of $^1O_2$, heterogeneity is no issue. In such cases, the signal is a superposition of signals from different homogeneous regions or a weighted average of all of them, respectively. It turns out that in most cases none of the simple cases applies in cells (vide infra).

15.2.1 DIFFUSION RANGE OF $^1O_2$ IN CELLS

If at position $x = 0$ and at time $t = 0$ a certain amount of $^1O_2$ is generated, its spatial distribution $C(x, t)$ will widen with time in dependence on the diffusion coefficient D. If diffusion is discussed related to imaging, then 1D diffusion is of interest rather than 3D. Does a $^1O_2$ molecule diffuse far enough to show up in another pixel or can it manage to cross a flat membrane (with a dimension on the scale of $^1O_2$ diffusion) in the time it takes to be detected by a sensor outside the cell (like shown in Figure 15.1b). In such cases, just one direction is of interest.

Let us start with the well-known diffusion equation. However, since $^1O_2$ decays, the equation has to include a term to describe that, which results in

$$\frac{\partial C(x,t)}{\partial t} = D \frac{\partial^2 C(x,t)}{\partial x^2} - \frac{1}{\tau_\Delta} C(x,t)$$ (15.1)

As a stationary solution for $^1O_2$ being continuously generated at $x = 0$, we get

$$C_{cw,Norm}(x) = \frac{1}{\sqrt{4D\tau_\Delta}} \cdot e^{-|x|/\sqrt{D\tau_\Delta}}$$ (15.2)

$C_{cw,Norm}$ represents as well the time integral of the spatial distribution of the decaying $^1O_2$ or the integrated presence probability, which decays exponentially with distance. The full calculation can be found in (Hackbarth et al. 2015a). The average absolute displacement is

$$\langle |x| \rangle = \sqrt{D\tau_\Delta}$$ (15.3)

The relative impact (RI) describes the probability for a $^1O_2$ molecule to reach at least a certain minimum distance l:

$$RI(l) = 1 - \int_{x=-l}^{l} C(x)_{cw,Norm} \, dx$$ (15.4)

RI also decays by a factor of 1/e for each multiple of $\sqrt{D\tau_\Delta}$. Note that this term accounts for both forward and backward diffusion. In many cases, for example, $^1O_2$ leaving a cell or not, just one sense of direction is of interest. In such cases RI has to be divided by 2.

About 95% of the generated $^1O_2$ is quenched before reaching $3\sqrt{D\tau_\Delta}$, which is around 250 nm in case of water. For the diffusion constant in cells, the reported values range from $1.8 \cdot 10^{-6}$ cm^2 s^{-1} to $2.7 \cdot 10^{-5}$ cm^2 s^{-1} depending on the cell type (Dutta and Popel 1995). These values were given for "intact" cells, including intracellular transportation pathways for oxygen via lipids or myoglobin (Sidell 1998). For diffusion outside of such channels, it appears likely that rather smaller values apply, at least smaller than the value for water; let us assume $1 \cdot 10^{-5}$ cm^2 s^{-1} would be a good choice for this estimation. Using the shortest so far reported $^1O_2$ decay times in cells for membrane-located PSs (0.3 µs), 95% of the generated $^1O_2$ is then quenched within a range of just around 50 nm. For water-soluble PSs in the cytoplasm, the diffusion range will be bigger; on one hand, longer $^1O_2$ decay times have been reported (~1.5 µs; Jiménez-Banzo et al. 2008b), while on the other hand, the diffusion constant will be closer to that of water. Still, this results in a 95% limit of not more than 160 nm. Such diffusion ranges are bigger than natural membranes that have 4–12 nm thickness (Bielka and Escherich 1985; Freitas 1999), which means it is highly probable that $^1O_2$, due to diffusion, encounters more than one type of environment. On the other hand, there will be no kinetic averaging across the cell as the diffusion length is way too small for that to occur. As a consequence, $^1O_2$ detection is very sensitive to the localization of the PS.

15.2.2 How $^1O_2$ diffusion limits the quantitative accuracy of $^1O_2$ imaging

On the upside, diffusion of $^1O_2$ is too small to affect the optical resolution for imaging. On the downside, it makes any quantitative measurement very difficult. Though having the same reason, the complications arising from it are distinct for PET sensors and $^1O_2$ luminescence detection and will therefore be discussed separately.

Assuming a sensor molecule is located at a certain distance from the PS, for example, behind a phase boundary, only a fraction of the generated $^1O_2$ reaches the sensor. Based on the earlier estimated parameter sets for membrane-located or water-soluble PS, the relative detectable intensity vs. distance is shown in Figure 15.2. In the vicinity of membranes, a separation of PS and sensor of 20 nm reduces the detected amount of $^1O_2$ by

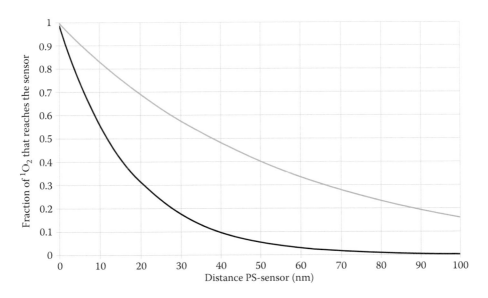

Figure 15.2 Relative amount of $^1O_2$ that can be detected by a sensor molecule depending on the distance between PS and sensor for diffusion coefficients and $^1O_2$ decay time as that reported for membrane-localized PS (black) and for PS in the cytoplasm (gray).

a factor of 3 or more. A parameter of 20 nm is just about twice the thickness of a native cellular membrane and an order of magnitude below optical resolution of any microscope in the visible range. If a PS localizes inside of a cell compartment larger than the $^1O_2$ diffusion length and the sensor remains outside, then the detected amount of $^1O_2$ further reduces by a factor of 2—remember half of $^1O_2$ diffuses in the other direction. Due to the heterogeneity of biological material, every sensor molecule has a distribution pattern—as shown for the Aarhus sensor green (ASG) probe, in the presence of the PS, this distribution pattern might even change (Pedersen et al. 2014). Since this pattern is observable on a microscopic scale, the resulting distances between PS and sensor inside cells might be bigger than the diffusion range of $^1O_2$, thus preventing any reaction ab initio. Such an effect was reported by Shen et al. (2011), who observed great differences in SOSG activation after photosensitization of cells with PS that localize at very different subcellular structures. SOSG was in the surrounding medium in this experiment, Protoporphyrin IX localized in the cell plasma membrane produced SOSG fluorescence after illumination, while for TMPyP located in the nucleus (thus more than 500 nm away from the plasma membrane), no reaction at all was visible even after extended illumination time.

Colocalization turns out to be the major issue that affects all indirect detection methods of $^1O_2$. Distances between the PS and the sensor molecule below the optical resolution limit may completely inhibit the detection.

The second method that will be discussed, that is, direct $^1O_2$ luminescence detection of $^1O_2$, is also affected by diffusion. Quantitative measurements in biological environments suffer from the fact that the radiative rate constant of $^1O_2$ is strongly dependent on the local environment (Scurlock et al. 1995; Hackbarth et al. 2010, 2012). This constant is estimated to be higher in biological systems than it is in water (Schweitzer and Schmidt 2003). A factor of around 3 for the relative magnitude of the rate constants of lipids and water was reported recently (Hackbarth and Röder 2015c). Hence, a PS displacement way below the resolution of the imaging system can cause huge changes in luminescence intensity. As a consequence, the $^1O_2$ luminescence intensity alone cannot give reliable information about the amount of generated $^1O_2$ in cells, and therefore time-resolved detection is required. The analysis of the kinetics may reveal the existence of phase borders in the vicinity of the PS and thus give additional information on the exact location of $^1O_2$ generation that helps to quantify the detected signals.

15.2.3 INFLUENCE OF $^1O_2$ DIFFUSION ON THE LUMINESCENCE INTENSITY

Whenever diffusion of $^1O_2$ occurs near a phase boundary (e.g., near membranes), the $^1O_2$ may move between areas with different radiative rate constants or decay times, and this will influence the signal kinetics.

This effect has been addressed by different authors several years ago. In 1983 Lee and Rodgers described changes in $^1O_2$ luminescence decay times for rose bengal in inverted micelles due to heterogeneity (Lee and Rodgers 1983), but they were not able to identify diffusion effects. Baker and Kanofsky published the first diffusion model to describe the kinetics of membrane-localized PS in cells (Baker and Kanofsky 1993). The very first (to my knowledge) experiment giving evidence for diffusion effects was performed by Oelckers et al. using pheophorbide-a in erythrocyte ghosts in a deuterated buffer (Oelckers et al. 1997). A clear deviation from the normal biexponential luminescence kinetics was attributed to backward diffusion of $^1O_2$ into the ghost membrane with a shorter $^1O_2$ decay time.

However, the most illustrative experiment was done by Snyder et al. (2004), when the influence of $^1O_2$ diffusion across a D_2O/CS_2 interface on the steady-state luminescence intensity was investigated. The experimental setup and the result is illustrated in Figure 15.3. $^1O_2$ was generated by a water-soluble PS in the D_2O phase only; however, the lifetime (Rodgers 1983), solubility (Battino et al. 1983), and radiative rate constant of $^1O_2$ (Poulsen et al. 1998) are greater in CS_2. Of course, even if none of the $^1O_2$ was generated there, $^1O_2$ diffuses into CS_2. Detection of $^1O_2$ luminescence with an InGaAs line array through a microscope objective recorded the strongest signal in CS_2 directly next to the phase boundary. The detected signal had nothing in common with the spatial distribution of $^1O_2$ generation or interaction. The interactions that generated this discrepancy require a short explanation:

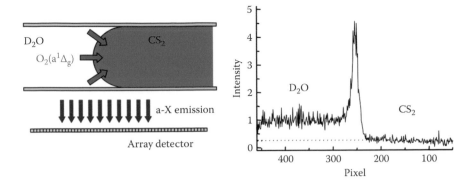

Figure 15.3 Stationary spatially resolved $^1O_2$ luminescence at the phase boundary of water and CS_2. (Reprinted from Snyder, J.W. et al., *Acc. Chem. Res.*, 37, 894.)

The radiative rate constant and decay time of $^1O_2$ is much bigger in CS_2 compared to D_2O. This means the same $^1O_2$ concentration results in a nearly 50 times bigger signal from CS_2. On the other hand, the solvent interaction is around three times lower for CS_2 compared to D_2O; the $^1O_2$ decay time in this experiment is mainly determined by the solvent. Both effects acting together mean that the same luminescence signal from both phases leads to more than 100 times less solvent interaction of $^1O_2$ in the CS_2 phase compared to D_2O.

This is probably the most impressive demonstration that steady-state luminescence detection in microscopically heterogeneous environment is of no use for imaging of active processes.

15.2.4 INFLUENCE OF $^1O_2$ DIFFUSION ON THE LUMINESCENCE KINETICS

$^1O_2$ diffusion reduces the concentration in one phase and increases it in another. While it acts just like a quenching process in the phase of origin, it appears like a source of $^1O_2$ in the other phase. Consequently, the kinetics in both phases are different. The sum of both signal components reveals this diffusion, if the radiative rate constants or the lifetimes in both phases are different.

An example of a clear identification of the location of $^1O_2$ generation in liposomes with an accuracy way below the diffraction limit was published recently. Liposomes are a good choice for this proof-of-principle experiment. They have a very simple spherical symmetric geometry and their size can be determined independently by dynamic light scattering. Therefore, the generation, diffusion, and decay of $^1O_2$ can be described accurately using a spherical symmetric diffusion model in polar coordinates.

$$\frac{\partial C(r,t)}{\partial t} = \frac{1}{r^2}\frac{\partial}{\partial r}\left[r^2 \cdot D(r)\frac{\partial C(r,t)}{\partial r}\right] - \frac{C(r,t)}{\tau_\Delta(r)} + \frac{T(r,t)}{\tau_T(r)} \tag{15.5}$$

The lipid bilayer is then represented by a certain interval of the radius (r_{min}, r_{max}). T is the concentration of PS in the triplet state, which decays with τ_T. The concentration C must be corrected for the partition coefficient. However, when approximated by a step function, the partition coefficient has to be taken into account only at the phase boundaries. D and τ_Δ and τ_T are the functions of radius as they may differ in different phases, but they are constant within each phase. $^1O_2$ is generated in direct vicinity of the PS. If the PS is distributed spherical symmetric, then the amount of generated $^1O_2$ also depends on r and t only.

If the PS is localized in the water phase only, then $T(r,t)=0$ for $r_{min} \leq r \leq r_{max}$. In such a case, the time-resolved luminescence follows the well-known biexponential kinetics, as the distance of the thin lipid bilayer (e.g., ~4 nm for DPPC; Nagle and Tristram-Nagle 2000; Cordeiro 2014) can be neglected. The concentration in the membrane will nearly instantly follow the concentration of the $^1O_2$ in the surrounding water.

In the other extreme case for PS localized exclusively in the membrane, it is also the small radial dimension of the bilayers that allows us to assume an immediate averaging of the $^1O_2$ concentration inside the bilayer according to the local solubility of $^1O_2$. However, in this case the kinetics inside the lipid bilayer is different from the kinetics outside. All the $^1O_2$ is generated inside the membrane and the radiative rate constant is bigger than it is in water. Emission from inside the bilayer thus will be overemphasized shortly after excitation.

If, regardless of the diffusion, the signal is fitted biexponentially, both the determined times would be wrong. The shorter one of the fitted decay times is shortened and the longer one is prolonged. If any of the parameters is known from an independent measurement, for instance, the PS triplet lifetime, then the different results from both measurements could reveal the membrane localization.

The localization of the PS pheophorbide-a (Pheo) and TMPyP relative to the lipid bilayer could be determined by a combination of $^1O_2$ luminescence and flash photolysis. As explained earlier, Pheo generation of $^1O_2$ within the membrane with different $^1O_2$ decay times and radiative constants compared to the surrounding water results in deviations of the luminescence kinetics (Figure 15.4), while generation everywhere in the water for TMPyP results in a perfect two exponential luminescence kinetics. Besides the poor quality of the biexponential fit in the case of Pheo, the determined decay times differed markedly from the PS triplet decay

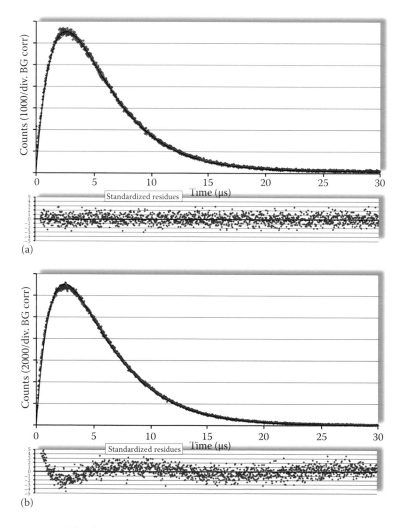

Figure 15.4 Biexponential fit of $^1O_2$ luminescence signals from two different PSs in SUV solution. For TMPyP (a) the residues show a good fit quality. For Pheo (b), the residues show a significant aberration. (Reprinted from Hackbarth, S. and Röder, B., *Photochem. Photobiol. Sci.*, 2015c.)

time that was determined by flash photolysis. Running a numerical simulation of $^1O_2$ kinetics and diffusion based on Equation 15.5 and the spherical symmetric diffusion model, good correlation to the experimental results could be obtained (not shown here) (Hackbarth and Röder 2015c). The positioning of Pheo near the membrane of the liposomes could be proved. However, data do not tell whether the PS is in the center of the membrane or closer to its surface.

Here the triplet decay of the PS may give additional information. The concentration of oxygen near the head groups of the lipids is much lower than between the lipophilic fatty acid tails, even lower than in the water outside, as was calculated for DOPC (Figure 15.5; Cordeiro 2014). It is highly probable that the faster the PS triplet decay time, the closer the PS is to the center of the membrane. In cells the geometry is not as simple as it is in liposomes, but $^1O_2$ decays fast and as described earlier, the $^1O_2$ diffusion length is very short. Therefore, membranes can be regarded as being infinite in two dimensions. Using this approximation the diffusion near a membrane can be described with 1D diffusion (Hackbarth et al. 2010).

The influence of the inner membrane signal on the overall signal of a membrane-localized PS is stronger in cells compared to that in liposomes. Natural membranes are thicker than merely lipid bilayers and the $^1O_2$ decay time is generally shorter in cells. This causes even stronger overemphasis shortly after excitation and the rising flank of the luminescence signal appears even faster compared to that with a water-soluble PS.

Both signal components, from inside and outside the membrane, are determined by the triplet PS decay. It is the second parameter that causes the difference in signal shape. In membranes $^1O_2$ is generated with τ_T, and the decay is mainly caused by its diffusion out of the membrane. As seen from the outside, the majority of $^1O_2$ leaves the membrane nearly immediately after generation, which means it enters the outer phase following τ_T, but it decays mainly determined by τ_Δ. The shorter the τ_Δ, the more similar both signal components and the smaller and earlier the deviation from the biexponential shape. This makes it less obvious during measurements in cells, since the time range shortly after excitation is often masked by measurement artifacts.

The difference in kinetics depending on the PS localization and the consequences thereof can be illustrated by comparing $^1O_2$ luminescence and phototoxicity of chlorin e_6 (Ce6) and pheophorbide-a (Pheo) after just 30 min of incubation in LNCaP cells (Hackbarth et al. 2015b). For Ce6 a much stronger $^1O_2$ luminescence signal was measured from inside the cells compared to Pheo (Figure 15.6); however, the latter PS is much more phototoxic. Both PSs are very similar in molecular structure but only differ due to the opening of the Phorbin ring in the case of Ce6, resulting in a partly water-soluble PS. This seems to result in a delayed accumulation of the PS close to cellular membranes. The $^1O_2$ decay time of Ce6 is bigger than the one of Pheo, which indicates less chemical quenching by cell components resulting in lower phototoxicity. While the luminescence signal of Ce6 could be fitted biexponentially, for the signal of Pheo a 1D diffusion fit was necessary, indicating different localizations.

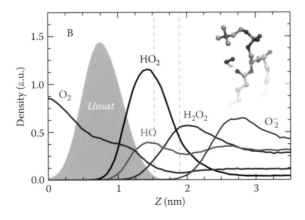

Figure 15.5 Local concentration of various ROS near membranes of DOPC. The z-axis represents a path vertical to the lipid bilayer with 0 being in the very center of it. (Reprinted from Cordeiro, R., *Biochim. Biophys. Acta*, 1838, 438, 2014.)

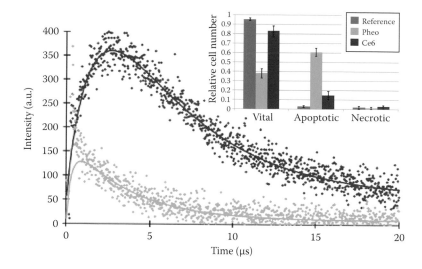

Figure 15.6 While the intensity of the $^1O_2$ luminescence signal of Ce6 is bigger than that of Pheo after incubation of Jurkat cells for 30 min, the treatment impact is lower for Ce6 (inset). (Reprinted from Hackbarth, S. et al., Chapter 26: Singlet oxygen in heterogeneous systems, in *Singlet Oxygen : Applications in Biosciences and Nanosciences*, Vol. 2, ed. S. Nonell, pp. 27–42, Comprehensive Series in Photochemical and Photobiological Sciences, Royal Society of Chemistry, 2015a; Hackbarth, S. et al., *Photon. Lasers Med.*, 4, 299, 2015b.)

For membrane-localized PS, the information about subcellular localization is encoded in the luminescence kinetics, which is an effect caused by $^1O_2$ diffusion out of the membrane. Even though this analysis is not an imaging method, it reveals details of the PS localization at distances below optical resolution.

Time-resolved luminescence detection can identify differences in the local quencher concentration and is therefore the most reliable method to detect $^1O_2$. Especially in combination with an independent method to determine the PS triplet decay—PS phosphorescence (Jiménez-Banzo et al. 2008b) or flash photolysis (Hackbarth et al. 2010)—it may even allow quantitative detection of $^1O_2$ in cells in the future.

However, this statement is only valid as long as the PS accumulates in places within the cell that all experience similar conditions.

15.3 INTERACTION OF $^1O_2$ WITH CELLULAR QUENCHERS

The electronic transition from $^1O_2$ to its ground state is triple forbidden, resulting in an extremely long natural lifetime (>ms). This is fundamentally the reason why the luminescence of $^1O_2$ is so very weak. Many bimolecular interactions do quench $^1O_2$ at a much higher rate and so the decay time is nearly exclusively determined by the solvent. In a biological environment, water can deactivate $^1O_2$ by vibrational interaction (physical quenching). For pure water, decay times between 3.5 ± 0.5 μs (Baier et al. 2005) and 3.7 ± 0.2 μs (Hackbarth et al. 2010) have been reported.

15.3.1 $^1O_2$ IN LIVING CELLS: THE MAJORITY IS DEACTIVATED BY CELLULAR QUENCHERS

In most biological materials, water represents the majority of the overall volume on weight basis. This observation thus defines in most cases an upper limit of the $^1O_2$ decay time. The only exception so far reported is the $^1O_2$ decay measured in the stratum corneum (Schlothauer et al. 2012). Due to the large amount of keratin, the corneocytes contain water-free areas that exceed the diffusion length of $^1O_2$ and allow decay times as long as 12.5 ± 0.5 μs. However, all normal living cells do contain a lot of water and therefore the aforementioned upper limit applies. Additionally, quenchers like proteins, nucleic acids, and polyunsaturated fatty acids will further shorten this decay time (Castano et al. 2004; Redmond and Kochevar 2006). Cells express several enzymes, of which many are able to react with $^1O_2$, like catalase or superoxide dismutase. Heat shock protein HSP32 initiates the production of bilirubin, which is an effective $^1O_2$ quencher (Kondo et al. 2007).

Several investigators have made estimations for the decay time of $^1O_2$ within cells (Baker and Kanofsky 1992; Snyder et al. 2005; Hackbarth et al. 2010; Jarvi et al. 2011). Most of them found a very short decay time of 0.5 µs or less, which means that the vast majority of $^1O_2$ is quenched (physically or chemically) in cells by molecules other than water. However, these short decay times were reported for hydrophobic molecules, thus representing decay times near membranes, where the local concentration of proteins is high. For water-soluble PSs, longer decay times (~1.5 µs) have been reported (Jiménez-Banzo et al. 2008b), which points to a lower quencher concentration at their place of accumulation. Similar values have been measured recently for $^1O_2$ generated by Ce6, 2 h after subcutaneous injection into the back of a nude mouse. Ce6 is not taken up by cells very efficiently (Bastien et al. 2015) and will just be distributed in the local area of the tissue. Still the determined $^1O_2$ decay time was as short as 1.7 ± 0.2 µs (Pfitzner et al. 2016). This observation leads to an important conclusion. The majority of singlet oxygen in biomaterial is deactivated by cellular components and the majority thereof is quenched chemically, which is fundamentally the reason for the photodynamic effect resulting in cell death. Most of these quenchers are proteins and other molecules essential for cell survival and are destroyed by reaction with $^1O_2$.

15.3.2 How measurement of $^1O_2$ changes the object under investigation

Unlike physical quenching, chemical quenching consumes both the quencher and the oxygen. As a consequence, the quencher concentration decreases with time and the singlet oxygen decay time gets longer. This effect was first observed for Jurkat cells, incubated with Pheo (Schlothauer et al. 2009; Hackbarth et al. 2010). Later it was found for other PSs and other cell types as well (Ogilby 2010; Hackbarth et al. 2012). An interesting finding was that the observed $^1O_2$ decay times for membrane-localized PSs were altered even at very low light doses (Figure 15.7).

As shown in Figure 15.7 for Pheo in Jurkat cells and ongoing illumination, the $^1O_2$ decay time starts far below 0.4 µs and rises fast, while at higher doses of light the increase slows down.

At the beginning of the experiment, mainly the quenchers in the direct vicinity of the PS are being consumed, while with ongoing illumination, the generated $^1O_2$ has to diffuse even further to find a quenching molecule. The longer this movement takes, the more probable physical quenching becomes as opposed to chemical quenching. Continuing illumination will probably bring the $^1O_2$ decay time close to the values determined in water due to the consumption of all the chemical quenchers in the vicinity of the PS, unless disintegration of the cell happens earlier.

Watson et al. carried out Monte Carlo simulations to describe the consumption of quenchers for two different scenarios: (1) Quencher and $^1O_2$ can freely move. (2) $^1O_2$ can move while the quenchers are fixed in a 3D lattice structure within the cell (Weston and Patterson 2014). The development of $^1O_2$ decay times with ongoing illumination was then simulated. The first scenario failed, and no realistic parameters could be found to account for the experimental results. The second scenario was more successful and will be therefore discussed in more detail.

$^1O_2$ molecules were placed in the center of a quencher lattice to go on a random walk (Figure 15.8). To keep the modeling process tractable, the movement of the $^1O_2$ molecule was limited to steps along the lattice in all three directions. Encounter with a quencher yielded a certain probability of interaction. Every time quenching occurred, the affected quencher was taken out of the lattice before placing the next $^1O_2$ molecule. With time the lattice becomes pitted (full of holes) and the $^1O_2$ decay time increases. The parameters of the simulation could be adapted to account for the experimental results shown in Figure 15.7 (Hackbarth et al. 2010). However, the authors had to limit the final $^1O_2$ lifetime to 1.2 µs to get a good match of the model with the experimental data. That value is much shorter than the value of around 3 µs, as reported by Snider et al.

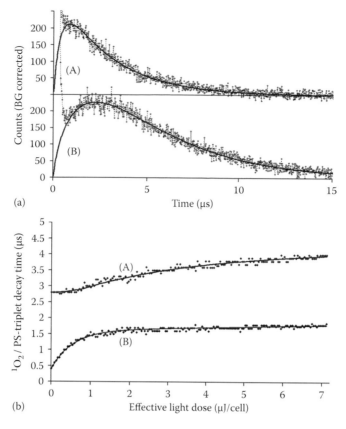

(a)

(b)

Figure 15.7 (a) $^1O_2$ luminescence decay from Pheo in Jurkat cells excited at 670 nm. (A) Fresh and (B) after illumination with 7 µJ/cell. (b) Triplet decay times of Pheo in Jurkat cells (A) and $^1O_2$ decay times in cells outside the membrane (B) as determined for consecutive measurements of the time-resolved $^1O_2$ luminescence from Pheo in Jurkat cells. (Reprinted from Hackbarth, S. et al., *J. Photochem. Photobiol. B*, 98, 173, 2010.)

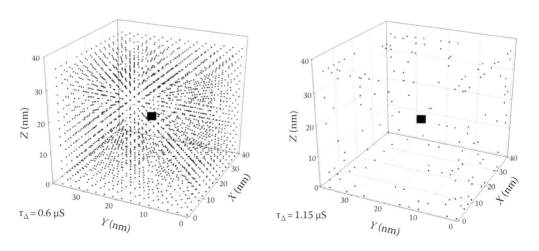

Figure 15.8 $^1O_2$ quencher distribution (dots) around a PS molecule (square) after different amounts of $^1O_2$ had been generated during PDT simulations in which [PS] = 26.7 µM. The amount of $^1O_2$ generated during the simulations was 46.5 and 353.6 mM, which corresponds to $^1O_2$ lifetimes of 0.6 and 1.15 µs, respectively. (Reprinted from Weston, M.A. and Patterson, M.S., *Photochem. Photobiol. Sci. Off. J. Eur. Photochem. Assoc. Eur. Soc. Photobiol.*, 13, 112, 2014.)

for the $^1O_2$ decay in a single cell (Snyder et al. 2005). However, illumination dose used in both experiments was very different with 180 mJ for the single cell measurement of Snyder et al. compared to just 7 µJ/cell at a maximum in the ensemble measurement of Hackbarth et al.

A possible explanation for the discrepancy between decay times is the existence of the different types of quenchers in cells with different reaction constants, while the simulation of Weston and Patterson was based on only one quencher type. The situation in cells is rather a mixture of fixed and floating quenchers. A great number of essential proteins are localized or fixed in and near membranes, but without many other proteins floating around and being mobile, cell biochemistry would not work efficiently. Unlike fixed quenchers, the floating quenchers can be replaced by others that diffuse in from all over the cytoplasm. As observed in the time scale when the simulation was run in, this situation appears to be a steady state. Hence, the assumption of the final lifetime as reported by Weston and Patterson (2014) seems correct, although it might just not be determined by physical quenching but by floating quenchers. Further illumination then only slowly increases the $^1O_2$ decay time until—after much higher light doses—finally the state of pure physical quenching is reached.

15.3.3 APPLYING CHANGES IN $^1O_2$ KINETICS AS SENSOR FOR CELL VITALITY

On one hand, the self-induced changes in $^1O_2$ kinetics limit the illumination dose for imaging, and on the other hand, this may offer an opportunity for direct observation of a PDT treatment, especially for membrane-localized PSs.

From the PDT standpoint, choosing PSs with a high affinity for membranes would seem to be the first choice. Recently published results have suggested that membrane-localized PSs show higher phototoxicity and thus have a higher PDT impact on cells than water-soluble PSs that would not be in membranes (Bacellar et al. 2014). This is important for two reasons. First, even though imaging cannot resolve the subcellular localization of the PS, kinetics analysis should be able to tell whether a PS is membrane bound or not. Second, all reported $^1O_2$ decay times for membrane-localized PSs that have so far been determined in cell suspensions are in the range of 0.5 µs. For several of those, a fast increase of the $^1O_2$ decay times after illumination was reported. It seems highly likely that this decay time can act as monitor for cell viability during PDT treatment without the necessity of adding any extra sensor molecule. Initial supporting results for this assumption have been reported (Hackbarth et al. 2015b).

15.4 DETECTION LIMITS IN LIVING CELLS

15.4.1 DIRECT OBSERVATION IN VITAL SINGLE CELLS

In Hackbarth et al. (2012), the question was addressed whether the pioneering work to detect $^1O_2$ luminescence from a single cell can be used to gain information about subcellular PS activity. Unfortunately, the number of photons that can be emitted from $^1O_2$ in one average cell in vitro, before around half of the chemical quenchers in the vicinity of a membrane-located PS have reacted with the $^1O_2$ and thus the kinetics of the $^1O_2$ is changed beyond acceptable limits (Figure 15.7), is way too low.

For cells comparable in size to Jurkat or LNCaP cells, this limit is reached after the generation of around 10^{10} $^1O_2$ molecules. From those, only around 1 out of 10^7 molecules or more is able to emit a photon. The dramatic shortening of the $^1O_2$ lifetime in the presence of cellular quenchers affecting the luminescence is the main reason for this low number. Therefore, just around 330 photons will be emitted from $^1O_2$ per single living cell, before the limit is exceeded. This is almost a "death sentence" for $^1O_2$ luminescence detection from single cells. Even if all the photons coming from a single cell could be collected and detected, the signal would barely match the noise background (Schlothauer et al. 2015).

In reality, both collection and detection are limited by the size and sensitivity of the detector. The PMT H10330 of HAMAMATSU reaches up to 5% sensitivity with a sensitive area of 1.6 mm in diameter.

Single quantum detectors reach a higher sensitivity. In Gemmell et al. (2013) a figure of 15% has been reported, but their active area is just a few µm in diameter and it is fiber coupled limiting the detector aperture. As a result, in reality not more than 1 photon per cell can be detected in average within the illumination limit.

What about the luminescence kinetics that have been estimated for single neurons incubated with TMPyP (Snyder et al. 2005)? The results gained in single cell experiments significantly differ from those determined with measurements in suspensions of millions of cells and the reason for that is obvious. The dose applied during such a single cell measurement using the high flux density in the focus of a microscope is around 200 times above the limit. Therefore, it is likely that in single cell experiments all chemical quenchers are destroyed during the measurement and only physical quenching remains. Unfortunately, though being fascinating, the results gained with single cell experiments have not much in common with the situation in a living cell.

15.4.2 FLUORESCENT PROBES IN VITAL CELLS

Among chemical $^1O_2$ quenchers, dimethylanthracene (DMA) and DBPF are regarded to be the molecules that react fastest with bimolecular rate constants of nearly 10^9 mol^{-1} s^{-1} (Tanaka et al. 2001). None of them does fluorescent and DBPF is not even $^1O_2$ specific, but DMA and many derivatives are able to control the fluorescence intensity of a covalently linked xanthene dye via PET. Reaction with $^1O_2$ and formation of an anthracene endoperoxide disables the PET and the linked dye molecule can emit fluorescent photons. Fluorescent probes, once activated, are much easier to detect than $^1O_2$ itself. Their fluorescence quantum yields range from 0.4 to 1 (Lin et al. 2013; Ruiz-González et al. 2013; Pedersen et al. 2014). However, a certain emission is observable also in the so-called off state. The PET is not fast enough to really switch off fluorescent emission (Gollmer et al. 2011). Besides that, in biological material the localization of such probes is far from being homogeneously distributed.

Now one can argue which change of signal intensity can be regarded as significant for $^1O_2$ detection and what more quantitative information apart from the published confirmation studies (Figure 15.1) can be gained. Let us do a rough estimation. The aforementioned maximum illumination dose for killing cells corresponds to a $^1O_2$ concentration of 0.03 M after delta pulse excitation. This $^1O_2$ interacts with the sensor molecules during a time interval, as determined by the decay time of $^1O_2$, that is, 0.3 µs for membrane-localized PS (Hackbarth et al. 2012). The bimolecular rate constant for the reaction of $^1O_2$ and sensor was reported as 1.7–2.5 · 10^7 M^{-1} s^{-1} (Lin et al. 2013; Ruiz-González et al. 2013). Hence, the sensors get switched on at a rate of around 8 · 10^5 s^{-1}, which finally means that about 20% of the molecules do react.

ASG has a fluorescence intensity ratio between on and off state of just 10 (Pedersen et al. 2014). This means that in case of good colocalization of PS and ASG, $^1O_2$ confirmation might be gained, but not more. For SOSG the on/off ratio is only slightly better with a value of 48 (Gollmer et al. 2011). However, all sensor molecules face the earlier mentioned diffusion problem in combination with a nonhomogeneous distribution, so completely quantitative measurements are probably an illusion. The sensitivity is limited to just confirmation of $^1O_2$ generation in the best case. The published results support this statement.

15.4.3 DIRECT OBSERVATION DISREGARDING CELL VITALITY

For some investigations, like testing if $^1O_2$ is generated at all, it is not really necessary to keep the cells alive. Most cells keep their general shape even subjected to much higher light doses than the limit for measurements in vital cells. Of course, PSs that are localized in the outer cell membrane could more likely cause a membrane rupture than those localized in the nucleus. However, it is known that PSs that mainly localize "far away" from the outer membrane compromise the cells (Hatz et al. 2007). Images using organelle stains are more blurry than in vital cells. In short, the cell will be somewhat homogenized in the surrounding of the PSs.

Ongoing illumination will destroy the vast majority of all chemical quenchers. Therefore, the $^1O_2$ decay time will become similar all over the remains of the formerly living cell. Consequently, the diffusion length of $^1O_2$ increases in a less and less structured environment. This will at least partly compensate for the differences in radiative rate constants. As a result, the images captured this way will somehow reflect the amount of generated $^1O_2$. However, in the case of direct observation of the $^1O_2$ luminescence, the resolution is compromised due to the damaged cell.

In the case of fluorogenic sensors, the resolution is even more uncertain due to the mobility of such sensors in compromised cells. As an example, Figure 15.1b shows complete flooding of cells by SOSG after membrane rupture.

The question is whether a simple fluorescence lifetime image (FLIM) of the PSs in cells can give an estimation of the generated $^1O_2$ much easier. Therefore, for completeness, the related method, although known for a long time, will briefly be mentioned in Section 15.4.5.

15.4.4 $^1O_2$ LUMINESCENCE KINETICS IN CELL ENSEMBLES

If just one photon can be detected from a single vital cell within the illumination limit, then all we need to get a reliable $^1O_2$ luminescence kinetics is around 100,000 cells—actually, most authors used a million or more cells (Niedre et al. 2002; Baier et al. 2005; Jiménez-Banzo et al. 2008b; Vyklický et al. 2013). However, besides signal intensity also a sufficient signal to noise ratio (SNR) is a prerequisite for a detailed analysis of the kinetics. In 2008 the first setup with sufficient sensitivity and SNR to detect changes in the kinetics during the measurement as described in Section 15.3.2 was built (Schlothauer et al. 2009).

Up to that time the standard fit for $^1O_2$ kinetics in cells still was just biexponential, even if the idea to include the diffusion of $^1O_2$ into the fitting process was described already years ago (Baker and Kanofsky 1993; Oelckers 1999) and even if in some cases an obviously wrong time shift of the fit to negative values was necessary.

The improvement of SNR of $^1O_2$ luminescence detection achieved recently has allowed time measurements with LED excitation instead of lasers (Figure 15.9; Hackbarth et al. 2013b). Decay times, even in cells, could be determined with an accuracy of 0.1 µs. However, this method is limited by the selectivity of the PS under investigation. More complex systems like in vivo ensembles of cells may comprise different cell types. The PS might accumulate not just in one location, but in several cell types/locations with different conditions. Also it has turned out that the PS phosphorescence may become an issue (see Section 4.2.1 [Pfitzner]). In short, $^1O_2$ luminescence measurements in cell assemblies are very sensitive to the selectivity of PS localization. In each case, additional information about the intracellular PS location and triplet decay is needed for analysis.

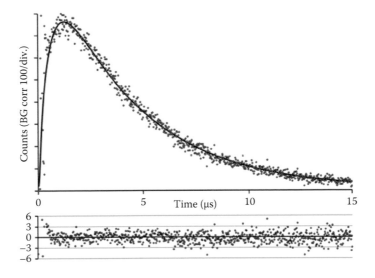

Figure 15.9 $^1O_2$ luminescence signal of HL60 cells in PBS ($5 \cdot 10^6$ m L^{-1}) incubated with Pheo (24 h, 3 µM) as determined with the LED setup, fitted with 1D diffusion model. The PS triplet decay and the $^1O_2$ decay time outside the membrane could be determined as τ_{Trip} = 4.0 µs and τ_Δ = 0.6 µs. (Reprinted from Hackbarth, S. et al., *Laser Phys. Lett.*, 10, 125702, 2013b.)

15.4.5 ESTIMATING $^1O_2$ IN CELLS BASED ON PS FLUORESCENCE AND TRIPLET KINETICS

In principle, one can expect, that $^1O_2$ generation and PS fluorescence are colocalized, yet their intensities might not correlate, since parameters like the triplet quantum yield Φ_T of the PS may strongly depend on the local environment. However, knowledge about the fluorescence decay times may allow a good estimation of the PS environment. Of course, the optical resolution of FLIM is not sufficient to discriminate a membrane from its surroundings, but, depending on the PS, the fluorescence decay time may provide that information. This way the triplet quantum yield of the PS in the cell may be estimated. Here we come to the limit of this method. The reliability of the correlation between fluorescence lifetime and triplet quantum yield limits the accuracy of all the measurement.

To determine which percentage of these PS molecules in the triplet state finally generates $^1O_2$, the triplet decay time can be determined in the presence and in the absence of oxygen (e.g., with flash photolysis). The average $^1O_2$ quantum yield Φ_Δ can be calculated with only a few prerequisites.

Since the rate of Dexter energy transfer kET to the oxygen is zero in the absence of oxygen, it can be stated that

$$\Phi_\Delta = \Phi_{ISC} \cdot \tau_{T,O} \cdot k_{ET} = \Phi_{ISC} \cdot \tau_{T,O} \cdot \left[\frac{1}{\tau_{T,O}} - \frac{1}{\tau_{T,\ominus}} \right] = \Phi_{ISC} \cdot \left[1 - \frac{\tau_{T,O}}{\tau_{T,\ominus}} \right] \qquad (15.6)$$

where

$\tau_{T,O}$ is the PS triplet decay time
$\tau_{T,\ominus}$ in the absence of oxygen

The only assumption used in such measurements is an exclusive type II photosensitization for all interactions of the PSs in the triplet state with oxygen, but according to (Bensasson et al. 1993; Schweitzer and Schmidt 2003), this assumption holds true for many PSs.

This method can give information about the location and the amount of generated $^1O_2$, but not about the interaction of the generated $^1O_2$ with the cellular material and the photosensitization resulting from it.

15.5 CONCLUSIONS

Subcellular imaging of PS activity comes along with a lot of problems: $^1O_2$ has a weak emission; it easily diffuses and may react with many biological molecules.

The latter problem limits the illumination dose and, together with the extremely weak emission, it makes direct imaging of $^1O_2$ in single living cells impossible. The interaction of the generated $^1O_2$ with cell components very soon kills the cell and changes the $^1O_2$ decay far beyond acceptable limits.

However, if killing of cells is aspired, e.g. during a PDT treatment, $^1O_2$ kinetics can be used to monitor the cell viability without the necessity of any additional sensor.

Diffusion of $^1O_2$ in cells is very short ranged. Therefore, colocalization is a serious issue for any indirect imaging method based on fluorogenic sensors. Measurements of many cells assembled together might allow to identify the place of PS localization encoded in the luminescence signal, due to $^1O_2$ diffusion.

As of the moment, the best option for PS activity imaging at the cellular scale seems to be time-resolved $^1O_2$ luminescence measurements in cell ensembles in combination with flash photolysis (or time-resolved phosphorescence) and FLIM.

REFERENCES

Baker, A. and J. R. Kanofsky. 1992. Quenching of singlet oxygen by biomolecules from L1210 leukemia cells. *Photochem. Photobiol.* **55** (4): 523–528. doi:10.1111/j.1751-1097.1992.tb04273.x.

Bacellar, I. O. L., C. Pavani, E. M. Sales, R. Itri, M. Wainwright, and M. S. Baptista. 2014. Membrane damage efficiency of phenothiazinium photosensitizers. *Photochem. Photobiol.* **90** (4): 801–813. doi:10.1111/php.12264.

Baier, J., M. Maier, R. Engl, M. Landthaler, and W. Bäumler. 2005. Time-resolved investigations of singlet oxygen luminescence in water, in phosphatidylcholine, and in aqueous suspensions of phosphatidylcholine or HT29 cells. *J. Phys. Chem. B* **109** (7): 3041–3046. doi:10.1021/jp0455531.

Baker, A. and J. R. Kanofsky. 1993. Time-resolved studies of singlet-oxygen emission from L1210 Leukemia cells labeled with 5-(N-Hexadecanoyl)amino eosin. A comparison with a one-dimensional model of singlet oxygen diffusion and quenching. *Photochem. Photobiol.* **57** (4): 720–727. doi:10.1111/j.1751-1097.1993.tb02944.x.

Bastien, E., R. Schneider, S. Hackbarth, D. Dumas, J. Jasniewski, B. Röder, L. Bezdetnaya, and H.-P. Lassalle. 2015. PAMAM G4.5-chlorin e6 dendrimeric nanoparticles for enhanced photodynamic effects. *Photochem. Photobiol. Sci. Off. J. Eur. Photochem. Assoc. Eur. Soc. Photobiol.* **14** (12): 2203–2212. doi:10.1039/c5pp00274e.

Battino, R., T. R. Rettich, and T. Tominaga. 1983. The solubility of oxygen and ozone in liquids. *J. Phys. Chem. Ref. Data* **12** (2): 163. doi:10.1063/1.555680.

Bensasson, R. V., E. J. Land, and T. G. Truscott. 1993. *Excited States and Free Radicals in Biology and Medicine: Contributions from Flash Photolysis and Pulse Radiolysis*. Oxford, U.K.: Oxford University Press/Oxford Science Publications.

Bielka, H. and K. Escherich, eds. 1985. *Molekularbiologie: Mit 81 Tabellen. Lizenz des Fischer-Verl., Jena.* Stuttgart, Germany: Fischer.

Castano, A. P., T. N. Demidova, and M. R. Hamblin. 2004. Mechanisms in photodynamic therapy: Part one-photosensitizers, photochemistry and cellular localization. *Photodiagn. Photodyn.* **1** (4): 279–293. doi:10.1016/S1572-1000(05)00007-4.

Cavalcante, R. S., H. Imasato, V. S. Bagnato, and J. R. Perussi. 2009. A combination of techniques to evaluate photodynamic efficiency of photosensitizers. *Laser Phys. Lett.* **6** (1): 64–70. doi:10.1002/lapl.200810082.

Cordeiro, R. M. 2014. Reactive oxygen species at phospholipid bilayers: Distribution, mobility and permeation. *Biochim. Biophys. Acta* **1838** (1 Pt B): 438–444. doi:10.1016/j.bbamem.2013.09.016.

Dutta, A. and A. S. Popel. 1995. A theoretical analysis of intracellular oxygen diffusion. *J. Theor. Biol.* **176** (4): 433–445. doi:10.1006/jtbi.1995.0211.

Flors, C., M. J. Fryer, J. Waring, B. Reeder, U. Bechtold, P. M. Mullineaux, S. Nonell, M. T. Wilson, and N. R. Baker. 2006. Imaging the production of singlet oxygen in vivo using a new fluorescent sensor, Singlet Oxygen Sensor Green. *J. Exp. Bot.* **57** (8): 1725–1734. doi:10.1093/jxb/erj181.

Freitas, R. A. 1999. *Nanomedicine*. Austin, TX: Landes Bioscience.

Gemmell, N. R., A. McCarthy, B. Liu, M. G. Tanner, S. D. Dorenbos, V. Zwiller, M. S. Patterson, G. S. Buller, B. C. Wilson, and R. H. Hadfield. 2013. Singlet oxygen luminescence detection with a fiber-coupled superconducting nanowire single-photon detector. *Opt. Express* **21** (4): 5005–5013. doi:10.1364/OE.21.005005.

Gollmer, A., J. Arnbjerg, F. H. Blaikie, B. W. Pedersen, T. Breitenbach, K. Daasbjerg, M. Glasius, and P. R. Ogilby. 2011. Singlet oxygen sensor green (R): Photochemical behavior in solution and in a mammalian cell. *Photochem. Photobiol.* **87** (3): 671–679. doi:10.1111/j.1751-1097.2011.00900.x.

Hackbarth, S., T. Bornhütter, and B. Röder. 2015a. Chapter 26: Singlet oxygen in heterogeneous systems. In *Singlet Oxygen: Applications in Biosciences and Nanosciences*, Vol. 2, eds. S. Nonell, pp. 27–42. Comprehensive Series in Photochemical and Photobiological Sciences. Royal Society of Chemistry, Cambridge, London.

Hackbarth, S., A. Preuss, T. Perna, J. Schlothauer, and B. Röder. 2013a. LEDs as excitation source for time resolved singlet oxygen luminescence detection in cell suspensions. In *SPIE 8568, Optical Methods for Tumor Treatment and Detection: Mechanisms and Techniques in Photodynamic Therapy XXII*, Bellingham, WA, 85680W SPIE. doi:10.1117/12.2008185.

Hackbarth, S. and B. Röder. 2015c. Singlet oxygen luminescence kinetics in heterogeneous environment— Identification of the photosensitizer localization in small unilamellar vesicles. *Photochem. Photobiol. Sci.* **14** (2): 329–334. doi:10.1039/C4PP00229F.

Hackbarth, S., J.C. Schlothauer, A. Preuss, C. Ludwig, and B. Röder. 2012. Time resolved sub-cellular singlet oxygen detection—Ensemble measurements versus single cell experiments. *Laser Phys. Lett.* **9** (6): 474–480. doi:10.7452/lapl.201110146.

Hackbarth, S., J. C. Schlothauer, A. Preuss, and B. Röder. 2010. New insights to primary photodynamic effects—Singlet oxygen kinetics in living cells. *J. Photochem. Photobiol. B* **98** (3): 173–179. doi:10.1016/j.jphotobiol.2009.11.013.

Hackbarth, S., J. C. Schlothauer, A. Preuss, and B. Röder. 2013b. Highly sensitive time resolved singlet oxygen luminescence detection using LEDs as the excitation source. *Laser Phys. Lett.* **10** (12): 125702. doi:10.1088/1612-2011/10/12/125702.

Hackbarth, S., J. C. Schlothauer, A. Preuss, and B. Röder. 2015b. First Sino-German Symposium on Singlet molecular oxygen and photodynamic effects: [1.01] Time-resolved singlet oxygen luminescence detection under PDT-relevant light doses. *Photon Lasers Med.* **4** (4): 299–301.

Han, S. K., T.-M. Hwang, Y. Yoon, and J.-W. Kang. 2011. Evidence of singlet oxygen and hydroxyl radical formation in aqueous goethite suspension using spin-trapping electron paramagnetic resonance (EPR). *Chemosphere* **84** (8): 1095–1101. doi:10.1016/j.chemosphere.2011.04.051.

Hatz, S., J. D. C. Lambert, and P. R. Ogilby. 2007. Measuring the lifetime of singlet oxygen in a single cell: Addressing the issue of cell viability. *Photochem. Photobiol. Sci.* **6** (10): 1106–1116. doi:10.1039/b707313e.

Jamnongwong, M., K. Loubiere, N. Dietrich, and G. Hébrard. 2010. Experimental study of oxygen diffusion coefficients in clean water containing salt, glucose or surfactant: Consequences on the liquid-side mass transfer coefficients. *Chem. Eng. J.* **165** (3): 758–768. doi:10.1016/j.cej.2010.09.040.

Jarvi, M. T., M. J. Niedre, M. S. Patterson, and B. C. Wilson. 2011. The influence of oxygen depletion and photosensitizer triplet-state dynamics during photodynamic therapy on accurate singlet oxygen luminescence monitoring and analysis of treatment dose response. *Photochem. Photobiol.* **87** (1): 223–234. doi:10.1111/j.1751-1097.2010.00851.x.

Jarvi, M. T., M. S. Patterson, and B. C. Wilson. 2012. Insights into photodynamic therapy dosimetry: Simultaneous singlet oxygen luminescence and photosensitizer photobleaching measurements. *Biophys. J.* **102** (3): 661–671. doi:10.1016/j.bpj.2011.12.043.

Jiménez-Banzo, A., X. Ragas, P. Kapusta, and S. Nonell. 2008a. Time-resolved methods in biophysics. Photon counting vs. analog time-resolved singlet oxygen phosphorescence detection. *Photochem. Photobiol. Sci.* **7** (9): 1003–1010. doi:10.1039/b804333g.

Jiménez-Banzo, A., M. L. Sagristà, M. Mora, and S. Nonell. 2008b. Kinetics of singlet oxygen photosensitization in human skin fibroblasts. *Free Radic. Biol. Med.* **44** (11): 1926–1934. doi:10.1016/j.freeradbiomed.2008.02.011.

Juzeniene, A., Q. Peng, and J. Moan. 2007. Milestones in the development of photodynamic therapy and fluorescence diagnosis. *Photochem. Photobiol. Sci.* **6** (12): 1234. doi:10.1039/b705461k.

Kanofsky, J. R. 2011. Measurement of singlet-oxygen in vivo: Progress and pitfalls. *Photochem. Photobiol.* **87** (1): 14–17. doi:10.1111/j.1751-1097.2010.00855.x.

Kondo, R., K. V. Gleixner, M. Mayerhofer, A. Vales, A. Gruze, P. Samorapoompichit, K. Greish et al. 2007. Identification of heat shock protein 32 (Hsp32) as a novel survival factor and therapeutic target in neoplastic mast cells. *Blood* **110** (2): 661–669. doi:10.1182/blood-2006-10-054411.

Krumova, K. and G. Cosa. 2013. Fluorogenic probes for imaging reactive oxygen species. In *Photochemistry*. Vol. 41, eds. A. Albini and E. Fasani, pp. 279–301. Cambridge, U.K.: Royal Society of Chemistry.

Lee, P. C. and M. A. J. Rodgers. 1983. Singlet molecular oxygen in micellar systems. 1. Distribution equilibriums between hydrophobic and hydrophilic compartments. *J. Phys. Chem.* **87** (24): 4894–4898. doi:10.1021/j150642a027.

Li, B., H. Lin, D. Chen, B. C. Wilson, and G. Ying. 2013. Singlet oxygen detection during photosensitization. *J. Innov. Opt. Health Sci.* **06** (01): 1330002. doi:10.1142/S1793545813300024.

Lin, H., Y. Shen, D. Chen, L. Lin, B. C. Wilson, B. Li, and S. Xie. 2013. Feasibility study on quantitative measurements of singlet oxygen generation using singlet oxygen sensor green. *J. Fluoresc.* **23** (1): 41–47. doi:10.1007/s10895-012-1114-5.

Nagle, J. F., and S. Tristram-Nagle. 2000. Structure of lipid bilayers. *Biochim. Biophys. Acta* **1469** (3): 159–195.

Niedre, M. J., M. S. Patterson, and B. C. Wilson. 2002. Direct near-infrared luminescence detection of singlet oxygen generated by photodynamic therapy in cells in vitro and tissues in vivo. *Photochem. Photobiol.* **75** (4): 382–391. doi:10.1562/0031-8655(2002)0750382DNILDO2.0.CO2.

Oelckers, S. 1999. *Singulett-Sauerstoff im Modellsystem photosensibilisierte Erythrozyten-Ghost-Suspensionen: Apparative Entwicklungen und zeitaufgelöste spektroskopische Untersuchungen.* 1. Aufl. Berlin, Germany: Mensch-und-Buch-Verl.

Oelckers, S., M. Sczepan, T. Hanke, and B. Röder. 1997. Time-resolved detection of singlet oxygen luminescence in red cell ghost suspensions. *J. Photochem. Photobiol. B Biol.* **39** (3): 219–223. doi:10.1016/S1011-1344(97)00011-0.

Ogilby, P. R. 2010. Singlet oxygen: There is still something new under the sun, and it is better than ever. *Photochem. Photobiol. Sci. Off. J. Eur. Photochem. Assoc. Eur. Soc. Photobiol.* **9** (12): 1543–1560. doi:10.1039/c0pp00213e.

Pedersen, St. K., J. Holmehave, F. H. Blaikie, A. Gollmer, T. Breitenbach, H. H. Jensen, and P. R. Ogilby. 2014. Aarhus sensor green: A fluorescent probe for singlet oxygen. *J. Org. Chem.* **79** (7): 3079–3087. doi:10.1021/jo500219y.

Pfitzner, M., J. C. Schlothauer, S. Hackbarth, and B. Röder. 2016. Prospects of singlet oxygen luminescence monitoring after administration of PS in living mice. *Photodiag. Photodyn. Ther.* **14**: 204–210.

Poulsen, T. D., P. R. Ogilby, and K. V. Mikkelsen. 1998. Solvent effects on the O_2 (a 1 Δ g) - O_2 (X 3 Σ g-) radiative transition: Comments regarding charge-transfer interactions. *J. Phys. Chem. A* **102** (48): 9829–9832. doi:10.1021/jp982567w.

Price, M., J. J. Reiners, A. M. Santiago, and D. Kessel. 2009. Monitoring singlet oxygen and hydroxyl radical formation with fluorescent probes during photodynamic therapy. *Photochem. Photobiol.* **85** (5): 1177–1181. doi:10.1111/j.1751-1097.2009.00555.x.

Redmond, R. W. and I. E. Kochevar. 2006. Spatially resolved cellular responses to singlet oxygen. *Photochem. Photobiol.* **82** (5): 1178–1186. doi:10.1562/2006-04-14-IR-874.

Rodgers, M. A. J. 1983. Solvent-induced deactivation of singlet oxygen: Additivity relationships in nonaromatic solvents. *J. Am. Chem. Soc.* **105** (20): 6201–6205. doi:10.1021/ja00358a001.

Ruiz-González, R., R. Zanocco, Y. Gidi, A. L. Zanocco, S. Nonell, and E. Lemp. 2013. Naphthoxazole-based singlet oxygen fluorescent probes. *Photochem. Photobiol.* **89** (6): 1427–1432. doi:10.1111/php.12106.

Schlothauer, J. C., S. Hackbarth, L. Jäger, K. Drobniewski, H. Patel, S. M. Gorun, and B. Röder. 2012. Time-resolved singlet oxygen luminescence detection under photodynamic therapy relevant conditions: Comparison of ex vivo application of two photosensitizer formulations. *J. Biomed. Opt.* **17** (11): 115005. doi:10.1117/1.JBO.17.11.115005.

Schlothauer, J. C., S. Hackbarth, and B. Röder. 2009. A new benchmark for time-resolved detection of singlet oxygen luminescence—Revealing the evolution of lifetime in living cells with low dose illumination. *Laser Phys. Lett.* **6** (3): 216–221. doi:10.1002/lapl.200810116.

Schlothauer, J. C., S. Hackbarth, and B. Röder. 2015. First Sino-German Symposium on Singlet molecular oxygen and photodynamic effects: [1.03] Current prospects of detectors for high performance time-resolved singlet oxygen luminescence detection. *Photon. Lasers Med.* **4** (4): 303–306.

Schweitzer, C. and R. Schmidt. 2003. Physical mechanisms of generation and deactivation of singlet oxygen. *Chem. Rev.* **103** (5): 1685–1757. doi:10.1021/cr010371d.

Scurlock, R. D., S. Nonell, S. E. Braslavsky, and P. R. Ogilby. 1995. Effect of solvent on the radiative decay of singlet molecular oxygen (a1.DELTA.g). *J. Phys. Chem.* **99** (11): 3521–3526. doi:10.1021/j100011a019.

Shen, Y., H. Lin, Z. F. Huang, D. F. Chen, B. Li, and S. Xie. 2011. Indirect imaging of singlet oxygen generation from a single cell. *Laser Phys. Lett.* **8** (3): 232–238. doi:10.1002/lapl.201010113.

Sidell, B. D. 1998. Intracellular oxygen diffusion: The roles of myoglobin and lipid at cold body temperature. *J. Exp. Biol.* **201** (Pt 8): 1119–1128.

Snyder, J. W., E. Skovsen, J. D. C Lambert, and P. R. Ogilby. 2005. Subcellular, time-resolved studies of singlet oxygen in single cells. *J. Am. Chem. Soc.* **127** (42): 14558–14559. doi:10.1021/ja055342p.

Snyder, J. W., I. Zebger, Z. Gao, L. Poulsen, P. K. Frederiksen, E. Skovsen, S. P. McIlroy, M. Klinger, L. K. Andersen, and P. R. Ogilby. 2004. Singlet oxygen microscope: From phase-separated polymers to single biological cells. *Acc. Chem. Res.* **37** (11): 894–901. doi:10.1021/ar040075y.

Spiller, W., H. Kliesch, D. Woehrle, S. Hackbarth, B. Röder, and G. Schnurpfeil. 1997. Singlet oxygen quantum yields of different photosensitizers in polar solvents and micellar solutions. Accessed August 15, 2014.

St-Denis, C. E. and C. J. D Fell. 1971. Diffusivity of oxygen in water. *Can. J. Chem. Eng.* **49** (6): 885. doi:10.1002/cjce.5450490632.

Tanaka, K., T. Miura, N. Umezawa, Y. Urano, K. Kikuchi, T. Higuchi, and T. Nagano. 2001. Rational design of fluorescein-based fluorescence probes. Mechanism-based design of a maximum fluorescence probe for singlet oxygen. *J. Am. Chem. Soc.* **123**(11): 2530–2636. doi:10.1021/ja0035708.

Vyklický, V., R. Dedic, N. Curkaniuk, and J. Hála. 2013. Spectral- and time-resolved phosphorescence of photosensitizers and singlet oxygen: From in vitro towards in vivo. *J. Luminescence* **143**: 729–733.

Wang, K. K.-H., J. C. Finlay, T. M. Busch, S. M. Hahn, and T. C. Zhu. 2010. Explicit dosimetry for photodynamic therapy: Macroscopic singlet oxygen modeling. *J. Biophotonics* **3** (5–6): 304–318. doi:10.1002/jbio.200900101.

Weston, M. A. and M. S. Patterson. 2014. Effect of $^1O_2$ quencher depletion on the efficiency of photodynamic therapy. *Photochem. Photobiol. Sci. Off. J. Eur. Photochem. Assoc. Eur. Soc. Photobiol.* **13** (1): 112–121. doi:10.1039/c3pp50258a.

White, C. J., C. T. Elliott, and J. R. White. 2010. Micro-electron spin resonance (ESR/EPR) spectroscopy. In *SPIE Defense, Security, and Sensing*, eds. M. A. Druy, C. D. Brown, and R. A. Crocombe, pp. 76800O–76800O-11. SPIE Proceedings

Zebger, I., J. W. Snyder, L. K. Andersen, L. Poulsen, Z. Gao, J. D. C. Lambert, U. Kristiansen, and P. R. Ogilby. 2004. Direct optical detection of singlet oxygen from a single cell. *Photochem. Photobiol.* **79** (4): 319–322.

Bioluminescence imaging for monitoring the effectiveness of photodynamic therapy for infections in animal models

PAWEL MROZ AND MICHAEL R. HAMBLIN

16.1 PHOTODYNAMIC THERAPY FOR INFECTIONS

Photodynamic therapy (PDT) combines visible light illumination and certain nontoxic dyes known as photosensitizers (PS) [1]. When PS are irradiated by light of appropriate wavelength, the absorbed energy carried by photons leads to the activation of the PS from the ground state to the excited singlet state (Figure 16.1). This excited singlet state may then undergo intersystem crossing to the slightly lower energy but longer-lived triplet state [2]. The latter may then react further by one or both of two pathways. Type I pathway leads to electron transfer reactions to produce radicals, while type II pathway leads to energy transfer reactions to produce excited-state, singlet molecular oxygen. Both of these processes are oxygen dependent and lead to the production of highly toxic reactive oxygen species (ROS). The ROS can readily react with biological molecules such as proteins, lipids, and nucleic acids and therefore can lead to their oxidation, subsequent damage, and activation of apoptosis [3].

The advantage of PDT over other therapies is that it has dual selectivity: not only the PS may preferentially target the diseased tissue, but also the selective delivery of light to the specific area augments the selectivity of therapy and protects uninvolved tissues.

Although PDT was initially developed as an anticancer therapy, it has recently been successfully applied to treat other conditions including microbial infections [4–8].

In the 1990s, it was observed that fundamental differences in susceptibility to PDT exist between Gram-positive and Gram-negative bacteria. This was explained by differences in their morphology: in Gram-positive bacteria the cytoplasmic membrane is surrounded by a thick layer of only peptidoglycan and lipoteichoic acid that is relatively porous, while the Gram-negative bacteria have a somewhat more intricate, nonporous cell wall structure consisting of an inner cytoplasmic membrane and an outer membrane, which are separated by the thin peptidoglycan-containing periplasm. It was discovered that in general, neutral or

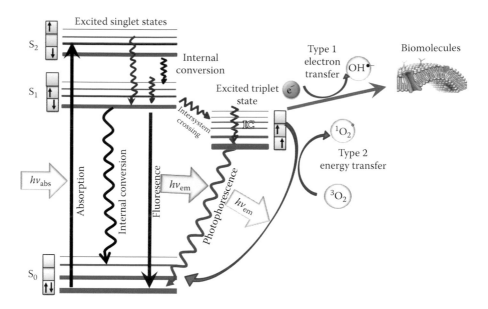

Figure 16.1 Jablonski diagram.

anionic PS molecules bind more efficiently to Gram-positive bacteria and therefore they are more effective at PDI, whereas photodynamic inactivation (PDI) of Gram-negative bacteria requires the penetration of PS inside the cell, making Gram-negative bacteria a more challenging target [5]. Several techniques have been developed to allow for better intracellular uptake of PS by bacteria and to improve the treatment outcomes, including the use of agents that are capable of increasing the permeability of the cell outer membrane (poly-myxin B nonapeptide, or EDTA) [9–12], the use of PS with an intrinsic positive charge, or the polycationic PS conjugates formed from polymers such as polylysine.

The ability of PDI to efficiently destroy multiple classes of microorganisms, together with concern about the rapidly increasing emergence of antibiotic resistance among pathogenic bacteria, has suggested that PDT may be a useful tool to combat infectious diseases [13]. Several studies have shown that antibiotic-resistant bacteria are as susceptible to PDI as their naïve counterparts. The nature of the PDI-induced damage that involves oxidative modification of vital cellular constituents suggests that bacteria will not easily be able to develop resistance mechanisms, and one study has shown that resistance to PDI does not occur. Moreover, it is not necessary to microbiologically identify the infectious microorganisms before administering PDT, as in the case when prescribing antibiotics, which means that treatment can be started sooner.

Nevertheless, there are several limitations to PDI. Because the delivery of visible light is almost by definition a localized process, PDT for infections is likely to be applied exclusively to localized disease, as opposed to systemic infections such as bacteremia. The key issues to be addressed with PDT are the effectiveness of the treatment in destroying sufficient numbers of the disease-causing pathogens; the selectivity of the PS for the microbes, thus avoiding an unacceptable degree of PDT damage to host tissue in the area of infection; and the avoidance of regrowth of the pathogens from a few survivors in the time following the treatment. In vivo studies would provide many answers to these questions. However, despite the considerable number of reports on in vitro PDI of microorganisms, in vivo studies on infection models are rare. One of the reasons for this is probably the difficulty in monitoring the development of an infection and its response to treatment. Standard microbiological techniques used to follow infections in animal models frequently involve sacrifice of the animals, removal of the infected tissue, homogenization, serial dilution, plating, and colony counting. These assays use a large number of animals, are time consuming, and often are not statistically reliable.

Bioluminescence imaging (BLI) therefore has been recently successfully explored as an efficient way to monitor the effectiveness of PDT in murine models of microbial infections [14,15].

16.2 BIOLUMINESCENCE

Various living organisms are able to emit light. The enzymes involved in this process, named luciferases, are oxygenases that utilize molecular oxygen to oxidize a substrate molecule (luciferin, coelenterazine, or decanal), with the formation of a product molecule in an excited state that emits the light. Several different luciferases and substrates from several organisms are known, many of which have different light emission spectra [15]. Three luciferases have been successfully cloned and their chemistries characterized to a point where they can be used routinely in the laboratory [16]. These include the luciferases from firefly (coleoptera) [17], jellyfish and sea pansies (cnidaria), and bacteria (*Vibrio* spp. and *Photorhabdus luminescens*) [18]. Representatives of each of these types of luciferases have been used for imaging in living laboratory animals.

The luciferases from firefly, click beetles, and railroad worms take the form of a single protein related to the CoA ligase family of enzymes and use a benzothiazole luciferin substrate along with ATP and oxygen to generate light [19]. The gene encoding firefly luciferase has been cloned, and the coding sequence has been optimized for mammalian expression. Cells expressing this enzyme, when provided with luciferin, will emit a yellow-green light with an emission peak at 560 nm using cellular ATP as the energy source.

The luciferases from sea pansy *Renilla* and jellyfish *Aequorea* use coelenterazine as the substrate, and unlike the firefly or bacterial luciferases, neither enzyme requires a cellular energy source [20] because the coelenterazine substrate itself provides the necessary energy. The different spectra of light emission of the firefly and coelenterazine-utilizing luciferases and their mutually exclusive substrate specificity have allowed both reporters to be used in the same cell to monitor the expression of two different tagged genes.

Bacterial luciferases are heterodimeric proteins and use oxygen, long-chain fatty aldehydes (e.g., decanal), and reduced flavin mononucleotide ($FMNH_2$) as substrates to produce a blue-green light with emission peak at 490 nm [21]. In both marine and terrestrial bioluminescent bacteria, a five-gene operon (*luxCDABE*) encodes the luciferase and biosynthetic enzymes necessary for the synthesis of the aldehyde substrate and light production. The genes *luxA* and luxB encode the alpha and beta subunits of the luciferase, with *luxC*, *luxD*, and *luxE* encoding proteins for aldehyde production [22]. The *lux* operon from *P. luminescens* has been shown to be ideally suited for the study of pathogens in mammalian animal models as the enzyme retains significant activity at 37°C.

The first demonstration of detection and monitoring of light emission from small mammals was performed in 1995 using a bioluminescent genetically engineered Gram-negative bacteria expressing the full bacterial lux operon [23,24]. Although bacterial bioluminescent reporters have been limited to use in prokaryotic systems and emit blue light, they have the advantages of being well expressed in bacteria and not requiring the exogenous addition of a substrate.

The luxCDABE operon from *P. luminescens* can be expressed successfully in a wide range of Gram-negative bacteria, including *Escherichia coli* and *Salmonella* spp. [25]. However, for expression in Gram-positive bacteria (such as *Staphylococcus aureus*) [26], the operon had to be redesigned with Gram-positive ribosome binding sites (Shine–Dalgarno sites) at the start of each gene for optimal expression and bioluminescence at temperatures above 35°C [27]. The gene order was also changed from *luxCDABE* to *luxABCDE* in these constructs.

16.2.1 BIOLUMINESCENCE IMAGING

For optimal detection of light emitted by bioluminescence reporter genes in animal models, a CCD-based imaging system has been successfully employed [23,28,29]. These systems consist of a light-tight chamber in which the animal subjects are placed, a sensitive CCD camera to detect the light emitted, and a computer controller to acquire the image and allow analysis of the data. Typically, a grayscale reference image of the animal is acquired under weak illumination, and then the bioluminescent signal is captured in complete darkness. This process may take from a few seconds to several minutes, depending on the brightness of the bioluminescent signal, the depth within the tissue from which it arises, and the sensitivity of the detector.

The signal intensity is then represented as a pseudocolor image and superimposed on the grayscale reference image. The magnitude of the signal can then be measured from specified regions of the animals using a "region of interest" function.

Different CCD cameras may have different sensitivities for varying wavelengths of light that can be important for in vivo BLI since blue and green lights (shorter wavelengths) are largely absorbed by tissues, while red light (longer wavelengths) penetrates deeper. The primary absorber in the body in the visible region of the spectrum (400–600 nm) is hemoglobin. At wavelengths of 600 nm and above, scattering of photons becomes a more significant attenuation factor than absorption. Other pigments such as melanin (in animals with dark skin and fur) can also influence the efficiency of BLI. This can be avoided by using hairless or nude animals or by breeding dark mouse strains into albino backgrounds. The thickness of the tissue is also important: the more tissue between the reporter and the detector, the more light is lost as a result of the combination of light absorption and scattering. Therefore, the use of smaller animals (e.g., mice and rats) for BLI is preferable [30].

BLI can be used to either track the course of an infection or monitor the efficacy of antimicrobial therapies. Small animals are routinely used to model both human infections and the effects of antibiotics against pathogens. In such studies, groups of animals have typically been infected with the pathogenic organism and, at defined time points, subsets of these are sacrificed, and tissues are excised for the determination of pathogen numbers and localization. The effects of antimicrobial drugs on the infection have been determined by measuring changes in this pathogen burden or, alternatively, by the prolonged survival of the animal after a lethal dose of the pathogen. Such approaches have traditionally required large numbers of animals and potentially time-consuming processing of animal tissue to locate and quantify the infections. The use of pathogens that have been engineered to express luciferase and the imaging of their location and cell number have streamlined these studies and refined these animal models as the necessity to sacrifice the animals to access the data has essentially been eliminated. Bacterial pathogenesis appeared to be unaffected by the presence of the luciferase genes, and bioluminescence can be detected throughout the study period in animals. Further, the intensity of the bioluminescence measured from the living animal correlated well with the bacterial burden subsequently determined by standard protocols [28–30]. Subsequent studies have used transposon-mediated integration of the luciferase operon into the bacterial chromosome to improve stability and to create strains that remain bioluminescent in the absence of drug selection. This means that reduction of luminescence from sites of infection in animals can be attributed to reduction of bacterial numbers rather than loss of plasmids.

In our initial studies we used Gram-negative bacterial species *E. coli* and *Pseudomonas aeruginosa* that had been transformed by electroporation with a plasmid, pCGSL1, containing the entire *P. luminescens* lux operon, which also confers resistance to ampicillin (carbenicillin) on the bacteria. This plasmid is a ColE1 replicon containing the *luxCDABE* operon from *P. luminescens* and an ampicillin resistance marker. Because the highest levels of luminescence occur in the exponential phase of growth, we used cells from cultures at a density of about 10^8 cells/mL. We subsequently used the Gram-positive *S. aureus* that had been stably engineered to express bioluminescence. This was done by using a luxABCDE transposon cassette, Tn4001 luxABCDE Km(r), that allows random integration of lux genes onto the bacterial chromosome.

16.2.2 PROCEDURE FOR BIOLUMINESCENCE MONITORING OF PDI OF INFECTIONS

First, ascertain that the luminescence signal measured in a tube luminometer is linearly proportional to bacterial colony-forming units (CFUs) as determined by serial dilution and plating from 10^3 to 10^7 organisms. The signal saturates at large bacterial numbers, that is, $>10^7$. In addition to counting the colonies, imaging the plates using the photon-counting camera is another way to accumulate data.

In vitro measure the light from bacterial suspensions using a tube luminometer or on a 96-well luminescence plate reader. In vivo imaging can be done using the Hamamatsu photon-counting camera controlled by ARGUS software. The system consists of an ICCD camera fitted with a f1.2 50 mm lens and mounted in a light-tight specimen chamber. In a photon-counting mode, capture an image of the emitted light using an integration time of 2 min at a maximum setting on the image intensifier control module. Using ARGUS software presents the luminescence image as a false-color image superimposed on top of the grayscale reference image.

For the light source for PDT, use a diode laser providing up to 1 W of light through an SMA coupled fiber and lens that provides a uniform spot ranging from 1 to 3 cm in diameter for both in vitro and in vivo experiments.

Next, in order to verify that killing the bacteria, as demonstrated by loss of CFUs, correlates with loss of luminescence, carry out in vitro PDI experiments. Measure the loss of viability by CFU and by loss of luminescence as a function of applied light dose. In our experience the CFU assay has a limit of sensitivity of six orders of magnitude in reduction of viability, while the bioluminescence assay has a limit of three orders of magnitude. Loss of luminescence should show the same dose–response curves as loss of CFU but the absolute reductions are 1–3 logs less. We believe that the reason for this is most likely to be due to the limit of sensitivity of the camera, which is only capable of measuring a 3 log reduction in signal, as compared to a 6 log reduction in viability measurable by CFU plating. Nevertheless, it is important to note that luminescent measurements can be achieved in minutes, as opposed to several hours from a combination of overnight incubation followed by laborious and time-consuming counting of CFU. The mechanism by which luminescence decreases after PDI is uncertain, but may be due to exhaustion of $FMNH_2$ supplies from the bacteria (needed for the luciferase enzyme to make luminescence) and cannot be replenished if the cells are fatally damaged.

Next, move on to the animal model of infection by inoculating an aliquot of a midlog culture of bioluminescent bacteria into an excisional wound on the mouse. The inoculum should give a sufficiently bright luminescence signal from the wound to allow at least two logs of signal reduction to be accurately followed. Apply PS and perform PDT treatment after the predetermined drug-light interval.

Capture images at several time points at several bit ranges in order to ensure that a set of images at the same bit range for the different time points of the whole experiment are generated in order to make a set of composite images in which the bioluminescence signals could be directly compared (even if some images have saturated pixels). For the ARGUS quantification to be accurate however, it is important to analyze images that contain no saturated pixels, hence the need to capture many images at each time point.

For quantitative data, calculate the mean luminescence values in a region of interest drawn on the experimental animal using the imaging software.

16.2.3 EXAMPLES OF PDT OF INFECTIONS MONITORED BY BIOLUMINESCENCE IMAGING

The first study is concerned on the PDT of excisional wounds on the mouse back that were infected with bioluminescent E. coli DH5α (Figure 16.2) [30]. The PS employed was a covalent conjugate between the polycationic polymer poly-L-lysine and chlorin (e6) called pL-ce6 [5]. Because this particular strain of E. coli is noninvasive, the infection is self-limiting and multiple wounds could be constructed on a single mouse to allow the testing of a treatment such as antimicrobial PDT with four separate wounds on each mouse acting as appropriate controls. It can be seen that only the wounds that received the combination of pL-ce6 and 165 J/cm² of 660 nm light had a total loss of bioluminescent signal indicating bacterial eradication. The next study went on to show that mouse excisional wounds infected by a virulent strain of bioluminescent P. aeruginosa could also be successfully treated with a PDT, saving mice from death due to sepsis [31] (Figure 16.3). Because this was a highly invasive strain of P. aeruginosa, we were only able to use a single wound on each mouse. Subsequent studies went on to study excisional wounds infected with bioluminescent Proteus mirabilis or P. aeruginosa, treated with a PDT mediated by a cationic fullerene and white light activation [32].

We then developed two different models of infected skin abrasions to study the effect of a PDT. The first model consisted of an overlapping series of needle scratches that could develop an infection by topically applied methicillin-resistant S. aureus (MRSA) cells [33]. In order for the infection to become established, the mice needed to be rendered temporarily neutropenic. This was accomplished by administering two successive

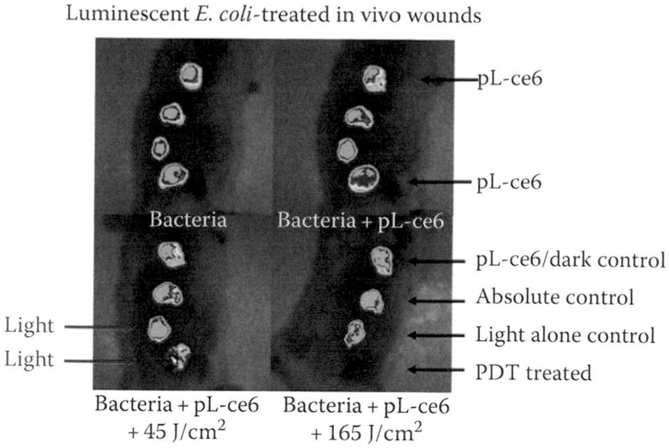

Luminescent *E. coli*-treated in vivo wounds

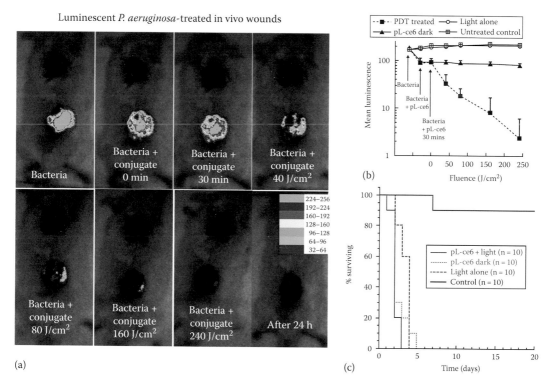

Figure 16.2 Photodynamic therapy of mouse excisional wounds infected with bioluminescent *E. coli*. Successive overlaid bioluminescence images of a mouse with four excisional wounds infected with equal numbers of luminescent *E. coli*. Wounds 1 (nearest tail) and 4 (nearest head) received topical application of pL-ce6. Wounds 1 and 2 (two nearest tail) were then illuminated with successive fluences (40–160 J/cm²) of 665 nm light.

Figure 16.3 Photodynamic therapy of mouse excisional wounds infected with bioluminescent *P. aeruginosa*. (a) Successive bioluminescence images of a mouse bearing an excisional wound infected with 5 × 10 [6] luminescent *P. aeruginosa* and treated by the addition of pL-ce6, followed by illumination with 660 nm light up to 240 J/cm² and 24 h after PDT. (b) Mean pixel values of luminescence signals from defined areas in infected wounds determined by image analysis. The four groups comprised absolute control, light-alone control, dark pL-ce6 conjugate control, and PDT treated. Data points are means of values from the wounds on 10 mice per group and bars are SD. (c) Kaplan–Meier survival plot for the four groups of mice.

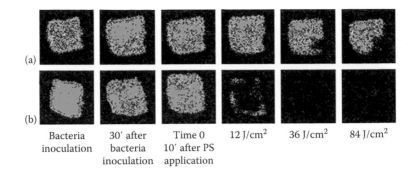

Figure 16.4 Photodynamic therapy of mouse partial thickness skin abrasions infected with bioluminescent MRSA. Successive bioluminescence images of a representative mouse skin scratch model infected with 10 [8] CFU MRSA treated with (a) light alone and (b) PDT using RLP068/Cl (40 μL of 75 μM solution) at 30 min after bacterial inoculation +15 min from PS application. PDT was carried out with 84 J/cm² red light.

IP injections of cyclophosphamide, the first of 100 mg/kg 4 days before wounding and the second of 150 mg/kg 1 day before wounding. Topical application of a tetracationic phthalocyanine (RLP068) (40 μL of a 75 μM solution) and irradiation with up to 84 J/cm² of 690 nm light led to a light dose-dependent reduction of luminescence signal (Figure 16.4).

The second model involved removal of a superficial layer of epidermis by scraping with a scalpel blade or by using "sandpaper" that could be infected with *Candida albicans* [34].

16.3 CONCLUSIONS

BLI has revolutionized the approach to monitoring bacterial infections and allowed for much faster and precise monitoring of therapeutic effects of a range of antimicrobial therapies. In the case of PDI, the loss of bioluminescence signal during the PDT correlated well with delivered fluence and with photosensitizer concentration that collectively determines the "PDT dose." BLI can be used to check the reproducibility of the added bacterial inoculum and to monitor the progress of the infection over time and the response to the treatment over the succeeding days.

REFERENCES

1. Agostinis P, Berg K, Cengel KA, Foster TH, Girotti AW, Gollnick SO et al. Photodynamic therapy of cancer: An update. *CA Cancer J Clin.* 2011; **61**(4):250–281.
2. Castano AP, Mroz P, Hamblin MR. Photodynamic therapy and anti-tumour immunity. *Nat Rev Cancer.* 2006; **6**(7):535–545.
3. Mroz P, Bhaumik J, Dogutan DK, Aly Z, Kamal Z, Khalid L et al. Imidazole metalloporphyrins as photosensitizers for photodynamic therapy: Role of molecular charge, central metal and hydroxyl radical production. *Cancer Letters.* 2009; **282**(1):63–76.
4. Malik Z, Ladan H, Nitzan Y. Photodynamic inactivation of Gram-negative bacteria: Problems and possible solutions. *J Photochem Photobiol B.* 1992; **14**(3):262–266.
5. Hamblin MR, O'Donnell DA, Murthy N, Rajagopalan K, Michaud N, Sherwood ME et al. Polycationic photosensitizer conjugates: Effects of chain length and Gram classification on the photodynamic inactivation of bacteria. *J Antimicrob Chemother.* 2002; **49**(6):941–951.
6. Soukos NS, Ximenez-Fyvie LA, Hamblin MR, Socransky SS, Hasan T. Targeted antimicrobial photochemotherapy. *Antimicrob Agents Chemother.* 1998; **42**(10):2595–2601.

7. Lauro FM, Pretto P, Covolo L, Jori G, Bertoloni G. Photoinactivation of bacterial strains involved in periodontal diseases sensitized by porphycene-polylysine conjugates. *Photochem Photobiol Sci.* 2002; **1**(7):468–470.

8. Rovaldi CR, Pievsky A, Sole NA, Friden PM, Rothstein DM, Spacciapoli P. Photoactive porphyrin derivative with broad-spectrum activity against oral pathogens In vitro. *Antimicrob Agents Chemother.* 2000; **44**(12):3364–3367.

9. Nitzan Y, Gutterman M, Malik Z, Ehrenberg B. Inactivation of gram-negative bacteria by photosensitized porphyrins. *Photochem Photobiol.* 1992; **55**(1):89–96.

10. Bertoloni G, Rossi F, Valduga G, Jori G, van Lier J. Photosensitizing activity of water- and lipid-soluble phthalocyanines on *Escherichia coli. FEMS Microbiol Lett.* 1990; **59**(1–2):149–155.

11. Merchat M, Bertolini G, Giacomini P, Villanueva A, Jori G. Meso-substituted cationic porphyrins as efficient photosensitizers of gram-positive and gram-negative bacteria. *J Photochem Photobiol B.* 1996; **32**(3):153–157.

12. Minnock A, Vernon DI, Schofield J, Griffiths J, Parish JH, Brown SB. Mechanism of uptake of a cationic water-soluble pyridinium zinc phthalocyanine across the outer membrane of *Escherichia coli. Antimicrob Agents Chemother.* 2000; **44**(3):522–527.

13. Hamblin MR, Hasan T. Photodynamic therapy: A new antimicrobial approach to infectious disease? *Photochem Photobiol Sci.* 2004; **3**(5):436–450.

14. Hamblin MR, Zahra T, Contag CH, McManus AT, Hasan T. Optical monitoring and treatment of potentially lethal wound infections in vivo. *J Infect Dis* 2003; **187**(11):1717–1726.

15. Doyle TC, Burns SM, Contag CH. In vivo bioluminescence imaging for integrated studies of infection. *Cell Microbiol.* 2004; **6**(4):303–317.

16. Hastings JW. Chemistries and colors of bioluminescent reactions: A review. *Gene.* 1996; **173**(1 Spec No):5–11.

17. de Wet JR, Wood KV, DeLuca M, Helinski DR, Subramani S. Firefly luciferase gene: Structure and expression in mammalian cells. *Mol Cell Biol.* 1987; **7**(2):725–737.

18. Viviani VR. The origin, diversity, and structure function relationships of insect luciferases. *Cell Mol life Sci CMLS.* 2002; **59**(11):1833–1850.

19. Hart RC, Matthews JC, Hori K, Cormier MJ. *Renilla reniformis* bioluminescence: Luciferase-catalyzed production of nonradiating excited states from luciferin analogues and elucidation of the excited state species involved in energy transfer to Renilla green fluorescent protein. *Biochemistry.* 1979; **18**(11):2204–2210.

20. Parsons SJ, Rhodes SA, Connor HE, Rees S, Brown J, Giles H. Use of a dual firefly and Renilla luciferase reporter gene assay to simultaneously determine drug selectivity at human corticotrophin releasing hormone 1 and 2 receptors. *Anal Biochem.* 2000; **281**(2):187–192.

21. Meighen EA. Molecular biology of bacterial bioluminescence. *Microbiol Rev.* 1991; **55**(1):123–142.

22. Meighen EA. Bacterial bioluminescence: Organization, regulation, and application of the lux genes. *FASEB J Off Publ Feder Am Soc Exp Biol.* 1993; **7**(11):1016–1022.

23. Contag CH, Contag PR, Mullins JI, Spilman SD, Stevenson DK, Benaron DA. Photonic detection of bacterial pathogens in living hosts. *Mol Microbiol.* 1995; **18**(4):593–603.

24. Contag PR, Olomu IN, Stevenson DK, Contag CH. Bioluminescent indicators in living mammals. *Nat Med.* 1998; **4**(2):245–247.

25. Rocchetta HL, Boylan CJ, Foley JW, Iversen PW, LeTourneau DL, McMillian CL et al. Validation of a noninvasive, real-time imaging technology using bioluminescent *Escherichia coli* in the neutropenic mouse thigh model of infection. *Antimicrob Agents Chemother.* 2001; **45**(1):129–137.

26. Francis KP, Joh D, Bellinger-Kawahara C, Hawkinson MJ, Purchio TF, Contag PR. Monitoring bioluminescent *Staphylococcus aureus* infections in living mice using a novel luxABCDE construct. *Inf Immun.* 2000; **68**(6):3594–3600.

27. Francis KP, Yu J, Bellinger-Kawahara C, Joh D, Hawkinson MJ, Xiao G et al. Visualizing pneumococcal infections in the lungs of live mice using bioluminescent Streptococcus pneumoniae transformed with a novel gram-positive lux transposon. *Inf Immun.* 2001; **69**(5):3350–3358.

28. Contag CH, Bachmann MH. Advances in in vivo bioluminescence imaging of gene expression. *Ann Rev Biomed Eng.* 2002; **4**:235–260.

29. Contag CH, Spilman SD, Contag PR, Oshiro M, Eames B, Dennery P et al. Visualizing gene expression in living mammals using a bioluminescent reporter. *Photochem Photobiol.* 1997; **66**(4):523–531.

30. Demidova TN, Gad F, Zahra T, Francis KP, Hamblin MR. Monitoring photodynamic therapy of localized infections by bioluminescence imaging of genetically engineered bacteria. *J Photochem Photobiol B.* 2005; **81**(1):15–25.

31. Hamblin MR, Zahra T, Contag CH, McManus AT, Hasan T. Optical monitoring and treatment of potentially lethal wound infections in vivo. *J Inf Dis.* 2003; **187**(11):1717–1725.

32. Lu Z, Dai T, Huang L, Kurup DB, Tegos GP, Jahnke A et al. Photodynamic therapy with a cationic functionalized fullerene rescues mice from fatal wound infections. *Nanomedicine.* 2010; **5**(10):1525–1533.

33. Dai T, Tegos GP, Zhiyentayev T, Mylonakis E, Hamblin MR. Photodynamic therapy for methicillin-resistant *Staphylococcus aureus* infection in a mouse skin abrasion model. *Lasers Surg Med.* 2010; **42**(1):38–44.

34. Dai T, Bil de Arce VJ, Tegos GP, Hamblin MR. Blue dye and red light, a dynamic combination for prophylaxis and treatment of cutaneous *Candida albicans* infections in mice. *Antimicrob Agents Chemother.* 2011; **55**(12):5710–5717.

PART 6

CLINICAL IMAGING

Imaging of photosensitizers in skin

MARICA B. ERICSON, DANNI WANG, DESPOINA KANTERE,
JOHN PAOLI, AND ANN-MARIE WENNBERG

17.1 INTRODUCTION

This chapter will focus on the clinical applications of fluorescence imaging of photosensitizers in skin, in particular, the imaging of photosensitizers in connection with photodynamic therapy (PDT). It is possible to divide this topic into three main objectives: (1) fluorescence imaging with the aim to provide skin cancer diagnostics, (2) fluorescence monitoring to predict clinical outcome of PDT, and (3) the implementation of fluorescence techniques in the discovery of new photosensitizers to improve clinical PDT. Since these topics are closely connected, and it is impossible to introduce one without touching upon the other, this chapter will cover all the mentioned topics by presenting the clinical applications of imaging photosensitizers in skin and the available techniques for fluorescence imaging.

Fluorescence imaging of skin is the digital detection of fluorescence exhibited by photosensitizers upon excitation with light of a specific wavelength. The emission is generally recorded in the red spectral region, while excitation is most frequently performed in the blue spectral region; however, other means are possible as will be revealed in this chapter. There are many different technical approaches that enable imaging of photosensitizers in skin. This chapter will cover the available methods ranging from macroscopic imaging to more advanced optical microscopy techniques. Depending on the purpose, the choice of technique will differ; thus each presented technique will also be illustrated with some examples. The chapter intends to give an illustrative overview of how imaging of photosensitizers in skin can be performed, and hopefully serve as inspiration for future discoveries in the field.

17.2 CLINICAL APPLICATIONS OF FLUORESCENCE IMAGING

It was discovered early that fluorescence could be employed to visualize tissue abnormalities, particularly in the field of dermatology (Policard, 1924; Margarot and Devèze, 1925). Thus, by monitoring the fluorescence, it was possible to explore the accumulation of fluorophores in tissue in a noninvasive fashion. Initially, UV light obtained from a so-called Wood's lamp (filtered low-output mercury light source) was used as an excitation source with the fluorescence detected by simple visual examination. However, with the development of digital cameras and high-energy light sources, the process has been refined and digitized.

In parallel with the development of PDT and photosensitizers designed for PDT, the approach to visualize fluorescence has evolved. Pottier and Kennedy demonstrated in 1986, by spectroscopic measurement, that protoporphyrin IX (PpIX) accumulated in tissue after the application of aminolevulinic acid (ALA) (Pottier et al., 1986). Thus, topical delivery of ALA was early applied to induce PpIX accumulation in skin and visualized by monitoring fluorescence. The group of Andersson-Engels and Svanberg pioneered this research by adopting fluorescence monitoring of photosensitizers for clinical purposes (Andersson-Engels et al., 1989, 1990a,b). It was later verified that the accumulation of PpIX is higher in skin tumors compared to healthy skin after application of ALA and a mechanism was proposed (Moan et al., 2001), laying down grounds for adopting ALA-induced fluorescence as a technique for tumor diagnostics.

17.2.1 SKIN CANCER DEMARCATION

Nonmelanoma skin cancers and precancerous lesions such as actinic keratoses are increasing health concerns, particularly with the aging population (Lomas et al., 2012). Of particular concern are the increasing numbers of basal cell carcinomas. The invasive growth pattern of aggressive basal cell carcinomas can make surgery complicated, particularly when located in the facial region. Mohs micrographic surgery has evolved as an important surgical technique to ensure complete removal of the tumor (Neville et al., 2007), but the approach is highly labor intensive. Thus, attempts have been made to implement fluorescence diagnosis as a tool to improve tumor demarcation before and in connection to surgery (Stenquist et al., 2006).

Previous work by Wennberg et al. demonstrated a good correspondence between ALA-induced fluorescence and the histopathologic extension of tumor borders (Wennberg et al., 1999). In this study, the Wennberg factor was discovered for describing the contrast threshold suitable for tumor demarcation. This factor was further validated by Ericson et al. in a follow-up study, also investigating the kinetics of the PpIX contrast in the tumor regions (Ericson et al., 2003a; Figure 17.1).

The most prominent limiting factor when it comes to applying fluorescence imaging as a diagnostic tool for tumor demarcation is the degree of contrast obtained by the sensitizer applied. In addition to optimizing the imaging optical setup and the image analysis process, the localization of the sensitizer dictates the imaging contrast. Despite promising results, ALA-induced PpIX fluorescence has been demonstrated to suffer from poor tumor selectivity (Martin et al., 1995), predominantly due to a high accumulation in surrounding normal tissue.* Methyl aminolevulinate (MAL) was introduced as an alternative prodrug with improved pharmacodynamics compared to ALA, focusing on its properties for PDT. Figure 17.2 shows a comparison in

---

* The primary reason for lack of tumor contrast was most likely attributed to the fact that a 20% (w/w) ALA cream has a very low pH (around 2.5), severely affecting the skin barrier and, thus, enhancing the uptake in normal tissue. Since MAL-cream has a higher pH (around 5), the selective uptake in the tumor due to its comprised skin barrier is preferable.

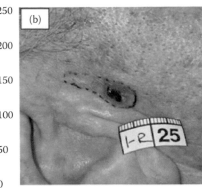

Figure 17.1 (a) Fluorescence image of a morphoeic BCC lesion located on the cheek after exposure to ALA (excitation: 365, 405 nm, emission: >610 nm). (b) Photography of the same lesion. The wound is due to a tissue biopsy. The false color scale is implemented to highlight areas with fluorescence 1.4× fluorescence in ALA-treated surrounding tissue. (Reprinted from *J. Photochem. Photobiol. B*, 69, Ericson, M.B., Sandberg, C., Gudmundson, F., Rosén, A., Larkö, O., and Wennberg, A.M., Fluorescence contrast and threshold limit: Implications for photodynamic diagnosis of basal cell carcinoma, 121–127. Copyright 2003a; with permission from Elsevier.)

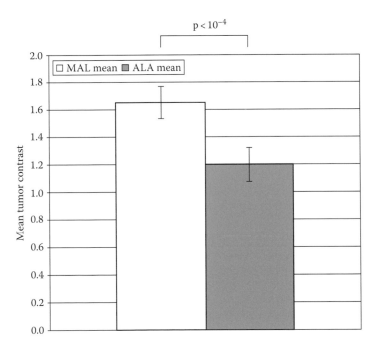

Figure 17.2 Fluorescence data of basal cell carcinomas (BCCs) exposed to MAL (open bar) (n = 32) compared to ALA (filled bar) (n = 15). The values correspond to the mean fluorescence contrast in the tumor area. Error bars are 95% confidence intervals. (Reprinted from Sandberg, C. et al., *Acta Dermato-Venereologica*, 91, 398, Copyright 2011. With permission.)

the tumor contrast acquired with ALA and MAL (Sandberg et al., 2011). As shown by the figure, it was demonstrated that higher tumor contrast could be obtained using MAL compared to ALA. Thus, for diagnostics purposes, the use of MAL is recommended in order to provide higher tumor contrast when performing fluorescence imaging of nonmelanoma skin cancer.

17.2.2 OTHER APPLICATIONS

In addition to skin cancer demarcation, imaging of photosensitizers in the skin has other clinical applications. For example, fluorescence monitoring of ALA- or MAL-induced PpIX for optimizing topical drug delivery systems has been explored in preclinical research (Bender et al., 2005; Evenbratt et al., 2013). Since ALA and MAL are low molecular weight compounds with different chemical properties, they are used as model compounds for pharmaceutical active ingredients. This allows for noninvasive monitoring of local delivery of active compounds, which can be utilized for optimizing topical delivery systems in a more general context and not just restricted to protocols for PDT. Fluorescence imaging has also been applied clinically to investigate the effect of pretreating skin with an ablative fractional laser to facilitate topical delivery of ALA and MAL (Haedersdal et al., 2014). Fluorescence imaging of photosensitizers can also be used for cutaneous wound assessment in skin (Paul et al., 2015), which has significant implications in regenerative medicine and tissue engineering. One of the most important applications of fluorescence imaging is in conjunction to optimization of PDT protocols, which will be covered in the subsequent section.

17.2.3 PHOTODYNAMIC THERAPY

Imaging of photosensitizers in skin has been demonstrated to be an important tool in monitoring clinical efficacy of PDT. Of particular interest are the applications of fluorescence imaging to monitor accumulation of photosensitizer to predict clinical outcome and in order to acquire noninvasive monitoring of sensitizer photobleaching during treatment. Both these topics will be discussed later.

17.2.3.1 PREDICTION OF CLINICAL OUTCOME

In order for PDT to be effective, the photosensitizer has to have accumulated in the tissue. Here, fluorescence imaging has been shown to provide valuable information when assessing the dosage and distribution of the accumulated photosensitizer. Fluorescence imaging has also been used to not only optimize treatment protocols, particularly related to ALA/MAL protocols (Wiegell et al., 2003, 2008; Lerche et al., 2015), but also for other sensitizers, such as a chlorin-based photosensitizer (Gamayunov et al., 2015). Finally, fluorescence imaging can also be applied for monitoring treatment outcome. Figure 17.3 demonstrates an example from a study where fluorescence monitoring was performed at follow-up for patients undergoing MAL-PDT (Truchuelo et al., 2014). The authors found a positive correlation between the posttreatment fluorescence and the histopathological evaluations, indicating that fluorescence imaging could avoid unnecessary posttreatment biopsies during in clinical follow-up of nonmelanoma skin cancer treated with PDT.

PDT is also being explored as a potential treatment modality for acne. Moderate acne is often treated with oral antibiotics, in most instances with tetracyclines, but there are increasing problems with antibiotic resistance. In addition, tetracyclines may pose an environmental hazard as they are difficult to degrade in nature. Consequently, there is a need for other therapeutic regimens. Although PDT has been shown to be effective against acne (Hongcharu et al., 2000; Hörfelt et al., 2006; Wiegell and Wulf, 2006; Hörfelt et al., 2009; Dong et al., 2016), unwanted side effects such as severe inflammatory responses and pain during treatment have limited its applicability so far. Potentially, innovative treatment protocols can minimize these adverse effects.

The suggested mode of action during PDT of acne is that PpIX accumulates in rapidly proliferating sebocytes after application of ALA or MAL. Thus, the photosensitized sebocytes are targeted during light exposure. Recently, derivatives other than ALA have been explored, such as indocyanine green and indole-3-acetic acid (Jang et al., 2011). In order to optimize PDT protocols for acne, fluorescence imaging

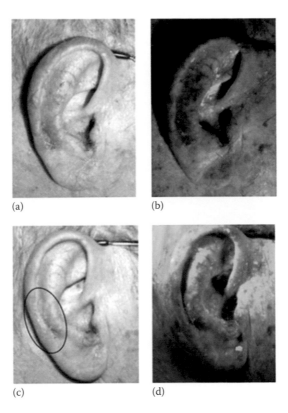

(a) (b)

(c) (d)

Figure 17.3 Photos (a, c) and fluorescence images (b, d) of Bowen's disease (a precancerous non-melanoma skin cancer lesion) on the ear pre-PDT (a, b) and post-PDT (c, d). Absence of fluorescence post-PDT (d) correlated with histopathological complete response, highlighting MAL-induced fluorescence imaging as a post-PDT procedure to avoid unnecessary biopsies when monitoring treatment response. (Reprinted from Truchuelo, M.T., Pérez, B., Fernández-Guarino, M., Moreno, C., Jaén-Olasolo, P.: Fluorescence diagnosis and photodynamic therapy for Bowen's disease treatment. *J. Eur. Acad. Dermatol. Venereol.* 2014. 28. 86–93. Copyright Wiley-VCH Verlag GmbH & Co. KGaA. Reproduced with permission.)

has demonstrated to be valuable for assessing the amount of PpIX in tissue (Wiegell and Wulf, 2006; Hörfelt et al., 2009). PpIX was found to be accumulated mostly in inflammatory acne lesions after application of ALA or MAL. In addition, due to the presence of endogenous porphyrins produced by the commensal bacteria *Propionibacterium acnes*, fluorescence can be observed from sebaceous glands where the bacteria accumulate, as illustrated in Figure 17.4. So far, it is unclear to what extent the porphyrins from commensal bacteria contribute to the effect when treating acne with PDT. Thus, the interplay between commensal bacteria and inflammatory conditions should be studied further. In the future, fluorescence imaging is expected to be an important tool in the PDT of acne to fully elucidate the mode of action, in order to optimize treatment protocols, and be able to predict and monitor the therapeutic outcome.

17.2.3.2 MONITORING PHOTOBLEACHING

The clinical outcome of PDT is related not only to the presence of sensitizer in the tissue and the light delivery, but also to the concentration of oxygen in the tissue. Therefore, there is a need for tools to monitor tissue oxygen concentration. Direct measurements of oxygen levels or formation of singlet oxygen during illumination would be ideal but is experimentally challenging. Therefore, in a clinical context, indirect measurement of oxygen concentration is a more promising and practical approach.

It is well known that during the illumination phase of PDT, the photosensitizer is bleached due to photo-oxidative processes. The photosensitizer itself is consumed, by reacting with the singlet oxygen produced

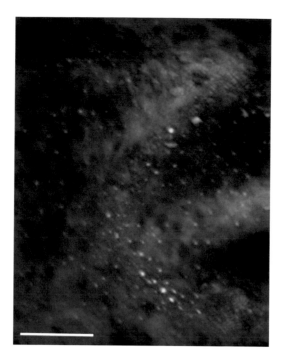

Figure 17.4 Fluorescence image of the alar rim of the nose, demonstrating the presence of porphyrin formed by commensal Propionibacterium acnes accumulating in the sebaceous glands of the skin. Scale bar = 1 cm.

in the photodynamic process. Since photobleaching is an oxygen-dependent process, it can be used as a noninvasive tool to "track" oxygen levels *in vivo*. By spectroscopic measurements of photosensitizer levels during PDT, the rate of photobleaching can be determined (Johansson et al., 2006; Cottrell et al., 2008; Tyrrell et al., 2010b). Ericson et al. (2004) were the first to demonstrate the relevance of monitoring photobleaching during PDT in order to predict clinical outcome. Figure 17.5 shows a typical series of sequential fluorescence images in a study on actinic keratosis treated with PDT. As shown by the figure, the predominant part of the photobleaching takes place during the initial phase of the treatment. In addition, the bleaching rate was found to positively correlate with clinical outcome. Other groups have confirmed that PpIX photobleaching is indicative of the cellular damage of PDT and predictive for clinical outcome in patients followed up after treatment of nonmelanoma skin cancers (Tyrrell et al., 2010b; Piffaretti et al., 2013). Thus, the possibility of noninvasively monitoring photobleaching provides an interesting means for predictive assessment of clinical outcome.

17.3 FLUORESCENCE IMAGING TECHNIQUES

An optical system for fluorescence imaging requires a light source matching the excitation of the photosensitizer and a spectrally filtered detector allowing for detection of the emitted fluorescence. When choosing the optical system, there is a general trade-off between imaging depth, resolution, field of view, and speed. Macroscopic imaging allows for a large field of view, which is preferable in, for example, clinical imaging or for preclinical studies using whole animal imaging, but is limited in resolution. With microscopic imaging techniques, cellular resolution can be achieved at the cost of significantly limited field of view and imaging depth. While all techniques have their advantages and drawbacks, each can be implemented to focus on different aspects depending on the scientific questions asked. The following sections will introduce the basic principles of the different techniques used for macroscopic and microscopic fluorescence imaging and discuss their applications for imaging photosensitizers in skin.

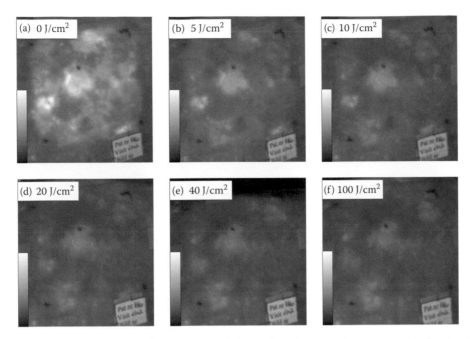

Figure 17.5 Fluorescence images of actinic keratosis located on the scalp during PDT: (a) before treatment, (b–e) during treatment at the cumulative light doses 5–40 J/cm² and (f) after treatment. The ALA-treated area is within the four black marks. The areas with high fluorescence most likely correspond to the lesions. As can be seen, the PpIX fluorescence in these areas decreases rapidly up to a cumulative treatment dose of 0–10 J/cm². Thereafter, no further photobleaching was detected, but some fluorescence remained. Similar behavior was found in all 33 actinic keratoses in the study. (Reprinted from Ericson, M.B., Sandberg, C., Stenquist, B., Gudmundson, F., Karlsson, M., Ros, A.-M., Rosén, A., Larkö, O., Wennberg, A.-M., and Rosdahl, I.: Photodynamic therapy of actinic keratosis at varying fluence rates: Assessment of photobleaching, pain, and primary clinical outcome. *Br. J. Dermatol.* 2004. 151. 1204–1212. Copyright Wiley-VCH Verlag GmbH & Co. KGaA. Reproduced with permission.)

17.3.1 MACROSCOPIC FLUORESCENCE IMAGING

The methods for detecting macroscopic fluorescence from photosensitizers in skin can be divided into laser-based point monitoring systems and noncoherent imaging systems, but are sometimes incorrectly grouped together as laser-induced fluorescence (Drakaki et al., 2014). The point monitoring systems have the advantage of giving multispectral information and have been applied by several investigators (Pottier et al., 1986; Sterenborg et al., 1994; Brancaleon et al., 2001; Na et al., 2001; Van Leeuwen-Van Zaane et al., 2014). The drawback is the difficulty of obtaining information from larger areas for which the noncoherent imaging techniques are superior (Wennberg et al., 1999; Ericson et al., 2005; Tyrrell et al., 2010a; Truchuelo et al., 2014). The basic setup for macroscopic fluorescence imaging includes an excitation light source, a detector, and a spectral filter for wavelength selection, as exemplified by Figure 17.6. The excitation and emission wavelengths are selected depending on the photosensitizer of choice. For example, when imaging ALA- or MAL-induced PpIX fluorescence, the excitation generally targets the Soret peak at 405 nm, while the emission is recorded at its maximum around 630 nm (Box 17.1).

The wavelength of the light source has to match the absorption of the sensitizer. Most frequently, light in the blue-UV region is used, since most photosensitizers have their principal absorption in this region. Both lasers and filtered spectral lamps have been used for fluorescence investigations of basal cell carcinoma (BCC). For example, nitrogen lasers in combination with dye lasers tuned to 405 nm have been used (Sterenborg et al., 1994), having the advantage of narrow wavelength distribution and high powers. Among noncoherent light sources, Hg (mercury) lamps have been most widely used (Wennberg et al., 1999; Ericson et al., 2005).

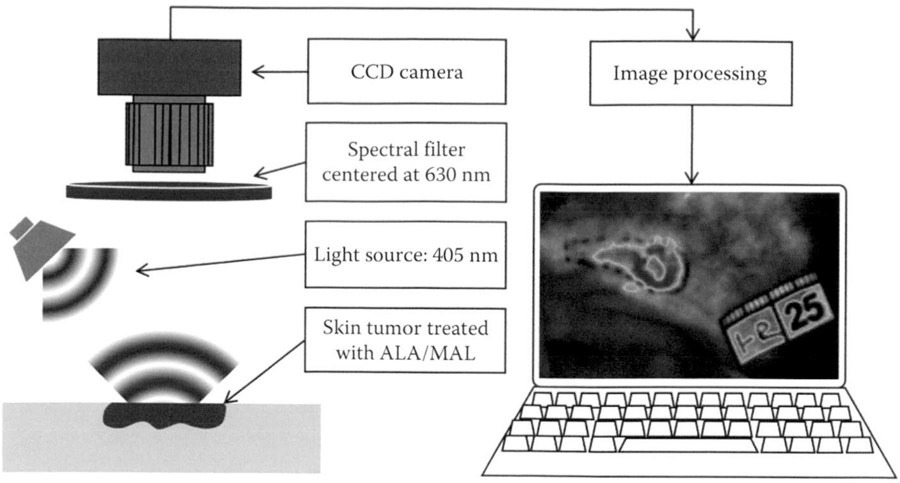

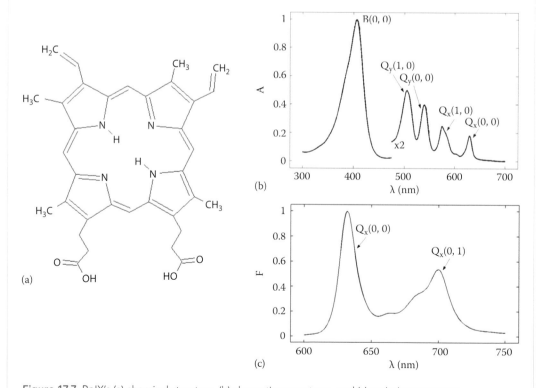

Figure 17.6 Schematic illustration of the setup required for macroscopic imaging of ALA- or MAL-induced PpIX fluorescence in skin.

BOX 17.1: Spectral characteristics of protoporphyrin IX

Protoporphyrin IX is a free-base porphyrin, exhibiting a five-banded visible absorption spectrum, as seen in Figure 17.7. The intense Soret band (also called B-band) between 380 and 420 nm corresponds to transitions from the second excited singlet state ($S_0 \rightarrow S_2$), and the Q-bands correspond to the first singlet excitation transitions ($S_0 \rightarrow S_1$). The difference in the molar extinction coefficient between the two

Figure 17.7 PpIX's (a) chemical structure, (b) absorption spectrum, and (c) emission spectrum.

(Continued)

BOX 17.1 (*Continued*): Spectral characteristics of protoporphyrin IX

types of transitions implies that the Soret transition is strongly allowed, whereas the Q-transitions are quasi allowed. However, all bands (both Soret and Q-bands) are interpreted as being $\pi \rightarrow \pi^*$ transitions.

The splitting of the Q-band into four is caused by the presence of two free-base hydrogens in the center of the ring that reduce the symmetry from fourfold to twofold symmetry, that is, D_{2h}. The result of the symmetry is a splitting of the first excited singlet Q(0, 0) band and its vibronic overtone Q(1, 0) into $Q_x(0, 0)$, $Q_y(0, 0)$, $Q_x(1, 0)$, and $Q_y(1, 0)$. A dramatic effect on the absorption spectra of PpIX is obtained by reducing one or more of the exo-pyrrole double bonds, resulting in a chlorin, that is, a structure similar to the heterocyclic base structure of chlorophyll. This ring reduction produces a characteristic far-red absorption band, which is also the reason why grass (containing chlorophyll) is green while blood (containing heme with a porphyrin structure) is red.

While the fluorescence quantum yield of PpIX is relatively low, that is, approximately 6%, PpIX is preferably deactivated by triplet formation. It is in fact the high triplet yield that makes PpIX a good photosensitizer, since the quenching of triplet state is generally obtained by the formation of singlet oxygen, the crucial component for PDT. Despite the low fluorescence quantum yield, the emission of PpIX can be detected, and preferably acquired from the two peaks $Q_x(0, 0)$, and $Q_x(0, 1)$, where the primary emission is centered around 630 nm, as illustrated in Figure 17.7c.

When using Hg lamps, it should be noted that the largest contribution (~95%) to the excitation comes from the 365 nm peak of Hg, with a small contribution (<5%) from the spectral line at 405 nm. This has proved advantageous since the same light source can be used to excite both tissue autofluorescence and Pp IX fluorescence (Ericson et al., 2005). Other sources of incoherent light have been employed, for example, filtered Xe (xenon) arc lamps (Sterenborg et al., 1994; Tyrrell et al., 2010a). With the development of intense LEDs (light-emitting diodes) operating in the blue spectral region, it is expected that these will take over as illumination light sources as they can provide energy efficient narrow band and wide-area illumination.

The main drawback of using short wavelengths for excitation is the poor optical penetration into tissue. Using wavelengths at around 400 nm, the light attenuation is high in tissue, resulting in a decrease of the incident light energy to ~37% at a depth of 90 μm (Anderson and Parrish, 1981). Near-UV light allows for the visualization of fluorescence from the epidermis (the outer layer of the skin which is approximately 100 μm thick) and the very upper part of the dermis (the middle layer of the skin). This is sufficient for fluorescence imaging of superficial BCCs since they grow in this area of the skin, but for tumors infiltrating deeper parts of the dermal layer or even lower, light penetration will pose a challenge. The use of longer excitation wavelengths (red and near infrared, NIR) for fluorescence imaging has been proposed as an alternative to increase imaging depth (Fischer et al., 2001a,b). When exciting at 635 nm, for example, the fluorescence is recorded at 710 nm, which corresponds to the $Q_x(0, 1)$ peak of Pp IX (Box 17.1); however, because of the lower emission at this wavelength and the generally poor quantum efficiency of PpIX fluorescence, this approach is challenging.

One of the most common types of detectors for fluorescence imaging is a CCD (Charged Coupled Device) camera in which the spatial intensity distribution is recorded for larger areas in a monochrome fashion and the desired wavelength region is chosen using appropriate filters (Wennberg et al., 1999; Ericson et al., 2005). The data consist of gray-scale images, where each pixel value corresponds to the measured intensity value. Alternatively, an RGB camera can be used, where the photosensitizer emission usually appears in the red (R) channel, whereas the green (G) and blue (B) channels serve as controls (Tyrrell et al., 2010a; Truchuelo et al., 2014). The advantage of the RGB setup is the simultaneous detection of different spectral regions, where the red (R) channel corresponds to the PpIX emission. The drawback is that the spectral properties are not easily controlled, as they are inherent to the camera.

Image processing can be performed so that the regions of interest (ROIs), for example, the tumor, can be highlighted by false coloring. By implementing the Wennberg factor, a threshold based on 1.4 times the surrounding baseline fluorescence, areas with abnormalities can be highlighted (Wennberg et al., 1999; Ericson et al., 2003a). An alternative semiautomatic thresholding algorithm has been explored (Sandberg et al., 2011) allowing for a more dynamic image assessment insensitive to varying imaging conditions, such as background illumination, or illumination irregularities during acquisition.

Ratiometric fluorescence imaging (Andersson-Engels et al., 2000; Ericson et al., 2005) has been proposed to enhance contrast between the sensitizer fluorescence and autofluorescence by defining

$$Z_{P/A} = \frac{P - kP_0}{A} \tag{17.1}$$

where
P is the red spectral image when photosensitizer has been applied
P_0 is the baseline red image
A is the autofluorescence image acquired in green

The parameter k is introduced to account for intensity differences between P and P_0 (Ericson et al., 2003b). A representative ratiometric multispectral fluorescence image highlighting a BCC after the application of ALA is presented in Figure 17.8. The PpIX fluorescence is higher in the tumor region after ALA application, in contrast to the autofluorescence, which is lower. The resulting ratio image demonstrates high contrast between the tumor and normal skin. Due to the nonsimultaneous recording of different spectral regions, distortion is introduced into the fluorescence images. These distortions can be corrected by using the so-called image warping, where the images are matched before calculating the $Z_{P/A}$ ratio image. In addition to simple thresholding of gray scale images, more advanced pattern recognition in combination with discriminant analysis can be implemented to improve the training of the algorithm (Ericson et al., 2005).

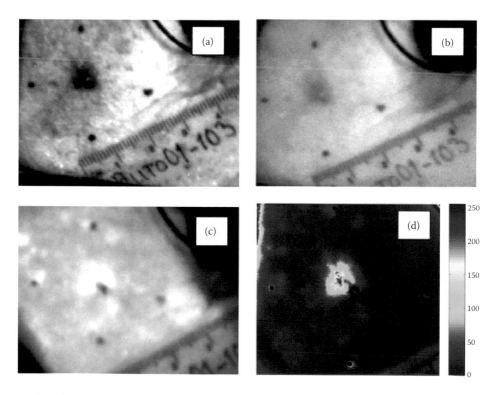

Figure 17.8 Multispectral fluorescence images of a basal cell carcinoma after ALA application where (a) shows the autofluorescence image, A; (b) is the background PpIX image, P_0, before ALA application; (c) shows the PpIX image after ALA application, P, and (d) is the $Z_{P/A}$ image in false color. (Reprinted from Ericson, M.B. et al., *SPIE Proc.*, 5141, 114. Copyright 2003b, with permission from SPIE Publication.)

17.3.2 Microscopic fluorescence imaging

Due to the limited resolution of macroscopic imaging modalities, optical microscopy is necessary to visualize the distribution of photosensitizers on a cellular or subcellular level. Traditionally, in this context, optical microscopy is performed on cell cultures or tissue sections due to the inherently dense optical properties of skin. However, with the development of laser-scanning optical microscopy, there are now tools allowing for noninvasive microscopic fluorescence imaging.

17.3.2.1 CONVENTIONAL WIDE-FIELD FLUORESCENCE MICROSCOPY

Conventional wide-field fluorescence microscopy in skin is restricted to thin tissue sections of skin biopsies, limiting its use to investigative studies for cellular distribution of photosensitizers with limited clinical applicability. Utilizing a simple optical design (Figure 17.9a), the optical magnification of the thin tissue sample is imaged directly onto the detector, allowing for rapid, superficial imaging. Wide-field microscopy is capable of surveying a large field of view on the specimen, thus providing an overview that can help identify the regions of interest; however, wide-field microscopes lack the ability for optical sectioning. In order to perform wide-field fluorescence microscopy of, for example, PpIX, the optical setup should be chosen so that the excitation is obtained using 405 nm light, and the emission detected in the red spectral region around 630 nm. For studies on skin, wide-field microscopy has been adapted in a proof-of-principle study for topical delivery of nanoparticle-conjugated photosensitizers (Da Silva et al., 2013). Wide-field microscopy has also been applied to elucidate the cellular localization of PpIX formation after application of ALA. Figure 17.9b and c demonstrate an example where PpIX fluorescence was compared to a mitochondria stain, illustrating that the cellular accumulation of PpIX corresponds to the location of mitochondria (Ji et al., 2006).

17.3.2.2 CONFOCAL LASER SCANNING MICROSCOPY

Confocal laser scanning microscopy (CLSM) is considered to be one of the most important advances in optical imaging, and has, since its inception by Marvin Minsky in the late 1950s (Minsky, 1961), become an essential tool in biological sciences and medical diagnostics. The fundamental principle behind CLSM is described in Box 17.2. Confocal images are generally acquired in a point-by-point fashion as the focal spot is scanned in two or three dimensions and stitched together (Diaspro, 2001; Pawley, 2006). The various design modifications to increase imaging speed of CLSM such as line-scanning and spinning-disk confocal microscopes will not be discussed in this chapter. In connection to the conventional single-axis setup, a dual-axis confocal

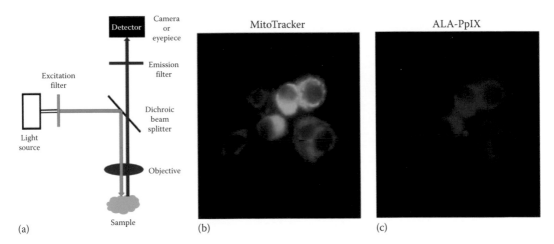

Figure 17.9 (a) Schematic drawing of wide-field fluorescence microscopy; (b and c) show squamous cell carcinoma cells incubated with ALA in which the green label (b) corresponds to mitochondria using a MitoTracker stain, and the red channel (c) corresponds to PpIX emission. (Panels b and c: Reprinted from *J. Photochem. Photobiol. B Biol.*, 84, Ji, Z., Yang, G., Vasovic, V., Cunderlikova, B., Suo, Z., Nesland, J.M., and Peng, Q., Subcellular localization pattern of protoporphyrin IX is an important determinant for its photodynamic efficiency of human carcinoma and normal cell lines, 213–220. Copyright 2006, with permission from Elsevier.)

BOX 17.2:   Confocal laser scanning microscopy

In a confocal microscope (Diaspro, 2001; Pawley, 2006), light from a point source is focused into the specimen of interest, using an optical setup illustrated in Figure 17.10. Generally, the illumination is focused to a point in the specimen and the confocal image is constructed in a point-by-point fashion as the focal spot is scanned in 2D or 3D within the specimen, and the microscope is called a point-scanned confocal microscope. The emitted fluorescence is typically collected by the same objective lens in a setup referred to as the single-axis configuration. A collection pinhole is required to remove the out-of-focus signal, which is one of the key components of the confocal microscope. Some reconstruction software, typically a frame grabber, is used to obtain the 2D images and 3D image stacks.

Since the illumination and collection light travel the same path between the beam splitter and the sample in the conventional single-axis confocal configuration, the rejection of out-of-focus and multiply scattered photons is challenging. This is particularly problematic as imaging depth increases, limiting the conventional confocal microscope to superficial imaging and optically thin specimens. While the conventional confocal microscope remains immensely useful in basic science research, the miniaturization process, a crucial step in translational research, is difficult and costly due to the short working distance and bulky nature of the high numerical aperture (NA) of the focusing objective. To address the limitations of the single-axis confocal, a dual-axis confocal microscope has been developed (Liu et al., 2008), utilizing off-axis illumination and collection with low NA objectives, allowing for more efficient background rejection and increasing imaging depth. In the dual-axis configuration, single-mode fibers are used as spatial filters instead of illumination and collection pinholes.

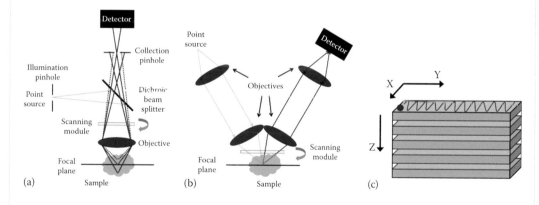

Figure 17.10 Schematic illustrations of confocal laser scanning microscopy (CLSM). (a) Conventional single-axis confocal setup, (b) dual-axis confocal setup designed for improved *In vivo* imaging conditions, and (c) illustration of the sequential buildup of 2D images that by changing focus depth enables generation of 3D imaging stacks.

microscope has been developed (Liu et al., 2008) utilizing off-axis illumination and collection, allowing for more efficient background rejection and, in turn, increasing imaging depth.

As part of the characterization process of novel photosensitizers, conventional CLSM has been utilized for investigating the cellular localization of photosensitizers in cell cultures (Castano et al., 2004). It has also been used for studying the photosensitizer metabolism in skin homogenates and *in vivo* accumulation in animal models (De Rosa et al., 2004). Conventional CLSM has also been applied to visualize photosensitizers applied to skin, predominantly on thin tissue sections of biopsies, for example, to explore cutaneous delivery of the second-generation photosensitizer silicon phthalocyanine PC4 (Lam et al., 2011).

The dual-axis confocal system is still in its prototyping stage but has nevertheless been miniaturized to a handheld form to enable point-of-care investigations (Liu et al., 2010). One of the primary applications for the dual-axis confocal point-of-care system is the monitoring of topically delivered fluorescent probes used for tumor demarcation or therapeutics. Skin penetration of NIR dye (Figure 17.11) and siRNA (small interfering RNA) probes has been

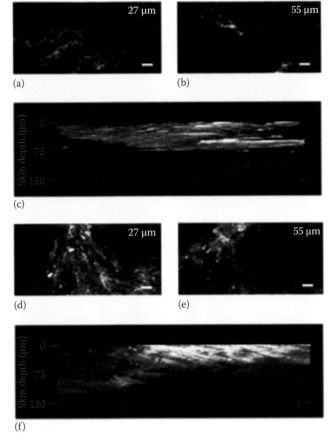

Figure 17.11 *In vivo* imaging using dual-axis confocal microscopy demonstrating topical delivery of NIR dye applied to two different anatomical sites of human volunteer, corresponding to calf skin (a, b, c) and calloused skin (d, e, f). *En face* images (a, b, d, e) acquired at depth of 27 and 55 μm, scale bar = 50 μm. Full 3D volumes (e, f) corresponding to 650 × 320 × 150 μm³. (Reproduced by permission Macmillan Publishers Ltd. *J. Invest. Dermatol.*, Ra, H., Piyawattanametha, W., Gonzalez-Gonzalez, E., Mandella, M.J., Kino, G.S., Solgaard, O., Leake, D., Kaspar, R.L., Oro, A., and Contag, C.H., *In vivo* imaging of human and mouse skin with a handheld dual-axis confocal fluorescence microscope, Copyright 2010.)

investigated (Ra et al., 2011) to improve understanding of topical drug delivery in order to optimize the development of fluorescent probes, including photosensitizers, to precisely penetrate specific regions within the skin.

Within the field of skin imaging, a technique based on reflectance confocal microscopy has emerged as an important clinical tool to noninvasively visualize tissue morphology of skin with cellular resolution down to depths of around 200 μm (Rajadhyaksha et al., 1999a,b). The miniaturized reflectance confocal microscopy has been commercialized as a medical device, the VivaScope (Caliber I.D.), and has since 2008 been approved for clinical use in Canada, Europe, Australia, the United States, and China. However, despite being an excellent tool for providing noninvasive 3D information of tissue morphology and intraoperative skin cancer imaging (Flores et al., 2015; Rossi et al., 2015), the reflectance-mode confocal microscope alone lacks the ability to provide functional information necessary for imaging photosensitizers in the skin and has to be combined with fluorescence-mode CLSM for this purpose.

17.3.2.3 MULTIPHOTON LASER SCANNING MICROSCOPY

Multiphoton microscopy (MPM) has rapidly evolved from a photonic novelty (Denk et al., 1990) to a well-established laboratory tool that allows for noninvasive 3D imaging of tissue (Diaspro, 2001; Zipfel et al., 2003). By operating in the "optical window" of biological tissue (corresponding to λ ~600–1300 nm), MPM is able to achieve an increased imaging depth compared to single photon excitation modalities (see Box 17.3).

BOX 17.3:   Multiphoton microscopy

Similar to confocal microscopy, multiphoton microscopy uses laser illumination and point-scanning image formation. Instead of utilizing a pinhole as a spatial filter to reject out-of-focus photons, MPM utilizes the multiphoton process, a nonlinear process which occurs when the photon flux is sufficiently high that the energy combined from multiple low-energy photons can be used to excite a fluorophore in the tissue (Diaspro, 2001; Zipfel et al., 2003), as illustrated by Figure 17.12. As the temporal window of this process is narrow, the photons have to arrive at the same location almost simultaneously; thus, a high repetition rate pico- or femtosecond-pulsed laser has to be used to ensure the delivery of the high peak power required for the process.

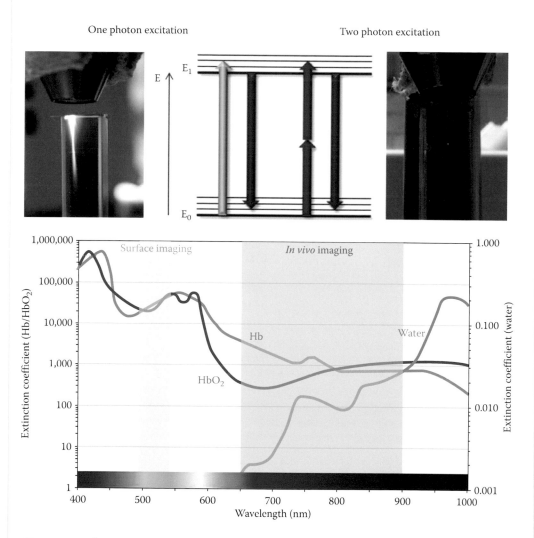

Figure 17.12 Illustration of the difference between one-photon excitation and two-photon excitation. Photos from experiments illustrate the inherent confocality of the two-photon excitation. MPM operates in the optical window of tissue where absorption is at its minimum. The optical setup is similar to single-axis CLSM; however, no pinhole is necessary as the excitation process in inherently confocal. (Spectrum reprinted with permission from Kobayashi, H., M. Ogawa, R. Alford, P.L. Choyke, and Y. Urano, (2010), New strategies for fluorescent probe design in medical diagnostic imaging. *Chemical Reviews* **110**: 2620–2640. Copyright 2010 American Chemical Society)

(Continued)

BOX 17.3 (*Continued*):   Multiphoton microscopy

In a MPM setup, the multiphoton process occurs most efficiently at the focal plane, generating negligible background fluorescence, achieving an "inherent confocality" without needing a physical pinhole. In addition, by illuminating with low energy (longer wavelength) photons with little tissue absorption, MPM allows for better light penetration in the specimen compared to its single-photon linear microscopy counterparts. Furthermore, since the fluorescence excitation only occurs at the focal plane, the photodamage from MPM is less than that of single-photon linear microscopy techniques such as CLSM. The most commonly implemented MPM setup utilizes two-photon excitation for fluorescence imaging.

MPM utilizes high intensity femtosecond-pulsed lasers for generating a high flux of excitation photons. This is necessary for multiphoton absorption, which is inherently nonlinear and only occurs at the focal plane (inherent confocality), allowing for optical sectioning and noninvasive tomographic scanning. Recent applications of MPM show high-impact advances within the field of life science and has been successfully implemented for experimental skin research (Yu et al., 2003; Bender et al., 2008). MPM has demonstrated potential for skin cancer diagnostics based on autofluorescence imaging (König and Riemann, 2003; Paoli et al., 2008, 2009). The technique has expanded its use on human skin in the clinics by the commercial setup DermaInspect (Jenlab, Germany) with approval from the European notified body for medical products.

MPM has been applied to study distribution of photosensitizers in some investigative reports (Kirejev et al., 2012, 2014b), but so far the clinical applications using MPM to visualize photosensitizers have been limited. Because of its successful implementation to visualize cell morphology, enabling *in vivo* histopathology, it comes as a natural step to also adopt MPM for investigative studies of photosensitizers in skin. However, MPM of PpIX fluorescence has proved to be challenging. Because of the electronic band structures of porphyrins, 2PE is not favored, as illustrated by Figure 17.13. In fact, we have demonstrated that

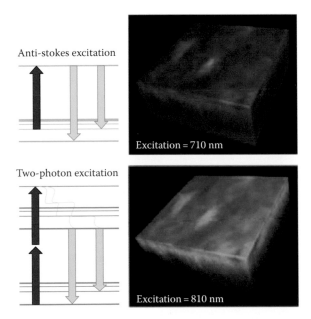

Figure 17.13 3D volume z-stacks acquired using MPM on basal cell carcinomas exposed to MAL. (a) Demonstrates elevated PpIX emission when excitation at 710 nm is used, targeting anti-Stokes excitation compared to (b) where 810 nm is targeting two-photon excitation. Thus, in order to visualize PpIX using MPM, anti-Stokes fluorescence should preferably be utilized. (From Kantere, D., Guldbrand, S., Paoli, J., Goksör, M., Hanstorp, D., Wennberg, A.M., Smedh, M., and Ericson, M.B.: Anti-stokes fluorescence from endogenously formed protoporphyrin IX—Implications for clinical multiphoton diagnostics. *J. Biophoton.* 2013. 6. 409–415. Copyright Wiley-VCH Verlag GmbH & Co. KGaA. Reproduced with permission.)

2PE for ALA- and MAL-induced PpIX fluorescence is not possible in tissue, as the PPIX fluorescence is overshadowed by the tissue autofluorescence (Kantere et al., 2013). By lowering the excitation wavelength, MPM can still be adopted for visualizing PpIX, but as the process is based on anti-Stokes fluorescence, rather than 2PE, the confocality is lost and the resolution is reduced. Nevertheless, MPM can provide several possibilities for visualizing photosensitizers in the skin, particularly in a more exploratory phase.

17.4 FUTURE DIRECTIONS

Fluorescence imaging of photosensitizers in skin has already proven its potential for nonmelanoma skin cancer diagnostics, as it has been discussed in this chapter. In addition, it serves as an important tool for mechanistic studies in combination to PDT of skin cancer and precancerous lesions. In connection to other indications for PDT, for example, for the treatment of acne, where treatment protocols need to be refined, fluorescence imaging will continue to serve as an important tool for optimizing treatment protocols and monitoring treatment outcome. Another interesting direction is the translation of PDT into regenerative medicine and tissue engineering (Paul et al., 2015), where fluorescence imaging is expected to be of importance.

When it comes to determining tumor margins, a consensus has not been reached for how fluorescence information can really assist in finding and outlining tumors in comparison to, for example, Mohs surgery. There are still several technical hurdles. As reflectance-mode confocal microscopy is making its way to become a more generally accepted medical device to assist in tumor diagnostics, it is likely that techniques extending the reflectance-mode confocal system will emerge that also allow for fluorescence registration. In fact, fluorescence-based CLSM in combination with reflectance-mode CLSM has already been applied for skin cancer demarcation (Larson et al., 2013; Bennàssar et al., 2014; Longo et al., 2014, 2015), after applying the fluorescent dye acridine orange to skin tissue. The combined technique has not yet been used for the visualization of photosensitizers however. Utilizing topical application of ALA/MAL prior to the excision to increase tumor contrast could possibly further improve the accuracy of the approach.

Nevertheless, with the development of novel photosensitizers, MPM remains a valuable tool in monitoring photosensitizer distribution in exploratory studies under *in vitro* and *ex vivo* conditions and extends its influence to *in vivo* preclinical studies. For example, MPM has recently been applied to visualize the distribution of a novel sensitizer system based on a carbon dot conjugate in intact tissue for targeting malignant melanoma (Beack et al., 2015). As well as being a tool for visualization, MPM may also play a role in the development of photosensitizers and protocols, utilizing its highly confined excitation for photoactivation purposes (Kirejev et al., 2014a). Novel photosensitizers based on the release of nitric oxide, to complement the more traditional singlet oxygen-based sensitizers, have been designed with multifunctionality to enable the monitoring of nitric oxide release. Also fluorescence lifetime imaging microscopy (FLIM) has demonstrated to be a powerful tool (Yeh et al., 2012; Kirejev et al., 2014b; Sanchez et al., 2015), as it is insensitive to the actual concentration of the fluorophore but rather dependent on the state and environment of the fluorophore. FLIM is preferably implemented in combination with the point-scanning fluorescence techniques, that is, CLSM or MPM. Although the technique is currently restricted to investigative studies, it demonstrates great potential in determining the mechanism of cellular accumulation of novel photosensitizers. The combination of "smart" sensitizers with the confined multiphoton excitation and FLIM expands the current exploration of a novel field of photosensitizers, and fluorescence imaging is expected to play an important role in their development.

Since individual imaging modalities have their drawbacks, when appropriate, combining complementary modalities can be designed to cater to specific diagnostic interests. Due to the trade-off between resolution and imaging depth as described earlier, and despite operating in the optical window of tissue, MPM is restricted to only the superficial part of the skin (up to 200 µm depth). Information from deeper tissue layers can be acquired by macroscopic fluorescence imaging, at the cost of loss of optical sectioning and cellular resolution. Techniques based on optical coherence tomography (OCT) (Fujimoto, 2003) provide a balanced alternative. Benefiting from the use of more penetrating NIR light and principles of coherence approach, mesoscopic fluorescence molecular tomography has demonstrated the potential to image skin at depths of several millimeters (~3–5 mm) with a relatively high resolution of ~100–200 μm (Ozturk et al., 2014). The combination of ultrasound imaging enabled the visualization of three-dimensional biodistribution of a novel pheophorbide-based photosensitizer in a preclinical skin cancer model.

Another interesting combination is multimodal reflectance confocal and multiphoton microscopy, which has been explored for imaging the cytoplasm rat esophageal epithelial cells and to monitor the metabolic state of the epithelium (Zhuo et al., 2008). The use of reflectance-mode CLSM and MPM in skin has been limited to the study of autofluorescence (Wang et al., 2013), but with appropriate photosensitizers, the use of this multimodal imaging technique can be expanded.

Photoacoustic imaging, a technique utilizing light illumination and acoustic wave collection, has been dominating the field of biomedical optics, particularly for *in vivo* neuroimaging (Wang et al., 2003). Photoacoustic imaging is versatile in that it can be combined with many other optical imaging modalities to supply multimodal feasibility. Porphyrin-based photosensitizers have been explored to enhance photoacoustic contrast when performing antibacterial PDT (Hirao et al., 2010). Since many well-characterized photosensitizers have low fluorescence quantum yields but relatively high singlet oxygen quantum yields, photoacoustic imaging has been proposed as an alternative or complementary technique to fluorescence imaging *in vivo* (Ho et al., 2014). Similar to how multimodal imaging can enable the monitoring of multiple aspects of the specimen, photosensitizers can be multiplexed or multifunctionalized. To enable NIR-induced imaging guided therapy, core-shell nanoparticulate systems have been proposed (Lv et al., 2015); these are not only photoactive but also can be made visible to multiple imaging modalities, for example, computer tomography, that can enable image-guided therapy.

So far, most studies dealing with oxygen consumption during PDT have been restricted to monitoring photobleaching. Another interesting direction is to monitor the formation of singlet oxygen directly (see Roede chapter in this book). By using NIR-sensitive detectors, luminescence from singlet oxygen can be monitored and is found to correlate with the generation of singlet oxygen to the microstructure of the skin (Schlothauer et al., 2013). A transgenic mouse model expressing ratiometric redox-sensitive green fluorescent protein has been developed (Wolf et al., 2014) for preclinical exploratory studies. This work is important as formation of singlet oxygen is the crucial parameter in PDT, and tools allowing for direct *in vivo* monitoring of singlet oxygen formation might be very helpful in optimizing PDT protocols.

Super-resolution optical microscopy techniques have not yet entered the arena when it could come close to imaging of photosensitizers in skin. This is likely due to the fact that the specific clinical questions related to PDT have not demanded such high spatial resolution as yet. However, with the development of more advanced and multifunctional photosensitizers, it is becoming more crucial to investigate the subcellular localization. Thus, it is very likely that super-resolution microscopy techniques will also be of great interest for visualizing photosensitizers in experimental skin research in the near future.

17.5 CONCLUSION

This chapter has demonstrated the potential of adopting fluorescence imaging for visualizing and exploring photosensitizers in the skin. Mainly, the focus has been on the topic of fluorescence from PpIX induced by application of ALA or MAL in order to enable mechanistic clinical studies in connection to PDT. In addition, this type of fluorescence has been explored in order to facilitate skin cancer diagnostics. Fluorescence imaging also plays an important role in the development of new photosensitizers and has been successfully implemented in several studies in exploratory studies.

When it comes to the techniques enabling fluorescence imaging, macroscopic fluorescence imaging is the most widely implemented approach especially with regard to clinical imaging thus far; however, with the advances of fluorescence microscopy, there are now interesting alternatives today allowing for microscopic fluorescence imaging *in vivo*. For example, the dual-axis confocal microscope holds potential for providing noninvasive imaging of photosensitizers in skin. In addition, MPM is an emerging technique for *in vivo* imaging; however, two-photon excitation of PpIX has demonstrated challenging, limiting the potential of

MPM in combination to ALA- or MAL-induced clinical fluorescence imaging. Thus, in order to acquire *in vivo* fluorescence imaging with cellular resolution, other alternatives and multimodal approaches should be considered.

Taken together, the data shows that fluorescence imaging is a powerful tool in order to provide mechanistic insights when exploring and optimizing treatment protocols for PDT. There are a variety of techniques that can be applied, and depending on study design, different techniques could preferably be implemented. This chapter intends to shed some light upon these considerations and potentially be a guide for future exploration of photosensitizers applied to skin.

ACKNOWLEDGMENTS

The authors thank Johan Borglin for image courtesy Figure 17.12, and acknowledge Centre for Skin Research, SkinResQU, at the University of Gothenburg and Chalmers University of Technology.

REFERENCES

Anderson RR, Parrish JA (1981) The optics of human skin. *Journal of Investigative Dermatology* **77**:13–19.

Andersson-Engels S, Canti G, Cubeddu R et al. (2000) Preliminary evaluation of two fluorescence imaging methods for the detection and the delineation of basal cell carcinomas of the skin. *Lasers in Surgery and Medicine* **26**:76–82.

Andersson-Engels S, Johansson J, Stenram U, Svanberg K, Svanberg S (1990b) Malignant tumor and atherosclerotic plaque diagnosis using laser-induced fluorescence. *IEEE Journal of Quantum Electronics* **26**:2207–2217.

Andersson-Engels S, Johansson J, Svanberg S, Svanberg K (1989) Fluorescence diagnosis and photochemical treatment of diseased tissue using lasers. 1. *Analytical Chemistry* **61**:A1367–A1373.

Andersson-Engels S, Johansson J, Svanberg S, Svanberg K (1990a) Fluorescence diagnosis and photochemical treatment of diseased tissue using lasers. 2. *Analytical Chemistry* **62**:A19–A27.

Beack S, Kong WH, Jung HS, Do IH, Han S, Kim H, Kim KS, Yun SH, Hahn SK (2015) Photodynamic therapy of melanoma skin cancer using carbon dot-chlorin e6—Hyaluronate conjugate. *Acta Biomaterialia* **26**:295–305.

Bender J, Ericson MB, Merclin N, Iani V, Rosén A, Engström S, Moan J (2005) Lipid cubic phases for improved topical drug delivery in photodynamic therapy. *Journal of Controlled Release* **106**:350–360.

Bender J, Simonsson C, Smedh M, Engström S, Ericson MB (2008) Lipid cubic phases in topical drug delivery: Visualization of skin distribution using two-photon microscopy. *Journal of Controlled Release* **129**:163–169.

Bennàssar A, Vilata A, Puig S, Malvehy J (2014) *Ex vivo* fluorescence confocal microscopy for fast evaluation of tumour margins during Mohs surgery. *British Journal of Dermatology* **170**:360–365.

Brancaleon L, Durkin AJ, Tu JH, Menaker G, Fallon JD, Kollias N (2001) *In vivo* fluorescence spectroscopy of nonmelanoma skin cancer. *Photochemistry and Photobiology* **73**:178–183.

Castano AP, Demidova TN, Hamblin MR (2004) Mechanisms in photodynamic therapy: Part one-photosensitizers, photochemistry and cellular localization. *Photodiagnosis and Photodynamics Therapy* **1**:279–293.

Cottrell WJ, Paquette AD, Keymel KR, Foster TH, Oseroff AR (2008) Irradiance-dependent photobleaching and pain in d-aminolevulinic acid-photodynamic therapy of superficial basal cell carcinomas. *Clinical Cancer Research* **14**:4475–4483.

Da Silva CL, Del Ciampo JO, Cristina Rossetti F, Badra Bentley MVL, Riemma Pierre MB (2013) PLGA nanoparticles as delivery systems for protoporphyrin ix in topical pdt: Cutaneous penetration of photosensitizer observed by fluorescence microscopy. *Journal of Nanoscience and Nanotechnology* **13**:6533–6540.

De Rosa FS, Lopez RF, Thomazine JA, Tedesco AC, Lange N, Bentley MV (2004) *In vitro* metabolism of 5-ALA esters derivatives in hairless mice skin homogenate and *in vivo* PpIX accumulation studies. *Pharmaceutical Research* **21**:2247–2252.

Denk W, Strickler JH, Webb WW (1990) 2-photon laser scanning fluorescence microscopy. *Science* **248**:73–76.

Diaspro A (2001) *Confocal and Two-Photon Microscopy: Foundations Applications and Advances*, Wiley. Inc., New York.

Dong Y, Zhou G, Chen J, Shen L, Jianxin Z, Xu Q, Zhu Y (2016) A new LED device used for photodynamic therapy in treatment of moderate to severe acne vulgaris. *Photodiagnosis and Photodynamics Therapy* **13**:188–195.

Drakaki E, Dessinioti C, Stratigos AJ, Salavastru C, Antoniou C (2014) Laser-induced fluorescence made simple: Implications for the diagnosis and follow-up monitoring of basal cell carcinoma. *Journal of Biomedical Optics* **19**:030901.

Ericson MB, Berndtsson C, Stenquist B, Wennberg A-M, Larkö O, Rosén A (2003b) Multispectral fluorescence imaging of basal cell carcinoma assisted by image warping. *SPIE Proceedings* **5141**:114–121.

Ericson MB, Sandberg C, Gudmundson F, Rosén A, Larkö O, Wennberg AM (2003a) Fluorescence contrast and threshold limit: Implications for photodynamic diagnosis of basal cell carcinoma. *Journal of Photochemical and Photobiological B* **69**:121–127.

Ericson MB, Sandberg C, Stenquist B, Gudmundson F, Karlsson M, Ros A-M, Rosén A, Larkö O, Wennberg A-M, Rosdahl I (2004) Photodynamic therapy of actinic keratosis at varying fluence rates: Assessment of photobleaching, pain and primary clinical outcome. *British Journal of Dermatology* **151**:1204–1212.

Ericson MB, Uhre J, Berndtsson C, Stenquist B, Larkö O, Wennberg A-M, Rosén A (2005) Bispectral fluorescence imaging combined with texture analysis and linear discrimination for correlation with histopathologic extent of basal cell carcinoma. *Journal of Biomedical Optics* **10**:034009.

Evenbratt H, Jonsson C, Faergemann J, Engstrom S, Ericson MB (2013) *In vivo* study of an instantly formed lipid-water cubic phase formulation for efficient topical delivery of aminolevulinic acid and methylaminolevulinate. *International Journal of Pharmaceutics* **452**:270–275.

Fischer F, Dickson EF, Kennedy JC, Pottier RH (2001b) An affordable, portable fluorescence imaging device for skin lesion detection using a dual wavelength approach for image contrast enhancement and aminolaevulinic acid-induced protoporphyrin IX. Part II. *In vivo* testing. *Lasers Medical Sciences* **16**:207–212.

Fischer F, Dickson EF, Pottier RH, Wieland H (2001a) An affordable, portable fluorescence imaging device for skin lesion detection using a dual wavelength approach for image contrast enhancement and aminolaevulinic acid-induced protoporphyrin IX. Part I. Design, spectral and spatial characteristics. *Lasers Medical Science* **16**:199–206.

Flores ES, Cordova M, Kose K, Phillips W, Rossi A, Nehal K, Rajadhyaksha M (2015) Intraoperative imaging during Mohs surgery with reflectance confocal microscopy: Initial clinical experience. *Journal of Biomedical Optics* **20**:61103.

Fujimoto JG (2003) Optical coherence tomography for ultrahigh resolution *in vivo* imaging. *Nature Biotechnology* **21**:1361–1367.

Gamayunov SV, Grebenkina EV, Ermilina AA et al. (2015) Fluorescent monitoring of photodynamic therapy for skin cancer in clinical practice. *Sovremennye Tehnologii v Medicine* **7**:75–81.

Haedersdal M, Sakamoto FH, Farinelli WA, Doukas AG, Tam J, Anderson RR (2014) Pretreatment with ablative fractional laser changes kinetics and biodistribution of topical 5-aminolevulinic acid (ALA) and methyl aminolevulinate (MAL). *Lasers in Surgery and Medicine* **46**:462–469.

Hirao A, Sato S, Saitoh D, Shinomiya N, Ashida H, Obara M (2010) *In vivo* photoacoustic monitoring of photosensitizer distribution in burned skin for antibacterial photodynamic therapy. *Photochemical and Photobiology* **86**:426–430.

Ho CJ, Balasundaram G, Driessen W, McLaren R, Wong CL, Dinish US, Attia AB, Ntziachristos V, Olivo M (2014) Multifunctional photosensitizer-based contrast agents for photoacoustic imaging. *Science Report* **4**:5342.

Hongcharu W, Taylor CR, Chang Y, Aghassi D, Suthamjariya K, Anderson RR (2000) Topical ALA-photodynamic therapy for the treatment of acne vulgaris. *Journal of Investigative Dermatology* **115**:183–192.

Hörfelt C, Funk J, Frohm-Nilsson M, Wiegleb Edström D, Wennberg AM (2006) Topical methyl aminolaevulinate photodynamic therapy for treatment of facial acne vulgaris: Results of a randomized, controlled study. *British Journal of Dermatology* **155**:608–613.

Hörfelt C, Stenquist B, Halldin CB, Ericson MB, Wennberg AM (2009) Single low-dose red light is as efficacious as methyl-aminolevulinate- photodynamic therapy for treatment of acne: Clinical assessment and fluorescence monitoring. *Acta Dermato-Venereologica* **89**:372–378.

Jang MS, Doh KS, Kang JS, Jeon YS, Suh KS, Kim ST (2011) A comparative split-face study of photodynamic therapy with indocyanine green and indole-3-acetic acid for the treatment of acne vulgaris. *British Journal of Dermatology* **165**:1095–1100.

Ji Z, Yang G, Vasovic V, Cunderlikova B, Suo Z, Nesland JM, Peng Q (2006) Subcellular localization pattern of protoporphyrin IX is an important determinant for its photodynamic efficiency of human carcinoma and normal cell lines. *Journal of Photochemistry and Photobiology B: Biology* **84**:213–220.

Johansson A, Johansson T, Thompson MS, Bendsoe N, Svanberg K, Svanberg S, Andersson-Engels S (2006) *In vivo* measurement of parameters of dosimetric importance during interstitial photodynamic therapy of thick skin tumors. *Journal of Biomedical Optics* **11**:34069.

Kantere D, Guldbrand S, Paoli J, Goksör M, Hanstorp D, Wennberg AM, Smedh M, Ericson MB (2013) Anti-stokes fluorescence from endogenously formed protoporphyrin IX—Implications for clinical multi-photon diagnostics. *Journal of Biophotonics* **6**:409–415.

Kirejev V, Gonçalves AR, Aggelidou C, Manet I, Mårtensson J, Yannakopoulou K, Ericson MB (2014b) Photophysics and *ex vivo* biodistribution of ß-cyclodextrin-meso- tetra(m-hydroxyphenyl) porphyrin conjugate for biomedical applications. *Photochemical and Photobiological Sciences* **13**:1185–1191.

Kirejev V, Guldbrand S, Borglin J, Simonsson C, Ericson MB (2012) Multiphoton microscopy—A powerful tool in skin research and topical drug delivery science. *Journal of Drug Delivery Science and Technology* **22**:250–259.

Kirejev V, Kandoth N, Gref R, Ericson MB, Sortino S (2014a) A polymer-based nanodevice for the photo-regulated release of NO with two-photon fluorescence reporting in skin carcinoma cells. *Journal of Materials Chemistry B* **2**:1190–1195.

Kobayashi H, Ogawa M, Alford R, Choyke PL, Urano Y (2010) New strategies for fluorescent probe design in medical diagnostic imaging. *Chemical Reviews* **110**:2620–2640.

König K, Riemann I (2003) High-resolution multiphoton tomography of human skin with subcellular spatial resolution and picosecond time resolution. *Journal of Biomedical Optics* **8**:432–439.

Lam M, Hsia AH, Liu Y et al. (2011) Successful cutaneous delivery of the photosensitizer silicon phthalocyanine 4 for photodynamic therapy. *Clinical and Experimental Dermatology* **36**:645–651.

Larson B, Abeytunge S, Seltzer E, Rajadhyaksha M, Nehal K (2013) Detection of skin cancer margins in Mohs excisions with high-speed strip mosaicing confocal microscopy: A feasibility study. *British Journal of Dermatology* **169**:922–926.

Lerche CM, Fabricius S, Philipsen PA, Wulf HC (2015) Correlation between treatment time, photobleaching, inflammation and pain after photodynamic therapy with methyl aminolevulinate on tape-stripped skin in healthy volunteers. *Photochemical and Photobiological Sciences* **14**:875–882.

Liu JT, Mandella MJ, Crawford JM, Contag CH, Wang TD, Kino GS (2008) Efficient rejection of scattered light enables deep optical sectioning in turbid media with low-numerical-aperture optics in a dual-axis confocal architecture. *Journal of Biomedical Optics* **13**:034020.

Liu JTC, Mandella MJ, Loewke NO, Haeberle H, Ra H, Piyawattanametha W, Solgaard O, Kino GS, Contag CH (2010) Micromirror-scanned dual-axis confocal microscope utilizing a gradient-index relay lens for image guidance during brain surgery. *Journal of Biomedical Optics* **15**:026029.

Lomas A, Leonardi-Bee J, Bath-Hextall F (2012) A systematic review of worldwide incidence of nonmelanoma skin cancer. *British Journal of Dermatology* **166**:1069–1080.

Longo C, Ragazzi M, Gardini S, Piana S, Moscarella E, Lallas A, Raucci M, Argenziano G, Pellacani G (2015) *Ex vivo* fluorescence confocal microscopy in conjunction with Mohs micrographic surgery for cutaneous squamous cell carcinoma. *Journal of the American Academy of Dermatology* **73**:321–322.

Longo C, Rajadhyaksha M, Ragazzi M et al. (2014) Evaluating *ex vivo* fluorescence confocal microscopy images of basal cell carcinomas in Mohs excised tissue. *British Journal of Dermatology* **171**:561–570.

Lv R, Zhong C, Li R, Yang P, He F, Gai S, Hou Z, Yang G, Lin J (2015) Multifunctional anticancer platform for multimodal imaging and visible light driven photodynamic/photothermal therapy. *Chemistry of Materials* **27**:1751–1763.

Margarot J, Devèze P (1925) Aspect de quelques dermatoses en lumière ultraparaviolette—Note préliminaire. *Bulletin of the Social Science and Medicine Montpellier* **6**:375–378.

Martin A, Tope WD, Grevelink JM, Starr JC, Fewkes JL, Flotte TJ, Deutsch TF, Anderson RR (1995) Lack of selectivity of protoporphyrin IX fluorescence for basal cell carcinoma after topical application of 5-aminolevulinic acid: Implications for photodynamic treatment. *Archives of Dermatological Research* **287**:665–674.

Minsky M (1961) Microscopy apparatus, US Patent 3013467.

Moan J, Van den Akker JTHM, Juzenas P, Ma LW, Angell-Petersen E, Gadmar OB, Iani V (2001) On the basis for tumor selectivity in the 5-aminolevulinic acid-induced synthesis of protoporphyrin IX. *Journal of Porphyrins and Phthalocyanines* **5**:170–176.

Na R, Stender IM, Wulf HC (2001) Can autofluorescence demarcate basal cell carcinoma from normal skin? A comparison with protoporphyrin IX fluorescence. *Acta Dermato Venereologica* **81**:246–249.

Neville JA, Welch E, Leffell DJ (2007) Management of nonmelanoma skin cancer in 2007. *Nature Clinical Practice Oncology* **4**:462–469.

Ozturk MS, Rohrbach D, Sunar U, Intes X (2014) Mesoscopic fluorescence tomography of a photosensitizer (HPPH) 3D biodistribution in skin cancer. *Academic Radiology* **21**:271–280.

Paoli J, Smedh M, Ericson MB (2009) Multiphoton laser scanning microscopy—A novel diagnostic method for superficial skin cancers. *Seminars in Cutaneous Medicine and Surgery* **28**:190–195.

Paoli J, Smedh M, Wennberg AM, Ericson MB (2008) Multiphoton laser scanning microscopy on nonmelanoma skin cancer: Morphologic features for future non-invasive diagnostics. *Journal of Investigative Dermatology* **128**:1248–1255.

Paul DW, Ghassemi P, Ramella-Roman JC, Prindeze NJ, Moffatt LT, Alkhalil A, Shupp JW (2015) Noninvasive imaging technologies for cutaneous wound assessment: A review. *Wound Repair and Regeneration* **23**:149–162.

Pawley J (2006) *Handbook of Biological Confocal Microscopy*, Springer, New York.

Piffaretti F, Zellweger M, Kasraee B, Barge J, Salomon D, Van Den Bergh H, Wagnières G (2013) Correlation between protoporphyrin IX fluorescence intensity, photobleaching, pain and clinical outcome of actinic keratosis treated by photodynamic therapy. *Dermatology* **227**:214–225.

Policard A (1924) Etudes sur les aspects offert par des tumeurs expérimentales examinées a la lumière de Wood. *C R Biology* **91**:1423–1424.

Pottier RH, Chow YFA, Laplante JP, Truscott TG, Kennedy JC, Beiner LA (1986) Noninvasive technique for obtaining fluorescence excitation and emission-spectra *in vivo*. *Photochemistry and Photobiology* **44**:679–687.

Ra H, Piyawattanametha W, Gonzalez-Gonzalez E, Mandella MJ, Kino GS, Solgaard O, Leake D, Kaspar RL, Oro A, Contag CH (2011) *In vivo* imaging of human and mouse skin with a handheld dual-axis confocal fluorescence microscope. *Journal of Investigative Dermatology* **131**:1061–1066.

Rajadhyaksha M, Anderson RR, Webb RH (1999a) Video-rate confocal scanning laser microscope for imaging human tissues *in vivo*. *Applied Optics* **38**:2105–2115.

Rajadhyaksha M, Gonzalez S, Zavislan JM, Anderson RR, Webb RH (1999b) *In vivo* confocal scanning laser microscopy of human skin II: Advances in instrumentation and comparison with histology. *Journal of Investigative Dermatology* **113**:293–303.

Rossi AM, Sierra H, Rajadhyaksha M, Nehal K (2015) Novel approaches to imaging basal cell carcinoma. *Future Oncology* **11**:3039–3046.

Sanchez W, Pastore M, Haridass I, König K, Becker W, Roberts M (2015) Fluorescence lifetime imaging of the skin. In: *Advanced Time-Correlated Single Photon Counting Applications* (Becker W ed.), pp. 457–508, Springer, Heidelberg, Germany.

Sandberg C, Paoli J, Gillstedt M, Halldin CB, Larko O, Wennberg AM, Ericson MB (2011) Fluorescence diagnostics of basal cell carcinomas comparing methyl-aminolaevulinate and aminolaevulinic acid and correlation with visual clinical tumour size. *Acta Dermato-Venereologica* **91**:398–403.

Schlothauer JC, Falckenhayn J, Perna T, Hackbarth S, Röder B (2013) Luminescence investigation of photosensitizer distribution in skin: Correlation of singlet oxygen kinetics with the microarchitecture of the epidermis. *Journal of Biomedical Optics* **18**:115001.

Stenquist B, Ericson MB, Strandeberg C, Mölne L, Rosén A, Larkö O, Wennberg A-M (2006) Bispectral fluorescence imaging of aggressive basal cell carcinoma combined with histopathologic mapping: A preliminary study indicating a possible adjunct to Mohs micrographic surgery. *British Journal of Dermatology* **154**:305–309.

Sterenborg HJCM, Motamedi M, Wagner RF, Duvic M, Thomsen S, Jacques SL (1994) *In-vivo* fluorescence spectroscopy and imaging of human skin tumors. *Lasers Medicine Science* **9**:191–201.

Truchuelo MT, Pérez B, Fernández-Guarino M, Moreno C, Jaén-Olasolo P (2014) Fluorescence diagnosis and photodynamic therapy for Bowen's disease treatment. *Journal of the European Academy of Dermatology and Venereology* **28**:86–93.

Tyrrell J, Campbell S, Curnow A (2010a) Validation of a non-invasive fluorescence imaging system to monitor dermatological PDT. *Photodiagnosis and Photodynamic Therapy* **7**:86–97.

Tyrrell JS, Campbell SM, Curnow A (2010b) The relationship between protoporphyrin IX photobleaching during real-time dermatological methyl-aminolevulinate photodynamic therapy (MAL-PDT) and subsequent clinical outcome. *Lasers in Surgery and Medicine* **42**:613–619.

Van Leeuwen-Van Zaane F, Gamm UA, Van Driel PBAA, Snoeks TJ, De Bruijn HS, Van Der Ploeg-Van Den Heuvel A, Sterenborg HJCM, Lowik CW, Amelink A, Robinson DJ (2014) Intrinsic photosensitizer fluorescence measured using multi-diameter single-fiber spectroscopy *in vivo*. *Journal of Biomedical Optics* **19**:015010.

Wang H, Lee AM, Frehlick Z, Lui H, McLean DI, Tang S, Zeng H (2013) Perfectly registered multiphoton and reflectance confocal video rate imaging of *in vivo* human skin. *Journal of Biophotonics* **6**:305–309.

Wang X, Pang Y, Ku G, Xie X, Stoica G, Wang LV (2003) Noninvasive laser-induced photoacoustic tomography for structural and functional *in vivo* imaging of the brain. *Natural Biotechnology* **21**:803–806.

Wennberg AM, Gudmundson F, Stenquist B, Ternesten A, Mölne L, Rosén A, Larkö O (1999) *In vivo* detection of basal cell carcinoma using imaging spectroscopy. *Acta Dermatol Venereology* **79**:54–61.

Wiegell SR, Skiveren J, Philipsen PA, Wulf HC (2008) Pain during photodynamic therapy is associated with protoporphyrin IX fluorescence and fluence rate. *British Journal of Dermatology* **158**:727–733.

Wiegell SR, Stender IM, Na R, Wulf HC (2003) Pain associated with photodynamic therapy using 5-aminolevulinic acid or 5-aminolevulinic acid methylester on tape-stripped normal skin. *Archives of Dermatology* **139**:1173–1177.

Wiegell SR, Wulf HC (2006) Photodynamic therapy of acne vulgaris using methyl aminolaevulinate: A blinded, randomized, controlled trial. *British Journal of Dermatology* **154**:969–976.

Wolf AM, Nishimaki K, Kamimura N, Ohta S (2014) Real-time monitoring of oxidative stress in live mouse skin. *Journal of Investigative Dermatology* **134**:1701–1709.

Yeh SC, Diamond KR, Patterson MS, Nie Z, Hayward JE, Fang Q (2012) Monitoring photosensitizer uptake using two photon fluorescence lifetime imaging microscopy. *Theranostics* **2**:817–826.

Yu B, Kim KH, So PTC, Blankschtein D, Langer R (2003) Visualization of oleic acid-induced transdermal diffusion pathways using two-photon fluorescence microscopy. *Journal of Investigative Dermatology* **120**:448–455.

Zhuo SM, Chen JX, Jiang XS, Lu KC, Xie SS (2008) Imaging rat esophagus using combination of reflectance confocal and multiphoton microscopy. *Laser Physics Letters* **5**:614–618.

Zipfel WR, Williams RM, Webb WW (2003) Nonlinear magic: Multiphoton microscopy in the biosciences. *Nature Biotechnology* **21**:1368–1376.

Brain tumor imaging with ALA

HERBERT STEPP AND OLIVER SCHNELL

18.1 INTRODUCTION

Brain tumors have an average annual age-adjusted incidence in adults of 21–22 cases per 100,000 population. They can be subdivided into primary brain tumors, which arise from glial or precursor cells of the brain itself, and secondary brain tumors or brain metastases, which originate from cancers outside the central nervous system (CNS). Brain metastases account for the majority of all malignant brain tumors (approximately 11/100,000/year) and are almost twice as common as primary brain tumors, with an incidence rate of 6–7/100,000 per year (Ostrom et al., 2014). Due to their cellular origin, primary brain tumors are often referred to as gliomas and the most common subtype, Glioblastoma multiforme (GBM), is also the most malignant primary brain tumor (15.7% of all tumors and 45.6% of malignant tumors). Despite extensive treatment with gross total tumor resection, radiochemotherapy followed by different salvage treatment options, its prognosis remains dismal, and the median overall survival is only 14–16 months (Stupp et al., 2005; Gilbert et al., 2013, 2014; Chinot et al., 2014).

The impact of surgery on the prognosis of malignant gliomas has been a matter of discussion for several decades since there are only a few retrospective and mostly single-center studies reporting a favorable outcome of gross total tumor resection in glioblastomas (Lacroix et al., 2001; Sanai and Berger, 2011). Moreover, due to their infiltrating growth pattern and often eloquent location (near or within functionally relevant areas of the brain), tumor resection of gliomas has to be considered with great care since subtotal resection may not have a significant prognostic impact, and too much tissue resection could damage normal brain function. Therefore, if surgical resection is intended, the major goal must be the complete removal of all contrast enhancement in MRI while preserving all functionally relevant eloquent areas (gross total resection [GTR]), meaning that the volume of residual contrast-enhancing tumor tissue in postoperative MRI is minimal (less than very few percent of the original volume), and the complete resection of enhancing tumor (CRET), meaning that no residual enhancement is detectable (Schucht et al., 2012).

In a multivariate analysis of fluorescence-guided surgery with 5-aminolevulinic acid (ALA) compared to white light tumor resection, this was achieved in the majority of malignant gliomas using ALA-induced fluorescence (AIF) guidance (Schucht et al., 2012), and gross total resection of all contrast-enhancing tumor in MRI led to a survival benefit for glioblastoma patients (Stummer et al., 2006,b). ALA leads to a tumor-selective accumulation of red fluorescent protoporphyrin IX (PpIX) by stimulating the intracellular heme biosynthesis as will be described in more detail. The advantage of this approach in comparison to other fluorescence-based techniques is the fact that the drug, which is applied to the patient (ALA) is itself not fluorescent. There is neither background fluorescence from circulating fluorochrome nor spilling of fluorochrome from injured blood vessels during surgery.

Another intriguing property of ALA-induced PpIX is its phototoxicity, meaning that it could be used for photodynamic therapy (PDT). Apart from showing fluorescence, excited PpIX can produce reactive oxygen species (ROS), mostly singlet oxygen ($^1O_2$). Cells harboring a sufficient amount of PpIX can be destroyed by prolonged irradiation with otherwise harmless visible light (photodynamic therapy [PDT]). By applying PDT after fluorescence-guided surgery, a further significant proportion of invading tumor cells might be destroyed. We will briefly address this topic, as it may potentially become very important in the management of GBM.

Since the approval of fluorescence-guided resection (FGR) of malignant glioma with ALA (Gliolan®) in the EU in 2007 (European Medicines Agency, 2007b), the clinical value has been investigated in a number of studies. A few recent review articles provide a comprehensive overview of clinical results and discussions (Zhao et al., 2013a; Barone et al., 2014; Ewelt et al., 2015; Hadjipanayis et al., 2015; Leroy et al., 2015; Moiyadi and Stummer, 2015). In this chapter, we will also focus on the technical aspects.

18.2 CURRENT SURGICAL TREATMENT STRATEGY FOR MALIGNANT GLIOMA

Complete surgical removal of gliomas is not possible due to their infiltrative growth pattern. Tumor cells are not just limited to the contrast-enhancing tumor areas, but they also present in decreasing amounts depending on the distance from the central tumor parts (Sahm et al., 2012; Wang and Jiang, 2013).

Moreover, it is usually not possible for the surgeon to differentiate tumor from infiltration zone and infiltration zone from the normal brain by simple visual assessment through the surgical microscope. Therefore, especially adjacent to eloquent regions of the brain, surgery has to be undertaken with great care, when approaching the tumor borders. If no additional tools are available, the surgeon may only estimate location and size of the tumor from preoperative MRI or CT scans. Under such conditions, GTR, as defined earlier, will hardly be achieved in more than 50% of cases (Sanai and Berger, 2008). However, GTR may not only prolong progression-free survival but also improve the efficacy of adjuvant therapies (Stummer et al., 2011, 2012) and may be associated with an improved quality of life (Brown et al., 2005). Moreover, GTR has been shown to be of a significant survival benefit, if more than 98% of contrast-enhancing tumor has been removed (Lacroix et al., 2001). Of note, subtotal surgical resection will not be relevant from an oncological point of view. This pure cytoreduction may however sometimes be an option to achieve tumor debulking in order to enable adjuvant therapy (Lacroix et al., 2001; Laws et al., 2003; Brown et al., 2005; Pichlmeier et al., 2008).

Since achieving GTR is of benefit for the patient, several surgical guidance tools have been developed in order to achieve maximal and safe resection by avoiding expansion of tumor resection into eloquent brain tissue. In this chapter, we briefly present the most important surgical tools (except AIF) that could be used in order to provide the neurosurgeon with intraoperative (and if possible real-time) information about (1) the anatomy of the brain and tumor, (2) biologically relevant tumor areas, and (3) cerebral functionality, and discuss the limitations of each. The comparison to AIF, as far as available, is also discussed.

18.2.1 Surgical guidance tools

18.2.1.1 NEURONAVIGATION

The aim of this technique is to support the surgeon in identifying the exact location during the current resection with respect to the preoperative imaging. A 3D set of MRI, CT, and/or PET images (or any overlay of these) is correlated with the position of a pointing pen or resection tool, the tip of which the surgeon has to place at the point of interest in the current resection cavity, then a display of that location in the 3D image is obtained. However, due to pressure changes and brain tissue movement during resection, the preoperatively determined positions of the tumor borders are not precisely preserved. This so-called brain-shift can be quite significant. Shifts of several millimeters are normal, and up to 2.5 cm must be considered possible (Trantakis et al., 2003; Willems et al., 2006). In terms of volumes, average resection cavity volumes on postoperative MRI of 29 cm^3 were measured, 84 cm^3 had effectively been resected (Schucht et al., 2014). Moreover, the use of standard MRI-based neuronavigation with (Wu et al., 2007) or without (Willems et al., 2006) integrated diffusion-weighted imaging (DWI) demonstrated that tumor resection was more pronounced with additional use of the neuronavigation system, and even more with additional DWI, but there was only limited information about its prognostic impact and therefore not enough evidence to support its recommendation for everyday use (Barone et al., 2014). Since FET–PET may give some additional information about the biology of the tumor and especially the most active tumor parts that are crucial for histopathological appraisal, this imaging modality should be imported into the neuronavigation system, at least if the tumor borders are particularly diffuse (Popperl et al., 2007; Kunz et al., 2011).

18.2.1.2 INTRAOPERATIVE MRI

Being aware of the limitations of neuronavigation, intraoperative MRI (iMRI) may appear to be an ideal solution, as it should allow for immediate control and localization of any residual contrast-enhancing tumor. CRET should be achieved in all cases, where resection of contrast-enhancing tumor is possible without compromising safety. In a monocentric, randomized controlled trial, the extent of resection was significantly improved and gross total resection was achieved in up to 96% of patients operated on with iMRI compared to 68% in patients in the control arm without additional iMRI (Senft et al., 2011). Additionally, glioblastoma patients who had complete resection of their tumors showed significantly longer progression-free survival (PFS) (218 days) compared to patients with subtotal resection (110 days). Interestingly, this difference did not persist after stratification for patients who had undergone surgery with iMRI and those without iMRI, which leads to the conclusion that the extent of resection but not use of iMRI itself was prognostic. Moreover, both treatment arms showed higher gross total resection rates than previously reported (Stummer et al., 2008b), which may be due to a certain selection bias toward patients with more resectable tumors in this study. Cost and complexity of performing iMRI are practical limitations. As AIF is less costly, much simpler to implement, and more compatible with the intraoperative workflow, it must be considered an alternative (Kubben et al., 2011), and it is critically compared with iMRI in Section 18.3.6.

18.2.1.3 INTRAOPERATIVE ULTRASOUND

Although easily adapted to intraoperative applications, ultrasound imaging is as yet not broadly accepted as a guidance tool for glioma surgery. It appears especially valuable for the delineation of low-grade gliomas, where it approaches the accuracy of iMRI (Gerganov et al., 2011; Coburger et al., 2015b). Limitations are concerned with the judgment of residual tumor in the resection cavity. For high-grade glioma patients, similar limitations have been reported: In Gerganov et al. (2009), it was found difficult to identify residual tumor in the resection cavity by 2D ultrasound, if the lesion was less than 1 cm in diameter, and also a blood clot and peritumoral parenchyma were misinterpreted as tumor tissue. Even with 3D ultrasound, a poor specificity during GBM resection (42%) and a disappointing sensitivity when judging the resection cavity (26%) were found (Rygh et al., 2008). One should mention, however, that recent improvements in the intraoperative ultrasound technique and the use of contrast-enhancing agents may improve its reliability in identifying brain tumor tissue: In Coburger et al. (2015a) linear array transducers were shown to be clearly superior to conventional ultrasound, although the specificity of the technique was still only 58% in their collective data. A comparison of microbubble-enhanced ultrasound with iMRI in a rat model has shown promising results (Yang et al., 2015). The technique was also applied in GBM patients, and it was concluded that this relatively economic and accurate tool might contribute to maximized tumor resection (Prada et al., 2014).

18.2.1.4 CORTICAL FUNCTIONAL MAPPING

The increasing use of various neurosurgical techniques has certainly contributed to the improvement of surgical resection and the reduction of surgical risks. However, these techniques do not provide information about the integrity of brain functions during tumor resection. Due to large intraindividual differences in the anatomical and functional localization, direct electrophysiological brain mapping and intraoperative monitoring on cortical and subcortical stimulation (either under general anesthesia or in awake patients) remains the gold standard to obtain reliable information about the functionally relevant areas of the brain (Duffau et al., 2008; Sanai et al., 2008; Hervey-Jumper et al., 2015). Our understanding of certain brain functions, such as language and its regional distribution, has greatly improved due to new findings by these intraoperative stimulation techniques (Duffau et al., 2008; Sanai et al., 2008). Brain mapping and intraoperative monitoring (IOM) should always be combined with the different imaging methods described so far, at least, if the resection must be performed near or within eloquent areas. This was demonstrated recently in a large meta-analysis of more than 8000 patients who had a surgical glioma resection with or without the use of intraoperative monitoring. The extent of resection was larger if these neurophysiological techniques were used (De Witt Hamer et al., 2012). Both groups had a high rate of eloquently located tumors (99.9% in IOM group and 95.8% in patients without IOM application), and while the rate of early postoperative neurological deterioration was higher in the IOM group (47.9% versus 7.5%), there was a significant reduction after 3 months of 8.2%–3.5%. Moreover, complete resection was achieved in 75% of patients compared to only 58% if no IOM was used. Therefore, cortical or subcortical mapping can be performed during glioma surgery in order to prevent injury to functional brain. This method is not a guidance tool to discriminate brain tumor from the normal brain, but it discriminates functionally relevant and intact brain areas from nonfunctional parts and may therefore be regarded as a safety tool for functional integrity. Even though intraoperative seizures have been reported in some cases, this method is easy to use and fast. Nevertheless, when aiming for CRET in the proximity of eloquent regions, cortical functional mapping should be seriously considered.

18.2.1.5 FLUORESCENCE GUIDANCE AND OTHER METHODS

Apart from the surgical guidance tools described, some largely experimental new approaches are briefly described in the following section. Most of them are optics based, which make them potentially well suited for intraoperative application. ALA-induced fluorescence guidance is the topic of the next main section, however.

According to the currently widely accepted standard, CRET is the ultimate goal one can achieve in glioma surgery. Consequently, intraoperative contrast-enhanced MRI should guarantee the highest possible success rate. However, the infiltrative nature of malignant glioma and the persistent low cure rates even with CRET under iMRI guidance clearly indicate that CRET is not sufficient and more sensitive detection tools may be necessary to further improve clinical outcome. One strategy to go beyond iMRI is based on a more microscopic tissue characterization.

Mass spectrometry analysis is one of such tools. It is frequently used in laboratory research for the molecular characterization of tissue and recently was also suggested to guide brain tumor surgery by analyzing tiny tissue samples (Santagata et al., 2014).

Optical coherence tomography (OCT) provides ultrasound-like images with improved resolution (ca. 20 μm), albeit with less depth penetration (ca. 1 mm), delivering structural information in real time (Bizheva et al., 2005). Adaption to surgical microscopes is available and may soon allow for scanning the entire resection cavity surface (Finke et al., 2012).

Confocal laser endomicroscopy (CLE) provides even higher resolution, albeit at the cost of penetration depth. In order to generate sufficient signal and to obtain good structural contrast, systemic or topical fluorochromes are usually applied (Martirosyan et al., 2014; Mooney et al., 2014). In human brain tumor samples, CLE was performed after staining with four different fluorophores, and excellent agreement with histopathological staining was reported (Foersch et al., 2012). CLE can be easily adapted to more target-specific fluorescent molecules (Hoetker and Goetz, 2013). The main drawback is that the field of view is limited to a few hundred microns. A red-flag technique with very high sensitivity—such as AIF—is therefore needed to identify appropriate sites to probe with CLE.

Two-photon endomicroscopy (TPE) further extends the possibilities to obtain contrast even without endogenous fluorophores in high resolution tissue imaging. In preclinical experiments, cell densities determined with TPE correlated well with histopathology (Kantelhardt et al., 2009).

Photoacoustics has the intriguing potential of providing functional information (e.g., oxygen saturation) with high resolution in 3D or with less resolution from depths of several millimeters. It employs the combination of optics and ultrasound where a short laser pulse causes absorbing structures (e.g., blood vessels) to suddenly expand and emit an acoustic wave. Recent progress of the technique was demonstrated to allow for tomographic imaging of the blood oxygenation in capillaries with a lateral resolution of up to 3 μm and a depth of a few 100 μm in mouse brains (Yao et al., 2015). As with ultrasound, direct contact with the tissue is required, limiting the field of view to a few millimeters.

Fluorescence lifetime imaging (FLI) or fluorescence lifetime spectroscopy of tissue autofluorescence demonstrated the potential for label-free delineation of malignant tissue (Butte et al., 2011; Papour et al., 2013). Fluorescence lifetime is a measure of the average delay time between an exciting light pulse and the emission of a fluorescent photon (the lifetime of the electronically excited singlet state of a fluorochrome molecule). This lifetime depends on the microenvironment of a fluorochrome and not on its relative concentration. It therefore provides a type of contrast, which indirectly maps conditions like pH, polarity, or the presence of quenchers in the immediate vicinity of the fluorochrome. These properties are potentially different between normal and adjacent malignant tissue and are otherwise difficult to visualize. Autofluorescence intensity mapping itself was also considered to have a high discrimination potential (Croce et al., 2003; Toms et al., 2007) but has not been investigated in clinical studies.

Various *exogenous fluorochromes* have been investigated for their brain tumor selectivity. Probably the first fluorochrome to be applied clinically was sodium fluorescein. Moore et al. (1948) suggested the use of the fluorescein technique to "confirm the complete removal of infiltrating gliomas." For many years, sodium fluorescein was used by a few neurosurgeons at a high concentration and visualized even without dedicated spectral filtering of its fluorescence emission, probably observing the color change of the tissue rather than its fluorescence (Shinoda et al., 2003; Koc et al., 2008). As ALA-based AIF is not yet approved in the United States, fluorescein mapping has experienced an astonishing revival, when surgical microscope manufacturers implemented a fluorescence mode in their instruments (Babu and Adamson, 2012; Acerbi et al., 2014). How this fluorescence mode compares to AIF will be discussed in Section 18.3.7. Indocyanine green (ICG) fluorescence has long been used as a test of liver function, but has recently been recognized as allowing intraoperative guidance for a variety of applications, including aneurysm surgery (Roessler et al., 2014). ICG is an interesting fluorochrome, as it operates in the near infrared. Both wavelengths (excitation at around 780 nm and fluorescence emission at around 820 nm) are in the range where light penetration into tissue is highest and background autofluorescence is negligible. Furthermore, if ICG is injected intravenously, it binds tightly to plasma (lipo) proteins and is therefore helpful for fluorescence angiography. ICG is metabolized in the liver within minutes, enabling repetitive investigations of perfusion dynamics. Concerning glioma surgery, the reports in the literature are rare, although as early as 1993, promising results were reported (Hansen et al., 1993; Haglund et al., 1996). The disturbed blood–brain barrier in malignant glioma leaks ICG and its fluorescence can be imaged as soon as the vessel-confined ICG has been cleared. Thus, 15 min after a bolus injection, ICG fluorescence shows contrast in regions with a deficient blood–brain barrier (Martirosyan et al., 2011). In a mouse model, ICG enabled deep tomographic imaging of the vessel architecture of inoculated U87 glioma cells by multispectral optoacoustic tomography (Burton et al., 2013). An ICG nanoemulsion for functional MRI and combined photodynamic and photothermal therapy was also proposed (Wang et al., 2013). Last but not least, the photosensitizers in use or proposed for PDT of malignant glioma also show fluorescence, which can potentially be used for surgical guidance as well, for instance, as described for mTHPC (Zimmermann et al., 2001) or hypericin (Ritz et al., 2012).

The fluorochromes that have been used in the earlier methods rely on a more or less passive kind of targeting of malignant brain tissue. Their tumor selectivity can mostly be ascribed to the deficient blood–brain barrier and they may fail as soon as it becomes necessary to judge tumor invasion at the single cell level. The techniques used for their detection, however, can mostly be adapted to more target-specific drugs, as long as they carry a fluorescent tag. This more "active" kind of targeting can be obtained by labeled antibodies, functionalized nanoparticles, or "smart probes" that respond to enzymatic reactions or that recognize specific RNA sequences. For the fluorescent labeling of antibody-based targeting moieties, near-infrared dyes are preferred, as tissue autofluorescence background is minimal and light penetration into tissue is maximal. One such dye is ICG bound to chlorotoxin that showed high affinity to human glioblastoma tissue (Butte et al., 2014). Another fluorescent dye (called IRDye 800CW), which was developed for flexible binding to any antibody, is available and has been tested—coupled to cetuximab—for fluorescence-guided resection of glioblastoma in an animal model (Warram et al., 2015). As its fluorescence properties are very similar to ICG, the same equipment can be used for its intraoperative imaging without further modification. One downside of this type of labeling is the unspecific tissue staining during circulation of the fluorochrome and the nonspecific binding of the antibody. Although the target-specific fluorescence technology is already quite advanced, these imaging agents will probably not enter clinical evaluations in the very near future. The reader is referred to reviews (Pogue et al., 2010; Hoetker and Goetz, 2013) to learn more about this.

18.3 ALA-BASED FLUORESCENCE-GUIDED RESECTION

The unique feature of AIF is that the drug applied is not itself the fluorochrome, which is finally detected. All other passively targeting fluorescence-based approaches rely on a target-specific accumulation of a preformed fluorochrome, which is usually applied systemically. As a consequence, there is at least an initial phase of nonspecific presence of the fluorochrome in the circulation or in the interstitial space, so that fluorescence accumulates not only within the target tissue but in other parts of the brain. Especially with malignant glioma, preoperative diffusion with edema or intraoperative leakage from injured blood vessels is a potential source of false-positive staining. ALA, on the other hand, is not fluorescent itself and will not cause unspecific fluorescence during the systemic distribution in the patient's body. The fluorochrome is only produced intracellularly after metabolism has taken place. This enables high fluorescence contrast potentially even with cellular resolution.

In this chapter, we describe the biological background as well as the clinical results. The limitations and comparison with other techniques are discussed, as well as possible improvements.

18.3.1 HEME BIOSYNTHESIS

Heme is not only synthesized in early erythrocytes to form hemoglobin but is required by all cells as the essential functional component in cytochromes and many heme-containing enzymes. Its synthesis starts with the formation of ALA inside mitochondria, is continued in the cytosol until coproporphyrinogen III, which is transported back into the mitochondria, where protoporphyrin IX (PpIX) is formed, which is finally chelated with bivalent iron to form heme (Figure 18.1, Collaud et al., 2004; Layer et al., 2010).

The only photoactive molecule in the heme biosynthesis pathway is PpIX. Its photophysical and photochemical properties (fluorescence and phototoxicity) are mediated by the conjugated bonds of the tetrapyrrolic porphyrin skeleton, forming a large π-electron system. Upon insertion of the ferrous ion (Fe^{2+}), these properties are lost.

A lot of enzymes are involved in heme biosynthesis, and the rate-limiting enzymes have been identified as PBG-D and ferrochelatase. The activity of the enzyme, which is responsible for the synthesis of ALA, ALA synthase, is governed by the concentration of free heme in the mitochondrion in a feedback-control manner. For this reason, under normal conditions, none of the intermediate molecules accumulates. For a more complete understanding of the pharmacokinetics of heme synthesis, one also has to consider the membrane transporters responsible for the transmembrane transport of ALA and the other intermediate products. The known ones are indicated in Figure 18.1 and play a pivotal role in the tumor selectivity of PpIX accumulation as discussed next (Table 18.1).

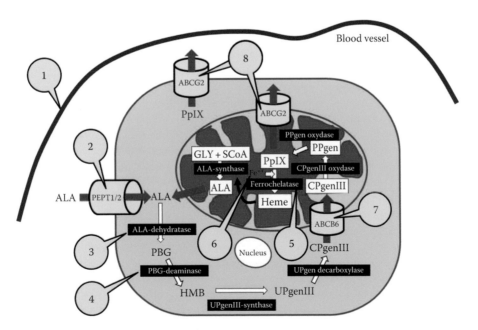

Figure 18.1 Simplified schematic of the biosynthesis of heme. The numbers indicate potential reasons for a tumor selectivity of PpIX accumulation (cmp. Table 18.1). GLY, glycine; SCoA, Succinyl-Coenzyme A; PBG, Porphobilinogen; HMB, Hydroxymethylbilane; UPgenIII, Uroporphyrinogen III; CPgenIII, Coproporphyrinogen III; PPgen, Protoporphyrinogen.

Table 18.1 Potential reasons for a tumor selectivity of PpIX accumulation

	Source of selectivity	Effect	Reference
1.	Blood–brain barrier leakage in glioma	Normal brain fairly protected from ALA	Ennis et al. (2003)
2.	Increased activity of pepT1, pepT2 transporter	Uptake of ALA in glioma cell increased	Zimmermann and Stan (2010)
3.	Increased activity of ALA-D	More of PpIX-precursor PBG synthesized	Navone et al. (1990)
4.	Increased activity of PBG-D	More of PpIX-precursor HMB synthesized	Hinnen et al. (1998)
5.	Reduced ferrochelatase activity	Accumulation of PpIX as one of the substrates of this step	Teng et al. (2011)
6.	Reduced availability of Fe^{2+}	Accumulation of PpIX as the other substrate of this step	Krieg et al. (2000)
7.	ABCB6-transporter	Transport of CPgenIII into mitochondria	Zhao et al. (2013b)
8.	ABCG2-transporter	Transport of PpIX from mitochondria into the cytosol, but also loss of PpIX through the plasma membrane	Kobuchi et al. (2012)

Notes: ALA-D, ALA-dehydrogenase; PBG, Porphobilinogen; PBG-D, Porphobilinogen-deaminase; HMB, hydroxymethylbilane; CPgenIII, coproporphyrinogen III. Numbers cmp. Figure 18.1.

18.3.2 TUMOR SELECTIVITY OF PpIX ACCUMULATION IN MALIGNANT GLIOMA

For an understanding of the potential sensitivity and specificity of ALA-based fluorescence detection of malignant glioma, it is essential to understand the mechanisms underlying the selective accumulation of PpIX in the tumor cells. Unfortunately, these multifactorial elements that govern PpIX accumulation have not been fully elucidated (Collaud et al., 2004).

Before intracellular heme synthesis can operate after ALA has been systemically administered, the ALA has to leave the blood vessels, diffuse through the interstitial space, and be taken up by the cells. At the level of the blood vessels, the blood–brain barrier (BBB) of the normal brain represents a fairly effective barrier against ALA, even though ALA is a small molecule. The wall of the blood vessels in the normal brain consists of endothelial cells, which are tightly connected with each other. In the normal brain, the molecules in the blood mostly reach the interstitial space by active transport across the endothelial barrier. In contrast, the neovessels induced by malignant glioma show defects both in the function and morphology of this endothelial layer, and molecules may leak through these vessels. This leaky vasculature constitutes the mechanism by which gadolinium-diethylenetriaminepentaacetic acid (Gd-DTPA) enables contrast-enhanced MRI of brain tumors (Galldiks et al., 2010). After intravenous injection of radioactively labeled ALA in mice, ALA uptake could be detected only in brain structures, which were connected to the cerebral spinal fluid via periventricular structures, such as the choroid plexus, where the capillaries have a reduced barrier function (Terr and Weiner, 1983). The protective function of the BBB against ALA transport is lost, if ALA is encapsulated into liposomes, leading to a measurable porphyrin accumulation in the normal brain (Fukuda et al., 1992). The relative tightness of the normal brain capillaries for ALA was also shown (Ennis et al., 2003). These authors found a very low influx rate except at the choroid plexus, confirming the results of Terr and Weiner (1983). As a conclusion, the normal brain is fairly well protected from ALA and PPIX accumulation.

One source of unspecific PpIX accumulation in the normal brain may however be the photosensitization of the endothelial cells themselves. In one study (Madsen and Hirschberg, 2010), a transient and localized opening of the BBB was shown to be inducible in normal rat brains after delivery of ALA followed by a moderate dose of light, implying a previous accumulation of at least some PpIX in the endothelial cells. As the volume percentage of endothelial cells within the entire brain tissue is in the order of 1%, this PpIX accumulation will be hardly detectable macroscopically as long as the rest of the brain remains protected from ALA.

Infiltrating glioma cells may have traveled sufficiently far into brain tissue that still possesses an intact BBB and might no longer be within the range of ALA diffusion. In a rat tumor model, the existence of dimly fluorescent or nonfluorescent isolated tumor cell nests around the bulk of the inoculated tumor were demonstrated (Madsen et al., 2006). On the other hand, it was also demonstrated that PpIX accumulation may extend into parts of the tumor that are contrast-MRI negative. In Samkoe et al., (2011), it was shown that PpIX accumulation in transplanted U251 glioma cells, which were transfected with green fluorescent protein (GFP), correlated better with GFP fluorescence and histology than contrast MRI.

Once having leaked through the deficient BBB in the tumor, ALA is present in the interstitial fluid and can diffuse a certain distance before it will be taken up by the tumor cells. This uptake occurs actively via peptide transporters PEPT1 or PEPT2 (Doring et al., 1998), a second potential source for tumor selectivity, if the expression of these transporters should be specifically upregulated in tumor compared to normal brain. Indeed, in different tumor systems, including glioma, four different groups (Hagiya et al., 2012; Chung et al., 2013; Hagiya et al., 2013; Suzuki et al., 2013; da Rocha Filho et al., 2015) have reported on a close correlation of the expression of these transporters and PpIX accumulation, although not as the only factor governing the tumor selectivity.

Once inside the cell, selective PpIX accumulation will occur if the enzyme activity needed for PpIX synthesis is upregulated, or if the enzyme ferrochelatase, which incorporates the bivalent iron into the PpIX-molecule is downregulated, or if the availability of free iron is reduced. Many investigations have been performed on ferrochelatase, clearly describing its decisive role for tumor selectivity (Van Hillegersberg et al., 1992; Hinnen et al., 1998; Krieg et al., 2000, 2002). Low iron availability will increase the PpIX concentration, as demonstrated by coincubation of cells with ALA and iron chelators (Berg et al., 1996; Blake and Curnow, 2010). A reduced expression of ferrochelatase in human GBM tissue samples could indeed be verified (Teng et al., 2011). The reason for the tumor-specific downregulation of ferrochelatase may partly lie in the indirect influence of tumor-suppressor proteins on the ferrochelatase activity, such as has been reported for the p53-dependent activity of mitochondrial frataxin (Sawamoto et al., 2013). Another key enzyme that is responsible for tumor-selective PpIX accumulation is porphobilinogen deaminase (PBG-D) (Navone et al., 1990; Hinnen et al., 1998). Interestingly, PBG-D was unexpectedly found in the nuclei of glioma cells and ascribed a role in cell proliferation, independent of its role in heme synthesis (Greenbaum et al., 2002, 2003).

A further factor influencing the intracellular PpIX concentration is the transport of intermediate compounds across membranes: coproporphyrinogen III into the mitochondrion, protoporphyrin IX into the cytosol and eventually across the plasma membrane. The transporters involved have not yet been unambiguously identified. Previous reports on the peripheral benzodiazepine receptor being responsible for mitochondrial transport of PPIX (Collaud et al., 2004) may have to be reconsidered in the light of reports that ABCB6 was the main transport protein responsible for coproporphyrinogen III influx (Krishnamurthy et al., 2006; Kobuchi et al., 2012; Zhao et al., 2013b). Increased expression of ABCB6 in malignant glioma, correlating with intraoperative PpIX-fluorescence, was found in tissue sampled during clinical AIF-guided resection (Zhao et al., 2013b). For the efflux of PpIX from mitochondria as well as for the efflux through the plasma membrane, the protein ABCG2 has been identified (Ishikawa et al., 2010; Ogino et al., 2011; Kobuchi et al., 2012). This finding may have little influence on the diagnostic aspect of PpIX accumulation, but may be worthwhile to keep in mind for the therapeutic application, as it potentially leads to the resistance of cells expressing (or overexpressing) ABCG2 to PDT-mediated cell death. As ABCG2 expression is associated with stem cell properties and has also been described for glioma stem cells (Jin et al., 2009), the small, but decisive fraction of tumor stem cells able to cause a recurrence may potentially escape therapy.

Finally, cadherin13 overexpression was found to be negatively correlated with PpIX accumulation in tissue specimens from glioblastoma patients (Suzuki et al., 2013). In cadherin13 knock-down cells, ABCG2 was downregulated and pepT1 was upregulated, which would readily explain the observation. The underlying mechanisms could not be clarified, however.

Under practical considerations for clinical AIF, one can summarize the mechanisms of selectivity as follows:

- The drug delivered to the patient, ALA, is not a fluorochrome. There is no unspecific background during systemic distribution.
- ALA does not easily penetrate the BBB. Normal brain does not accumulate measurable concentrations of PpIX with the recommended dose of ALA delivered.
- Leaky tumor neovasculature is a first source for tumor selectivity.
- Cellular uptake of ALA by peptide transporters is another potential source of tumor cell selectivity.
- Intracellular PpIX synthesis via tumor selectively up- (PBG-D) or downregulated (ferrochelatase) enzyme activities contributes to tumor selectivity.
- Intracellular redistribution or efflux of PpIX may also occur tumor selectively.

PpIX accumulation can be expected to be at least as tumor selective as contrast MRI, as both methods share a deficient BBB as a decisive factor for tissue penetration. As PpIX accumulation additionally depends on tumor-selective intracellular enzyme activities, it may be concluded that PpIX fluorescence imaging correlates better with PET imaging of brain tumors than with contrast MRI (see Section 18.3.6).

Reports on systematic investigations of possible correlations of PpIX accumulation with prognostic factors, such as MGMT or IDH mutation status or Ki67 index are rare. As the vast majority of glioblastomas shows strong PpIX fluorescence, a dependence on MGMT status as a determining single factor can be ruled out. For grade III gliomas, in a genetically engineered cell line IDH1 mutation was identified to correlate positively with PpIX fluorescence (Kim et al., 2015), whereas others (Hickmann et al., 2015) found nonfluorescent recurrent gliomas were more often IDH mutated. Ki67 index is a proliferation marker and PpIX accumulation has at least some correlation with the cell division rate (Iinuma et al., 1994). It is therefore not astonishing that Ki67 index measured in slides from malignant glioma samples correlates reasonably well with intraoperative PpIX fluorescence intensity (Johansson et al., 2010; Idoate et al., 2011; Valdes et al., 2011a). A more systematic assessment of predictors for "ALA-positivity" in 166 nonglioblastoma tumors (8 being atypical GBMs) identified an ^{18}F-FET-PET uptake ratio of >1.85 as predictive for fluorescence apart from Ki67 (Jaber et al., 2016). MGMT, IDH1, and 1p19q codeletion did not correlate with fluorescence in these tumors. Interestingly, of 82 WHO grade II tumors, 15.9% did reveal intraoperative fluorescence, whereas 16.7% of enhancing grade III tumors did not show fluorescence.

18.3.3 IMAGING WITH THE SURGICAL MICROSCOPE

AIF can easily be integrated into the clinical workflow. ALA (Gliolan®, medac, Wedel) is recommended to be dissolved in 50 ml of drinking water at a concentration of 20 mg/kg body weight and applied orally 3–4 h before anesthesia (Figure 18.2) (European Medicines Agency, 2007b). The surgery is planned using preoperative CT, MRI, and PET-imaging (Figure 18.3). No special arrangements with the exception of reducing ambient light are necessary to switch between white light and fluorescence modes when using one of the commercial surgical microscopes (Zeiss, Göttingen, Germany; Leica, Wetzlar, Germany; Möller-Wedel, Wedel, Germany). As a measure of precaution to avoid skin erythema and retinal injury, the patient is protected from sunlight or bright indoor light for 24 h after drug delivery. During resection the neurosurgeon has to distinguish the different parts of the heterogeneous tumor and to decide where continued resection starts to pose a risk by inducing functional deficits. AIF can support this goal by clearly showing residual bulk tumor tissue by its strong fluorescence (Figure 18.4). In the infiltration zone, the fluorescence intensity will gradually decrease with the decreasing density of tumor cells. There will not be a sharp border between the tissue needing to be resected and the tissue needing to be preserved. Ultimately, the resection limits will depend on the tumor location with respect to eloquent regions. If tumor infiltration penetrates deep into functional brain, PpIX may still be detectable, but surgery has to stop. The sensitivity of fluorescence imaging should therefore be adjusted to a reasonable value, where bulk tumor can be distinguished from the onset of the infiltration zone rather than highlighting lowest tumor cell densities to not mislead the surgeon to undue extension of the resection volume.

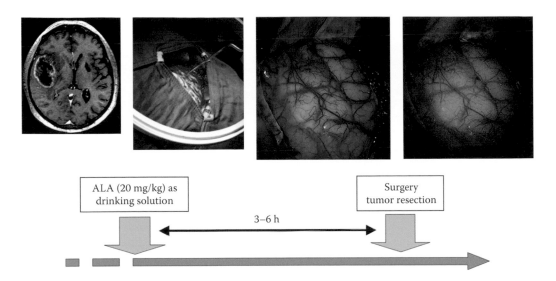

Figure 18.2 Application of ALA is 3–6 h prior to surgery (2–4 h prior to induction of anesthesia (EuropeanMedicinesAgency, 2007a)). Top row: clear suspicion of a GBM in contrast MRI, prepared surgical site, same through the surgical microscope in white light and fluorescence mode. Red fluorescent PpIX from the tumor tissue is visible even prior to onset of resection.

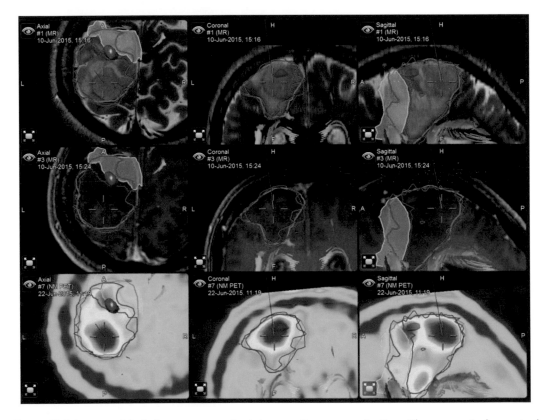

Figure 18.3 Image-guided glioma surgery using intraoperative neuronavigation with preoperatively acquired MRI (top row: T2-weighted MRI, middle row: T1-weighted MRI with gadolinium enhancement, bottom row: FET–PET. Objects of interest (tumor as depicted in T2w MRI = green; tumor as outlined in FET–PET = pink; suspected FET–PET "hot spot" area = violet; left precentral gyrus = brown; presumed resectable tumor = red), and relevant fiber tracts (left corticospinal tract = blue; fibers adjacent to tumor = green) are shown in the different planes (left column = axial, middle column = coronal; right column = sagittal).

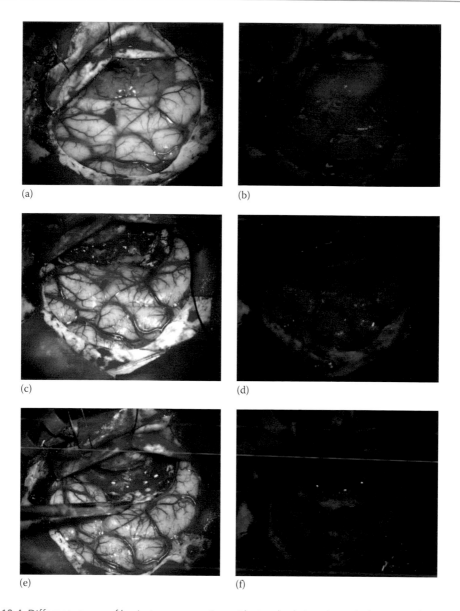

Figure 18.4 Different stages of brain tumor resection with standard view through the surgical microscope in white light (left column) and fluorescence mode (right column). First row: red fluorescent tumor extends to the cortical surface until right underneath the prepared dura mater (a, b). Middle row: during resection, red fluorescence correlates with white light impression (c, d). Bottom row: toward the end of resection no suspicion of residual tumor in white light (e), whereas red fluorescence clearly depicts residual tumor (f).

The approach realized by major manufacturers of AIF surgical microscopes is similar to the approach that previously had been successfully established for the endoscopic fluorescence imaging of bladder cancer (Jocham et al., 2008). The excitation of the tissue is achieved by switching a short-pass filter into the light path of the microscope light source. The filter fully transmits all light with wavelengths shorter than 430 nm (violet) and thereby covers the main PpIX absorption band at 380–430 nm (FWHM) (Figure 18.5). At the 1% level, this filter also transmits blue light until 460 nm before it more or less completely blocks all longer wavelengths. All light that is reflected or emitted from the tissue under investigation has to pass a long-pass filter, which transmits only wavelengths longer than 440 nm (blue, green, yellow, red) before it can be visualized by a camera or by the surgeon. All excitation light is thus blocked from being observed. From the light

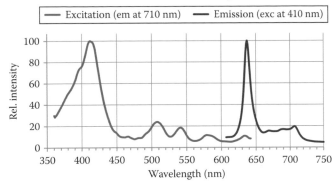

Figure 18.5 Excitation and emission spectra of freshly resected glioblastoma tissue after delivery of 20 mg/kg bw of ALA.

source, only the small peak between 440 and 460 nm, which is diffusely reflected from the tissue surface, will be transmitted to the observer and make the nonfluorescent tissue look blue. Since the blood absorption spectrum has a local minimum at this wavelength range, blood vessels appear darker and clearly visible. Hence, details in the tissue are clearly displayed. Tissue autofluorescence has its maximum intensity in the green wavelength range, but also extends into the red spectral range. By illuminating the tissue with the low intensity blue light, this tissue autofluorescence is only recognized by a change of the hue of the blue light (shift to greenish blue), but normal brain still appears blue. PpIX-positive tissue leads to a switch in perceived color from blue to red. This is true for bulk tumor, where the intensity of red PpIX fluorescence is much larger than reflected blue light and often described as "strong" or "solid" fluorescence. In the infiltration zone, where tumor cell density decreases, the ratio of red fluorescence versus blue reflection is reduced and the perceived color becomes more and more purple and darker, sometimes described as "vague" fluorescence. As soon as PpIX fluorescence intensity is as low as the red part of tissue autofluorescence, it can no longer be perceived as red. Explicitly, this means that fluorescent tumor cells may still be present, but the system will not display the tissue as "positive" to avoid progressive resection into the infiltration zone, where the risk of inducing functional deficits would increase.

The cameras used in these surgical microscopes must also be modified to fulfill the requirements of fluorescence imaging. First of all, the available light intensity is very low and the cameras will be switched simultaneously with the light source to a gain setting, which may produce some noise but enables imaging in real time, or use frame integration to produce high-quality imaging, albeit with a short time delay. The gain settings of the different color channels is also preset and fixed in the fluorescence mode. Additionally, the infrared filtering of the camera sensor chips is modified to improve the sensitivity in the PpIX fluorescence wavelength range (600–710 nm).

The wavelength range in the violet to blue, which is used to excite the PpIX fluorescence, is also absorbed by blood. The blood absorption is indeed strong enough to completely screen the PpIX fluorescence even if only very thin layers cover the tissue (Figure 18.6). Careful rinsing and cleaning of the tissue surface is absolutely mandatory for a reliable visualization of residual fluorescence, especially toward the end of the resection process. When investigating the resection cavity in fluorescence mode at the end of surgery, all areas appearing black or very dark cannot be judged properly, because they are covered by liquid or dried blood. If there was any underlying fluorescent tissue, it would not be visible.

Another issue to keep in mind is the low penetration depth of the excitation light of only a few 100 μm. This implies (1) that a fluorescent tissue layer, even if strongly fluorescent may already be very thin and (2) fluorescent tumor cell nests buried underneath nonfluorescent tissue will be invisible.

Of some concern is also the fact that fluorescence of PpIX is unstable over time; with prolonged light irradiation, the fluorescence gradually fades. This process is called photobleaching. Under normal conditions,

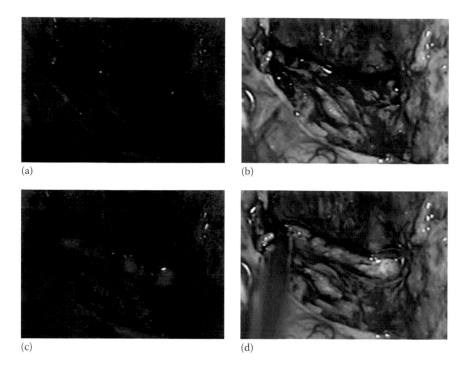

(a)   (b)

(c)   (d)

Figure 18.6 Blood conceals PpIX fluorescence completely. Top row: a layer of blood has filled the floor of the resection cavity (a: fluorescence mode, b: corresponding white light image). PpIX positivity can only be judged after careful rinsing and cleaning of the tissue surface (bottom row, c and d).

however, there is no restriction with respect to investigation time, as photobleaching occurs in minutes, not in seconds (Stummer et al., 1998). During resection, there is always previously unexposed tissue being exposed on the operating surface, which, due to the low light penetration depth, has not yet experienced photobleaching.

Practical use of the equipment with a more detailed explanation of how to avoid potential pitfalls is provided by a review article (Tonn and Stummer, 2008). We discuss in Section 18.3.5.3 how and under which conditions more sensitive and deeper penetrating fluorescence detection may be possible and useful.

18.3.4 AIF-GUIDED BIOPSY

The high positive predictive value found for PpIX staining of viable high-grade glioma tissue (see Section 18.3.5.2) may offer a chance for significant improvement of stereotactic biopsy sampling. The usefulness has been shown as proof of principle in a few studies, investigating the fluorescence of biopsy specimens ex situ with the surgical microscope (Moriuchi et al., 2011; von Campe et al., 2012; Widhalm et al., 2012). The concept of how the procedure can be implemented into a medical device and into the clinical workflow was presented in (Stepp et al., 2012). The first clinical case with intraoperative AIF guidance, demonstrating suitable equipment, was reported (Gobel et al., 2012; Eigenbrod et al., 2014).

18.3.5 CLINICAL RESULTS

The European approval of Gliolan®-based AIF was obtained after completion of a phase III trial (Stummer et al., 2006). This trial was a prospective, randomized, multicenter trial demonstrating safety and efficacy of AIF in high-grade glioma cases. Ninety-seven percent of the 139 patients, who received the study drug, were grade IV tumors, only 3 were grade III. In general, grade I and II tumors are considered as not being "ALA positive", except for the intriguing possibility to detect anaplastic foci (as defined by "hot spots" in FET–PET imaging) intraoperatively by their circumscribed fluorescence (Engh, 2010; Widhalm et al., 2010, 2013; Ewelt et al., 2011; Jaber et al., 2016). This is true for the currently employed equipment (surgical microscope equipped with "blue light" or "400" fluorescence mode). More sensitive spectroscopic equipment may be able to also detect low-grade tumors (Valdes et al., 2015). In this section, we will focus on high-grade gliomas, of which glioblastoma multiforme (GBM) represents the vast majority.

18.3.5.1 PROGRESSION-FREE AND OVERALL SURVIVAL

Even if there is still no level I evidence in the literature to recommend microsurgical tumor resection (Olson et al., 2009), results from the multivariate analysis of fluorescence-guided surgery with 5-aminolevulinic acid (5-ALA) compared to white light tumor resection demonstrated that total resection of all the tumor mass showing contrast enhancement in MRI leads to a survival benefit for glioblastoma patients (Stummer et al., 2006, 2008b). In the multicenter phase III study published by Stummer (Stummer et al., 2006) the primary end points were "complete resection of contrast-enhancing tumor" and "6-month progression-free survival." The study compared the outcomes of 139 high-grade glioma patients operated on using AIF guidance with 131 patients operated on with the standard procedure under white light. Complete tumor resections under white light were achieved in 36% of cases, whereas in the fluorescence arm, 65% of complete tumor resections could be achieved. Progression-free survival was also significantly longer in the fluorescence arm versus the white light arm (41% vs. 21%). The study was not powered to show significantly increased overall survival and, indeed, the survival advantage for the fluorescence arm (15.2 vs. 13.5 months) was not statistically significant. If, however, the overall survival times of patients with complete resections (disregarding the study arm) were compared with the overall survival of the patients with residual contrast enhancement, the difference was significant (Stummer et al., 2008b; 17.9 vs. 12.9 months). No significant difference in side effects was noted for the study arms. This was the first study with level 2b evidence that "complete resection" is superior to noncomplete resection.

The phase III trial by Stummer et al. is still the largest trial evaluating survival benefit. Trials involving more than 100 patients have been published by two other independent groups (Slotty et al., 2013; Diez Valle et al., 2014). The Spanish multicenter VISIONA trial (Diez Valle et al., 2014) showed a significant advantage of AIF guidance for complete resection rate (67% vs. 45%) and 6-month progression-free survival (69% vs. 48%). Interestingly, in this trial, cost-effectiveness was calculated (Slof et al., 2015), resulting in costs of 4550 Euros per additional complete resection, or 9021 Euros per QALY (quality adjusted life year), gained. These data were very similar to the 9100 Euros per QALY calculated by Esteves et al. (2015). Another larger trial (Slotty et al., 2013) compared median overall survival between standard surgery and AIF-guided resection, and showed an advantage for AIF guidance (20.1 vs. 16.6 months), but this difference was not statistically significant. Several reviews with clinical outcome data can be found (Zhao et al., 2013a; Barone et al., 2014; Leroy et al., 2015).

The benefit of partial tumor resection compared to not performing surgery at all seems to be very limited, even if some authors advocate tumor debulking to reduce the existing tumor mass in order to allow external beam ionizing radiation, and to avoid the risk for brain herniation in the course of the radiation therapy (Quigley and Maroon, 1991; Kelly and Hunt, 1994). External beam radiation has been one of the cornerstones in the treatment of malignant gliomas for more than 30 years (Walker et al., 1980) and technical improvements have led to a reduction in radiogenic complications. Therefore, until recently, the standard therapy for patients with newly diagnosed GBM either after microsurgical tumor resection or via stereotactical biopsy, consisted of radiotherapy alone (Kleinberg et al., 1997), consisting of 54–60 Gy delivered in 1.8–2.0 Gy fractions over a 6-week time period at regional fields with a margin around the contrast-enhancing lesion of about 2 cm (Laperriere et al., 2002; Roa et al., 2009). Median survival times of 7–8 months even in patients older than 70 years have been reported with acceptable toxicity (Mohan et al., 1998; Villa et al., 1998). However, the EORTC/NCIC trial provided class I evidence for concomitant radiochemotherapy with temozolomide (TMZ) followed by six adjuvant cycles of TMZ alone and led to a change in standard cancer care for GBM (Stupp et al., 2005). In the initial report there was an increase in the median survival of 2.5 months from 12.1 to 14.6 months due to additional use of TMZ. Moreover, the 2-year survival rate was increased from 10.4% to as much as 26.5% for radiotherapy with TMZ. Subanalysis of these patients revealed that epigenetic silencing of the O6-methylguanine methyl-transferase (MGMT) by hypermethylation of its gene promoter led to a significantly better progression-free survival (PFS) as well as overall survival (OS). This was seen irrespective of treatment modality but even more if they received combined treatment (Hegi et al., 2005). The final analysis of these patients now revealed an overall survival for combined treatment with TMZ of 9.8% in contrast to 1.9% for radiotherapy alone after 5 years (Stupp et al., 2009).

18.3.5.2 LIMITATIONS

Ideally, PpIX fluorescence would unambiguously stain all malignant cells and be completely absent in the normal brain. Even in this case, however, resection cannot continue until the last single tumor cell has been removed as there will inevitably be injury to the functional brain or to blood vessels supplying the normal brain long before this aim could be achieved. The macroscopic nature of surgery is thus the first limitation in AIF. We briefly describe in Section 18.3.9, how the photosensitizing property of PpIX might be exploited to perform some kind of "photochemical microsurgery" to continue treatment beyond the surgical limit.

PpIX staining does not address a specific molecular target on the tumor cell. It rather relies on systematic differences in cellular metabolism between tumor cells and normal cells. In addition, tissue availability of ALA depends on a deficient blood–brain barrier. It is therefore not surprising that sensitivity and specificity of PpIX staining of GBM are not 100%. In the following, we describe and discuss clinical observations, which outline the limitations of AIF.

18.3.5.2.1 Heterogeneity of PpIX fluorescence

PpIX fluorescence intensity was shown to vary considerably even within nonnecrotic, vital parts of coalescent histologically identical tumor tissue from the same patient (Moiyadi and Sridhar, 2015). It is speculated that the PpIX variability may reflect some biological variability, which is not immediately apparent histologically. This assumption is supported by the finding of Piccorillo et al. (2012) that tumor-initiating cells (TICs) within the tumor mass behave differently depending on whether they are isolated from PpIX-positive or PpIX-negative tumor tissue.

Intra- and interpatient variability of PpIX accumulation has been reported before (Eleouet et al., 2000; Johansson et al., 2010). The absolute value of PpIX fluorescence intensity may contain some biologically relevant information, but as a guide for resection, the unpredictable fluorescence intensity represents a limitation. The neurosurgeon will have to individually adjust the intensity of bulk tumor fluorescence to correctly estimate the regions of infiltrative tumor. In practice, this is not a problem.

18.3.5.2.2 False-negative PpIX fluorescence

Of more concern is tumor which does not show any PpIX fluorescence. If the entire tumor is void of red fluorescence, the application or the dose of ALA applied should be questioned as a possible reason. Among 47 patients with GBM, Hefti et al. (2008) found only 1 tumor completely nonfluorescent. Tsugu et al. (2011) reported a higher failure rate of 3 out of 20 GBMs being nonfluorescent, but this group used nonstandard equipment. In our own assessment (Stepp et al., 2012), 2 of 19 patients showed no PpIX fluorescence in representative biopsy samples. As a conclusion, one has to expect that the vast majority of, but not absolutely all, high-grade gliomas accumulate detectable amounts of PpIX.

On a per-biopsy basis, the sensitivities reported for high-grade gliomas range above 75%, that is, false-negative fluorescence is observed in a nonnegligible number of cases. From the preclinical findings reported earlier, this has to be expected (Madsen et al., 2006). In the first clinical report on the method (Stummer et al., 1998), a sensitivity of 85% was found. However, of the 9 false-negative samples, 4 were predominantly necrotic and 5 showed a low density of infiltrating tumor. Another group (Roberts et al., 2011) reported a sensitivity of 75% for visual assessment of PpIX fluorescence. Later, the same group (Valdes et al., 2011b) compared quantitative spectroscopy with visual inspection and demonstrated a sensitivity of 95% for high-grade glioma, when using the more sensitive spectroscopic method. A sensitivity of >91% was found by Panciani et al. (2012a,b), where the false-negative samples showed a low density of tumor cells histologically. In an earlier study (Stummer et al.,

2000), a biopsy-based sensitivity of 89% was found, where only 5 nonfluorescent samples out of 237 histologically positive ones contained solid tumor, the other 21 samples showed only diffuse infiltration of tumor. Finally, in a more recent evaluation of 33 patients with high-grade glioma, tumor infiltration was detected in 60 of 100 biopsies gathered from nonfluorescent tissue as judged through the surgical microscope (Stummer et al., 2014).

The discussion of the consequences of the less than 100% sensitivity for AIF only makes sense when it is put in context with alternatives, such as neuronavigation or interventional MRI, which we discuss later. What one can state here is that most of the reports of negative fluorescence concern samples obtained from the borders of the resection cavity, and most of the false-negative samples contained a low tumor cell density. These samples are thus part of the infiltration zone, where it is questionable whether resection should have continued anyway.

18.3.5.2.3 False-positive PpIX fluorescence

False-positive findings imply there is a risk of resecting normal brain tissue and should therefore ideally never occur. Compared to other fluorescent photosensitizers, ALA carries no risk of unspecific staining during systemic delivery and biodistribution, because ALA is not fluorescent. PpIX accumulation, however, may occur nonspecifically, as has been reported for its diagnostic application for the detection of bladder cancer (Jocham et al., 2008). PpIX may also potentially leak from tumor into surrounding edema and thus stain normal brain tissue. As this represents a considerable risk factor, the issue has been given some attention in the literature.

The statistically relevant value to judge the rate of false positives is the "positive predictive value" (ppv) rather than the specificity, because the latter depends a lot on the sampling rate of true negatives, which could be driven to high numbers, thus keeping specificity arbitrarily high. The ppv, on the other hand, judges only fluorescence-positive samples and, if the ppv is high, guarantees correct prediction of tumor wherever there is fluorescence. Stummer et al. (2014) in a recent study on 33 patients reported that there was a ppv of 100% for strong fluorescence, and a ppv of 92% (biopsy based) or 83% (patient based) for weak fluorescence as observed through the surgical microscope. All these samples had been obtained in close proximity to the tumor margin, and none from remotely sampled tissue. In the first clinical report in 1998, no false-positive samples were collected among 53 fluorescent biopsies (Stummer et al., 1998). In an investigation on 36 patients, the strong fluorescence in 72 samples predicted tumor with a ppv of 100%, and only 2 samples from vaguely fluorescent tissue (n = 72) were histopathologically specified as normal (Diez Valle et al., 2011). The question of false positives was also investigated with recurrent tumors (Nabavi et al., 2009); in 12 of 354 fluorescent biopsies (3.4%), mostly weakly fluorescent tissue was judged normal. Similar observations on newly diagnosed GBM were reported by Roberts et al. (2011) with only one of 86 fluorescent samples containing only normal tissue, whereas the other 3 false positives showed signs of necrosis or abnormal vasculature. Of 212 fluorescent samples, Stummer et al. (2000) found only a single sample not showing tumor. From the data published in Hefti et al. (2008) one can calculate a ppv for strong fluorescence of 100% and for weak fluorescence of 91%. Similar data were also published by Idoate et al. (2011) in 30 patients with GBM, where they found a ppv of 100% for strong and 97% for weak fluorescence. Finally, in Ando et al. (2011), fluorescence spectroscopy on tissue sections was described, where false-positive areas could be discriminated from true-positive ones by their increased autofluorescence.

With regard to the reasons for false-positive fluorescence, it was mostly found in recurrent cases of malignant glioma in peritumoral edema and inflammatory cell and reactive astrocyte infiltration (Utsuki et al., 2007b). Kamp et al. (2015) retrospectively identified 13 of 313 patients with suspicion of recurrent GBM with no active tumor in the resected tissue. In all but one of these 13 cases, heterogeneous strong or vague fluorescence had been detected intraoperatively. All samples demonstrated reactive changes, so were not classified as normal functional brain. One might consider that the main reason for false-positive PpIX fluorescence could be the diffusion of PpIX from adjacent brain tumor into an area of edema. However, there is a report on strong false-positive fluorescence detected around a nonfluorescent metastasis of a malignant melanoma in tissue showing simple gliosis only (Schucht et al., 2011). Hence, local nonspecific synthesis of PpIX must be considered at least in this case. This, in turn, implies that the diffusion of 5-ALA into regions with effective BBB could be relevant.

In Section 18.3.2, we have mentioned that ALA may reach the cerebral spinal fluid via periventricular structures that lack a classical BBB. PpIX fluorescence in (normal) ventricle ependyma has been reported in an animal model (Hebeda et al., 1998). In our own experience, the ventricular wall, even when distant to the opening, usually exhibits a weak but clearly visible fluorescence without apparent tumor infiltration. However, a more systematic investigation on 65 patients with GBM and ventricle wall opening showed that the fluorescence did not always extend over the entire wall (Tejada-Solis et al., 2012). Whether the extent of ventricle wall fluorescence has any useful information will have to be investigated further. In the study by Tejada-Solis et al. the fluorescence was not a predictor for complications or survival. On the other hand, tumor cell infiltration into the ependyma was reported in six out of seven cases with fluorescent (but visually normal) ventricle wall (Hayashi et al., 2010). These authors speculated that "5-ALA fluorescence of the ventricular wall may be predictive of postoperative hydrocephalus associated with CSF dissemination even in cases without evidence of CSF dissemination on MR imaging studies before surgery."

In conclusion, the risk of inducing functional deficits by resecting false-positive fluorescent tissue is very low, as the positive predictive values reported are almost 100% for strongly fluorescent tissue. The somewhat lower values for weak fluorescence are still mostly correlated with the immediate peritumoral zone or demonstrate reactive changes. Therefore, resection of weakly fluorescent tissue should be considered carefully, especially in close vicinity to functionally eloquent areas. The reasons for unspecific PpIX staining have not been completely clarified.

18.3.5.3 IMPROVEMENTS

Improvements in AIF may address the performance of PpIX staining (improved drug delivery or accumulation) or the equipment (improved visualization device).

18.3.5.3.1 Improvement of the accuracy of PpIX staining

The positive predictive value of PpIX fluorescence is already very high, especially if only strongly fluorescent tissue is considered. One may therefore first focus on false negatives and discuss attempts to improve PpIX accumulation.

One possibility to increase intracellular PpIX levels is to directly modulate cellular heme synthesis. One promising target in this regard is the enzyme ferrochelatase, which transforms fluorescent PpIX into nonfluorescent heme. That the inhibition of this enzyme does indeed increase PpIX levels was shown by Teng et al. (2011). Iron chelators, such as desferrioxamine have also been shown to increase PpIX levels (Chang et al., 1997; Blake and Curnow, 2010; Fukuhara et al., 2013).

Another possibility had been identified that involves modifying cell differentiation with some pharmacological agents. Indirectly, this approach may also interfere with heme synthesis, as it has been observed that coproporphyrin oxidase activity is enhanced in more differentiated cancer cells. An increase in PpIX levels and improvement of PDT effectiveness of squamous carcinoma cells was demonstrated, when the cells were pretreated with calcitriol (Vitamin D) (Cicarma et al., 2009). The mechanisms of differentiation-induced expression of coproporphyrin oxidase have been addressed by Anand et al. (2013). In vitro investigations presented by Chen et al. (2014) demonstrated similar effects on glioma cells and also indicated that a PpIX increase may occur in a tumor-selective manner by pretreatment with calcitriol.

Clinically, the combination of ALA and the delivery of a PpIX modifying drug have not yet been reported and would represent a significant challenge, as one has to exclude that the attempt to increase PpIX levels in brain tumor also produces PpIX in normal brain. It may however be the case that some glioma patients may be on Vitamin D medication, which is prescription free.

18.3.5.3.2 Improvement of PpIX detection

Most clinical papers are based on fluorescence observation using one of the dedicated commercial surgical microscopes (Zeiss, Göttingen, Germany; Leica, Wetzlar, Germany; Möller-Wedel, Wedel, Germany) (Colditz et al., 2012).

Three problems are associated with this technology: (1) you can only see where you look. The presence of PpIX fluorescence can only be detected within the field of view of the optical instrument. The surgeon must be able to direct the microscope reasonably perpendicularly to the investigated tissue surface. This may be difficult with deep-seated tumors. (2) Strong blood absorption: These surgical microscopes all excite the PpIX fluorescence with filtered white light at around 390–450 nm. In this spectral range, and especially at the excitation maximum of PpIX fluorescence at 405–415 nm, blood absorption is also maximal. Consequently, any diffuse bleeding within the resection cavity may lead to a complete elimination of any fluorescence from underlying tissue. In fact, a single layer of erythrocytes completely absorbs the excitation light. Even diluted blood may therefore easily prevent clear visibility of PpIX-containing tissue. Thorough rinsing and removal of any blood-containing liquid on top of the investigated tissue is mandatory. This is illustrated in Figure 18.6, where a thin layer of blood has covered the floor of the resection cavity. Only after thorough rinsing and aspiration of spilled blood, the fluorescence of the underlying tumor tissue was unveiled. (3) The optical filters are designed for high specificity, rather than high sensitivity by transmitting blue remitted light and green autofluorescence, which intentionally suppress very weak red PpIX fluorescence. (4) Ambient light must be sufficiently dimmed to not interfere with fluorescence imaging. In the worst case, some reflections from room lighting may make non-PpIX-containing tissue look seemingly fluorescence positive.

The first problem of visual accessibility may be solved by using side-view endoscopes equipped with similar technology, as demonstrated by different groups (Tamura et al., 2007; Ritz et al., 2011; Cornelius et al., 2013; Rapp et al., 2014).

The second problem of blood absorption is not a crucial issue for neurosurgeons with experience in AIF. The only restriction is that buried microinvasions, which might have accumulated PpIX, may be missed, due to the very limited penetration depth of the short-wavelength excitation light. It has been demonstrated, however, that PpIX fluorescence at 705 nm can be excited with red light at 633 nm, which penetrates much deeper into tissue and especially through thicker layers of diluted blood (Johansson et al., 2013; Potapov et al., 2013). So far, this red excitation has been demonstrated only with spectroscopic point detection of the 705 nm emission, but there is no reason in principle why it should not be feasible in an imaging mode. With appropriate filtering, the neurosurgeon can be protected from the intense excitation light needed and the fluorescence should still be visible or at least be captured by a sensitive camera and displayed in a false color overlay to the regular white light image. With such a system, the final judgment of the resection cavity might be more reliable than with violet light excitation and might even uncover buried microinvasions.

The approach to the third problem has to be performed with considerable caution as increasing sensitivity is always connected with the risk of simultaneously reducing specificity, that is, generating false positives. One means of detecting very low concentrations of PpIX is fluorescence spectroscopy. The spectral shape of tissue autofluorescence is uncharacteristic, showing decreasing intensity with increasing wavelength. On top of this curve, PpIX exhibits two characteristic peaks at 635 and 705 nm (Figure 18.5), which can be detected easily at low concentrations, where standard fluorescence imaging is no longer able to detect the presence of PpIX (Stummer et al., 2014). Indeed, sensitivity of GBM detection can be increased, but at the cost of specificity, as demonstrated by Stummer et al. (2014). PpIX fluorescence spectroscopy also provides access to a more quantitative judgment of the fluorescence intensity. In a simple approach, the height of the PpIX fluorescence peak at 635 nm can be quantitatively determined, which gives it an objective numerical value, in contrast to the subjective judgment of visual fluorescence as "strong," "weak" or "vague," or "none." Such an approach was presented by Haj-Hosseini et al. (2010). One might, however, also be interested in determining the absolute concentration of PpIX. Although the fluorescence peak intensity is of course proportional to the PpIX concentration, it also depends on tissue absorption and scattering. A number of approaches have been proposed to disentangle all the influencing factors; see, for example, Hoy et al. (2013) and Middelburg et al. (2015). A simple algorithm considering tissue backscattering at certain wavelengths to correct for tissue optical properties was demonstrated by Valdes et al. (2011b). With their system, the diagnostic accuracy could be significantly improved over visual inspection from 66% to 87%, but again at the expense of specificity, which was reduced from 100% to 92%. The high sensitivity may be beneficial to identify low-grade brain tumors by PpIX fluorescence, where the current assessment with standard surgical microscopes is "nonfluorescent." In a recent report, with their highly sensitive spectroscopic system, Valdes et al. (2015) indeed could show low but specific PpIX accumulation in 6 out of 12 low-grade tumors. A similar algorithm was used for an imaging system (Valdes et al., 2013).

The fourth problem may be overcome by using pulsed light sources for fluorescence excitation and synchronized gated camera systems (Sexton et al., 2013). However, this problem has hardly ever been stressed in clinical reports. Hence, it is obviously easily handled in clinical routine. With the development of LED or laser diode-based light sources for AIF, a simple and cost-effective implementation may be possible and should then seriously be considered. It would also allow for a quasi-simultaneous display of white light and fluorescence images.

The fluorescence imaging systems discussed so far employ color cameras, which may be equipped with some frame integration to increase brightness and fixed gain settings for the three color channels, but otherwise display simple real color fluorescence images, where the red channel brightness should indicate the presence of PpIX. Different approaches on how to improve fluorescence imaging with multispectral excitation or detection have been published (Yang et al., 2003; Bogaards et al., 2004; Gebhart et al., 2007; Leblond et al., 2011).

An intriguing possibility to determine the thickness of a fluorescent layer or the depth of a buried fluorescent lesion is by using structured light excitation. By changing the spatial frequency of the excitation light pattern, the depth sensitivity of this approach was nicely demonstrated (Mazhar et al., 2010). For AIF, especially if combined with two excitation wavelengths (405 and 633 nm), one could support surgery by indicating where there is still much bulk tumor and where the strongly fluorescent layer becomes thin or one might be able to discover buried microinvasion.

Fluorescence imaging usually is two-dimensional, even if some depth information can be extracted, as just described. With an ultrasound supported dedicated fluorescence tomography system, quantitative 3D distribution of PpIX to a depth of a few mm could be demonstrated (Flynn et al., 2013).

Whether any of these improved fluorescence-imaging systems will be commercialized certainly depends on the clinical need. A "high-sensitivity mode" may be useful for imaging of low-grade brain tumors.

18.3.6 COMPARISON WITH iMRI

It is not at present clear if iMRI is a competing or complementary tool that could be combined with 5-ALA fluorescence, or if either one can be used "interchangeably," depending on the availability. CRET may most reliably be achieved when contrast MRI can be performed during surgery. It has been demonstrated by Roder et al. (2014) that since the establishment of iMRI in their clinic, the rate of CRET could be increased from 13% (white light) to 74% in GBM patients with intended total resection. With FGR, the rate of CRET in their setting was significantly lower at 46%. This is astonishing, given the high sensitivity of 5-ALA-guided surgery. Especially when comparing the volumes of preoperative cMRI and the tumor mass resected under fluorescence guidance, where, for instance, Schucht et al. (2014) have found that 5-ALA enables safe resection of twice the volume indicated by cMRI, resulting in the conclusion that "…5-ALA also stains MRI non-enhancing tumor tissue. Use of 5-ALA may thus enable extension of coalescent tumor resection beyond radiologically evident tumor." The publication of Roder et al. was consequently commented upon by this group (Schucht et al., 2015) as well as by a group in Spain (Diez-Valle and Tejada, 2014), questioning the validity of their data.

In a study on 200 patients testing the usefulness of iMRI (55 pts) and ALA (113 pts) Schatlo et al., (2015) found that the low field iMRI used could not show a significant independent advantage in GTR (odds ratio 1.36) in a multivariate analysis, whereas the use of ALA was associated with a significant odds ratio of 3.19 for achieving GTR. GTR, on the other hand, was highly predictive of prolonged overall survival. Whether the use of low-field MRI (0.15 T) in this study contributed to the only limited benefit remains to be evaluated. A smaller study with the same equipment demonstrated iMRI positivity in 11 of 12 cases after complete resection using AIF guidance, but found more than 35% nontumor tissue in biopsies from such tissue (Hauser et al., 2016).

From a practical point of view, iMRI certainly does not fit as well into the surgical workflow as does AIF and requires considerably more investment into purchasing the equipment (Hadjipanayis et al., 2015).

18.3.7 COMPARISON WITH FLUORESCEIN FLUORESCENCE IMAGING

As mentioned before, the fluorochrome PpIX is synthesized intracellularly from the nonfluorescent precursor, which has been administered to the patient. Hence, the fluorochrome is produced inside the tumor and fluorescence only occurs outside the tumor if other cells unspecifically also produce detectable levels of PpIX, or smaller amounts of PpIX might diffuse out of the tumor with edema into the surrounding tissue. Fluorescein, on the other hand, is a fluorochrome, which is intravenously injected as such and will therefore cause unspecific staining during distribution in the circulation and inside tissues, wherever it leaks. As fluorescein is highly water soluble, it diffuses easily into and with edema. These reasons for potential unspecific fluorochrome localization are also the major concerns of neurosurgeons using AIF. Indeed, there is a heavy dispute concerning the question whether fluorescein fluorescence imaging can compete against AIF or not. A recent experimental and clinical report concludes that fluorescein is not tumor specific on a cellular basis, but localizes in extracellular "tumor cell-rich locations" (Diaz et al., 2015). In 12 patients investigated by these investigators, a biopsy-based sensitivity of 91% and specificity of 82% for fluorescein-guided surgery was found. The only report of using simultaneous staining with ALA and fluorescein was by Schwake et al. (2015), who showed much better selectivity for ALA guidance. However, the equipment used for fluorescein imaging and the timing of fluorescein administration were questioned by Acerbi et al. (2015), who defended fluorescein guidance. A critical comment on this report (Stummer, 2015) provoked a reply (Brawanski et al., 2015). The neurosurgical community will therefore have to wait for further clarification by properly designed comparative trials.

If not for high-grade glioma, fluorescein guidance might still be beneficial for metastasis as reported in (Schebesch et al., 2015) or for low-grade tumors, where standard AIF often fails.

18.3.8 OTHER BRAIN TUMORS

Apart from high-grade gliomas, AIF has been tested in various brain metastases, spinal cord tumors, and meningiomas. The number of patients investigated is still limited, however, and definite conclusions remain uncertain.

18.3.8.1 OTHER PRIMARY BRAIN TUMORS

Reports on AIF in nonglial brain tumors are rare and comprise a chordoma that was PPIX fluorescent (Potapov et al., 2008) (two further chordomas, one fluorescent, and one nonfluorescent are listed in Marbacher et al., [2014]), nine cases of hemangioblastoma (Utsuki et al., 2011), where in 3 cases AIF revealed tumor cells in the peritumoral cyst wall, lymphomas (Yamaguchi et al., 2007, 2015; Eljamel, 2009; Moriuchi et al., 2011; Grossman et al., 2014), and pituitary adenomas (Eljamel, 2009; Eljamel et al., 2009; Marbacher et al., 2014). A few cases of schwannoma, medulloblastoma, neurocytoma, hemangioma, and gangliocytoma showed no fluorescence in a report by Marbacher et al. (2014).

18.3.8.2 METASTASES

In their single-center retrospective experience on AIF, Marbacher et al. (2014) included 65 patients with brain metastases, of which 52% showed visible PpIX fluorescence. There is no definite conclusion which kind of tumor metastases are likely to be PpIX positive and which are not: among each histological type and each origin, there are cases that are PPIX positive as well as some with negative fluorescence, provided that more than four cases were investigated. Qualitatively, this finding is confirmed by all other reports on AIF with brain metastases.

In a study to compare iMRI with AIF, some brain metastases (8 adenocarcinomas, of which 3 were nonfluorescent and 3 squamous cell carcinomas) were included, and from 13 samples taken at the tumor borders one sample was found false-negative and one false-positive (Coburger et al., 2014). In Utsuki et al. (2007a), 9 of 11 metastases were reported to be fluorescent. A retrospective study included 52 patients with brain metastases of different origin (mainly nonsmall cell lung cancer and breast cancer) and different histology (mainly adenocarcinoma) (Kamp et al., 2012). Sixty-two percent of these tumors showed visible intraoperative fluorescence, although inhomogeneous. In 42 cases, the tumor bed was examined in both white light and fluorescence. In 57% of these, PpIX fluorescence was positive, but in only 33% of biopsies from such tissue, infiltrative metastasis could be histologically confirmed. The authors described two cases of weak fluorescence in the metastatic tumor tissue but strong fluorescence in adjacent nonmalignant brain tissue, similar to the case of a malignant melanoma metastasis reported by Schucht et al. (2011). Although a considerable number of false positives can be found during AIF-guided surgery on metastases, it is still considered valuable by the present authors, as some cases of metastatic infiltration would otherwise have been missed.

Additional cases of brain metastases resected with the guidance of AIF were reported in Morofuji et al. (2007), Valdes et al. (2011b), Eljamel et al. (2013), Potapov et al. (2008), Aziz et al. (2009) and Zilidis et al. (2008), who additionally performed PDT of the tumor bed.

Overall, fluorescence of brain metastases presents heterogeneous results: only approximately half of them (independent of their histology or origin) show intraoperative fluorescence, and this has mostly been reported to be patchy within the tumor. Moreover, false-positive staining outside the tumor is comparably frequently detected, sometimes even with the tumor itself being nonfluorescent or only weakly fluorescent. Keeping this in mind, AIF can still be regarded beneficial, as it provides a chance of detecting infiltrative parts of the metastasis.

18.3.8.3 SPINAL CORD TUMORS

A large series of 55 different spinal cord tumors resected under AIF guidance was reported in (Millesi et al., 2014). The investigators found all of 12 ependymomas, 12 meningiomas, 3 hemangiopericytomas, and 2 drop metastases fluorescent, whereas none of the 8 neurinomas, 5 metastases, and 3 primary spinal gliomas exhibited PpIX fluorescence. In at least 4 cases, AIF led to the additional resection of malignant tissue. In Ewelt et al. (2010) AIF was considered very useful in carefully resecting malignant glioma during a cordectomy. Shevelev et al. (2011) presented a poster describing 12 out of 16 ependymomas that showed visible fluorescence, while the remaining 4 could still be detected using sensitive spectral PpIX detection. In their investigation, two of three myxopapillary ependymomas showed visible fluorescence, one of four pilocytic astrocytomas showed moderate fluorescence, and two hemangioblastomas showed no fluorescence. Two cases of GBM exhibited strong fluorescence.

18.3.8.4 MENINGIOMA

Although meningiomas are mostly benign, their surgical removal can be challenging, and in cases of cranial bone invasion or in the proximity of vessels and nerves, recurrences are often observed, probably due to incomplete surgical resection. As meningiomas are the second most common primary brain tumors after gliomas, such difficult cases are not rare and intraoperative guidance with AIF has been studied by many groups, of which we only reference reports including several patients as opposed to single case reports. Many authors (Kajimoto et al., 2007; Coluccia et al., 2010; Valdes et al., 2011a,b; Cornelius et al., 2014; Della Puppa et al., 2014; Motekallemi et al. 2015) have critically reviewed the literature and conclude that overall AIF is not as reliable for meningioma as it is for GBM. PpIX fluorescence in meningiomas is usually very heterogeneous and false-negatives and false-positives appear to occur more frequently than with GBM. Nevertheless, most studies reviewed report that "fluorescence did lead to an extension of the resection and to the removal of additional tumor." Studies that compared AIF imaging with quantitative and sensitive AIF spectroscopy (Bekelis et al., 2011; Valdes et al., 2011b, 2014) showed a higher sensitivity and accuracy for AIF spectroscopy. AIF imaging, which has been developed for GBM, might have to be adapted for meningioma imaging to highlight lower concentrations of PpIX. With the current equipment, it is concluded that "5-ALA in intracranial meningioma surgery should only be used in a prospective protocol and a long-term study" (Motekallemi et al., 2015).

It may be surprising that meningiomas, although being mostly benign, frequently show strong PpIX fluorescence. There is little obvious reasoning, why this should be the case. An early study on the susceptibility of some meningioma cell lines to ALA-based PDT showed only a moderate response and hence a probably low accumulation of PpIX in these cells (Tsai et al., 1999). A more recent report on in vitro results with meningioma cell lines showed a differential response of the two cell lines compared and demonstrated that the more PDT-susceptible cell line accumulated higher concentrations of PpIX and had a lower activity of ferrochelatase (Hefti et al., 2011). Meningioma cells grown as primary cell cultures from freshly resected human meningioma were all susceptible to PDT and must therefore have accumulated sufficient concentrations of PpIX (El-Khatib et al., 2015).

18.3.9 PHOTODYNAMIC THERAPY

An article about ALA-based management of GBM is incomplete, if it fails to mention the photosensitizing properties of the accumulated PpIX. PpIX not only acts as a fluorochrome but can also transfer part of the absorbed light energy to ground state molecular oxygen to produce singlet oxygen, which in turn can destroy the function of proteins or the integrity of lipid membranes. Cells containing a sufficient concentration of PpIX that are exposed to a sufficient dose of light will undergo apoptotic or necrotic cell death pathways. More details on photodynamic therapy (PDT) can be read in review articles (Bechet et al., 2014; Mroz et al., 2011a). For the PDT treatment of brain tumors, usually laser light is employed to excite the PPIX. The laser light intensities applied are low enough to avoid heating of the tissue to more than 2 degrees above body temperature. Therefore, this type of laser application is nonthermal and would not lead to tissue damage in the absence of a photosensitizer.

Especially for the treatment of brain tumors, PDT relies on the intracellular tumor-selective presence of the photosensitizer (PPIX) and therefore is restricted to the tumor volume, even if normal brain received a full dose of light. It potentially enables "microsurgical" destruction of invading tumor cells within eloquent brain, if the photosensitizer staining is sufficiently selective. Some minor concentration of PpIX in normal cells would not be detrimental, as photobleaching will destroy the photosensitizer, before a lethal dose of reactive oxygen species (ROS) (mostly singlet oxygen in the case of PpIX-sensitization) is produced (Johansson et al., 2009).

18.3.9.1 CONCEPTS

Generally, in order to achieve a maximal penetration of tissue necrosis, red light (as opposed to violet light used to excite fluorescence) is used for PDT. For PpIX excitation, the longest wavelength that can be used is 633 nm, where the light penetration depth into brain tumor tissue is in the order of 3 mm (Beck et al., 2003, 2007). The depth of necrosis can be extended a bit further by increasing the light dose, so that an effective treatment depth of approximately 5 mm is feasible (Beck et al., 2007; Johansson et al., 2009; Bechet et al., 2014).

There is no published clinical experience with ALA-based PDT to the resection cavity except an initial report on safety issues and photobleaching (Stepp et al., 2005, 2007), although this is the most straightforward strategy. If one intends to perform the most radical but safe cytoreduction, AIF-guided surgical resection would first be performed as much as safely possible. A focal irradiation of residual strongly fluorescent tumor tissue or an integral irradiation of the entire resection cavity might then enable the destruction of part of the residual tumor tissue or invaded tumor cell nests. Superficial light doses of up to 200 J/cm^2 were found to be safe and reliably photobleached PpIX to below 5% of the initial fluorescence at the same dose of ALA as used for AIF-guided resection (20 mg/kg body weight).

In cases of recurrent or inoperable tumors, the stereotactic interstitial placement of cylindrical light diffuser fibers offers another intriguing possibility to treat tumors with ALA-based PDT. As the tumor mass is not removed in this case, the well-known immune stimulatory effects of PDT can be fully exploited as briefly discussed next.

18.3.9.2 CLINICAL EXPERIENCE

Most clinical experience with PDT for GBM has been obtained with classical photosensitizers, above all with Photofrin (Krishnamurthy et al., 2000; Stylli and Kaye, 2006; Eljamel et al., 2008). The overall conclusion with these sensitizers is that PDT may offer a significant survival advantage with occasional long-term survivors (Stylli et al., 2005), but that precise light dosimetry is needed to protect normal brain from photodynamic damage (Krishnamurthy et al., 2000). We believe that this considerable limitation can be overcome with the use of ALA-PPIX, because the selectivity of photosensitizer accumulation is higher than other photosensitizers and photobleaching limits the damage of the normal brain to sublethal levels, regardless of the light dose applied. Instead of carefully avoiding the exposure of normal brain to high doses of light, we try to make sure that PpIX is photobleached completely throughout the contrast-enhancing volume. The clinical results obtained so far are promising (Beck et al., 2007; Stummer et al., 2008a; Johansson et al., 2013). It even appears that by measuring transmission of laser light and fluorescence between fibers, one can predict the clinical response (Johansson et al., 2013). Currently, the results of interstitial PDT on newly diagnosed inoperable GBM performed on 15 patients are being summarized to be presented in the 2015 meeting of the Society for Neuro-Oncology (Schwartz et al., 2015). In brief, compared to a group of GBM patients with optimal surgery ("complete tumor resection"), iPDT proved significantly better with a median PFS of 16 vs. 10.2 months, $p < 0.001$, and a 3 year survival of 56% vs. 21%, $p < 0.01$. Six out of fifteen patients of the iPDT group experienced long-term progression free survival >30 months (range: 32–68 months). Transient morbidity was seen in 7 out of 15 iPDT patients (transient aphasia, pulmonary embolism).

18.3.9.3 OUTLOOK

The sensitivity of PpIX staining on a biopsy basis is well below 100%. It must therefore be concluded that some tumor cells, especially in the infiltration zone, will not be sensitized and tumor cell destruction will not be complete by PDT. Surviving tumor cells will then almost inevitably cause recurrence. The observed long-term survivors (Stummer et al., 2008a; Johansson et al., 2013) are difficult to be explained by the action of phototoxic cell damage alone. The phenomenon of immune stimulation has been described for PDT in general (Mroz et al., 2011b), and some preclinical results for ALA-based immune stimulation on glioma cells have also been acquired. Indeed, sublethal 5-ALA-based PDT can induce the expression of a series of proteins that are relevant to stimulation of the immune response, including heatshock-protein 70 (HSP-70) among others, which is known to contribute to dendritic cell maturation (Etminan et al., 2011; Kammerer et al., 2011). Given the potent immune stimulatory effect of PDT, it might be an intriguing concept to combine PDT with immune checkpoint inhibitors (Preusser et al., 2015) to further boost the antitumor immune response.

Another matter of debate and concern is the effectiveness of any kind of therapeutic intervention to identify and eliminate stem-like cancer cells, the so-called cancer stem cells or tumor-initiating cells (TICs). There is not yet a clear and reliable picture of how TICs and ALA-induced PpIX accumulation and phototoxicity are related. Piccirillo et al. (2012) found TICs both in fluorescent as well as in nonfluorescent tumor tissue, with TICs isolated from fluorescent tissue showing self-renewing behavior in vivo and in vitro, whereas TICs from nonfluorescent tissue were self-renewable only in vivo. Rampazzo et al. (2014) found that most CD133(+) cells (a marker associated with stem-like quality) in the tumor mass are PpIX positive, but this also means that a considerable proportion of TICs would not be efficiently stained. TICs are known to express particular membrane transport proteins, such as ABCG2 (multidrug efflux pumps), that pump out chemotherapeutic drugs and also PpIX, from the cytoplasm, potentially rendering the cancer stem cells resistant to therapy. If TICs should therefore be resistant to ALA-based PDT, established blockers or inhibitors of ABCG2, such as sorafenib (Mazard et al., 2013) or gefitinib, might reestablish the susceptibility of such cells to PDT cell damage (Ishikawa et al., 2015).

Even without blocking ABCG2 and without boosting antitumor immune response, ALA-based PDT has already showed intriguing impressive effectiveness in our single-center experience. Based on the availability of dedicated equipment (multiport laser, cylindrical diffuser fibers, treatment planning software for interstitial PDT), multicenter clinical studies aimed to gain regulatory approval are warranted.

18.4 CONCLUSIONS

Surgical resection for treatment of glioma patients must be considered with great care. In almost every part of the brain, a tumor biopsy can be performed with low risk and provides not only information on the histopathological diagnosis, but also the molecular and genetic profile of the lesion. Tumor resection, however, is usually associated with a higher risk of neurological deterioration, which in turn can have a negative impact on both quality of life and on other treatment options. Therefore, both prognostic utility and absolute life expectancy, but also the preservation of the quality of life and the risk of postoperative neurological dysfunction, need to be critically assessed. In order to achieve maximal safe tumor resection without harming normal brain, there are various instruments available, which should be used freely, either alone or in combination with each other. These include not only the ALA fluorescence-guided resection for malignant gliomas but also neuronavigation, including integration of metabolic imaging, such as FET–PET. In addition, intraoperative imaging methods such as iMRI and iUS may help to update the navigation data sets, while the intraoperative mapping and monitoring with direct or indirect cortical and subcortical stimulation especially in eloquent areas are used to ensure the safety and quality of tumor resection of gliomas.

As far as the added value of ALA-PPIX imaging in glioblastoma management is concerned, we conclude the following:

- The current technological implementation in surgical microscopes is simple to use and fits perfectly in the workflow of GBM surgery. It is an approved procedure in many countries.
- The positive predictive value of "strong fluorescence" is very high. "Vaguely fluorescent" tissue biopsies sometimes may be void of tumor cells histologically and resection should therefore only be continued, if functional brain is not at risk.
- Side effects due to the systemic application of the moderate dose ALA are restricted to a transient elevation of liver enzymes with a few patients and skin sensitivity to bright light for a maximum of 48 h.
- AIF may correctly indicate significantly larger tumor volumes than contrast MRI.
- The rates of "complete resection" in comparison to previous standard are elevated in all corresponding clinical trials.
- Data on the benefit for the patient in terms of progression-free and overall survival are still rare and require larger dedicated trials.
- It is unlikely that surgery alone (AIF guided or not) will ever be able to cure even a small fraction of GBM patients, but the larger tumor cell reduction achievable with AIF guidance may support the effectiveness of adjuvant therapies.
- The mechanisms by which PpIX accumulation occurs in a tumor-selective manner are not yet fully understood. It can only partly be explained why GBMs produce PpIX in very different concentrations and very inhomogeneously, but possibilities to increase both the degree and the selectivity of PpIX accumulation can be suggested.
- Technological limitations are the short penetration depth of the fluorescence imaging, the sensitivity to ambient light, the immediate obstruction of fluorescence by blood, the subjective interpretation of fluorescence quality, and the rather low and fixed sensitivity to detect PpIX. These limitations may all be overcome by technical measures, such as pulsed fluorescence excitation and detection, excitation in the red wavelengths, modern image processing algorithms, addition of spectroscopic detection, and similar approaches. However, caution is indicated, because a large increase in the sensitivity of PpIX detection may result in a decrease in its specificity.
- Fluorescence guidance may also be very helpful for stereotactic biopsy sampling.

AIF guidance has also been tried for brain tumors other than high-grade gliomas, mainly metastases and meningiomas. Although many of these reports are very promising, the adaptation of the procedure must be done carefully. There is no approval for these indications and the equipment may need considerable modification in order to fulfill the clinical requirements of a reliable detection of residual pathological tissue.

Photodynamic therapy is an intriguing possibility to either further improve cytoreduction after AIF-guided surgery or to use as a replacement for surgery in cases of recurrent or inoperable tumor. There are indications that an effective stimulation of an antitumor immune response is initiated by PDT and that the worrisome tumor-initiating cells are either sufficiently susceptible to PDT directly or can be made susceptible by short-term blocking of some membrane transporters.

REFERENCES

Acerbi F, Broggi M, Broggi G, Ferroli P (2015) What is the best timing for fluorescein injection during surgical removal of high-grade gliomas? *Acta Neurochir* (*Wien*).

Acerbi F et al. (2014) Is fluorescein-guided technique able to help in resection of high-grade gliomas? *Neurosurg Focus* **36**:E5.

Anand S, Hasan T, Maytin EV (2013) Mechanism of differentiation-enhanced photodynamic therapy for cancer: Upregulation of coproporphyrinogen oxidase by C/EBP transcription factors. *Mol Cancer Ther* **12**:1638–1650.

Ando T, Kobayashi E, Liao H, Maruyama T, Muragaki Y, Iseki H, Kubo O, Sakuma I (2011) Precise comparison of protoporphyrin IX fluorescence spectra with pathological results for brain tumor tissue identification. *Brain Tumor Pathol* **28**:43–51.

Aziz F, Telara S, Moseley H, Goodman C, Manthri P, Eljamel MS (2009) Photodynamic therapy adjuvant to surgery in metastatic carcinoma in brain. *Photodiagn Photodyn Ther* **6**:227–230.

Babu R, Adamson DC (2012) Fluorescence-guided malignant glioma resections. *Curr Drug Discov Technol* **9**:256–267.

Barone DG, Lawrie TA, Hart MG (2014) Image guided surgery for the resection of brain tumors. *Cochrane Database Syst Rev* **1**:CD009685.

Bechet D, Mordon SR, Guillemin F, Barberi-Heyob MA (2014) Photodynamic therapy of malignant brain tumors: A complementary approach to conventional therapies. *Cancer Treat Rev* **40**:229–241.

Beck TJ, Beyer W, Pongratz T, Stummer W, Waidelich R, Stepp H, Wagner S, Baumgartner R (2003) Clinical determination of tissue optical properties in vivo by spatially resolved reflectance measurements. *Photon Migr Diffuse Light Imaging* **5138**:96–105.

Beck TJ, Kreth FW, Beyer W, Mehrkens JH, Obermeier A, Stepp H, Stummer W, Baumgartner R (2007) Interstitial photodynamic therapy of nonresectable malignant glioma recurrences using 5-aminolevulinic acid induced protoporphyrin IX. *Lasers Surg Med* **39**:386–393.

Bekelis K, Valdes PA, Erkmen K, Leblond F, Kim A, Wilson BC, Harris BT, Paulsen KD, Roberts DW (2011) Quantitative and qualitative 5-aminolevulinic acid-induced protoporphyrin IX fluorescence in skull base meningiomas. *Neurosurg Focus* **30**:E8.

Berg K, Anholt H, Bech O, Moan J (1996) The influence of iron chelators on the accumulation of protoporphyrin IX in 5-aminolaevulinic acid-treated cells. *Br J Cancer* **74**:688–697.

Bizheva K et al. (2005) Imaging ex vivo healthy and pathological human brain tissue with ultra-high-resolution optical coherence tomography. *J Biomed Opt* **10**:11006.

Blake E, Curnow A (2010) The hydroxypyridinone iron chelator CP94 can enhance PpIX-induced PDT of cultured human glioma cells. *Photochem Photobiol* **86**:1154–1160.

Bogaards A, Varma A, Collens SP, Lin A, Giles A, Yang VX, Bilbao JM, Lilge LD, Muller PJ, Wilson BC (2004) Increased brain tumor resection using fluorescence image guidance in a preclinical model. *Lasers Surg Med* **35**:181–190.

Brawanski A, Acerbi F, Nakaji P, Cohen-Gadol A, Schebesch KM (2015) Poor man-rich man fluorescence. Is this really the problem? *Acta Neurochir* (*Wien*).

Brown PD, Maurer MJ, Rummans TA, Pollock BE, Ballman KV, Sloan JA, Boeve BF, Arusell RM, Clark MM, Buckner JC (2005) A prospective study of quality of life in adults with newly diagnosed high-grade gliomas: The impact of the extent of resection on quality of life and survival. *Neurosurgery* **57**:495–504; discussion 495–504.

Burton NC et al. (2013) Multispectral opto-acoustic tomography (MSOT) of the brain and glioblastoma characterization. *Neuroimage* **65**:522–528.

Butte PV, Mamelak A, Parrish-Novak J, Drazin D, Shweikeh F, Gangalum PR, Chesnokova A, Ljubimova JY, Black K (2014) Near-infrared imaging of brain tumors using the Tumor Paint BLZ-100 to achieve near-complete resection of brain tumors. *Neurosurg Focus* **36**:E1.

Butte PV, Mamelak AN, Nuno M, Bannykh SI, Black KL, Marcu L (2011) Fluorescence lifetime spectroscopy for guided therapy of brain tumors. *Neuroimage* **54**(Suppl. 1):S125–S135.

Chang SC, MacRobert AJ, Porter JB, Bown SG (1997) The efficacy of an iron chelator (CP94) in increasing cellular protoporphyrin IX following intravesical 5-aminolaevulinic acid administration: An in vivo study. *J Photochem Photobiol B* **38**:114–122.

Chen X et al. (2014) Calcitriol enhances 5-aminolevulinic acid-induced fluorescence and the effect of photodynamic therapy in human glioma. *Acta Oncol* **53**:405–413.

Chinot OL et al. (2014) Bevacizumab plus radiotherapy-temozolomide for newly diagnosed glioblastoma. *N Engl J Med* **370**:709–722.

Chung CW, Kim CH, Lee HM, Kim do H, Kwak TW, Chung KD, Jeong YI, Kang DH (2013) Aminolevulinic acid derivatives-based photodynamic therapy in human intra- and extrahepatic cholangiocarcinoma cells. *Eur J Pharm Biopharm* **85**:503–510.

Cicarma E, Tuorkey M, Juzeniene A, Ma LW, Moan J (2009) Calcitriol treatment improves methyl aminolaevulinate-based photodynamic therapy in human squamous cell carcinoma A431 cells. *Br J Dermatol* **161**:413–418.

Coburger J, Engelke J, Scheuerle A, Thal DR, Hlavac M, Wirtz CR, Konig R (2014) Tumor detection with 5-aminolevulinic acid fluorescence and Gd-DTPA-enhanced intraoperative MRI at the border of contrast-enhancing lesions: A prospective study based on histopathological assessment. *Neurosurg Focus* **36**:E3.

Coburger J, Scheuerle A, Kapapa T, Engelke J, Thal DR, Wirtz CR, Konig R (2015a) Sensitivity and specificity of linear array intraoperative ultrasound in glioblastoma surgery: A comparative study with high field intraoperative MRI and conventional sector array ultrasound. *Neurosurg Rev* **38**:499–509.

Coburger J, Scheuerle A, Thal DR, Engelke J, Hlavac M, Wirtz CR, Konig R (2015b) Linear array ultrasound in low-grade glioma surgery: Histology-based assessment of accuracy in comparison to conventional intraoperative ultrasound and intraoperative MRI. *Acta Neurochir (Wien)* **157**:195–206.

Colditz MJ, Leyen K, Jeffree RL (2012) Aminolevulinic acid (ALA)-protoporphyrin IX fluorescence guided tumor resection. Part 2: Theoretical, biochemical and practical aspects. *J Clin Neurosci* **19**:1611–1616.

Collaud S, Juzeniene A, Moan J, Lange N (2004) On the selectivity of 5-aminolevulinic acid-induced protoporphyrin IX formation. *Curr Med Chem Anti-Cancer Agents* **4**:301–316.

Coluccia D, Fandino J, Fujioka M, Cordovi S, Muroi C, Landolt H (2010) Intraoperative 5-aminolevulinic-acid-induced fluorescence in meningiomas. *Acta Neurochir (Wien)* **152**:1711–1719.

Cornelius JF, Slotty PJ, Kamp MA, Schneiderhan TM, Steiger HJ, El-Khatib M (2014) Impact of 5-aminolevulinic acid fluorescence-guided surgery on the extent of resection of meningiomas—With special regard to high-grade tumors. *Photodiagnosis Photodyn Ther* **11**:481–490.

Cornelius JF, Slotty PJ, Stoffels G, Galldiks N, Langen KJ, Steiger HJ (2013) 5-aminolevulinic acid and (18) F-FET-PET as metabolic imaging tools for surgery of a recurrent skull base meningioma. *J Neurol Surg B Skull Base* **74**:211–216.

Croce AC, Fiorani S, Locatelli D, Nano R, Ceroni M, Tancioni F, Giombelli E, Benericetti E, Bottiroli G (2003) Diagnostic potential of autofluorescence for an assisted intraoperative delineation of glioblastoma resection margins. *Photochem Photobiol* **77**:309–318.

da Rocha Filho HN, da Silva EC, Silva FR, Courrol LC, de Mesquita CH, Bellini MH (2015) Expression of genes involved in porphyrin biosynthesis pathway in the human renal cell carcinoma. *J Fluoresc*.

De Witt Hamer PC, Robles SG, Zwinderman AH, Duffau H, Berger MS (2012) Impact of intraoperative stimulation brain mapping on glioma surgery outcome: A meta-analysis. *J Clin Oncol* **30**:2559–2565.

Della Puppa A et al. (2014) Predictive value of intraoperative 5-aminolevulinic acid-induced fluorescence for detecting bone invasion in meningioma surgery. *J Neurosurg* **120**:840–845.

Diaz RJ, Dios RR, Hattab EM, Burrell K, Rakopoulos P, Sabha N, Hawkins C, Zadeh G, Rutka JT, Cohen-Gadol AA (2015) Study of the biodistribution of fluorescein in glioma-infiltrated mouse brain and histopathological correlation of intraoperative findings in high-grade gliomas resected under fluorescein fluorescence guidance. *J Neurosurg* **122**:1360–1369.

Diez Valle R, Slof J, Galvan J, Arza C, Romariz C, Vidal C, VISIONA study researchers (2014) Observational, retrospective study of the effectiveness of 5-aminolevulinic acid in malignant glioma surgery in Spain (The VISIONA study). *Neurologia* **29**:131–138.

Diez Valle R, Tejada Solis S, Idoate Gastearena MA, Garcia de Eulate R, Dominguez Echavarri P, Aristu Mendiroz J (2011) Surgery guided by 5-aminolevulinic fluorescence in glioblastoma: Volumetric analysis of extent of resection in single-center experience. *J Neurooncol* **102**:105–113.

Diez-Valle R, Tejada S (2014) Results expected in 5-ALA-guided resection of glioblastoma. *Eur J Surg Oncol* **40**:1021–1022.

Doring F, Walter J, Will J, Focking M, Boll M, Amasheh S, Clauss W, Daniel H (1998) Delta-aminolevulinic acid transport by intestinal and renal peptide transporters and its physiological and clinical implications. *J Clin Invest* **101**:2761–2767.

Duffau H, Peggy Gatignol ST, Mandonnet E, Capelle L, Taillandier L (2008) Intraoperative subcortical stimulation mapping of language pathways in a consecutive series of 115 patients with Grade II glioma in the left dominant hemisphere. *J Neurosurg* **109**:461–471.

Eigenbrod S et al. (2014) Molecular stereotactic biopsy technique improves diagnostic accuracy and enables personalized treatment strategies in glioma patients. *Acta Neurochir (Wien)* **156**:1427–1440.

Eleouet S, Rousset N, Carre J, Vonarx V, Vilatte C, Louet C, Lajat Y, Patrice T (2000) Heterogeneity of delta-aminolevulinic acid-induced protoporphyrin IX fluorescence in human glioma cells and leukemic lymphocytes. *Neurol Res* **22**:361–368.

Eljamel MS (2009) Which intracranial lesions would be suitable for 5-aminolevulenic acid-induced fluorescence-guided identification, localization, or resection? A prospective study of 114 consecutive intracranial lesions. *Clin Neurosurg* **56**:93–97.

Eljamel MS, Goodman C, Moseley H (2008) ALA and Photofrin fluorescence-guided resection and repetitive PDT in glioblastoma multiforme: A single centre Phase III randomized controlled trial. *Lasers Med Sci* **23**:361–367.

Eljamel MS, Leese G, Moseley H (2009) Intraoperative optical identification of pituitary adenomas. *J Neurooncol* **92**:417–421.

Eljamel S, Petersen M, Valentine R, Buist R, Goodman C, Moseley H (2013) Comparison of intraoperative fluorescence and MRI image guided neuronavigation in malignant brain tumors, a prospective controlled study. *Photodiagnosis Photodyn Ther* **10**:356–361.

El-Khatib M, Tepe C, Senger B, Dibue-Adjei M, Riemenschneider MJ, Stummer W, Steiger HJ, Cornelius JF (2015) Aminolevulinic acid-mediated photodynamic therapy of human meningioma: An in vitro study on primary cell lines. *Int J Mol Sci* **16**:9936–9948.

Engh JA (2010) Improving intraoperative visualization of anaplastic foci within gliomas. *Neurosurgery* **67**:N21–N22.

Ennis SR, Novotny A, Xiang J, Shakui P, Masada T, Stummer W, Smith DE, Keep RF (2003) Transport of 5-aminolevulinic acid between blood and brain. *Brain Res* **959**:226–234.

Esteves S, Alves M, Castel-Branco M, Stummer W (2015) A pilot cost-effectiveness analysis of treatments in newly diagnosed high-grade gliomas: The example of 5-aminolevulinic Acid compared with white-light surgery. *Neurosurgery* **76**:552–562; discussion 562.

Etminan N, Peters C, Lakbir D, Bunemann E, Borger V, Sabel MC, Hanggi D, Steiger HJ, Stummer W, Sorg RV (2011) Heat-shock protein 70-dependent dendritic cell activation by 5-aminolevulinic acid-mediated photodynamic treatment of human glioblastoma spheroids in vitro. *Br J Cancer* **105**:961–969.

European Medicines Agency (2007a) Gliolan scientific discussion. http://www.ema.europa.eu/docs/en_GB/document_library/EPAR_-_Scientific_Discussion/human/000744/WC500021788.pdf.

European Medicines Agency (2007b) Gliolan approval records. http://www.ema.europa.eu/ema/index.jsp?curl=pages/medicines/human/medicines/000744/human_med_000807.jsp&mid=WC000740b000701ac058001d000124.

Ewelt C, Floeth FW, Felsberg J, Steiger HJ, Sabel M, Langen KJ, Stoffels G, Stummer W (2011) Finding the anaplastic focus in diffuse gliomas: The value of Gd-DTPA enhanced MRI, FET-PET, and intraoperative, ALA-derived tissue fluorescence. *Clin Neurol Neurosurg* **113**:541–547.

Ewelt C, Nemes A, Senner V, Wolfer J, Brokinkel B, Stummer W, Holling M (2015) Fluorescence in neurosurgery: Its diagnostic and therapeutic use. *Rev Lit J Photochem Photobiol B* **148**:302–309.

Ewelt C, Stummer W, Klink B, Felsberg J, Steiger HJ, Sabel M (2010) Cordectomy as final treatment option for diffuse intramedullary malignant glioma using 5-ALA fluorescence-guided resection. *Clin Neurol Neurosurg* **112**:357–361.

Finke M, Kantelhardt S, Schlaefer A, Bruder R, Lankenau E, Giese A, Schweikard A (2012) Automatic scanning of large tissue areas in neurosurgery using optical coherence tomography. *Int J Med Robot* **8**:327–336.

Flynn BP, AV DS, Kanick SC, Davis SC, Pogue BW (2013) White light-informed optical properties improve ultrasound-guided fluorescence tomography of photoactive protoporphyrin IX. *J Biomed Opt* **18**:046008.

Foersch S, Heimann A, Ayyad A, Spoden GA, Florin L, Mpoukouvalas K, Kiesslich R, Kempski O, Goetz M, Charalampaki P (2012) Confocal laser endomicroscopy for diagnosis and histomorphologic imaging of brain tumors in vivo. *PLoS One* **7**:e41760.

Fukuda H, Paredes S, Batlle AM (1992) Tumor-localizing properties of porphyrins. In vivo studies using free and liposome encapsulated aminolevulinic acid. *Comp Biochem Physiol B* **102**:433–436.

Fukuhara H, Inoue K, Kurabayashi A, Furihata M, Fujita H, Utsumi K, Sasaki J, Shuin T (2013) The inhibition of ferrochelatase enhances 5-aminolevulinic acid-based photodynamic action for prostate cancer. *Photodiagnosis Photodyn Ther* **10**:399–409.

Galldiks N, Ullrich R, Schroeter M, Fink GR, Jacobs AH, Kracht LW (2010) Volumetry of [(11)C]-methionine PET uptake and MRI contrast enhancement in patients with recurrent glioblastoma multiforme. *Eur J Nucl Med Mol Imaging* **37**:84–92.

Gebhart SC, Thompson RC, Mahadevan-Jansen A (2007) Liquid-crystal tunable filter spectral imaging for brain tumor demarcation. *Appl Opt* **46**:1896–1910.

Gerganov VM, Samii A, Akbarian A, Stieglitz L, Samii M, Fahlbusch R (2009) Reliability of intraoperative high-resolution 2D ultrasound as an alternative to high-field strength MR imaging for tumor resection control: A prospective comparative study. *J Neurosurg* **111**:512–519.

Gerganov VM, Samii A, Giordano M, Samii M, Fahlbusch R (2011) Two-dimensional high-end ultrasound imaging compared to intraoperative MRI during resection of low-grade gliomas. *J Clin Neurosci* **18**:669–673.

Gilbert MR et al. (2013) Dose-dense temozolomide for newly diagnosed glioblastoma: A randomized phase III clinical trial. *J Clin Oncol* **31**:4085–4091.

Gilbert MR et al. (2014) A randomized trial of bevacizumab for newly diagnosed glioblastoma. *N Engl J Med* **370**:699–708.

Gobel W et al. (2012) Optical needle endoscope for safe and precise stereotactically guided biopsy sampling in neurosurgery. *Opt Express* **20**:26117–26126.

Greenbaum L, Gozlan Y, Schwartz D, Katcoff DJ, Malik Z (2002) Nuclear distribution of porphobilinogen deaminase (PBGD) in glioma cells: A regulatory role in cancer transformation? *Br J Cancer* **86**:1006–1011.

Greenbaum L, Katcoff DJ, Dou H, Gozlan Y, Malik Z (2003) A porphobilinogen deaminase (PBGD) Ran-binding protein interaction is implicated in nuclear trafficking of PBGD in differentiating glioma cells. 5221–5228.

Grossman R, Nossek E, Shimony N, Raz M, Ram Z (2014) Intraoperative 5-aminolevulinic acid-induced fluorescence in primary central nervous system lymphoma. *J Neurosurg* **120**:67–69.

Hadjipanayis CG, Widhalm G, Stummer W (2015) What is the surgical benefit of utilizing 5-aminolevulinic acid for fluorescence-guided surgery of malignant gliomas? *Neurosurgery.*

Hagiya Y et al. (2012) Pivotal roles of peptide transporter PEPT1 and ATP-binding cassette (ABC) transporter ABCG2 in 5-aminolevulinic acid (ALA)-based photocytotoxicity of gastric cancer cells in vitro. *Photodiagnosis Photodyn Ther* **9**:204–214.

Hagiya Y et al. (2013) Expression levels of PEPT1 and ABCG2 play key roles in 5-aminolevulinic acid (ALA)-induced tumor-specific protoporphyrin IX (PpIX) accumulation in bladder cancer. *Photodiagnosis Photodyn Ther* **10**:288–295.

Haglund MM, Berger MS, Hochman DW (1996) Enhanced optical imaging of human gliomas and tumor margins. *Neurosurgery* **38**:308–317.

Haj-Hosseini N, Richter J, Andersson-Engels S, Wardell K (2010) Optical touch pointer for fluorescence guided glioblastoma resection using 5-aminolevulinic acid. *Lasers Surg Med* **42**:9–14.

Hansen DA, Spence AM, Carski T, Berger MS (1993) Indocyanine green (ICG) staining and demarcation of tumor margins in a rat glioma model. *Surg Neurol* **40**:451–456.

Hauser SB, Kockro RA, Actor B, Sarnthein J, Bernays RL (2016) Combining 5-ALA fluorescence and intraoperative MRI in glioblastoma surgery: A histology-based evaluation. *Neurosurgery*.

Hayashi Y, Nakada M, Tanaka S, Uchiyama N, Kita D, Hamada J (2010) Implication of 5-aminolevulinic acid fluorescence of the ventricular wall for postoperative communicating hydrocephalus associated with cerebrospinal fluid dissemination in patients with glioblastoma multiforme: A report of 7 cases. *J Neurosurg* **112**:1015–1019.

Hebeda KM, Saarnak AE, Olivo M, Sterenborg HJ, Wolbers JG (1998) 5-Aminolevulinic acid induced endogenous porphyrin fluorescence in 9 L and C6 brain tumors and in the normal rat brain. *Acta Neurochir (Wien)* **140**:503–512.

Hefti M, Holenstein F, Albert I, Looser H, Luginbuehl V (2011) Susceptibility to 5-aminolevulinic acid based photodynamic therapy in WHO I meningioma cells corresponds to ferrochelatase activity. *Photochem Photobiol* **87**:235–241.

Hefti M, von Campe G, Moschopulos M, Siegner A, Looser H, Landolt H (2008) 5-aminolevulinic acid induced protoporphyrin IX fluorescence in high-grade glioma surgery: A one-year experience at a single institutuion. *Swiss Med Wkly* **138**:180–185.

Hegi ME et al. (2005) MGMT gene silencing and benefit from temozolomide in glioblastoma. *N Engl J Med* **352**:997–1003.

Hervey-Jumper SL, Li J, Lau D, Molinaro AM, Perry DW, Meng L, Berger MS (2015) Awake craniotomy to maximize glioma resection: Methods and technical nuances over a 27-year period. *J Neurosurg* **123**:325–339.

Hickmann AK, Nadji-Ohl M, Hopf NJ (2015) Feasibility of fluorescence-guided resection of recurrent gliomas using five-aminolevulinic acid: Retrospective analysis of surgical and neurological outcome in 58 patients. *J Neurooncol* **122**:151–160.

Hinnen P, de Rooij FW, van Velthuysen ML, Edixhoven A, van Hillegersberg R, Tilanus HW, Wilson JH, Siersema PD (1998) Biochemical basis of 5-aminolaevulinic acid-induced protoporphyrin IX accumulation: A study in patients with (pre)malignant lesions of the esophagus. *Br J Cancer* **78**:679–682.

Hoetker MS, Goetz M (2013) Molecular imaging in endoscopy. *United Eur Gastroent* **1**:84–92.

Hoy CL, Gamm UA, Sterenborg HJ, Robinson DJ, Amelink A (2013) Method for rapid multidiameter single-fiber reflectance and fluorescence spectroscopy through a fiber bundle. *J Biomed Opt* **18**:107005.

Idoate MA, Diez Valle R, Echeveste J, Tejada S (2011) Pathological characterization of the glioblastoma border as shown during surgery using 5-aminolevulinic acid-induced fluorescence. *Neuropathology* **31**:575–582.

Iinuma S, Farshi SS, Ortel B, Hasan T (1994) A mechanistic study of cellular photodestruction with 5-aminolaevulinic acid-induced porphyrin. *Br J Cancer* **70**:21–28.

Ishikawa T, Kajimoto Y, Inoue Y, Ikegami Y, Kuroiwa T (2015) Critical role of ABCG2 in ALA-photodynamic diagnosis and therapy of human brain tumor. *Adv Cancer Res* **125**:197–216.

Ishikawa T, Nakagawa H, Hagiya Y, Nonoguchi N, Miyatake S, Kuroiwa T (2010) Key role of human ABC transporter ABCG2 in photodynamic therapy and photodynamic diagnosis. *Adv Pharmacol Sci* **2010**:587306.

Jaber M, Wolfer J, Ewelt C, Holling M, Hasselblatt M, Niederstadt T, Zoubi T, Weckesser M, Stummer W (2016) The value of 5-ALA in low-grade gliomas and gigh-grade gliomas lacking glioblastoma imaging features: An analysis based on fluorescence, MRI, 18F-FET PET, and tumor molecular factors. *Neurosurgery*.

Jin Y, Bin ZQ, Qiang H, Liang C, Hua C, Jun D, Dong WA, Qing L (2009) ABCG2 is related with the grade of glioma and resistance to mitoxantone, a chemotherapeutic drug for glioma. *J Cancer Res Clin Oncol* **135**:1369–1376.

Jocham D, Stepp H, Waidelich R (2008) Photodynamic diagnosis in urology: State-of-the-art. *Eur Urol* **53**:1138–1148.

Johansson A, Faber F, Kniebuhler G, Stepp H, Sroka R, Egensperger R, Beyer W, Kreth FW (2013) Protoporphyrin IX fluorescence and photobleaching during interstitial photodynamic therapy of malignant gliomas for early treatment prognosis. *Lasers Surg Med* **45**(4):225–234.

Johansson A, Kreth FW, Stummer W, Stepp H (2009) Interstitial photodynamic therapy of brain tumors. *IEEE J Selected Top Quantum Electron.*

Johansson A, Palte G, Schnell O, Tonn JC, Herms J, Stepp H (2010) 5-Aminolevulinic acid-induced protoporphyrin IX levels in tissue of human malignant brain tumors. *Photochem Photobiol* **86**:1373–1378.

Kajimoto Y, Kuroiwa T, Miyatake S, Ichioka T, Miyashita M, Tanaka H, Tsuji M (2007) Use of 5-aminolevulinic acid in fluorescence-guided resection of meningioma with high risk of recurrence. *Case Report J Neurosurg* **106**:1070–1074.

Kammerer R, Buchner A, Palluch P, Pongratz T, Oboukhovskij K, Beyer W, Johansson A, Stepp H, Baumgartner R, Zimmermann W (2011) Induction of immune mediators in glioma and prostate cancer cells by non-lethal photodynamic therapy. *PLoS One* **6**:e21834.

Kamp MA, Felsberg J, Sadat H, Kuzibaev J, Steiger HJ, Rapp M, Reifenberger G, Dibue M, Sabel M (2015) 5-ALA-induced fluorescence behavior of reactive tissue changes following glioblastoma treatment with radiation and chemotherapy. *Acta Neurochir (Wien)* **157**:207–213; discussion 213–204.

Kamp MA, Grosser P, Felsberg J, Slotty PJ, Steiger HJ, Reifenberger G, Sabel M (2012) 5-aminolevulinic acid (5-ALA)-induced fluorescence in intracerebral metastases: A retrospective study. *Acta Neurochir (Wien)* **154**:223–228; discussion 228.

Kantelhardt SR, Leppert J, Kantelhardt JW, Reusche E, Huttmann G, Giese A (2009) Multi-photon excitation fluorescence microscopy of brain-tumor tissue and analysis of cell density. *Acta Neurochir (Wien)* **151**:253–262; discussion 262.

Kelly PJ, Hunt C (1994) The limited value of cytoreductive surgery in elderly patients with malignant gliomas. *Neurosurgery* **34**:62–66; discussion 66–67.

Kim JE et al. (2015) Mechanism for enhanced 5-aminolevulinic acid fluorescence in isocitrate dehydrogenase 1 mutant malignant gliomas. *Oncotarget*.

Kleinberg L, Slick T, Enger C, Grossman S, Brem H, Wharam MD, Jr. (1997) Short course radiotherapy is an appropriate option for most malignant glioma patients. *Int J Radiation Oncol Biol Phys* **38**:31–36.

Kobuchi H, Moriya K, Ogino T, Fujita H, Inoue K, Shuin T, Yasuda T, Utsumi K, Utsumi T (2012) Mitochondrial localization of ABC transporter ABCG2 and its function in 5-aminolevulinic acid-mediated protoporphyrin IX accumulation. *PLoS One* **7**:e50082.

Koc K, Anik I, Cabuk B, Ceylan S (2008) Fluorescein sodium-guided surgery in glioblastoma multiforme: A prospective evaluation. *Br J Neurosurg* **22**:99–103.

Krieg RC, Fickweiler S, Wolfbeis OS, Knuechel R (2000) Cell-type specific protoporphyrin IX metabolism in human bladder cancer in vitro. *Photochem Photobiol* **72**:226–233.

Krieg RC, Messmann H, Rauch J, Seeger S, Knuechel R (2002) Metabolic characterization of tumor cell-specific protoporphyrin IX accumulation after exposure to 5-aminolevulinic acid in human colonic cells381. *Photochem Photobiol* **76**:518–525.

Krishnamurthy PC, Du G, Fukuda Y, Sun D, Sampath J, Mercer KE, Wang J, Sosa-Pineda B, Murti KG, Schuetz JD (2006) Identification of a mammalian mitochondrial porphyrin transporter. *Nature* **443**:586–589.

Krishnamurthy S, Powers SK, Witmer P, Brown T (2000) Optimal light dose for interstitial photodynamic therapy in treatment for malignant brain tumors. *Lasers Surg Med* **27**:224–234.

Kubben PL, ter Meulen KJ, Schijns OE, ter Laak-Poort MP, van Overbeeke JJ, van Santbrink H (2011) Intraoperative MRI-guided resection of glioblastoma multiforme: A systematic review. *Lancet Oncol* **12**:1062–1070.

Kunz M et al. (2011) Hot spots in dynamic (18)FET-PET delineate malignant tumor parts within suspected WHO grade II gliomas. *Neuro Oncol* **13**:307–316.

Lacroix M et al. (2001) A multivariate analysis of 416 patients with glioblastoma multiforme: Prognosis, extent of resection, and survival. *J Neurosurg* **95**:190–198.

Laperriere N, Zuraw L, Cairncross G, Guideli CCOP (2002) Radiotherapy for newly diagnosed malignant glioma in adults: A systematic review. *Radiotherapy Oncol* **64**:259–273.

Laws ER, Shaffrey ME, Morris A, Anderson FA, Jr. (2003) Surgical management of intracranial gliomas— Does radical resection improve outcome? *Acta Neurochir Suppl* **85**:47–53.

Layer G, Reichelt J, Jahn D, Heinz DW (2010) Structure and function of enzymes in heme biosynthesis. *Protein Sci* **19**:1137–1161.

Leblond F, Ovanesyan Z, Davis SC, Valdes PA, Kim A, Hartov A, Wilson BC, Pogue BW, Paulsen KD, Roberts DW (2011) Analytic expression of fluorescence ratio detection correlates with depth in multi-spectral sub-surface imaging. *Phys Med Biol* **56**:6823–6837.

Leroy HA, Vermandel M, Lejeune JP, Mordon S, Reyns N (2015) Fluorescence guided resection and glioblastoma in 2015: A review. *Lasers Surg Med* **47**:441–451.

Madsen SJ, Angell-Petersen E, Spetalen S, Carper SW, Ziegler SA, Hirschberg H (2006) Photodynamic therapy of newly implanted glioma cells in the rat brain. *Lasers Surg Med* **38**:540–548.

Madsen SJ, Hirschberg H (2010) Site-specific opening of the blood–brain barrier. *J Biophotonics* **3**:356–367.

Marbacher S, Klinger E, Schwyzer L, Fischer I, Nevzati E, Diepers M, Roelcke U, Fathi AR, Coluccia D, Fandino J (2014) Use of fluorescence to guide resection or biopsy of primary brain tumors and brain metastases. *Neurosurg Focus* **36**:E10.

Martirosyan NL, Cavalcanti DD, Eschbacher JM, Delaney PM, Scheck AC, Abdelwahab MG, Nakaji P, Spetzler RF, Preul MC (2011) Use of in vivo near-infrared laser confocal endomicroscopy with indocyanine green to detect the boundary of infiltrative tumor. *J Neurosurg* **115**:1131–1138.

Martirosyan NL, Georges J, Eschbacher JM, Cavalcanti DD, Elhadi AM, Abdelwahab MG, Scheck AC, Nakaji P, Spetzler RF, Preul MC (2014) Potential application of a handheld confocal endomicroscope imaging system using a variety of fluorophores in experimental gliomas and normal brain. *Neurosurg Focus* **36**:E16.

Mazard T et al. (2013) Sorafenib overcomes irinotecan resistance in colorectal cancer by inhibiting the ABCG2 drug-efflux pump. *Mol Cancer Ther* **12**:2121–2134.

Mazhar A, Cuccia DJ, Gioux S, Durkin AJ, Frangioni JV, Tromberg BJ (2010) Structured illumination enhances resolution and contrast in thick tissue fluorescence imaging. *J Biomed Opt* **15**:010506.

Middelburg TA, Hoy CL, Neumann HA, Amelink A, Robinson DJ (2015) Correction for tissue optical properties enables quantitative skin fluorescence measurements using multi-diameter single fiber reflectance spectroscopy. *J Dermatol Sci* **79**:64–73.

Millesi M, Kiesel B, Woehrer A, Hainfellner JA, Novak K, Martinez-Moreno M, Wolfsberger S, Knosp E, Widhalm G (2014) Analysis of 5-aminolevulinic acid-induced fluorescence in 55 different spinal tumors. *Neurosurg Focus* **36**:E11.

Mohan DS, Suh JH, Phan JL, Kupelian PA, Cohen BH, Barnett GH (1998) Outcome in elderly patients undergoing definitive surgery and radiation therapy for supratentorial glioblastoma multiforme at a tertiary care institution. *Int J Radiat Oncol* **42**:981–987.

Moiyadi AV, Sridhar E (2015) Delta-aminolevulinic acid-induced fluorescence unmasks biological intratumoral heterogeneity within histologically homogeneous areas of malignant gliomas. *Acta Neurochir (Wien)* **157**:617–619.

Moiyadi AV, Stummer W (2015) Delta-Aminolevulinic acid-induced fluorescence-guided resection of brain tumors. *Neurol India* **63**:155–165.

Mooney MA, Zehri AH, Georges JF, Nakaji P (2014) Laser scanning confocal endomicroscopy in the neurosurgical operating room: A review and discussion of future applications. *Neurosurg Focus* **36**:E9.

Moore GE et al. (1948) The clinical use of fluorescein in neurosurgery: The localization of brain tumors. *J Neurosurg* **5**:392–398.

Moriuchi S, Yamada K, Dehara M, Teramoto Y, Soda T, Imakita M, Taneda M (2011) Use of 5-aminolevulinic acid for the confirmation of deep-seated brain tumors during stereotactic biopsy. Report of 2 cases. *J Neurosurg* **115**:278–280.

Morofuji Y, Matsuo T, Toyoda K, Takeshita T, Hirose M, Hirao T, Hayashi Y, Tsutsumi K, Abe K, Nagata I (2007) Skull metastasis of hepatocellular carcinoma successfully treated by intraoperative photodynamic diagnosis using 5-aminolevulinic acid: Case report. *No Shinkei Geka* **35**:913–918.

Motekallemi A, Jeltema HR, Metzemaekers JD, van Dam GM, Crane LM, Groen RJ (2015) The current status of 5-ALA fluorescence-guided resection of intracranial meningiomas—A critical review. *Neurosurg Rev* **38**:619–628.

Mroz P, Hashmi JT, Huang YY, Lange N, Hamblin MR (2011b) Stimulation of anti-tumor immunity by photodynamic therapy. *Expert Rev Clin Immunol* **7**:75–91.

Mroz P, Yaroslavsky A, Kharkwal GB, Hamblin MR (2011a) Cell death pathways in photodynamic therapy of cancer. *Cancers (Basel)* **3**:2516–2539.

Nabavi A, Thurm H, Zountsas B, Pietsch T, Lanfermann H, Pichlmeier U, Mehdorn M, Group ALARGS (2009) Five-aminolevulinic acid for fluorescence-guided resection of recurrent malignant gliomas: A phase ii study. *Neurosurgery* **65**:1070–1076; discussion 1076–1077.

Navone NM, Polo CF, Frisardi AL, Andrade NE, Battle AM (1990) Heme biosynthesis in human breast cancer—Mimetic "in vitro" studies and some heme enzymic activity levels. *Int J Biochem* 1407–1411.

Ogino T et al. (2011) Serum-dependent export of protoporphyrin IX by ATP-binding cassette transporter G2 in T24 cells. *Mol Cell Biochem* **358**:297–307.

Olson JJ, Fadul CE, Brat DJ, Mukundan S, Ryken TC (2009) Management of newly diagnosed glioblastoma: Guidelines development, value and application. *J Neurooncol* **93**:1–23.

Ostrom QT, Gittleman H, Liao P, Rouse C, Chen Y, Dowling J, Wolinsky Y, Kruchko C, Barnholtz-Sloan J (2014) CBTRUS statistical report: Primary brain and central nervous system tumors diagnosed in the United States in 2007–2011. *Neuro Oncol* **16**(Suppl 4):iv1–iv63.

Panciani PP, Fontanella M, Garbossa D, Agnoletti A, Ducati A, Lanotte M (2012a) 5-aminolevulinic acid and neuronavigation in high-grade glioma surgery: Results of a combined approach. *Neurocirugia (Astur)* **23**:23–28.

Panciani PP, Fontanella M, Schatlo B, Garbossa D, Agnoletti A, Ducati A, Lanotte M (2012b) Fluorescence and image guided resection in high grade glioma. *Clin Neurol Neurosurg* **114**:37–41.

Papour A, Taylor Z, Sherman A, Sanchez D, Lucey G, Liau L, Stafsudd O, Yong W, Grundfest W (2013) Optical imaging for brain tissue characterization using relative fluorescence lifetime imaging. *J Biomed Opt* **18**:60504.

Piccirillo SG, Dietz S, Madhu B, Griffiths J, Price SJ, Collins VP, Watts C (2012) Fluorescence-guided surgical sampling of glioblastoma identifies phenotypically distinct tumor-initiating cell populations in the tumor mass and margin. *Br J Cancer* **107**:462–468.

Pichlmeier U, Bink A, Schackert G, Stummer W (2008) Resection and survival in glioblastoma multiforme: An RTOG recursive partitioning analysis of ALA study patients. *Neuro Oncol* **10**:1025–1034.

Pogue BW, Gibbs-Strauss S, Valdes PA, Samkoe K, Roberts DW, Paulsen KD (2010) Review of neurosurgical fluorescence imaging methodologies. *IEEE J Sel Top Quantum Electron* **16**:493–505.

Popperl G, Kreth FW, Mehrkens JH, Herms J, Seelos K, Koch W, Gildehaus FJ, Kretzschmar HA, Tonn JC, Tatsch K (2007) FET PET for the evaluation of untreated gliomas: Correlation of FET uptake and uptake kinetics with tumor grading. *Eur J Nucl Med Mol Imaging* **34**:1933–1942.

Potapov AA et al. (2008) First experience in 5-ALA fluorescence-guided and endoscopically assisted microsurgery of brain tumors. *Med Laser Appl* **23**:202–208.

Potapov AA et al. (2013) Intraoperative combined spectroscopy (optical biopsy) of cerebral gliomas. *NN Burdenko J Neurosurg* **2**:3–10.

Prada F et al. (2014) Intraoperative cerebral glioma characterization with contrast enhanced ultrasound. *Biomed Res Int* **2014**:484261.

Preusser M, Lim M, Hafler DA, Reardon DA, Sampson JH (2015) Prospects of immune checkpoint modulators in the treatment of glioblastoma. *Nat Rev Neurol* **11**:504–514.

Quigley MR, Maroon JC (1991) The relationship between survival and the extent of the resection in patients with supratentorial malignant gliomas. *Neurosurgery* **29**:385–388; discussion 388–389.

Rampazzo E, Della Puppa A, Frasson C, Battilana G, Bianco S, Scienza R, Basso G, Persano L (2014) Phenotypic and functional characterization of Glioblastoma cancer stem cells identified through 5-aminolevulinic acid-assisted surgery [corrected]. *J Neurooncol* **116**:505–513.

Rapp M, Kamp M, Steiger HJ, Sabel M (2014) Endoscopic-assisted visualization of 5-aminolevulinic acid-induced fluorescence in malignant glioma surgery: A technical note. *World Neurosurg* **82**:e277–279.

Ritz R, Feigl GC, Schuhmann MU, Ehrhardt A, Danz S, Noell S, Bornemann A, Tatagiba MS (2011) Use of 5-ALA fluorescence guided endoscopic biopsy of a deep-seated primary malignant brain tumor. *J Neurosurg* **114**:1410–1413.

Ritz R et al. (2012) Hypericin for visualization of high grade gliomas: First clinical experience. *Eur J Surg Oncol* **38**:352–360.

Roa W, Xing JZ, Small C, Kortmann R, Miriamanoff R, Okunieff P, Shibamoto Y, Jeremic B (2009) Current developments in the radiotherapy approach to elderly and frail patients with glioblastoma multiforme. *Expert Rev Anticanc* **9**:1643–1650.

Roberts DW et al. (2011) Coregistered fluorescence-enhanced tumor resection of malignant glioma: Relationships between delta-aminolevulinic acid-induced protoporphyrin IX fluorescence, magnetic resonance imaging enhancement, and neuropathological parameters. *Clin Article J Neurosurg* **114**:595–603.

Roder C, Bisdas S, Ebner FH, Honegger J, Naegele T, Ernemann U, Tatagiba M (2014) Maximizing the extent of resection and survival benefit of patients in glioblastoma surgery: High-field iMRI versus conventional and 5-ALA-assisted surgery. *Eur J Surg Oncol* **40**:297–304.

Roessler K, Krawagna M, Dorfler A, Buchfelder M, Ganslandt O (2014) Essentials in intraoperative indocyanine green videoangiography assessment for intracranial aneurysm surgery: Conclusions from 295 consecutively clipped aneurysms and review of the literature. *Neurosurg Focus* **36**:E7.

Rygh OM, Selbekk T, Torp SH, Lydersen S, Hernes TA, Unsgaard G (2008) Comparison of navigated 3D ultrasound findings with histopathology in subsequent phases of glioblastoma resection. *Acta Neurochir (Wien)* **150**:1033–1041; discussion 1042.

Sahm F, Capper D, Jeibmann A, Habel A, Paulus W, Troost D, von Deimling A (2012) Addressing diffuse glioma as a systemic brain disease with single-cell analysis. *Arch Neurol* **69**:523–526.

Samkoe KS, Gibbs-Strauss SL, Yang HH, Khan Hekmatyar S, Jack Hoopes P, O'Hara JA, Kauppinen RA, Pogue BW (2011) Protoporphyrin IX fluorescence contrast in invasive glioblastomas is linearly correlated with Gd enhanced magnetic resonance image contrast but has higher diagnostic accuracy. *J Biomed Opt* **16**:096008.

Sanai N, Berger MS (2008) Glioma extent of resection and its impact on patient outcome. *Neurosurgery* **62**:753–764; discussion 264–756.

Sanai N, Berger MS (2011) Extent of resection influences outcomes for patients with gliomas. *Rev Neurol (Paris)* **167**:648–654.

Sanai N, Mirzadeh Z, Berger MS (2008) Functional outcome after language mapping for glioma resection. *N Engl J Med* **358**:18–27.

Santagata S et al. 2014) Intraoperative mass spectrometry mapping of an onco-metabolite to guide brain tumor surgery. *Proc Natl Acad Sci USA* **111**:11121–11126.

Sawamoto M, Imai T, Umeda M, Fukuda K, Kataoka T, Taketani S (2013) The p53-dependent expression of frataxin controls 5-aminolevulinic acid-induced accumulation of protoporphyrin IX and photodamage in cancerous cells. *Photochem Photobiol* **89**:163–172.

Schatlo B, Fandino J, Smoll NR, Wetzel O, Remonda L, Marbacher S, Perrig W, Landolt H, Fathi AR (2015) Outcomes after combined use of intraoperative MRI and 5-aminolevulinic acid in high-grade glioma surgery. *Neuro Oncol.*

Schebesch KM, Hoehne J, Hohenberger C, Proescholdt M, Riemenschneider MJ, Wendl C, Brawanski A (2015) Fluorescein sodium-guided resection of cerebral metastases-experience with the first 30 patients. *Acta Neurochir (Wien)* **157**:899–904.

Schucht P, Beck J, Abu-Isa J, Andereggen L, Murek M, Seidel K, Stieglitz L, Raabe A (2012) Gross total resection rates in contemporary glioblastoma surgery: Results of an institutional protocol combining 5-aminolevulinic acid intraoperative fluorescence imaging and brain mapping. *Neurosurgery* **71**:927–935; discussion 935–926.

Schucht P, Beck J, Raabe A (2015) Response to: Maximizing the extent of resection and survival benefit of patients in glioblastoma surgery: High-field iMRI versus conventional and 5-ALA-assisted surgery. *Eur J Surg Oncol* **41**:604–605.

Schucht P, Beck J, Vajtai I, Raabe A (2011) Paradoxical fluorescence after administration of 5-aminolevulinic acid for resection of a cerebral melanoma metastasis. *Acta Neurochir (Wien)* **153**:1497–1499.

Schucht P, Knittel S, Slotboom J, Seidel K, Murek M, Jilch A, Raabe A, Beck J (2014) 5-ALA complete resections go beyond MR contrast enhancement: Shift corrected volumetric analysis of the extent of resection in surgery for glioblastoma. *Acta Neurochir (Wien)* **156**:305–312; discussion 312.

Schwake M, Stummer W, Suero Molina EJ, Wolfer J (2015) Simultaneous fluorescein sodium and 5-ALA in fluorescence-guided glioma surgery. *Acta Neurochir (Wien)* **157**:877–879.

Schwartz C, Ruehm A, Tonn JC, Kreth S, Kreth FW (2015) Interstitial photodynamic therapy of de-novo glioblastoma multiforme WHO IV. *Meeting of the Society of Neuro-Oncology:SURG-25.*

Senft C, Bink A, Franz K, Vatter H, Gasser T, Seifert V (2011) Intraoperative MRI guidance and extent of resection in glioma surgery: A randomized, controlled trial. *Lancet Oncol* **12**:997–1003.

Sexton K, Davis SC, McClatchy D, 3rd, Valdes PA, Kanick SC, Paulsen KD, Roberts DW, Pogue BW (2013) Pulsed-light imaging for fluorescence guided surgery under normal room lighting. *Opt Lett* **38**:3249–3252.

Shevelev I et al. (October 9–14, 2011) 5-ALA-fluorescence diagnosis in surgery of spinal cord tumors. Poster presented at *European Congress of Neurosurgery*, Rome, Italy.

Shinoda J, Yano H, Yoshimura S, Okumura A, Kaku Y, Iwama T, Sakai N (2003) Fluorescence-guided resection of glioblastoma multiforme by using high-dose fluorescein sodium. Technical note. *J Neurosurg* **99**:597–603.

Slof J, Diez Valle R, Galvan J (2015) Cost-effectiveness of 5-aminolevulinic acid-induced fluorescence in malignant glioma surgery. *Neurologia* **30**:163–168.

Slotty PJ, Siantidis B, Beez T, Steiger HJ, Sabel M (2013) The impact of improved treatment strategies on overall survival in glioblastoma patients. *Acta Neurochir (Wien)* **155**:959–963; discussion 963.

Stepp H, Beck T, Pongratz T, Meinel T, Kreth FW, Tonn J, Stummer W (2007) ALA and malignant glioma: Fluorescence-guided resection and photodynamic treatment. *J Environ Pathol Toxicol Oncol* **26**:157–164.

Stepp H et al. (2005) Fluorescence guided resections and photodynamic therapy for malignant gliomas using 5-aminolevulinic acid. *Photonic Ther Diagn* **5686**:547–557.

Stepp H et al. (2012) Fluorescence guidance during stereotactic biopsy. *Proc. SPIE 8207, Photonic Therapeutics and Diagnostics VIII*, 82074H.

Stummer W (2015) Poor man's fluorescence? *Acta Neurochir (Wien)* **157**(8):1379–1381.

Stummer W, Meinel T, Ewelt C, Martus P, Jakobs O, Felsberg J, Reifenberger G (2012) Prospective cohort study of radiotherapy with concomitant and adjuvant temozolomide chemotherapy for glioblastoma patients with no or minimal residual enhancing tumor load after surgery. *J Neurooncol.*

Stummer W, Novotny A, Stepp H, Goetz C, Bise K, Reulen HJ (2000) Fluorescence-guided resection of glioblastoma multiforme by using 5-aminolevulinic acid-induced porphyrins: A prospective study in 52 consecutive patients. *J Neurosurg* **93**:1003–1013.

Stummer W, Pichlmeier U, Meinel T, Wiestler OD, Zanella F, Reulen H-J (2006) Fluorescence-guided surgery with 5-aminolevulinic acid for resection of malignant glioma: A randomized controlled multicentre phase III trial. *Lancet Oncol* **7**(5):392–401.

Stummer W, Stocker S, Wagner S, Stepp H, Fritsch C, Goetz C, Goetz AE, Kiefmann R, Reulen HJ (1998) Intraoperative detection of malignant gliomas by 5-aminolevulinic acid-induced porphyrin fluorescence. *Neurosurgery* **42**:518–525; discussion 525–516.

Stummer W, Tonn JC, Goetz C, Ullrich W, Stepp H, Bink A, Pietsch T, Pichlmeier U (2014) 5-Aminolevulinic acid-derived tumor fluorescence: The diagnostic accuracy of visible fluorescence qualities as corroborated by spectrometry and histology and postoperative imaging. *Neurosurgery* **74**:310–319; discussion 319–320.

Stummer W, van den Bent MJ, Westphal M (2011) Cytoreductive surgery of glioblastoma as the key to successful adjuvant therapies: New arguments in an old discussion. *Acta Neurochir (Wien)* **153**:1211–1218.

Stummer W et al. (2008a) Long-sustaining response in a patient with non-resectable, distant recurrence of glioblastoma multiforme treated by interstitial photodynamic therapy using 5-ALA: Case report. *J Neurooncol* **87**:103–109.

Stummer W et al. (2008b) Extent of resection and survival in glioblastoma multiforme: Identification of and adjustment for bias. *Neurosurgery* **62**:564–576; discussion 564576.

Stupp R et al. (2005) Radiotherapy plus concomitant and adjuvant temozolomide for glioblastoma. *N Engl J Med* **352**:987–996.

Stupp R et al. (2009) Effects of radiotherapy with concomitant and adjuvant temozolomide versus radiotherapy alone on survival in glioblastoma in a randomized phase III study: 5-year analysis of the EORTC-NCIC trial. *Lancet Oncol* **10**:459–466.

Stylli SS, Kaye AH (2006) Photodynamic therapy of cerebral glioma—A review. Part II—Clin studies.. *J Clin Neurosci* **13**:709–717.

Stylli SS, Kaye AH, MacGregor L, Howes M, Rajendra P (2005) Photodynamic therapy of high grade glioma—Long term survival. *J Clin Neurosci* **12**:389–398.

Suzuki T, Wada S, Eguchi H, Adachi J, Mishima K, Matsutani M, Nishikawa R, Nishiyama M (2013) Cadherin 13 overexpression as an important factor related to the absence of tumor fluorescence in 5-aminolevulinic acid-guided resection of glioma. *J Neurosurg* **119**:1331–1339.

Tamura Y, Kuroiwa T, Kajimoto Y, Miki Y, Miyatake S, Tsuji M (2007) Endoscopic identification and biopsy sampling of an intraventricular malignant glioma using a 5-aminolevulinic acid-induced protoporphyrin IX fluorescence imaging system. Technical note. *J Neurosurg* **106**:507–510.

Tejada-Solis S, Aldave-Orzaiz G, Pay-Valverde E, Marigil-Sanchez M, Idoate-Gastearena MA, Diez-Valle R (2012) Prognostic value of ventricular wall fluorescence during 5-aminolevulinic-guided surgery for glioblastoma. *Acta Neurochir (Wien)* **154**:1997–2002; discussion 2002.

Teng L, Nakada M, Zhao SG, Endo Y, Furuyama N, Nambu E, Pyko IV, Hayashi Y, Hamada JI (2011) Silencing of ferrochelatase enhances 5-aminolevulinic acid-based fluorescence and photodynamic therapy efficacy. *Br J Cancer* **104**:798–807.

Terr L, Weiner LP (1983) An autoradiographic study of delta-aminolevulinic acid uptake by mouse brain. *Exp Neurol* **79**:564–568.

Toms SA, Lin WC, Weil RJ, Johnson MD, Jansen ED, Mahadevan-Jansen A (2007) Intraoperative optical spectroscopy identifies infiltrating glioma margins with high sensitivity. *Neurosurgery* **61**:327–335; discussion 335–326.

Tonn JC, Stummer W (2008) Fluorescence-guided resection of malignant gliomas using 5-aminolevulinic acid: Practical use, risks, and pitfalls. *Clin Neurosurg* **55**:20–26.

Trantakis C, Tittgemeyer M, Schneider JP, Lindner D, Winkler D, Strauss G, Meixensberger J (2003) Investigation of time-dependency of intracranial brain shift and its relation to the extent of tumor removal using intra-operative MRI. *Neurol Res* **25**:9–12.

Tsai JC, Hsiao YY, Teng LJ, Chen CT, Kao MC (1999) Comparative study on the ALA photodynamic effects of human glioma and meningioma cells. *Lasers Surg Med* **24**:296–305.

Tsugu A, Ishizaka H, Mizokami Y, Osada T, Baba T, Yoshiyama M, Nishiyama J, Matsumae M (2011) Impact of the combination of 5-aminolevulinic acid-induced fluorescence with intraoperative magnetic resonance imaging-guided surgery for glioma. *World Neurosurg* **76**:120–127.

Utsuki S, Miyoshi N, Oka H, Miyajima Y, Shimizu S, Suzuki S, Fujii K (2007a) Fluorescence-guided resection of metastatic brain tumors using a 5-aminolevulinic acid-induced protoporphyrin IX: Pathological study. *Brain Tumor Pathol* **24**:53–55.

Utsuki S, Oka H, Kijima C, Miyajima Y, Hagiwara H, Fujii K (2011) Utility of intraoperative fluorescent diagnosis of residual hemangioblastoma using 5-aminolevulinic acid. *Neurol India* **59**:612–615.

Utsuki S, Oka H, Sato S, Shimizu S, Suzuki S, Tanizaki Y, Kondo K, Miyajima Y, Fujii K (2007b) Histological examination of false positive tissue resection using 5-aminolevulinic acid-induced fluorescence guidance. *Neurol Med Chir (Tokyo)* **47**:210–213; discussion 213–214.

Valdes PA, Bekelis K, Harris BT, Wilson BC, Leblond F, Kim A, Simmons NE, Erkmen K, Paulsen KD, Roberts DW (2014) 5-Aminolevulinic acid-induced protoporphyrin IX fluorescence in meningioma: Qualitative and quantitative measurements in vivo. *Neurosurgery* **10**(Suppl 1):74–82; discussion 82–73.

Valdes PA, Jacobs V, Harris BT, Wilson BC, Leblond F, Paulsen KD, Roberts DW (2015) Quantitative fluorescence using 5-aminolevulinic acid-induced protoporphyrin IX biomarker as a surgical adjunct in low-grade glioma surgery. *J Neurosurg* **123**:771–780.

Valdes PA, Jacobs VL, Wilson BC, Leblond F, Roberts DW, Paulsen KD (2013) System and methods for wide-field quantitative fluorescence imaging during neurosurgery. *Opt Lett* **38**:2786–2788.

Valdes PA, Kim A, Brantsch M, Niu C, Moses ZB, Tosteson TD, Wilson BC, Paulsen KD, Roberts DW, Harris BT (2011a) Delta-aminolevulinic acid-induced protoporphyrin IX concentration correlates with histopathologic markers of malignancy in human gliomas: The need for quantitative fluorescence-guided resection to identify regions of increasing malignancy. *Neuro Oncol* **13**:846–856.

Valdes PA et al. (2011b) Quantitative fluorescence in intracranial tumor: Implications for ALA-induced PpIX as an intraoperative biomarker. *J Neurosurg* **115**:11–17.

Van Hillegersberg R, Van den Berg JW, Kort WJ, Terpstra OT, Wilson JH (1992) Selective accumulation of endogenously produced porphyrins in a liver metastasis model in rats. *Gastroenterology* **103**:647–651.

Villa S, Vinolas N, Verger E, Yaya R, Martinez A, Gil M, Moreno V, Caral L, Graus F (1998) Efficacy of radiotherapy for malignant gliomas in elderly patients. *Int J Radiat Oncol* **42**:977–980.

von Campe G, Moschopulos M, Hefti M (2012) 5-Aminolevulinic acid-induced protoporphyrin IX fluorescence as immediate intraoperative indicator to improve the safety of malignant or high-grade brain tumor diagnosis in frameless stereotactic biopsies. *Acta Neurochir (Wien)*.

Walker MD et al. (1980) Randomized comparisons of radiotherapy and nitrosoureas for the treatment of malignant glioma after surgery. *N Engl J Med* **303**:1323–1329.

Wang Y, Jiang T (2013) Understanding high grade glioma: Molecular mechanism, therapy and comprehensive management. *Cancer Lett* **331**:139–146.

Wang YG, Kim H, Mun S, Kim D, Choi Y (2013) Indocyanine green-loaded perfluorocarbon nanoemulsions for bimodal (19)F-magnetic resonance/nearinfrared fluorescence imaging and subsequent phototherapy. *Quant Imaging Med Surg* **3**:132–140.

Warram JM, de Boer E, Korb M, Hartman Y, Kovar J, Markert JM, Gillespie GY, Rosenthal EL (2015) Fluorescence-guided resection of experimental malignant glioma using cetuximab-IRDye 800CW. *Br J Neurosurg* 1–9.

Widhalm G, Kiesel B, Woehrer A, Traub-Weidinger T, Preusser M, Marosi C, Prayer D, Hainfellner JA, Knosp E, Wolfsberger S (2013) 5-Aminolevulinic acid induced fluorescence is a powerful intraoperative marker for precise histopathological grading of gliomas with non-significant contrast-enhancement. *PLoS One* **8**:e76988.

Widhalm G, Wolfsberger S, Minchev G, Woehrer A, Krssak M, Czech T, Prayer D, Asenbaum S, Hainfellner JA, Knosp E (2010) 5-Aminolevulinic acid is a promising marker for detection of anaplastic foci in diffusely infiltrating gliomas with nonsignificant contrast enhancement. *Cancer* **116**:1545–1552.

Widhalm G et al. (2012) Strong 5-aminolevulinic acid-induced fluorescence is a novel intraoperative marker for representative tissue samples in stereotactic brain tumor biopsies. *Neurosurg Rev* **35**(3):381–391.

Willems PW, van der Sprenkel JW, Tulleken CA, Viergever MA, Taphoorn MJ (2006) Neuronavigation and surgery of intracerebral tumors. *J Neurol* **253**:1123–1136.

Wu JS, Zhou LF, Tang WJ, Mao Y, Hu J, Song YY, Hong XN, Du GH (2007) Clinical evaluation and follow-up outcome of diffusion tensor imaging-based functional neuronavigation: A prospective, controlled study in patients with gliomas involving pyramidal tracts. *Neurosurgery* **61**:935–948; discussion 948–939.

Yamaguchi F, Takahashi H, Teramoto A (2007) Photodiagnosis for frameless stereotactic biopsy of brain tumor. *Photodiagnosis Photodyn Ther* **4**:71–75.

Yamamoto T, Ishikawa E, Miki S, Sakamoto N, Zaboronok A, Matsuda M, Akutsu H, Nakai K, Tsuruta W, Matsumura A (2015) Photodynamic diagnosis using 5-aminolevulinic acid in 41 biopsies for primary central nervous system lymphoma. *Photochem Photobiol* **91**:1452–1457.

Yang C et al. (2015) Quantitative correlational study of microbubble-enhanced ultrasound imaging and magnetic resonance imaging of glioma and early response to radiotherapy in a rat model. *Med Phys* **42**:4762.

Yang VX, Muller PJ, Herman P, Wilson BC (2003) A multispectral fluorescence imaging system: Design and initial clinical tests in intra-operative Photofrin-photodynamic therapy of brain tumors. *Lasers Surg Med* **32**:224–232.

Yao J, Wang L, Yang J-M, Maslov KI, Wong TTW, Li L, Huang C-H, Zou J, Wang LV (2015) High-speed label-free functional photoacoustic microscopy of mouse brain in action. *Nat Methods* **12**:407–410.

Zhao S et al. (2013a) Intraoperative fluorescence-guided resection of high-grade malignant gliomas using 5-aminolevulinic acid-induced porphyrins: A systematic review and meta-analysis of prospective studies. *PLoS One* **8**:e63682.

Zhao SG et al. (2013b) Increased expression of ABCB6 enhances protoporphyrin IX accumulation and photodynamic effect in human glioma. *Ann Surg Oncol* **20**:4379–4388.

Zilidis G, Aziz F, Telara S, Eljamel MS (2008) Fluorescence image-guided surgery and repetitive photodynamic therapy in brain metastatic malignant melanoma. *Photodiagnosis Photodyn Ther* **5**:264–266.

Zimmermann A, Ritsch-Marte M, Kostron H (2001) mTHPC-mediated photodynamic diagnosis of malignant brain tumors. *Photochem Photobiol* **74**:611–616.

Zimmermann M, Stan AC (2010) PepT2 transporter protein expression in human neoplastic glial cells and mediation of fluorescently tagged dipeptide derivative beta-Ala-Lys-Nepsilon-7-amino-4-methyl-coumarin-3-acetic acid accumulation. *J Neurosurg* **112**:1005–1014.

PDT of non-muscle-invasive bladder cancer with Hexylester Aminolevulinate
Optimization of the illumination wavelengths by fluorescence spectroscopy and imaging

MATTHIEU ZELLWEGER, CLAUDE-ANDRÉ PORRET,
NORBERT LANGE, PATRICE JICHLINSKI, HUBERT VAN DEN BERGH,
AND GEORGES WAGNIÈRES

19.1 INTRODUCTION

Bladder cancer is the fourth most common cancer for men over 50 (Landis et al., 1999; Bray et al., 2002), the seventh most common cancer in men, and the 17th in women (2008 data, Babjuk et al., 2014). Approximately 75% of patients with bladder cancer present a disease confined to the mucosa (stage Ta, CIS) or submucosa (stage T1) upon admittance to hospital (Babjuk et al., 2014). These categories are grouped as non-muscle-invasive bladder cancers (NMIBC). Non-muscle-invasive has a high prevalence due to low progression rates and long-term survival in many cases. However, tumors associated with aggressive pathologic characters, such as presence of carcinoma in situ (CIS), can lead to death in 30% of the cases (Herr, 1997). Bladder cancer of various origins can develop at different rates and under various morphologies, going from flat to exophytic papillary lesions. As is the case for other epithelial cancers, superficial bladder cancer is a permanent disease of the urothelium and it can recur in up to 70% of the cases during the 3 years following the first treatment (Kurt et al., 2000).

The treatment of superficial bladder cancer is based on unique or iterative transurethral resections of the tumors, in association with different topical treatments based on chemo- or immunotherapeutic agents. Except BCG, no treatment modality is susceptible to limit the progression of CIS or aggressive tumors (Sylvester et al., 2002). The high tendency of superficial bladder cancer to recur is a concern (Holmäng et al., 1999), especially since long-term disease progression is correlated to the number of recurrences. Additionally, iterative treatments can impair bladder function and lead to cystectomy with bladder replacement (Pang and Catto, 2013). Thus, alternative treatment modalities are of high interest, especially if they allow the Urologist to treat the mostly occult in situ, residual or recurrent flat urothelial malignancies in superficial bladder cancer on nearly the entire bladder surface.

Protoporphyrin IX (PPIX)-based photodynamic therapy (PDT), following the instillation of 5-aminolaevu-linic Acid (5-ALA) or in particular its ester derivative Hexylester Aminolevulinate (HAL), is an interest-ing approach in this context (Krieg et al., 2000; Jichlinski and Leisinger, 2001). The reason for this is that HAL is approved, reimbursed, and clinically used in many western countries to detect early bladder can-cers (Wagnières et al., 2014) and leads to a selective production of PPIX in early NMIBC, thus preventing photodamage to deeper tissue layers of the bladder wall. In addition, the instillation time is significantly shorter with HAL than with 5-ALA. The broad absorption spectrum of PPIX, with peaks in the range of 390–660 nm, allows the use of various excitation wavelengths presenting different penetrations depths into the bladder wall, such as blue, green, or red alone, or a combination of those such as white-light illumination. Therefore, different clinical research protocols have been launched in different countries (Kriegmair et al., 1996; Waidelich et al., 2001; Shackley et al., 2002; Bader et al., 2013).

The aim of this study was to optimize the spectral design of PDT of non-muscle-invasive bladder cancer with HAL and to assess the usefulness of three illumination "colors" (405 nm, 635 nm, white) for this treat-ment approach. Initially, local illuminations were carried out in the bladder to assess the tissular effects and the safety of HAL-PDT. In parallel, the photodegradation (photobleaching) of PPIX during irradiation, as an indicator of the potency of these different spectral designs, was evaluated. With these results in mind, we determined key parameters, including the specifications of light delivery systems, for a next step, namely, a "whole bladder wall" PDT approach to treat all superficial NMIBC, invisible or not.

19.2 MATERIALS AND METHODS

19.2.1 LOCAL ILLUMINATIONS

19.2.1.1 PATIENTS

Eight patients (6 men/2 women) were included in this part of the study focusing on the assessment of the effects induced by local PDTs (average age: 68.5 y.o.; range: 59–83). All patients had a history of recurrent superficial bladder cancer and presented solitary (2 cases) or multifocal lesions (8 cases) (pTaG1-pTaG2). Inclusion criteria were as follows: male or female patients over 45 years old, not intending to be pregnant; patients with history of superficial bladder cancer (pTaG1-G2) at first or iterative recurrence of multifocal low-risk disease (defined as small papillary lesions, no larger than 5 mm in diameter); patients able to give written informed consent. Exclusion criteria were as follows: allergy to porphyrins/porphyria, pTaG3 or CIS disease, local chemo or immunotherapy less than 3 months before treatment, important hematuria. This study was approved by the ethics committee of Lausanne's CHUV Hospital. All patients were thoroughly informed verbally and in writing and signed an informed consent form. Local illuminations were carried out in the bladder to assess the tissular effects and the safety of HAL-PDT on a total of 10 lesions and on two additional sites of normal mucosa in two patients (hence a total of 4 normal sites in addition to the 10 lesions). Five lesions were treated with coherent red light (635 nm) and five lesions were treated with inco-herent white light (400–660 nm, see Figure 19.1). The photodegradation (photobleaching) of PPIX during

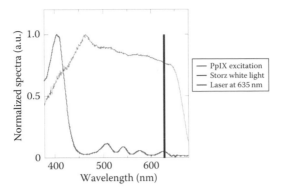

Figure 19.1 PPIX excitation spectrum; emission spectrum of the "white" light source used for this study; emission line of the red laser source used for this study.

these illuminations was evaluated on all fluorescent sites (10 lesions illuminated for PDT purposes, and one site on normal mucosa that was fluorescent, probably due to a local inflammation, hence 11 sites in total).

19.2.1.2 INSTILLATION

HAL powder (100 mg), synthesized as per Lange et al. (1999), was dissolved in 50 mL sterile phosphate buffered saline. The pH of the solution was adjusted to 5.7–6.2 with aqueous HCl for intravesical use. Nowadays, a similar formulation (Hexvix®) is commercially available (Ipsen Pharmaceuticals, Paris, France). This final solution of HAL (8 mM, or 0.2% w/w) was sterilized through a Millipore filter (0.22 μm Millex GS, Millipore, Millerica, Massachusetts). This solution was instilled into the patient's bladder during 2 h and followed by 2 h resting time, that is, the bladder was emptied 2 h before PDT, as suggested by the results of one of our previous studies (Lange et al., 1999; Marti et al., 2003).

19.2.1.3 LIGHT SOURCES

Red light at 635 nm was supplied from a Ceralas™ PDT 635 Laser Diode (635 nm, Ceramoptec, Bonn, Germany) for focal PDT trials. A frontal light distributor (Medlight SA, Ecublens, Switzerland, model FD1) was coupled to this laser diode to produce circular and homogenous light spots, as described in detail later. A 300 W PDD D-light-system (Karl Storz GmbH, Tuttlingen, Germany) delivering about 200 mW of white light (wavelength ranging from 400 to 660 nm) at the distal end of the cystoscope was used to perform the "white-light" focal illuminations of the bladder wall.

19.2.1.4 ENDOSCOPIC PROCEDURE

Prior to any treatment or measurement, a general examination of the bladder was performed under white-light illumination. Then, the illumination light of a commercially available system for photodynamic detection (PDD; D-Light, Karl Storz GmbH, Tuttlingen, Germany) was switched to fluorescence excitation mode (375–440 nm) to allow identification of PPIX fluorescent sites, PPIX fluorescence bleaching measurements, and local HAL-PDT. Papillary lesions larger than 5 mm in diameter were subject to transurethral resections of the bladder (TURB).

PPIX fluorescence emission spectra were then recorded with an optical fiber-based spectrofluorometer involving a filtered Xenon arc lamp and a Peltier-cooled CCD coupled to a spectrograph. This system is described in detail elsewhere (Zellweger et al., 1999). The distal end of the fiber was introduced into the bladder via the biopsy channel of the cystoscope, placed directly into contact with fluorescence positive tissues. Fluorescence spectra were acquired at regular intervals (0, 60, 120, 240, 360, 480, 600, and 1000 s) during illumination allowing the computation of the photobleaching decay constants. An aqueous solution of Rhodamine B was used as a reference to normalize the fluorescence spectra, thus enabling direct comparison of the intensities of spectra recorded at different times. Local illuminations of the bladder wall with red (635 nm) light were carried out by means of the FD1 frontal light distributor mentioned earlier.

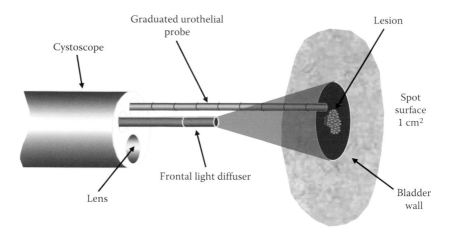

Figure 19.2 Schematic view of the local irradiation setup.

This frontal light distributor was introduced through one of the biopsy channels of the cystoscope. A graduated urothelial probe was introduced through the second biopsy channel in order to measure the distance between the bladder wall and the end of the frontal light diffuser. The knowledge of the power delivered by this light distributor and the use of this graduated probe allowed us to define the irradiance of the light homogeneously illuminating a circular spot of 1 cm^2 (see Figure 19.2).

This procedure allowed determination of the total incident light dose required to bleach the PPIX for the applied illumination parameters. A similar procedure was adopted to illuminate the bladder wall with white light (400–660 nm), except that the standard illumination fiber bundle of the cystoscope was used to guide and deliver the light.

The focal PDT treatments were used to generate information on the optimal light dose and spectroscopy for each set of illumination parameters, the comparative efficiency of the treatment, and its side effects. All lesions were irradiated with a light dose of 100 J/cm^2 (1 cm^2 spots), with both red or "white" light, and the normal mucosa sites with a light dose of 50 J/cm^2 (1 cm^2 spots). The incident fluence rate at the surface of the bladder was 100 mW/cm^2 for both illumination parameters and sites.

19.2.1.5 DETERMINATION OF THE PHOTOBLEACHING DECAY CONSTANT

The photobleaching data of ALA-induced PPIX were fitted with the following equation:

$$I(D) = I_0 e^{-D/k} + IB$$

where
   I_0 is the extrapolated signal above the background fluorescence at D = 0
   I(D) is the fluorescence signal after a given incident light dose D (J/cm^2) (see Figures 19.3 and 19.4)
   k is the photobleaching decay constant
   IB is a light dose-independent background fluorescence

All the data were normalized to the signals measured at D = 0.

19.2.1.6 FOLLOW-UP

Results (tissular effects and side effects of the illumination) were analyzed by means of a white-light cystoscopy at 48 h, 1–2 weeks, and 1 month. After 3 months, the patients underwent an additional HAL cystoscopic examination under white light and blue light (PDD fluorescence diagnosis) and a bladder washing cytology. We considered the absence of tumor and negative cytology a complete response; a reduced number of tumors and positive or negative cytology a partial response; a similar number of tumors and a positive or negative cytology a nonresponse. We considered that an increase in the number of tumors and of the tumor grade as disease

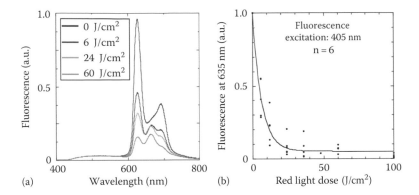

Figure 19.3 (a) Typical PPIX fluorescence emission spectra acquired during local illumination of the bladder wall with light at 635 nm, at various light doses. (a) Each individual fluorescence spectrum is normalized with an external reference (aqueous solution of Rhodamine B), allowing the operator to follow the fluorescence decay during a given illumination. (b) Fluorescence intensity (excitation wavelength: 405 nm) at 635 nm as a function of the light dose received during local illumination at 635 nm. The curve fit is drawn for visual support only.

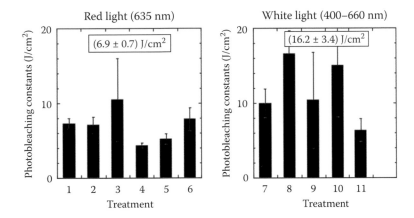

Figure 19.4 Photobleaching constants (J/cm²) measured on individual patients during local illuminations with red (635 nm, left, 6 lesions) or white (400–660 nm, right, 5 lesions) light. The error bars represent the 67% confidence interval.

progression. It is to be noted that in case the treatment is suboptimal or even unsuccessful, it does not result in any additional risk for the group of patients since they would otherwise receive the exact same follow-up.

19.3 RESULTS

19.3.1 LOCAL ILLUMINATIONS

19.3.1.1 LOCAL PDTs

A typical result of a local illumination at 635 nm (one lesion) is given in Figure 19.5.

All patients showed bullous erythema on the irradiation site, which disappeared progressively after 1 month. No ulceration or necrosis was noticed, nor was perforation of the bladder wall, or any kind of systemic side effect. All patients complained of a transient pollakiuria that resolved spontaneously in 1 week, except in one patient who complained about severe pollakiuria and leakage, which resolved spontaneously after 7–10 days. There were no serious side effects that could preclude further clinical testing. There was neither a restriction of bladder capacity nor a development of bladder shrinkage.

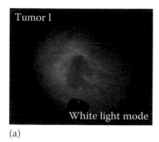

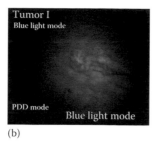

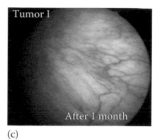

(a)   (b)   (c)

Figure 19.5 Tissular effect of local illumination at 635 nm seen with endoscopic views of the bladder wall before treatment under white light (a), violet fluorescence excitation light (b), or 1 month after treatment (c). The lesion is visible on the center of the images taken before treatment. After treatment, the lesion has disappeared and the urothelium is smooth and uncorrupted.

Table 19.1 Summary of clinical results of focal illuminations (local PDT) in the bladder and follow-up

Time of follow-up	Response	Red-light local PDT (635 nm, n = 5)	White-light local PDT (400–660 nm, n = 5)
1 month	Lost track	1/5	0/5
	No response	1/5	2/5
	Partial response	1/5	1/5
	Complete response	2/5	2/5
3 months	No recurrence	2/4	0/5
	Recurrence (on site)	2/4	4/5
	Recurrence (other site)	0/4	3/5

The bladders of both patients bearing solitary lesion (both illuminated with red light) healed completely at 3 months with no recurrence, negative fluorescence (PDD), and cytology. Results are more difficult to appreciate in patients with multiple disease sites since it was not always straightforward to locate the exact site of an earlier lesion during a follow-up cystoscopy 3 months later. However, a reduction of about 50% in the number of lesions was noticed in this subset of patients.

These experiments made it possible to estimate the bleaching process, both with red and "white" light, and gave information on the optimum light dose, the efficiency of the treatment (comparison between the efficiency of the red and white light), and the side effects. For a full summary of the patients and their treatment response, see Table 19.1. As can be seen, the approach that we describe is not entirely conclusive after 1 month. This applies to both wavelengths, although local treatments in the red might appear slightly better in terms of the number of patients who showed no response to the treatment. This must however be seen with some degree of caution, as the sample is very small, and each patient may thus bear a large impact on any tentative conclusion. At 3 months after the local PDT only in the group treated with red light one patient remained with no lesion but all patients in the white light group showed recurrences either at the treated spot or on another location.

19.3.1.2 PPIX PHOTOBLEACHING MEASUREMENTS

Photobleaching constants were derived from the measurements carried out preceding focal PDTs. They were calculated based on red-light (n = 6) and white-light treatments (n = 5). They were found to be 6.9 ± 0.7 J/cm^2 (red light) and 16.2 ± 3.4 J/cm^2 ("white" light as defined in Figure 19.1).

These results obtained on tumors in urinary bladders during focal illuminations for PDT purposes indicate that red light is two to three times more efficient than "white" light to photobleach PPIX at the surface. Since the penetration of red light in tissues is much better than that of the blue and green components of white light, it is very likely that this better potency of red light is more pronounced within the urothelium and submucosae.

Overall, our results show that HAL PDT has a high degree of tolerability in the bladder, that it results in a general desquamation of the treated area, which leaves the bladder clean, and that the phototoxic effects are well demonstrated, albeit with slightly inconsistent results, probably due to the irregular morphology of the papillomas. Additionally, red light seems to be advantageous (over white light) to achieve the desired tissular effect.

19.4 DISCUSSION

The aim of this study was to assess three illumination "colors" for PDT of NMIBC with Hexylester Aminolevulinate. These local illuminations were carried out in the bladder also to assess the safety of HAL-PDT and to evaluate the photodegradation (photobleaching) of PPIX during irradiation, as a light dosimetry indicator.

The results of these focal illuminations (both to measure the PPIX fluorescence bleaching decay and to treat localized lesions in a controlled manner) demonstrate that the concept can be used and that illuminations in the red domain are more efficient than broadband white-light illuminations. It is very likely that this difference in efficiency results from two main factors. First, in spite of the fact that the "white" light includes violet photons absorbed by the strong PPIX Soret absorption peak, the overall "product" of red laser light and PPIX absorption spectrum is larger. Second, the wavelength-dependent tissue optical properties of the bladder wall which partially impede the penetration of the green and violet part of the white light into deeper tissue layers, thus reducing the fluence rate underneath the urothelium as compared to red light. It is worth noting that the larger total reflectance of the bladder wall in the red increases the "integrating sphere" effect and, consequently, the fluence rate as well as the homogenization of the light in the bladder (van Staveren et al., 1996). It is also clear that recurrences at locations other than those treated do not indicate any kind of treatment failure, but the fact that no lesion was fully treated with white light is also in line with our cautious approach and clear decision to avoid overtreatment at all costs. These facts, combined with the reduced penetrations of the violet and green components of white light, explain why the dose of white light was too low to achieve convincing therapeutic results. Nonetheless, our results were positive and proved that focal HAL-PDT in the bladder is well tolerated, including with red light, with the exception of some transient pain experienced up to several days after the treatment, possibly due to a local inflammatory reaction, as also reported by others (Bader et al., 2013). Some treatment parameters would need refining in order to minimize the recurrences, but overall this approach is safe and efficient. Some degree of doubt will remain after local PDTs as to whether the possible appearance of a lesion at a location that was illuminated is a new lesion or a recurrence of a past lesion. This is especially the case in patients with field cancerization where disease is generally spread over the entire bladder mucosa. In spite of this difficulty, and providing the treatment parameters can be optimized further, this treatment modality appears promising.

We took exploratory steps to expand this concept to whole bladder PDTs with HAL, a concept already reported (with incoherent white light only) by Bader et al. (2013). Three additional patients were treated with an illumination of the entire bladder with red light (635 nm; Ceralas™ PDT 635 Laser Diode (Ceramoptec, Bonn, Germany); 10–40 J/cm²; 10–20 mW/cm²), three with white light (400–660 nm, PDD D-light-system, Karl Storz GmbH, Tuttlingen, Germany; 2–20 J/cm²; 4.5–12 mW/cm²), and one with violet light (407 and 413 nm, Kr-ion laser (Spectra-Physics; Model 171, Mountain View, CA, USA); 5.4 J/cm²; 1.5 mW/cm²), using an isotropic emitter fitted to a three-way Foley bladder catheter (Rüsch) (see Figure 19.6). All had a history of recurrent superficial bladder cancer and presented small lesions (pTaG1-pTaG3). They were thoroughly informed verbally and in writing, and signed an informed consent form. In addition, this study was approved by the ethics committee of Lausanne's CHUV Hospital. Before PDT, the bladder was filled to approximately 70% of its maximum capacity and the light diffuser was positioned in the center of the bladder under direct endoscopic vision and ultrasound monitoring. The bladder was emptied and refilled every 10 min during illumination to avoid absorption of light by urine and hemoglobin (Martoccia et al., 2014).

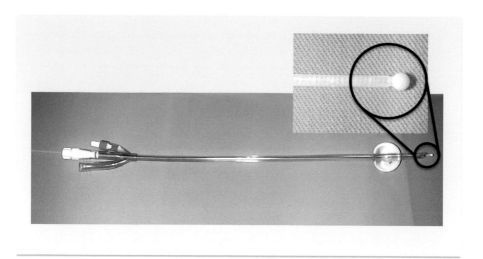

Figure 19.6 Close-up view of the isotropic diffuser (Medlight SA, Ecublens, Switzerland) used for the exploratory whole bladder illuminations. Its outer diameter is 3 mm and the core diameter of the fiber feeding is 1.5 mm.

In spite of the general safety of the PDT procedure, and in spite of the fact that the focal PDTs with higher light doses and light dose rates were found to be well tolerated and therapeutically efficient, patients treated with whole bladder illuminations with red light reported moderate to severe pain during the days following the procedure, which made it ethically difficult to pursue any kind of investigation with this set of parameters. This was reported for only one illumination after whole bladder illuminations with white light and not reported after illumination with violet light (in line with results reported by Bader et al. (2013) and others (Waidelich et al., 2001; Shackley et al., 2002) as well as with results reported in other organs (taking into account the differential absorption coefficient of PPIX in the violet and in the red parts of the spectrum) (Piffaretti et al., 2013). It should be noted that the conservative light doses chosen for whole bladder illuminations in the white (2–20 J/cm^2) are unlikely to be completely efficient, if any of the parameters can be extrapolated from (relatively inefficient) focal illuminations (100 J/cm^2) to whole bladder illuminations. Additionally, it is unlikely that suitable light doses could be achieved in the white range due to extended illumination durations. The use of more powerful white-light sources may help to solve this problem. However, the pain resulting from higher irradiances and doses of white light would have to be assessed.

On the other hand, whole bladder illuminations in the violet (405 nm) appear an interesting option: PPIX's absorption at this wavelength is 25 times higher than in the red (405 nm vs. 635 nm); tissular penetration of violet photons is very limited (several hundreds microns) and in line with the geometry of the lesions considered here; violet-light sources (LEDs, lasers, or filtered lamps) compatible with a clinical environment are widely available. This should make this option not only safe and pain free but also very therapeutically efficient for superficial lesions. A preliminary case of focal PDT is reported in Figure 19.7, showing complete PPIX photobleaching and good tissular reaction without damage to the bladder wall (filtered lamp, 375–440 nm, 190 mW/cm^2 to achieve 50 J/cm^2) or other adverse event/side effect. A follow-up cystoscopy carried out 1 month after treatment confirmed the complete elimination of the lesion.

It is noteworthy that this treatment modality avoids the major disadvantages observed with other modalities and could represent a suitable alternative option for prophylactic, potentially repeated "soft," whole bladder treatments, especially in the case of field-cancerized but non-muscle-invasive disease, thus possibly avoiding radical cystectomy for the patient.

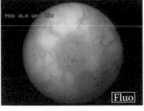 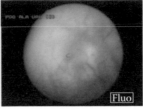 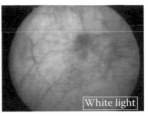

Before PDT PPIX fluorescence	End of PDT PPIX fluorescence photobleaching	After 2 weeks treated lesion zone
(a)	(b)	(c)

Figure 19.7 Endoscopic views of focal bladder illuminations with violet light (375–440 nm) before treatment (a), immediately after illumination with 190 mW/cm^2 to achieve 50 J/cm^2 (b) and 2 weeks after the illumination (c). The center image clearly shows the disappearance (bleaching) of the PPIX fluorescence initially seen on the illuminated site (a). The image at right shows residual inflammation with no lesion (confirmed by biopsy).

19.5 CONCLUSION

Our results open new doors to explore the possibility to realize whole bladder PDTs of superficial non-muscle-invasive bladder cancer with Hexylester Aminolevulinate. We demonstrated that this therapeutic approach needs optimization and showed that PPIX fluorescence decay is a good way to optimize this treatment. We explored the initial aspects of a possible set of treatment parameters (spectral design, irradiance, dose), which avoids risks and side effects otherwise observed when other illumination conditions are chosen. It would be interesting to further develop these concepts concomitantly to standard treatments, such as for instance during follow-up investigations of the bladder of patients who underwent another type of treatment for the very frequently observed recurrent flat lesions. Since this treatment can be repeated several times without known damage to the bladder wall, it could be envisioned as a good additional therapeutic modality.

REFERENCES

Babjuk M et al. (2014) Guidelines on non-muscle-invasive bladder cancer (Ta, T1 and CIS). *European Association of Urology*. http://uroweb.org/guideline/non-muscle-invasive-bladder-cancer/.

Bader MJ et al. (2013) Photodynamic therapy of bladder cancer—A phase I study using hexaminolevulinate (HAL). *Urologic Oncology: Seminars and Original Investigations* **31**(7):1178.

Bray F, Sankila R, Ferlay J, Parkin DM (2002) Estimates of cancer incidence and mortality in Europe in 1995. *European Journal of Cancer* **38**:99.

Herr HW (1997) Natural history of superficial bladder tumours: 10- to 20-year follow-up of treated patients. *World Journal of Urology* **15**:84.

Holmäng S, Hedelin H, Anderström C, Holmberg E, Busch C, Johansson S (1999) Recurrence and progression in low grade papillary urothelial tumors. *Journal of Urology* **162**:702.

Jichlinski P, Leisinger HJ (2001) Photodynamic therapy in superficial bladder cancer: Past. *Present and Future Urology Research* **29**:396.

Jichlinski P et al. (2000) Hexyl ester of ALA induced focal bladder PDT: A feasibility study on small transitional cell carcinoma. *BIOS 2000, SPIE Meeting*, San Jose, CA.

Krieg RC, Fickweiler S, Wolfbels O, Knuechel R (2000) Cell-type specific protoporphyrin IX metabolism in human bladder cancer in vitro. *Photochemistry and Photobiology* **72**(2):226.

Kriegmair M, Baumgartner R, Lumper W, Waidelich R, Hofstetter A (1996) Early clinical experience with 5-aminolevulinic acid for the photodynamic therapy of superficial bladder cancer. *British Journal of Urology* **77**:667.

Kurt KH et al. (2000) Treatment of superficial bladder tumors: Achievement and needs. *European Urology* **37**(Suppl 3):1.

Landis SH, Murray T, Borden S, Wingo PA (1999) Cancer statistics. *CA Cancer Journal of Clinical* **49**:8.

Lange N et al. (1999) Photodetection of early human bladder cancer based on the fluorescence of 5-aminolaevulinic acid hexylester-induced protoporphyrin IX: A pilot study. *British Journal of Cancer* **80**(1/2):185.

Marti A et al. (2003) Comparison of aminolevulinic acid and hexylester aminolevulinate induced protoporphyrin IX distribution in human bladder cancer. *The Journal of Urology* **170**:428.

Martoccia C, Zellweger M, Lovisa B, Jichlinski P, van den Bergh H, Wagnieres G (2014) Optical spectroscopy of the bladder washout fluid to optimize fluorescence cystoscopy with Hexvix®. *Journal of Biomedical Optics* **19**(9):1.

Pang KH, Catto JWF (2013) Bladder Cancer. *Surgery* **31**(10):523.

Piffaretti F et al. (2013) Correlation between protoporphyrin IX fluorescence intensity, photobleaching, pain and clinical outcome of actinic keratosis treated by photodynamic therapy. *Dermatology* **227**(3):214.

Shackley DC et al. (2002) Photodynamic therapy for superficial bladder cancer under local anaesthetic. *BJU International* **89**:665.

Sylvester RJ, van der Meijden APM, Lamm DL (2002) Intravesical *Bacillus* calmette-guerin reduces the risk of progression in patients with superficial bladder cancer: A meta-analysis of the published results of randomized clinical trials. *Journal of Urology* **168**:1964.

van Staveren HJ et al. (1996) Integrating sphere effect in whole-bladder-wall photodynamic therapy: III. Fluence multiplication, optical penetration and light distribution with an eccentric source for human bladder optical properties. *Physics in Medicine and Biology* **41**(4):579.

Wagnières G, Jichlinski P, Lange L, Kucera P, van den Bergh H (2014) Detection of bladder cancer by fluorescence cystoscopy: From bench to bedside—The Hexvix Story. In: *Handbook of Photomedicine* (Hamblin MR, Huang YY, Eds.), pp. 411–426, CRC Press/Taylor & Francis, Boca Raton, FL.

Waidelich R, Stepp H, Baumgartner R, Weninger E, Hofstetter A, Kriegmair M (2001) Clinical experience with 5-aminolevulinic acid and photodynamic therapy for refractory superficial bladder cancer. *Journal of Urology* **165**:1904.

Zellweger M, Grosjean P, Monnier P, van den Bergh H, Wagnières G (1999) Stability of the fluorescence measurement of Foscan® in the normal human oral cavity as an indicator of its content in early cancers of the esophagus and the bronchi. *Photochemical and Photobiology* **69**(5):605.

20

Endoscopic imaging and photodynamic therapy

HARUBUMI KATO, KINYA FURUKAWA, YASUFUMI KATO, JITSUO USUDA, KUNIHARU MIYAJIMA, AND KEISHI OHTANI

20.1 INTRODUCTION

Cancer is a leading cause of death throughout the world, but the early detection and treatment of cancer could save countless lives. Endoscopic cancer imaging is a useful technology for early detection and tumor localization. This technology has already been studied for half a century and continues to be a promising modality for future cancer diagnosis.

Some photosensitizers are known to possess an affinity to tumors and to fluoresce, in addition to exhibiting a photodynamic cytocidal effect upon light stimulation. The authors have studied these technologies for clinical use since 1978. In this chapter, the history of fluorescence bronchoscopy and photodynamic therapy (PDT) for lung cancer and the present status of these technologies and new trials for future endoscopic diagnosis and therapy for patients with lung cancer will be described.

PDT has gained considerable acceptance in many countries as a relatively new minimally invasive modality that can be used for the treatment of malignant tumors. PDT is a high-quality, safe, and inexpensive medical technology for patients. Since the early detection of lung cancer is extremely important, the authors will also discuss methodologies for the early detection and localization of tumors and the future possibility of this technology.

20.2 HISTORY OF FLUORESCENCE BRONCHOSCOPY AND PHOTODYNAMIC THERAPY FOR LUNG CANCER

20.2.1 FLUORESCENCE DIAGNOSIS

There have been several attempts to observe the in vivo fluorescence of hematoporphyrin derivatives (HPD) in order to localize tumors.[1–4] In the early 1970s when many people smoked cigarettes and the death rate from lung cancer was relatively high, x-ray examination and sputum cytology were experimentally introduced as part of lung cancer screening programs for the early detection of lung cancer in Japan. At that time, central-type lung cancers (CLC), consisting of mainly squamous cell carcinoma, could be detected by sputum cytology in the absence of x-ray abnormalities.[5] A bronchoscopy procedure was then indicated as the next step in the screening program for subjects requiring further examination. However, some patients may not have shown any abnormalities because the disease stage was too early to produce cancerous changes in the bronchial mucosa. Fluorescence bronchoscopy was thus developed to overcome these problems.

There are two kinds of endoscopic technologies involving cancer fluorescence: photodynamic diagnosis (PDD) using tumor-specific photosensitizers, and autofluorescence (AF) diagnosis (AFD). Tumor-specific photosensitizers are used for PDD. Historically, an arc lamp and a krypton ion laser were used to excite the photosensitizers. HPD was used as a photosensitizer in the late 1970s and in the 1980s. Several problems concerning the specificity of fluorescence at the tumor were encountered, as the fluorescence was difficult to observe with the naked eye because of its relative weakness. Furthermore, AF from normal mucosa as well as the nonspecific optical absorption of noncancerous tissues surrounding the cancer lesion, such as inflammatory tissue, produced difficulties. Therefore, it was necessary to use an image intensifier to magnify the weak fluorescence in the tumor, and spectroscopic analysis was needed to distinguish the AF of normal mucosa from the specific fluorescence of the photosensitizer in the cancer tissue, since the images were originally viewed in black and white at that time. The present PDD system utilizing a recent advanced spectroscopic technology has overcome the issues created by AF interference from normal mucosa. Since the excretion of drugs from normal tissue is faster than that from tumor tissue, the nonspecific absorption of normal tissue can be avoided by waiting for the excretion of the photosensitizer from normal tissue to occur, which requires approximately 48 h after the intravenous injection of the drug. Thus, the present PDD system has become practical for the detection of early-stage lung cancer including invisible superficial central-type early-stage lung cancer (CESLC) such as carcinoma in situ (*Cis*), and the area surrounding the superficial invasion can be seen more clearly than with white light (WL) bronchoscopy.

These imaging technologies can now be applied for the localization of superficial early-stage cancerous lesions and for making preoperative decisions regarding resection lines as well as for evaluating the response to PDT by visualizing the photobleaching of the photosensitizing drugs.

20.2.2 PRESENT EQUIPMENT FOR PDD AND AFD: THE PENTAX SAFE-3000 SYSTEM

The Pentax SAFE-3000 system (Tokyo, Japan) is a videoendoscopy-based AF system containing a full color CCD (Figure 20.1), and two light sources are available. One is a xenon lamp for white light (WL) imaging, and the other is a semiconductor laser diode that emits a 408-nm wavelength light for illumination. AF is collected using a single high-sensitivity color CCD sensor covering the fluorescence emission spectrum from 430 to 700 nm. In the AF mode, the excitation light illuminates the target from the tip of the scope and is reflected by a beam splitter and collected and transmitted by the light guide. The objective lens functions

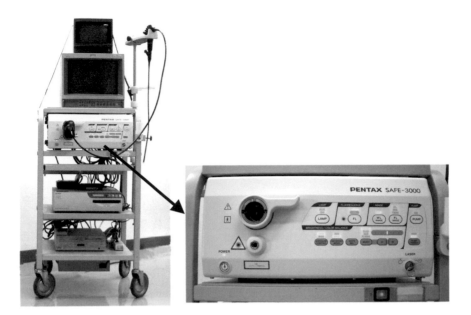

Figure 20.1 The SAFE-3000is a videoendoscopy-based AF system containing a full-color CCD. With this system, normal bronchial tissue emits an intense green autofluorescence when excited with blue light from a diode laser (408 nm), whereas abnormal tissue lacks the green autofluorescence because of differences in its tissue structure.

to eliminate the wavelength of excitation light and captures only the AF from the object. Normal bronchial mucosa shows a green AF when excited by a blue light from a diode laser (408 nm), while areas of cancer and dysplasia show a decreased AF, or defects in the AF (cold spots) that can be diagnosed as abnormal (positive) (Figure 20.2). The WL and AF modes can be easily changed using a hand-switch that makes it possible to alternate between WL and excitation light at a high speed, and also allows for real-time dual imaging, in which both the WL and AF images of the target can be displayed simultaneously on the monitor and both images can be recorded separately through one full-color CCD (Figure 20.3). However, areas with bleeding or hyperemia, since blood absorbs at 408-nm wavelength because of the high content of hemoglobin, can appear as false-positive findings.

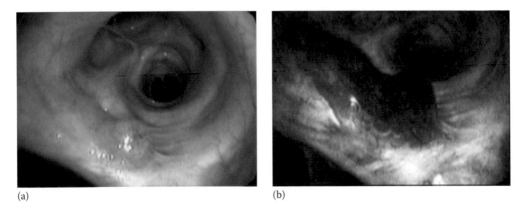

(a)   (b)

Figure 20.2 A 68-year-old man with a centrally located lung cancer in whom a bronchoscopy revealed a nodular lesion. (a) Nodular-type squamous cell carcinoma of the right B3 bronchus. (b) Negative autofluorescence was observed at the cancer lesion using the SAFE-3000 system.

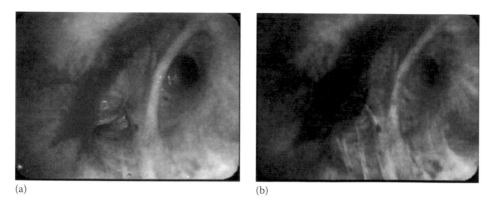

(a) (b)

Figure 20.3 A 72-year-old man. (a) Nodular-type squamous cell carcinoma in the left upper lobe bronchus. (b) Negative autofluorescence was observed at the tumor using the SAFE-3000 system.

20.2.3 PDD

Tumor localization is critically important for the success of PDT for diagnosing CESLC.[6-8] In addition to advances in fluorescence bronchoscopy (FB) and improved photosensitizers, the precise evaluation of the tumor borders and improved therapeutic techniques for CESLC can improve the therapeutic outcome of PDT.

The authors previously assessed the usefulness of a photodynamic diagnosis (PDD) for CESLC using the FB SAFE-3000 system and the photosensitizer talaporfin sodium (Laserphyrin®, or NPe6) as a means of accurately defining the tumor margins prior to PDT. As the tumor extent can be difficult to identify clearly using white light bronchoscopy, and in order to irradiate the tumor with the therapeutic laser accurately, the exact tumor area should be determined before PDT. PDD (SAFE-3000) was performed 4 h after the intravenous injection (i.v.) of Laserphyrin® (40 mg/m²) to observe the red fluorescence of Laserphyrin that had concentrated in the tumor tissue and that had been enhanced using a diode laser (408 nm). The fluorescence of Laserphyrin® can be clearly recognized in the tumor area (Figure 20.4b).

Immediately after PDT, the efficacy of the photosensitization caused by laser irradiation can be evaluated by observing the destruction of the fluorescence of Laserphyrin by photobleaching using this system (Figure 20.4c). If red fluorescence is still observed as a result of insufficient photobleaching, additional laser irradiation may be necessary. It is often difficult to decide whether additional laser irradiation in patients that have larger tumors is needed. In such cases, assessment using the photobleaching phenomenon might be helpful.

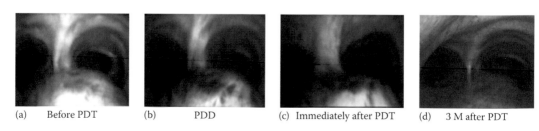

(a) Before PDT (b) PDD (c) Immediately after PDT (d) 3 M after PDT

Figure 20.4 A 63-year-old man. (a) WL bronchoscopy shows a superficial squamous cell carcinoma at the carina. (h) Photodynamic diagnosis showing the red fluorescence of Laserphyrin at the tumor just before PDT. (c) Photobleaching, or the loss of red fluorescence from the tumor, was confirmed using PDD with the SAFE-3000 system immediately after NPe6-PDT. (d) A CR was achieved 3 months after PDT.

These applications enable the indications for PDT to be better determined and provide more exact information regarding the area of treatment, as well as determining the optimal dose of laser illumination. The optimized procedures should be more effective for avoiding the possibility of local recurrence after PDT.

20.2.4 AFD

The detection of CESLC is impossible based on radiological findings alone. Bronchoscopy is an alternative modality for the early diagnosis of CESLC. Both advances in bronchoscopy and the expanding prevalence of sputum cytology have helped to increase the detection of CESLC.[5] However, conventional bronchoscopy is sometimes insufficient for the early localization of intraepithelial lesions. AFD has been increasingly adopted since the early 1990s, and several studies have shown that this technique improves the sensitivity of the detection of cancerous and precancerous lesions of the airway, compared with WL bronchoscopy, especially in cases of early intraepithelial stage lesions. AF bronchoscopy (AFB) has been widely used to detect subtle abnormal areas of the bronchial mucosa that sometimes cannot be recognized using conventional bronchoscopy.[9] AFB is based on the principle that the normal bronchial tissue emits green AF (500–600 nm) when excited by blue light, while malignant tissue lacks green AF.[10] Endogenous molecules that reportedly can cause AF upon light exposure include nicotinamide-adenine dinucleotide phosphate, and flavin adenine dinucleotide, as well as collagen and fibronectin.[11,12] Abnormal sites can therefore be discriminated from normal areas by examining differences in the intensity of green AF. AFB has been reported to have a higher sensitivity for *Cis* and dysplasia and to contribute to an objective diagnosis of the tumor extent on the bronchial surface.[9] The earlier AF systems were developed using fiberoptic bronchoscopes, the LIFE system, and the Pentax Safe 1000. With the advancement of charge-coupled device (CCD) sensor technology and the more widespread use of video bronchoscopy, AF systems with videobronchoscopes have now been developed.

20.3 OPTICAL COHERENCE TOMOGRAPHY FOR DEPTH DIAGNOSIS

Evaluating the depth of tumor invasion for the precise staging of lung cancer is also important particularly for *Cis*, which is well suited for PDT. Although two kinds of imaging technologies, endobronchial ultrasound (EBUS) and optical coherence tomography (OCT), are available, OCT produces much better images than EBUS. The initial OCT tools (Pentax SOCT-1000, Tokyo, 1998) are shown in Figure 20.5. The OCT probe is 1.5–0.75 mm in diameter, and the laser beam is used for excitation. Figure 20.6 shows that no abnormality is visible using bronchoscopy; however, AFB shows an abnormal AF defect. OCT imaging shows clear intraepithelial invasion, and a well-preserved basement membrane can be recognized. Carcinoma in situ was diagnosed by biopsy in the same area. PDT was regarded as being indicated for this case with the intention of achieving a complete cure.[9,13–17]

The authors concluded that OCT provides a clearer image of CESLC, such as the intraepithelial growth of the tumor (*Cis*), compared to images obtained using ultrasound echography. Recently, lung cancer screening using computed tomography (CT) has become widespread throughout the world. Peripheral small nodules, such as early-stage preinvasive adenocarcinoma and adenocarcinoma in situ, are easily detected using CT. Figure 20.7 shows a case of bronchioloalveolar cell carcinoma (BAC, adenocarcinoma in situ), including the CT findings showing ground glass opacity (GGO), the resected specimen, and the cytology and histology results. However, although a precise diagnosis is not always easy, the future application of OCT technology is promising for diagnosis using imaging because of its noninvasive nature. Figure 20.8 shows OCT images of the BAC tissue and the tissue of normal alveoli. A clear difference is apparent. The normal tissue has a regular honeycomb structure, while the BAC tissue shows irregular thickening of the alveolar wall, dilatation of the alveolar interstitial tissue, and an irregular alveolar cavity.

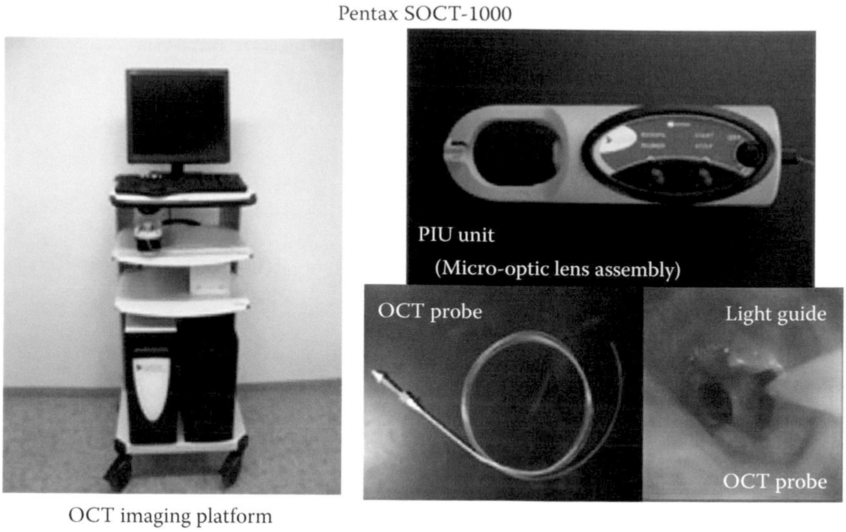

Pentax SOCT-1000

PIU unit
(Micro-optic lens assembly)

OCT probe

Light guide

OCT probe

OCT imaging platform

Figure 20.5 Tool used for OCT. Since the OCT probe is only 1.5–0.75 mm in diameter, it can be inserted into thin peripheral bronchi.

OCT findings of carcinoma in situ, squamous cell carcinoma

Right B1a and B1b spur, 68-year old man

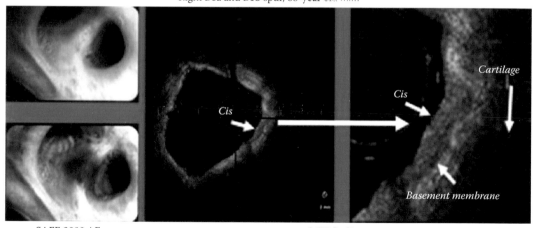

Cis

Cis

Cartilage

Basement membrane

SAFE 3000 AF

OCT findings

Figure 20.6 The left upper photo shows a white light image of a CESLC, which is difficult to recognize. The left lower photo is an autofluorescence image showing abnormal negative autofluorescence at the lesion. Optical coherent tomography (OCT) is effective for clarifying the depth of mucosal invasion. A well-preserved basement membrane is visible in this image. The histological specimen was found to be a carcinoma in situ.

Adenocarcinoma in situ (AIS)
1.5cm stage IA (pT1N0M0), 75-year old man

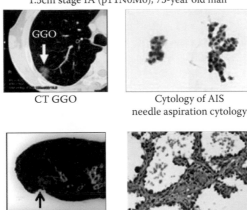

CT GGO

Cytology of AIS
needle aspiration cytology

Resected specimen of AIS

Histology of AIS

Figure 20.7 A peripheral-type, early-stage lung cancer that was identified as a bronchioloalveolar cell carcinoma (BAC, adenocarcinoma in situ). A computed tomography (CT) image shows ground-glass opacity (GGO) (left upper photo). The left lower photo shows the resected specimen, and the right photos show the cytological and histological features.

Possibility of definitive diagnosis by OCT

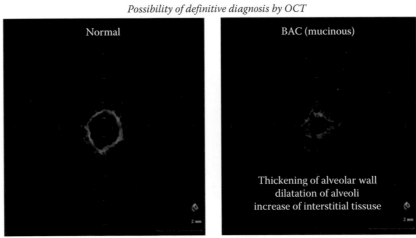

Pentax SOCT-2000

Figure 20.8 OCT images of BAC show differences between normal alveoli and cancerous alveoli. The normal alveoli have a honeycomb structure with uniform and thin walls. BAC shows uneven findings, such as a thickening of the alveolar wall, dilatation of the alveoli, and/or an increase in of interstitial tissue. Since the OCT procedure is noninvasive and produces a clear image, it is regarded as a promising technology.

20.4 PHOTODYNAMIC THERAPY

The presently used clinical applications of PDT were first reported in the 1970s by Thomas J. Dougherty et al. The effectiveness of PDT for the treatment of human metastatic breast cancer was first reported by Dougherty.[18] Since the beginning of its use in the late 1970s, international meetings concerning PDT have been held periodically, including both researchers and clinical doctors. These meetings were mainly held in North America, and many basic studies and clinical experiences have been discussed and disseminated internationally. In the early 1980s, HPD was used as the photosensitizer and an argon dye laser was used as the light source. In March 1980, a 74-year-old male patient with squamous CESLC detected by sputum cytology was successfully treated using PDT for the first time. The patient died at the age of 78 years, 4 years after the PDT, and an autopsy showed a complete cure (Figure 20.9).[9] An excimer dye laser and a YAG-OPO laser were also developed as laser light sources. Several kinds of new photosensitizers were also developed during these years. PDT has now been used clinically throughout the world as both an approved and as an investigational treatment for patients with malignant tumors.

The International Organization of PDT, International Photodynamic Association (IPA) was established by Professor Yoshihiro Hayata and Dr. Thomas J. Dougherty in Tokyo in 1986, and the 1st World Conference of IPA (WCIPA) was held in Tokyo in the same year; the WCIPA has since been held biennially. In 1988, a multicenter study on PDT for CESLC performed by the PDT cancer research group of the Ministry of Health and Welfare demonstrated that the rates of complete response (CR) were 77.3% (51/66 lesions) overall and 100% in cases with lesions of less than 1.0 cm in diameter (28 lesions); the recurrence rate was 15.7% (8/51 lesions).[13] Thereafter, the first prospective phase II multi-institutional study of PDT for early-stage, central-type lung cancer, esophageal cancer, gastric cancer, gynecological cervix cancer, and bladder cancer was conducted using porfimer sodium (HPD, Photofrin®; Wyeth Japan K.K., Tokyo, Japan) using either an argon dye laser (ADL) or an excimer dye laser (EDL) from June 1989 to February 1992.[16] The endpoint of these studies was the effectiveness of PDT, and an overall excellent PDT efficacy was demonstrated (CR rate: 84.8%, recurrence rate: 10.0%). The Japanese government approved the use of this modality using an EDL or ADL combined with porfimer sodium for early stage cancers of the lung, esophagus, stomach, and cervix in October 1994, and reimbursement through the National Health Insurance program began in April 1996.

First PDT case of early-stage lung cancer, 1980

74-year old man, Right B2b, squamous cell carcinoma

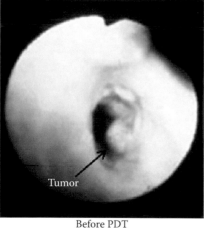

Before PDT

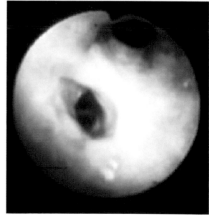

After PDT

Figure 20.9 A 74-year-old man. A tiny squamous cell carcinoma was detected using sputum cytology and was localized in the right B2b using a fiberoptic bronchoscope. A curative outcome was obtained using PDT performed with HPD and an argon dye laser in 1980. This was the first case of CESLC to be treated with PDT in the world.

As a second-generation drug, mono-l-aspartyl chlorin(e6) was developed by Japan Petrol Co. Ltd., Tokyo, Japan, in the mid-1980s after the completion of basic studies performed by Prof. David Kessel of Wayne State University. A phase II multi-institutional study for CESLC started in 1997, and the government approved its clinical use, enabling a better outcome, in 2003.[17] Regarding the absorption wavelength for Laserphyrin®, the longest absorption band is 664 nm, which is 34 nm longer than that of Photofrin; the extinction coefficient of Laserphyrin® at 664 nm is about 10 times higher than that of Photofrin, and it further has the advantage of avoiding the absorption band of hemoglobin. Furthermore, Laserphyrin® is rapidly eliminated from the skin, resulting in low photosensitivity to sunlight.

20.4.1 INDICATIONS FOR PDT FOR THE TREATMENT OF LUNG CANCER

The best candidates for PDT are lung cancer patients with CESLC because of the good endoscopic accessibility, and careful patient selection is important to achieve complete remission. Nagamoto et al.[14] demonstrated that no lymph node involvement was found in 59 cancers with a longitudinal extent of less than 20 mm, and another histological study using serial block sectioning showed that there was no nodal involvement in any CIS cases.[15] Furuse et al.[16] demonstrated that the length of the longitudinal tumor extent was the only independent predictor for a CR after PDT and that lesions less than 1.0 cm in diameter showed a 100% CR. According to these data, therapy for a CR requires the following endoscopic conditions: (1) no evidence of lymph node metastasis, (2) a superficial lesion with a maximum diameter of less than 1.0 cm, (3) no invasion into or beyond the cartilaginous layer, (4) a squamous cell carcinoma histology, and (5) the location of the lesion in a position that can be easily irradiated with a laser. The Japan Society of Lung Cancer Society set these criteria for PDT in 1995. Accordingly, 5 types of lesions were proposed to be candidates for treatment with PDT including: invisible type, flat type, nodular type, polypoid type, and mixed type.[19]

20.4.2 PDT USING PORFIMER SODIUM AND AN EXCIMER-DYE LASER FOR THE TREATMENT OF EARLY-STAGE LUNG CANCER

The laser light delivery system consists of an excimer laser, which emits a pulse laser beam, coupled to a dye laser (EDL; Hamamatsu Photonics Ltd., Hamamatsu, Japan).[20] The excimer laser uses a gas mixture containing 0.9% Xe, 0.1% HCl, and 99% helium at a pressure of 2 atm. The optimal performance of this laser is obtained at 30 mJ/pulse with a full width half maximum pulse duration of 10.9 ns at 308 nm. The XeCl excimer laser (308 nm) can be coupled to a pumped dye system, which contains 2 M Rhodamine B dye in ethanol, to convert the beam to 630 nm. The beams from the EDL are focused into 400-µm fused silica fibers (Moritex Ltd., Nagoya, Japan), the tips of which have been fitted with microlenses to improve the homogeneity of the light distribution throughout the treatment field. A total number of 145 patients with 191 endoscopic CESLC lesions underwent PDT using porfimer sodium and EDL during the period from February 1980 to April 2001 at Tokyo Medical University. The PDT procedures were performed using a combination of porfimer sodium, which is selectively taken up by tumor tissue, and an EDL. Laser irradiation was performed via a quartz fiber inserted through the biopsy channel of the endoscope at 48 h after the intravenous administration of 2.0 mg/kg of porfimer sodium. The total energy of the laser irradiation was 100 J/cm², and the use of energy levels in this range did not cause any heat damage or other adverse effects to the tissue. The required duration of irradiation was usually 10–20 min. Among the patients who underwent treatment, 93 patients with 114 lesions were followed up long term. The CR and 5-year survival rates of patients with initial lesions of less than 1.0 cm in diameter were 92.8% (77/83) and 57.9%; meanwhile, among patients with initial lesions of diameter of 1.0 cm or greater, the rates were 58.1% (18/31) and 59.3%, respectively. A significant difference in efficacy was observed between the 2 groups ($P < 0.001$). Next, the cases with initial tumors with a diameter of less than 1.0 cm that suffered recurrences after an initial CR were examined. Recurrences after a CR were observed in 9 of the 77 lesions (11.7%) that were less than 1.0 cm in diameter. To further reduce the recurrence rate, an accurate understanding of the tumor extent and the depth of the bronchogenic carcinoma prior to performing PDT is needed.

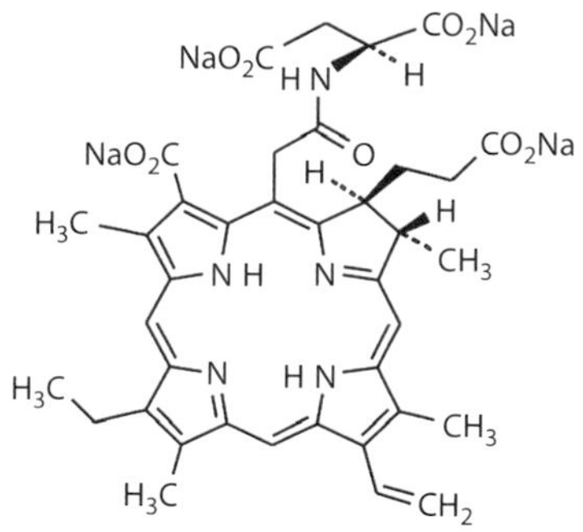

Figure 20.10 Chemical structure of talaporfin sodium (NPe6, Laserphyrin®). This compound is an effective photosensitizer with a major absorption band at 664 nm and a molecular weight of 799.69 (unit?).

20.4.3 PDT USING LASERPHYRIN® AND A DIODE LASER FOR CESLC

Talaporfin sodium has a molecular weight of 799.7, and its structure is shown in Figure 20.10. The characteristics of this photosensitizer include a low degree of skin photosensitivity[21] and a high degree of affinity for malignant tissues.[22] Kessel at al. demonstrated that the pharmakinetics kinetics of talaporfin sodium elimination from the plasma were consistent with a half-life (T1/2ß) of approximately 134 h,[23] which is much shorter than that for porfimer sodium (approximately 250 h); thus, Laserphyrin® is eliminated almost twice as rapidly as Photofrin. A diode laser system (Panalas 6405; Matsushita Industrial Equipment Co., Ltd., Osaka, Japan) was developed for PDT applications using Laserphyrin®.[24] The laser wavelength was adjusted to 664 nm, and the power output was variable within a range of 50–500 mW at the fiber tip in a continuous wave (CW) mode. The laser system weighs 20 kg and is portable. It runs on a 100-V current. This system generates a laser beam with a wavelength (664 ± 2 nm) suitable for the light activation of Laserphyrin®, providing a high therapeutic efficiency.

A phase I clinical study using Laserphyrin® and a diode laser (Panalas 6405) for CESLC was performed between April 1995 and December 1996 at Tokyo Medical University.[25] There were no serious abnormal subjective or objective adverse drug reactions as well as no abnormal laboratory findings, including skin photosensitivity.

20.5 PHASE II CLINICAL STUDY

A phase II clinical study was performed to investigate the antitumor effects and safety of Laserphyrin® PDT in patients with endoscopically evaluated CESLC[17] using an administration dosage, the safety and efficacy of which had been verified in a previous phase I clinical study. As mentioned before, a phase II clinical study on porfimer sodium performed by Furuse et al.[16] demonstrated that the longitudinal length of the tumor extent was the only independent predictor of a CR. Therefore, we decided that the tumor size should not be more than 2.0 cm in diameter and that the peripheral margin of these lesions must be accessible by observation so as to provide easy irradiation with the laser light. The study was a nationwide, multicenter study funded by the Ministry of Health and Welfare and was designed as an open-label clinical trial. A total of 10 institutions were enrolled and participated between October 1997 and March 2000. Based on the results of the phase I clinical study in patients with early-stage lung cancer (ESLC) (CR rate, 87.5%),[25] the expected efficacy rate of this study was set at 90.0%. Setting the range of the 95.0% confidence interval for the expected efficacy rate at 0.2, the required number of patients was calculated to be 35 cases. Furthermore, assuming that 10.0%–15.0% of the patients would be unable to complete the treatment, the planned number of patients was set at 40 cases. In the phase I clinical study, the optimal parameters for good safety and efficacy were suggested to be the intravenous administration of Laserphyrin® (40 mg/m²) followed by laser irradiation (100 J/cm²) using a diode laser apparatus at 4 h after administration.[25] Therefore, the dosage and administration were set accordingly. One vial of Laserphyrin® containing 100 mg was dissolved in 4 mL of physiological saline, and the defined dose (40 mg/m^2) was slowly injected intravenously. At 4 h after administration, a laser beam with a wavelength of 664 nm was used to irradiate the tumor site endoscopically using a directionally aimed quartz fiber (power density: 150 mW/cm^2, energy level: 100 J/cm^2). The output power and wavelength of the laser were determined before and after irradiation using a power meter to confirm the performance of the laser apparatus. The back of the hand was exposed to sunlight for 5 min to observe skin photosensitivity (e.g., erythema), followed by photography at 1 h after the exposure for inclusion in the medical record. This test was performed before administration and at 2 weeks after administration. If photosensitivity was observed, the test was repeated every several days until it disappeared; in the interim, the patient was asked to avoid direct sunlight and intense incandescent light. Among the 41 patients (46 lesions) who were registered in the trial, one patient refused to receive Laserphyrin®. Therefore, Laserphyrin® was administered to 40 patients (45 lesions) (Table 20.1). All the patients except one were male, and the median age was 67 years. The performance status was 0 or 1 for all but 1 patient. The histological type was squamous cell carcinoma in all the patients, and all the lesions were carcinomas in situ (CIS) or early invasive carcinomas. There were 19 cases of clinical stage 0 (CIS) (23 lesions) and 21 cases of stage I (22 lesions). Fifteen cases were not considered to be surgical candidates because of underlying cardiopulmonary dysfunction, and 25 cases refused surgery and wished to receive PDT. Twenty-one patients had received no previous therapy, and 15 patients had received surgery before PDT. The maximum tumor diameters were less than 1.0 cm for 33 lesions, more than 1.0 cm but less than 2.0 cm for 10 lesions, and more than 2.0 cm for 2 lesions. The evaluation committee judged 5 patients

Table 20.1 Backgrounds of the patients

Total number of patients treated	40 patients (45 lesions)		
Age	Mean: 65.9 years, Median: 67 years (48–77 years)		
Height	Mean: 162.3 cm (143.8–180 cm)		
Weight	Mean: 56.8 kg (39.0–76 kg)		
Sex	Male	39 patients	(44 lesions)
	Female	1	(1)
Performance status (ECOG PS)	0	26 patients	
	1	13	
	2	1	
Disease stage	0	19 patients	(23 lesions)
	I	21	(22)
Previous therapy for other lesion	None	21 patients	
	Surgery	9	
	Surg. + Rad. + Chemo.	1	
	Surg. + Chemo.	1	
	Surg. + Chemo. + PDT	2	
	Surg. + PDT	2	
	Rad.	1	
	PDT	2	
	Rad. + Chemo. + Electric cauterization	1	
Maximum tumor size	<0.5 cm	7 lesions	
	0.5–0.9 cm	26	
	1.0–1.4 cm	10	
	1.5–1.9 cm	0	
	2.0 cm	2	

Table 20.2 Antitumor effects by lesion and by patient

Classification	Eligible	CR	PR	NC	PD	NE	CR rate (%)	95.0% confidence rate (%)	Response rate (%)
Lesion	39	33	4	2	0	0	84.6	69.5–94.1	94.9
Patient	35	29	4	2	0	0	82.9	66.4–93.4	94.3

(6 lesions) to be ineligible for inclusion in the efficacy evaluation based on the inclusion criteria, so 35 eligible patients (39 lesions) were ultimately assessed. Among these patients, one patient who had two lesions was regarded as an eligible patient with one eligible lesion, since one of the two lesions that was treated with PDT was an eligible lesion, but the other lesion was ineligible because it was a benign tumor.

The antitumor effects classified according to lesion and according to patient characteristics are shown in Table 20.2. On a per lesion basis, the CR rate was 84.6% (33/39 lesions) and the overall response rate was 94.9% (37/39 lesions). On a per patient basis, the CR rate was 82.9% (29/35 patients) and the overall response rate was 94.3% (33/35 patients). Since the CR rate exceeded the lower limit of the expected CR rate (80.0%), the study supported the efficacy of Laserphyrin®. These encouraging results were similar to the data obtained in a previous phase II clinical study examining porfimer sodium (84.8% of lesions)[16] and data published by Tokyo Medical University (81.1% of cases)[26] (Figures 20.11 and 20.12). There were no serious adverse effects of grade 3 or more (Table 20.3). Only a few cases showed grade 2 adverse effects, such as an increased C-reactive protein level, increased sputum, coughing, fever, or neutropenia. These reactions seemed to be caused by the PDT procedure and by the repeated bronchoscopic examinations and were not considered to be directly related to the use of Laserphyrin® and diode laser irradiation. Among the grade 1 reactions, "itching of the forehead and the backs of both hands" occurred in 1 patient, since the patient had exposed himself to direct sunlight before the skin photosensitivity test. The results of the first skin photosensitivity test are shown in Table 20.4. Twenty-eight of the 33 patients (84.8%) in whom the first skin photosensitivity test was positive no longer exhibited photosensitivity at 14 days after drug administration. Five patients showed a reaction to light (minimal visible erythema in 3 patients; deep, clearly defined erythema in 1 patient, and blister formation in 1 patient), but the disappearance of the photosensitivity was confirmed in all 5 patients when a second test was performed within 7 days thereafter.

PDT for early-stage lung cancer

Left main bronchus, 63-year old man, squamous cell carcinoma

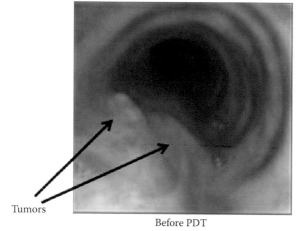

Tumors

Before PDT   3 months after PDT

Figure 20.11 A case of CESLC in the left main bronchus. The lesion was cured completely using PDT performed with Laserphyrin® and a diode laser.

PDT for early-stage lung cancer

Left B1 + 2 and 3 spur, 79-year old man, squamous cell carcinoma

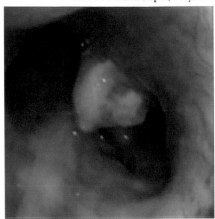 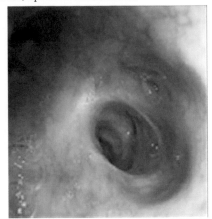

Before PDT   3 months after PDT

Figure 20.12 A case of CESLC at the spur of the left B1 + 2 and 3 bronchi. The lesion was a squamous cell carcinoma. A complete cure was obtained using PDT performed with Laserphyrin® and a diode laser.

Table 20.3 Adverse drug reactions (signs and symptoms)

Item	Number of patients evaluated	Incidence (%)	Grade			
			1	2	3	4
Pruritus cutaneous[a]	40	2 (5.0)	2	0	0	0
Itching of forehead and backs of both hands[a]	40	1 (2.5)	1	0	0	0
Blisters[a]	40	1 (2.5)	1	0	0	0
Coughing[b]	40	6 (15.0)	5	1	0	0
Increased sputum[b]	40	11 (27.5)	9	2	0	0
Bloody sputum[b]	40	10 (25.5)	10	0	0	0
Sorethroat[a]	40	2 (5.0)	2	0	0	0
Chest discomfort[a]	40	1 (2.5)	1	0	0	0
Fever[c]	40	4 (10.0)	3	1	0	0
Abnormal ECG	37	1 (2.5)	—	—	—	—

[a] These items were graded by the attending physician according to a 4-grade scale (Grade 1: mild, 2: moderate, 3: severe, 4: serious), since these items are not specified in the "Guidelines for Assessment of Adverse Drug Reactions" established by the Japan Society of Clinical Oncology.

[b] These items were graded according to the 4-grade scale specified in the protocol, since those are not specified in the "Guidelines for Assessment of Adverse Drug Reactions" established by the Japan Society of Clinical Oncology.

[c] The item was graded according to the "Guidelines for Assessment of Adverse Drug Reactions" established by the Japan Society of Clinical Oncology.

—, not graded.

In a phase II study using porfimer sodium,[16] a toxicity assessment showed grade 2 adverse reactions consisting of a transient elevation of alanine transaminase (ALT) (1.9%), allergic reaction (3.8%), pulmonary toxicity including exertional dyspnea and fever caused by bronchitis and obstructive pneumonia (7.7%), and sunburn (1.9%). The ALT elevations and allergic reactions might have been caused by the hydrophobic property of porfimer sodium, but our study showed no liver dysfunction and no allergic reactions of more than grade 2 proposed to be due to the hydrophilic property of Laserphyrin®. Grade 2 pulmonary

Table 20.4 Results of the first skin photosensitivity test

| Item | Days after administration (days) | | | | | | | | | | Total |
	9	10	11	12	13	14	15	16	17	18	
Number of patients tested	1	—	—	1	1	30	1	4	1	1	40
Negative reaction	1	—	—	1	0	26	1	4	1	1	35
Positive reaction	0	—	—	0	1	4	0	0	0	0	5

toxicity was seen in 7.5% (3 out of 40 cases) in our study, which was similar to the results of the study using porfimer sodium. The most frequent adverse effect of porfimer sodium was skin photosensitization, which was observed in 28.8% (grade 1) and 1.9% (grade 2) of the patients. However, our study showed a very low incidence of skin photosensitivity, with 10.0% (4 out of 40 cases) experiencing grade 1 and 0% experiencing grade 2 or higher photosensitivity. Furthermore, the photosensitive reactivity of the patients' skin to light had typically disappeared by 2 weeks after administration (84.8%) and had disappeared in the remaining patients by 3 weeks after administration. The number of days required for the disappearance of the reaction to light was consistent with the results obtained in the skin photosensitivity test conducted in the phase I clinical study. For PDT using Laserphyrin®, the incidence of hypersensitivity to light was very low and hyperpigmentation was not observed, while hypersensitivity to light was frequently observed in patients treated with porfimer sodium. Thus, the phase II clinical study demonstrated excellent antitumor effects and the safety of Laserphyrin® according to the administration dosage verified in the previous phase I clinical study, in patients with endoscopically evaluated ESLC. Therefore, the Japanese government approved second-generation PDT using a diode laser combined with talaporfin sodium (Laserphyrin) for the treatment of CESLC in October 2003, and reimbursement through the National Health Insurance program began in June 2004. Currently, second-generation PDT is the standard PDT modality for the treatment of central-type, early superficial squamous cell lung carcinoma in Japan. Figure 20.13 shows PDT taking place in a case with multiple primary early-stage squamous cell carcinomas.

20.5.1 PDT FOR ADVANCED LUNG CANCER

PDT for advanced lung cancer can be divided into three categories: palliative PDT, preoperative neoadjuvant PDT, and PDT in combination with chemo/radiotherapy. In patients complaining of dyspnea because of tracheobronchial obstruction or stenosis as a result of an advanced inoperable tumor, the opening of the bronchi is required as a palliative treatment to improve the patient's quality of life (QOL). Since 1980, advanced lung cancers have been treated using palliative laser therapy and with PDT, for the purpose of opening the tracheobronchial stenosis and the obstruction. Several papers have been published concerning the use of PDT in cases with advanced lung cancer.[27–29] The authors reported that an overall effective opening of the bronchi was achieved for 61 of 81 lesions (75%) treated using PDT, compared with 143 of 177 lesions (81%) treated using an Nd-YAG laser.[30] Thus, PDT seems to be useful for the treatment of obstructions in the lobar and segmental bronchi. PaO_2 data was evaluated before and after PDT in 15 cases, and the average PaO_2 before PDT was found to be 66 mmHg, while that after PDT had increased to 82 mmHg (Figure 20.14). In patients with advanced lung cancer, the improvement in the surgical results to reduce the resection volume and to increase the indications for resection when used in combination with PDT was evaluated.[31,32] In some cases, the need for a pneumonectomy performed using conventional surgery was revised downward to a lobectomy after PDT, and some inoperable patients with wide hilar invasion became treatable using a pneumonectomy or lobectomy (Figures 20.15 and 20.16). Thus, preoperative PDT is helpful for improving the patient's eligibility for surgical techniques.

PDT for multiple early stage lung cancer, squamous cell carcinoma

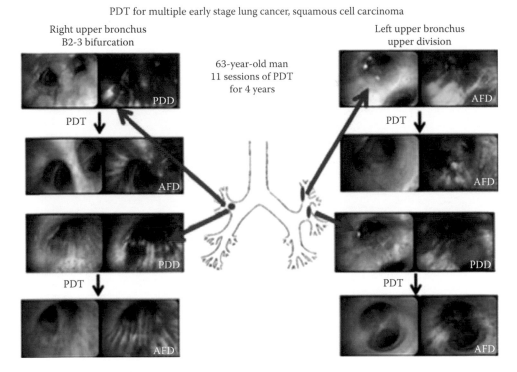

Right upper bronchus
B2-3 bifurcation

63-year-old man
11 sessions of PDT
for 4 years

Left upper bronchus
upper division

Figure 20.13 This case had multiple primary lesions. Therefore, this patient was not a candidate for surgery. Eleven sessions of PDT performed with Laserphyrin and a diode laser were completed over a period of 3 years, and a complete cure was nearly obtained. However, some lesions located in peripheral bronchi require further PDT.

PDT for advanced lung cancer improving QOL

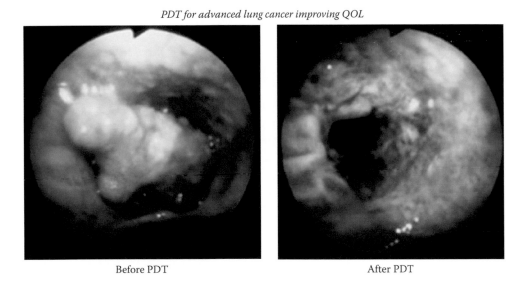

Before PDT   After PDT

Figure 20.14 The left main bronchus has been completely obstructed by the tumor. The bronchus was successfully opened using PDT performed with HPD and an argon dye laser.

Bronchoplasty after preoperative PDT

78-year old man, squamous cell carcinoma stage IIA (T1N1M0)

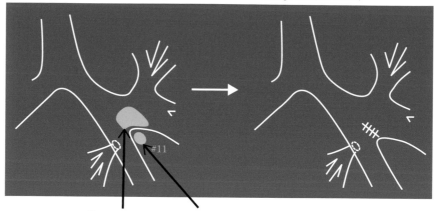

Primary tumor   Metastasis of No. 11 lymph node

Figure 20.15 PDT in combination with surgery was attempted in a patient with locally advanced lung cancer. The patient suffered dyspnea because of seriously poor pulmonary function. The tumor was located at the bifurcation of the left upper and lower bronchus, and the No. 11 lymph node was swollen. The resection of the left bifurcation between the upper lobe bronchus and the lower lobe bronchus and lymph node resection was performed after PDT.

Bronchoplasty after preoperative PDT

Resection of bifurcation between the left upper and lower lobe bronchi

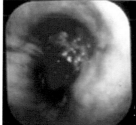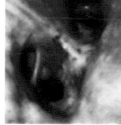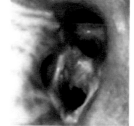

Before PDT   After PDT   After resection

Figure 20.16 The left photo shows the tumor before PDT. The middle photo shows the complete disappearance of the tumor after PDT. A thoracotomy was sequentially performed, and the bifurcation of the bronchus and the No. 11 lymph node were resected. The right photo shows the findings after surgery. The new bifurcation was constructed in a more peripherally located area.

The authors have investigated combination therapy of PDT with chemotherapy for the treatment of advanced lung cancer. The overall survival and QOL of patients with advanced lung cancers involving the obstruction or stenosis of a major bronchus were evaluated. Since 2010, 12 patients with 13 nonsmall cell lung cancers underwent PDT in combination with chemotherapy. Symptomatic patients with no significant extrinsic bronchial compression and patients with contraindicated curative operations were selected for this trial.

The median percentage of stenosis before treatment was 60% (range, 30%–00%); 1 week after treatment, this percentage had improved to 15% (range, 15%–99%), and it continued to remain at 15% at 1 month after treatment (range, 15% 60%). At 1 week after treatment, all the patients exhibited an improvement in their symptoms and their QOL and showed an objective response to the treatment, as

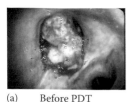
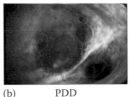
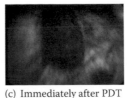
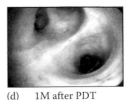

| (a) | Before PDT | (b) | PDD | (c) Immediately after PDT | (d) | 1M after PDT |

Figure 20.17 A 77-year-old man with a centrally located lung cancer. (a) A bronchoscopy revealed a 90% obstruction of the left B1 + 2 bronchus. (b) PDD performed with Laserphyrin and the Pentax SAFE-3000 system immediately before PDT shows red fluorescence at the cancerous lesion. (c) Quenching of the fluorescence produced by Laserphyrin was observed immediately after the PDT procedure. (d) The opening of the obstructed bronchus was confirmed 1 month after the PDT procedure.

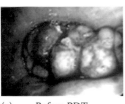
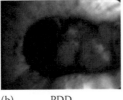
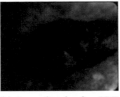
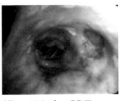

| (a) | Before PDT | (b) | PDD | (c) Immediately after PDT | (d) | 2M after PDT |

Figure 20.18 A 70-year-old man with squamous cell carcinoma. (a) A bronchoscopy showed the complete obstruction of the truncus intermediate bronchus. (b) PDD using a Pentax SAFE-3000 and Laserphyrin shows red fluorescence. (c) Photoquenching was observed immediately after PDT. (d) The opening of the obstructed bronchus was maintained for at least 6 months after PDT.

indicated by the substantial increase in the bronchial opening (Figures 20.17 and 20.18). This improvement was thought to reduce the likelihood of obstructive pneumonia. Thus, PDT in combination with chemotherapy was useful for alleviating obstructions of the bronchi and was recognized as a safe treatment.

Thus, the authors proposed the following inclusion criteria for patients with advanced lung cancer who might benefit from PDT: (1) dyspnea because of tumorous stenosis or obstruction of the central bronchus, (2) obstructive pneumonia or atelectasis, (3) possibility of extended surgery after PDT, (4) possibility of a reduction in the resection volume after PDT, (5) maintenance of QOL in combination with chemo/radiotherapy, (6) ECOG Performance Status of 0–2, (7) adequate organ function, (8) life expectancy of at least 12 weeks, and (9) written informed consent. The exclusion criteria were considered to be any serious comorbidities.

20.5.2 PDT FOR PERIPHERAL-TYPE LUNG CANCERS

Ground-glass opacification (GGO) nodules at the peripheral parenchyma of the lung noted at thin-section CT scan have shown to have a histopathologic relationship with atypical adenomatous hyperplasia (AAH) and adenocarcinoma (AIS) which is newly classified by International Association for the study of Lung Cancer (IASLC).[33] These preinvasive lesions, which correspond to type A or B adenocarcinoma according to Noguchi classification, have a favorable prognosis. The authors hypothesize that these early lung cancers in peripheral parenchyma such as AIS do not need surgical resection and may be cured by interventional approaches such as PDT. Recently, the authors reported that PDT using Laserphyrin, exerted a strong antitumor effect against cancer lesions >1.0 cm in diameter, which are assumed to involve extracartilaginous invasion and to be unsuitable for treatment with PDT using Photofrin.[34]

Peripheral-type early lung cancer cannot be detected using bronchoscopy nor be treated by conventional PDT. Therefore, the authors have developed a new minimally invasive laser device using a 1.0 mm diameter composite-type optical fiberscope (COF), which could transmit laser energy and obtain images in parallel, containing a laser Doppler blood-flow meter.[35] The use of COF technology was previously used in the field of atomic energy to observe inside nuclear reactors. It enables the acquisition of an image while simultaneously performing laser treatment such as PDT, measuring the blood flow, and estimating the distance between the laser and the tumor (Figure 20.19).

The authors aimed to develop a new endoscopic treatment for peripheral parenchymal cancer using Laserphyrin-PDT and a COF.

The changes in the normal peripheral parenchyma of the lung were observed using COF in pigs after irradiation with 664 nm laser (120 mW, 100 J) delivered 1 h after administration of Laserphyrin, 10 mg/kg. The authors were able to introduce the 1.0 mm COF into the peripheral parenchyma of the pig lungs safely and obtain clear images, and then NPe6-PDT was safely performed (Figure 20.20). The blood flow at the irradiated area was measured by COF during PDT, and the gradual disappearance of

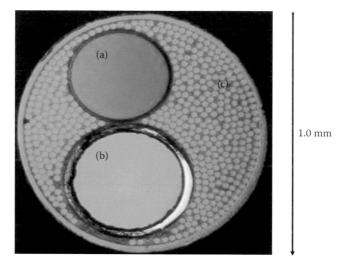

Figure 20.19 The tip of ultrathin composite type optical fiberscope (COF). The laser fiber (a), imaging (b), and illumination fibers (c).

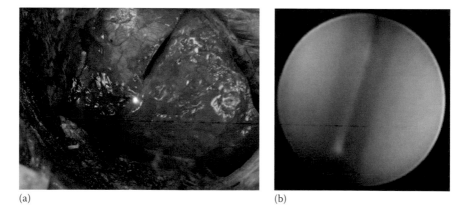

(a)　　　　　　　　　　　　　　　　(b)

Figure 20.20 Intrathoracic image of the pig lung and laser illumination (a) and bronchoscopical image by COF (b).

the blood-flow was observed. The pig lung was resected at 7 days after PDT and examined pathologically. Necrotic changes in the lung caused by PDT were observed using the new device, therefore the use of COF was validated. The mean diameter of necrosis in normal peripheral lung caused by Laserpyrin-PDT was 17 mm.

The 1.0 mm COF was a very useful device in carrying out Laserphyrin-PDT in the peripheral parenchyma of the lung. In the future, it is expected that Laserphyrin-PDT using COF for noninvasive adenocarcinoma such as AIS, will become one option for standard treatment and could play an important role in the treatment of synchronous or metachronous multiple primary lung cancer lesions.

20.6 NAVIGATION BRONCHOSCOPY

With the widespread use of CT scans in recent years, numerous small peripheral lung cancers have been detected. The diagnostic effectiveness of bronchoscopy for such peripheral pulmonary lesions (PPLs) has been reported only to a limited extent, since the use of accessible bronchial routes to identify small peripheral pulmonary nodules is often difficult. The American College of Chest Physicians (ACCP) guidelines have reported that the sensitivities for PPLs larger and smaller than 2 cm were 63% and 34%, respectively.[36] Therefore, several guided-bronchoscopy technologies have been developed to improve the yield of transbronchial biopsy for diagnosis of small pulmonary nodules, such as electromagnetic navigation bronchoscopy (ENB), virtual bronchoscopic navigation (VBN), and radial endobronchial ultrasound through a guide sheath (EBUS-GS).[37]

ENB and VBN can create virtual bronchoscopic images by reconstructing the CT images and identifying a pathway to the pulmonary nodule. The ENB system has been marketed mainly in Europe and in the United States and is an image-guided localization system designed to guide bronchoscopic instruments to predetermined points within the bronchial tree. The exact position of the steerable probe that contains a position sensor when placed within the electromagnetic field is depicted on the system monitor. Thus, it has the ability to guide bronchoscopy instruments to reach regions of the lung in a manner similar to how the global positioning system of an automobile can be used to navigate to a selected destination.[38] VBN is used to display three-dimensional images of the tracheal and bronchial lumens prepared from continuous volume data of helical CT images depicting them as though they were observed during bronchoscopy.[39] Bf-NAVI® (Cybernet System Inc., Tokyo, Japan) and LungPoint® (Broncus Medical Inc., Mountain View, Calif., USA) are two VBN systems that have been commercialized in Japan. Using the VBN images, a bronchoscope can be guided along a bronchial route to the peripheral lung nodule[40] (Figures 20.21 and 20.22). On the other hand, EBUS-GS allows the practitioner to visualize the peripheral lung nodule and to guide to a position in the periphery, enabling a biopsy to be taken.[41] The miniature EBUS probe with a guide sheath is inserted through

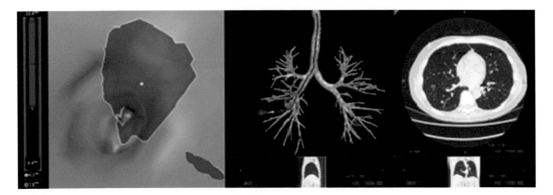

Figure 20.21 LungPoint® planning screen. A PPL is located in the right S[8] and it was set as the target (pink area) on the CT image (right image). The center image shows the path to the target through the entire bronchial tree. The left image is the virtual bronchoscopic image of the target.

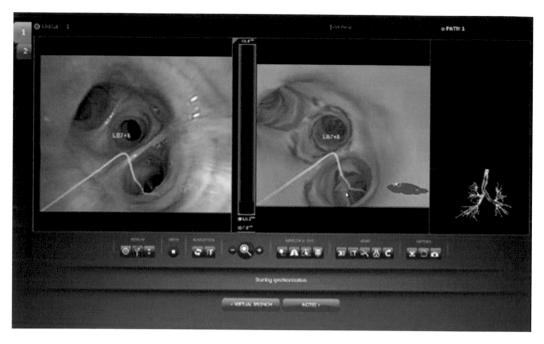

Figure 20.22 Real-time guidance using LungPoint®. VBN simultaneously shows the live (left image) and virtual views (right image); the path to the target is shown by the blue line.

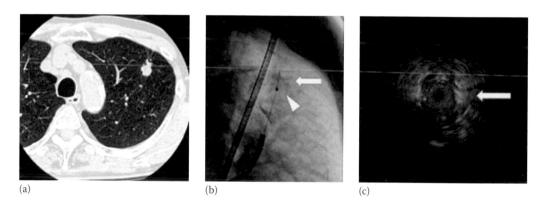

(a)　　　　　　　　　　　　　(b)　　　　　　　　　　　　　(c)

Figure 20.23 EBUS-GS for a PPL. (a) Chest CT shows a small PPL in the left segment 1 + 2. (b) Fluoroscopy image of TV brushing for the lesion (arrow). A bronchial brush was introduced into the lesion through a guide sheath (triangle). (c) The EBUS image shows a low echoic area with an irregularly margined lesion (arrow).

a biopsy channel of the bronchoscope into the bronchi leading to the target. Once the location of the lesion has been precisely identified using EBUS, the probe is removed and the guide sheath is left in place. Biopsy forceps can then be introduced through the guide sheath, and several biopsies can easily be performed at the same location (Figure 20.23).

Several investigators have reported that the combination of a navigation system and EBUS-GS can improve the diagnostic yield of peripheral lung nodules.[42–44] Asahina reported that the diagnostic yield of peripheral lung nodules less than 2 cm in diameter using VBN and EBUS-GS was 44.4%. Tamiya et al.[43] showed excellent results using the same method. Their diagnostic yield for malignant nodules ≤3 cm in diameter was 83.7%. Moreover, Ishida conducted a prospective multicenter study to examine the value of VBN-assisted EBUS for the diagnosis of small peripheral pulmonary lesions.[44] One hundred and ninety-nine patients with small peripheral pulmonary lesions (diameter, ≤3 cm) were randomly assigned to VBN-assisted (VBNA)

Medical expenses of PDT vs Surgery

PDT		¥760,000 ($8,444)
	DPC	249,430 (2,772)
	PDT procedure	87,100 (967)
	Laserphyrin	387,200 (4,302)
	Bronchoscopy	25,000 (277)
Surgery		¥1,700,000 (18,888)
	DPC	274,200 (3,046)
	Surgical procedure	1,050,000 (11,666)
	Anesthesia, drugs	300,000 (3,333)

H.Kato et al: analysis of the cost-effectiveness of PDT in early stage lung cancer, Diagnostic and therapeutic endoscopy; 6, 9–16, 1999

Figure 20.24 Cost-effectiveness of PDT. The difference in the medical cost between PDT and surgery was calculated using a QALY formula.

or non-VBN-assisted (NVBNA) groups. The diagnostic yield was higher for the VBNA group than for the NVBNA group (80.4% vs. 67.0%; $P = 0.032$).

These results suggest that instruments can be accurately guided to small peripheral lung lesions using a navigation system and EBUS-GS. Thus, these techniques may enable the navigation of a laser probe to deliver PDT to the sites of small peripheral lung cancers.

20.7 COST-EFFECTIVENESS OF PDT

The rapid increases in the expenses of medical care worldwide have created major problems. The authors have calculated the difference in medical costs between PDT and surgery using a quality-adjusted life year (QALY) formula. According to this calculation, PDT was about half the price of surgery in Japan. Since the therapeutic results are almost the same between these therapies for CESLC, PDT (which has been shown to be noninferior to surgery) is a promising approach[45] (Figure 20.24).

REFERENCES

1. Kinsey, J.H., Cortese, D.A., and Sanderson, D.R.: Detection of hematoporphyrin fluorescence during fiberoptic bronchoscopy to localize early bronchogenic carcinoma. *Mayo Clin Proc* 1978;**53**:594–600.
2. Profio, A.E., Doiron, D.R., and King, E.G.: Laser fluorescence bronchoscope for localization of occult lung tumor. *Med Phys* 1979;**6**:523–525.
3. Aizawa, K., Kato, H., Ono, J., Konaka, C., Kawate, N., and Hyata, Y.: New diagnostic system for malignant tumors using hematoporphyrin derivative, laser photoradiation and spectroscope. *Prog Clin Biol Res* 1984; **170**:227–238.
4. Hayata, Y., Kato, H., Konaka, C., Ono, J., Matsushima, Y., and Yoneyama, K.: Fiberoptic bronchoscopic laser photoradiation for tumor localization I lung cancer. *Chest* 1982;**82**:10–14.
5. Kato, H. and Horai, T.: *A Color Atlas of Endoscopic Diagnosis in Early Stage Lung Cancer*. London, U.K.: Wolfe, Aylesbury, 1992, p. 35.

6. Usuda, J., Kato, H., Okunaka, T. et al.: Photodynamic therapy for lung cancers. *J Thorac Oncol* 2006;**1**:489–495.

7. Furukawa, K., Kato, H., Konaka, C. et al.: Locally recurrent central-type early stage lung cancer <1.0 cm in diameter after complete remission by photodynamic therapy. *Chest* 2005;**128**:3269–3275.

8. Usuda J, Tsutsui H, Honda H, Ichinose S et al.: Photodynamic therapy for lung cancers based on novel photodynamic diagnosis using talaporfin sodium (NPe6) and autofluorescence bronchoscopy. *Lung Cancer* 2007;**58**:317–323.

9. Kato H, Konaka C, Kawate N et al.: Five-year disease-free survival of a lung cancer patient treated only by photodynamic therapy. *Chest* 1986;**90**:768–770.

10. Ikeda, N., Honda, H., Hayashi, A. et al.: Early detection of bronchial lesions using newly developed videoendoscopy- based autofluorescence bronchoscopy. *Lung Cancer* 2006;**52**:21–27.

11. Schomacker, K.T., Frisoli, J.K., Compton CC et al.: Ultraviolet laser-induced fluorescence of colonic tissue: Basic biology and diagnostic potential. *Lasers Surg Med* 1992;**12** 63–78.

12. Monici, M.: Cell and tissue autofluorescence research and diagnostic applications. *Biotechnol Annu Rev* 2005;**11**:227–256.

13. Kato, H.: Study on photodynamic therapy by laser. *Annual Report of the Cancer Research Ministry of Health and Welfare, National Cancer Center* 1988;**62–30**:255–261 (in Japanese).

14. Nagamoto, N., Saito, Y., Ohta, S. et al.: Relationship of lymph node metastasis to primary tumor size and microscopic appearance of roentgenographically occult lung cancer. *Am J Surg Pathol* 1989;**13**:1009–1013.

15. Nagamoto, N., Saito, Y., Sato, M. et al.: Clinicopathological analysis of 19 cases of isolated carcinoma in situ of the bronchus. *Am J Surg Pathol* 1993;**17**:1234–1243.

16. Furuse, K., Fukuoka, M., Kato, H. et al.: A prospective phase II study on photodynamic therapy with Photofrin II for centrally located early-stage lung cancer. *J Clin Oncol* 1993;**11**:1852–1857.

17. Kato, H., Furukawa, K., Sato, M. et al.: Phase II clinical study of photodynamic therapy using mono-L-aspartyl chlorin e6 and diode laser for early superficial squamous cell carcinoma of the lung. *Lung Cancer* 2003;**42**:103–111.

18. Dougherty, T.J., Lawrence, G., Kaufman, J.H. et al.: Photoradiation in the treatment of recurrent breast carcinoma. *J Natl Cancer Inst* 1978;**62**:231–237.

19. Classification of Lung Cancer. *The Japan Lung Cancer Society*. First English Edition, 2000, p. 35, Tokyo, Japan: Kanehara Co., Ltd.

20. Okunaka, T., Kato, H., Konaka, C. et al.: A comparison between argon-dye and excimer-dye laser for photodynamic effect in transplanted mouse tumor. *Jpn J Cancer Res* 1992;**83**:226–231.

21. Nelson, J., Roberts, W.G., and Berns, M.W.: In vivo studies on the utilization of mono-L-aspartyl chlorin (NPe6) for the photodynamic therapy. *Cancer Res* 1987;**47**:4681–4685.

22. Aizawa, K., Okunaka, T., Ohtani, T. et al.: Localization of mono-L-aspartyl chlorin e6 (NPe6) in mouse tissues. *Photochem Photobiol* 1987;**46**:789–794.

23. Kessel, D.: Pharmacokinetics of N-aspartyl chlorin e6 in cancer patients. *J Photochem Photobiol B* 1997;**39**:81–83.

24. Kaneda, A. and Ii, Y.: Diode laser for PDT. *J JSLSM* 1995;**16**:17–21 (in Japanese).

25. Furukawa, K., Okunaka, T., Tsuchida, T. et al.: A phase I clinical study of photodynamic therapy for early stage lung carcinoma using ME2906 and a diode laser system. *Porphyrins* 1998;**7**:199–206.

26. Kato, H.: Photodynamic therapy for lung cancer—A review of 19 years' experience. *J Photochem Photobiol B* 1998;**42**:96–99.

27. Hayata, Y., Kato, H., Konaka, C., Ono, J., and Takizawa, N.: Hematoporphyrin derivative and laser photoradiation in the treatment of lung cancer. *Chest* 1982;**81**:269–277.

28. Vincent, R.G., Dougherty, T.J., Rao, U., Boyle, D.G., and Potter, W.R.: Photoradiation therapy in advanced carcinoma of the trachea and bronchus. *Chest* 1984;**85**:29–33.

29. Moghissi, K., Dixon, K., Stringer, M.R. et al.: The place of bronchoscopic photodynamic therapy in advanced unresectable lung cancer: Experience of 100 cases. *Eur J Cardiothoracic Surg* 1995;**15**:1–6.

30. Furukawa, K., Okunaka, T., Yamamoto, H. et al.: Effectiveness of photodynamic therapy and Nd-YAG laser treatment for obstructed tracheobronchial malignancies. *Diagn Ther Endosc* 1999;**5**:161–166.

31. Kato, H., Konaka, C., Ono, J., Kawate, N., Nishimiya, K., Shinohara, H., Saito, M., Sakai, H., Noguchi, M., and Kito, T.: Preoperative laser photodynamic therapy in combination with operation in lung cancer. *J Thorac Cardiovasc Surg* 1985;**90**:420–429.

32. Okunaka, T., Hiyoshi, T., Furukawa, K., Yamamoto, H., Tsuchida, T., Usuda, J., Kumasaka, H., Ishida, J., Konaka, C., and Kato, H.: Lung cancers treated with photodynamic therapy and surgery. *Diagn Ther Endosc* 1999;**5**(3):155–160.

33. Travis, W.D., Brambilla, E., and Riely, G.: New pathologic classification of lung cancer: Relevance for clinical practice and clinical trials. *J Clin Oncol* 2013;**31**:992–1001.

34. Usuda, J., Ichinose, S., Ishizumi, T. et al.: Outcome of photodynamic therapy using NPe6 for bronchogenic carcinomas in central airways >1.0 cm in diameter. *Clin Cancer Res* 2010;**16**:2198–2204.

35. Oka, K., Seki, T., Naganawa, A., Kim, K., and Chiba, T.: A novel ultrasmall composite optical fiberscope. *Surg Endosc* 2011;**25**:2368–2371.

36. Rivera, M.P., Mehta, A.C., and Wahidi, M.M.: Establishing the diagnosis of lung cancer: Diagnosis and management of lung cancer, ed 3. American College of Chest Physicians evidencebased clinical practice guidelines. *Chest* 2013;**143**:e142S–e165S.

37. Wang Memoli, J.S., Nietert, P.J., and Silvestri, G.A.: Meta-analysis of guided bronchoscopy for the evaluation of the pulmonary nodule. *Chest* 2012:**142**:385–393.

38. Gildea, T.R., Mazzone, P.J., Karnak, D., Meziane, M., and Mehta, A.C.: Electromagnetic navigation diagnostic bronchoscopy: A prospective study. *Am J Respir Crit Care Med.* 2006;**174**:982–989.

39. Vining, D.J., Liu, K., Choplin, R.H., and Haponik, E.F.: Virtual bronchoscopy. Relationships of virtual reality endobronchial simulations to actual bronchoscopic findings. *Chest* 1996;**109**:549–553.

40. Asano, F., Matsuno, Y., Matsushita, T., and Seko, A.: Transbronchial diagnosis of a pulmonary peripheral small lesion using an ultrathin bronchoscope with virtual bronchoscopic navigation. *J Bronchol* 2002;**9**:108–111.

41. Kurimoto, N., Miyazawa, T., Okimasa, S., Maeda, A., Oiwa, H., Miyazu, Y., and Murayama, M.: Endobronchial ultrasonography using a guide sheath increases the ability to diagnose peripheral pulmonary lesions endoscopically. *Chest* 2004;**126**:959–965.

42. Asahina, H., Yamazaki, K., Onodera, Y., Kikuchi, E., Shinagawa, N., Asano, F., and Nishimura, M.: Transbronchial biopsy using endobronchial ultrasonography with a guide sheath and virtual bronchoscopic navigation. *Chest* 2005;**128**:1761–1765.

43. Tamiya, M., Okamoto, N., Sasada, S., Shiroyama, T., Morishita, N., Suzuki, H., Yoshida, E., Hirashima, T., Kawahara, K., and Kawase, I.: Diagnostic yield of combined bronchoscopy and endobronchial ultrasonography, under lungpoint guidance for small peripheral pulmonary lesions. *Respirology* 2013;**18**:834–839.

44. Ishida, T., Asano, F., Yamazaki, K., Shinagawa, N., Oizumi, S., Moriya, H., Munakata, M., and Nishimura, M.: Virtual bronchoscopic navigation combined with endobronchial ultrasound to diagnose small peripheral pulmonary lesions: A randomised trial. *Thorax* 2011;**66**:1072–1077.

45. Kato, H., Okunaka, T., Tsuchida, T., Shibuya, H., Fujino, S., and Ogawa, K.: Analysis of the cost-effectiveness of photodynamic therapy in early stage lung cancer. *Diag Ther Endosc* 1999;**6**:9–16.

Spectroscopic imaging in prostate PDT

ROZHIN PENJWEINI, BRIAN C. WILSON, AND TIMOTHY C. ZHU

21.1 INTRODUCTION

21.1.1 OVERVIEW

In the United States, prostate cancer is the second leading cause of death from cancer in men, after lung cancer [1–6]. Survival directly depends on the stage and grade of the disease at the time of diagnosis [1,4]. The main treatments for prostate cancer are surgery [2,3,7], radical prostatectomy [8,9], and radiation therapy [2,5,7], as well as hormone therapy and chemotherapy [7,10,11]. However, there are a myriad of potential complications associated with these therapies and many patients suffer from significant side effects [1,2]. The majority of prostate cancers currently diagnosed are of low/intermediate risk [2,5]. If minimally invasive treatment options could reliably cure or control low/intermediate-risk disease, then patients would likely select this option over the alternatives of active surveillance ("undertreatment") or radical prostatectomy and radiation therapy ("overtreatment"). Minimally invasive ablative treatments for both primary and recurrent (post radiotherapy failure) prostate cancer are under development [1,2]. In recent years, the most promising advances have come from interdisciplinary collaborations among physicists, chemists, biologists, and clinicians [4,12]. Preclinical and clinical trials of prostate photodynamic therapy (PDT) are examples of such collaborations. In this chapter, we discuss the fundamentals of PDT and its application to the treatment of prostate cancer. In particular, we explain the state of the art of spectroscopic imaging techniques used to quantify the key components for PDT dosimetry. The current clinical use of these methods in prostate PDT will also be presented.

21.1.2 CLINICAL PROSTATE PDT

PDT of prostate cancer is being developed in order to offer similar treatment efficacy to current therapies, while reducing the side effects [1,2,9,12–24]. Prostate PDT uses a photosensitizing drug that is injected intravenously and is distributed throughout the body. The photosensitizer is then activated in the prostate tissue by laser light delivered interstitially using optical diffusing fibers. The fibers are placed within needles inside the prostate, guided by transrectal ultrasound and a perineal template [4]. Following the absorption of light, the photosensitizer is transformed from its ground state (singlet state) into a relatively long-lived electronically excited state (triplet state) via a short-lived excited singlet state. The excited triplet can undergo two kinds of reactions [19,25]. In type I PDT, the excited triplet can react directly with a biological substrate, such as cell membranes, and transfer an electron to ground-state oxygen to form a charged superoxide, which in turn forms oxygen radicals, or reactive oxygen species, via secondary chemical reactions. These oxygen radicals can also interact with the biological substrate to produce oxygenated products [19,25]. In type II PDT, the triplet can transfer its energy directly to ground-state molecular oxygen, $^3O_2$, to form singlet oxygen ($^1O_2$) [19,25]. Both type I and type II reactions may occur simultaneously, and their relative contributions to the biological response depend on the type of photosensitizer and its concentration, the concentrations of substrate and $^3O_2$, as well as the binding affinity of the photosensitizer for the substrate. Following the activation of the photosensitizer and the formation of reactive oxygen species (ROS), necrotic or apoptotic cell death occurs at the site of interaction between the photosensitizer, light, and $^3O_2$. This may be the death of the tumor cells themselves or, in the case of vascular-targeted photosensitizers, the vascular endothelial cells, resulting in vascular shutdown and subsequent tumor necrosis.

Due to the high reactivity and short half-life of the ROS, only cells that are proximal to the area of the ROS production (areas of photosensitizer localization) are directly affected by PDT [25]. Hence, small-diameter optical fibers may be placed interstitially to deliver PDT light to either a portion of the prostate or the entire gland, using a variety of imaging techniques to achieve accurate positioning [26,27]. PDT may spare a sufficient amount of the neurovascular bundle so that sexual potency is preserved. Another advantage compared with other modalities where salvage therapy is limited is the ability to treat locally recurrent prostate cancer after prior radiation therapy [1,4,5,18], and PDT itself can be repeated several times if necessary. However, the PDT efficacy and the extent of photodamage and cytotoxicity is multifactorial, depending on the type of sensitizer, its extracellular and intracellular concentration and localization that depend also on the drug–light time interval, the total light dose delivered and local light fluence rate (ϕ), and the availability of molecular oxygen [1,2,4,9,12–18,25]. All of these factors are interdependent and may change dynamically during treatment.

There are different perspectives on what makes an ideal photosensitizer, either emphasizing photophysical properties such as high absorption coefficient and quantum yield of ROS generation or else concentrating on the biological behavior such as low systemic toxicity and high tumor selectivity. Nonetheless, there is general agreement that an ideal effective photosensitizer would meet the following criteria: a commercially available pure chemical, low dark toxicity but high photocytotoxicity, good selectivity toward target cells/tissues, long-wavelength absorption to achieve maximum treatment depth or volume, rapid clearance to minimize systemic toxicity, and ease of administration through various routes [28–31]. In addition, some degree of fluorescence of the photosensitizer is helpful for treatment guidance and monitoring. Although some photosensitizers satisfy some of these criteria, there are currently only a few photosensitizers that have received FDA approval for human use, and none to date has been approved for prostate cancer. Many studies of PDT for prostate cancer have been reported, both in tumor models and in clinical trials, using a variety of photosensitizers: hematoporphyrin derivative (porfirmer sodium, Photofrin) [4,32–37], BPD-MA (Verteporfin, Visudyne) [4,30,38–42], mTHPC (Foscan) [4,19–22,43], WST09 Pd-bacteriopheophorbide (TOOKAD) [4,7,44–47], WST11 padeliporfin (TOOKAD soluble) [4,48], Motexafin lutetium (MLu) [4,5,49], Talaporfin Sodium (LS-11) [4], silicon pthalocyanine 4 (PC-4) [4], and prodrugs such as ALA (Levulan) [4,50]. Each of these photosensitizers or prodrugs has different photophysical, pharmacokinetic, tumor targeting, and photodynamic efficacy characteristics. Table 21.1 presents typical dosages and systemic clearance times of these agents, as well as the drug–light interval and peak absorption wavelength commonly used for activation.

Table 21.1 Photosensitizers reported in preclinical and clinical trials for prostate PDT and typical treatment parameters

Photosensitizers	Drug dosage (mg kg⁻¹)	Drug–light interval	Clearance	Excitation (nm)
Photofrin [32–37]	2.5	48–150 h	4–6 weeks	630
ALA-PpIX (Levulan) [50]	20	14–18 h	2 days	635
BPD-MA (Verteporfin, Visudyne) [30,38–42]	0.5–1.0	15 min	5 days	689
mTHPC (Foscan) [19–22,43]	0.1–0.2	48–110 h	15 days	652
Motexafin lutetium (MLu) [5,49,51]	0.5–2	3–24 h	2 days	732
Pd-bacteriopheophorbide (WST09 TOOKAD) [7,44–47,52]	0.25–2	5–15 min	2 h	762
Padeliporfin (WST11 TOOKAD soluble) [48]	0.25–6	5–15 min	2 h	753

21.1.3 FUNDAMENTALS OF PDT TREATMENT PLANNING

PDT is inherently a dynamic process and all the key components (photosensitizer, light, and $^3O_2$) interact with each other in a time scale relevant to a single treatment. The spatial distribution of light is determined by the light source characteristics (wavelength and irradiation geometry), the tissue geometry (depth, lateral extent, volume), and the optical properties (primarily absorption and transport scattering coefficients at the treatment wavelength). The tissue optical properties, in turn, are affected by the concentration of the photosensitizer, as well as the concentration and oxygenation state of the blood in the tissue. The distribution of $^3O_2$ is altered by the photodynamic process, which consumes $^3O_2$, and in some cases also by changes in blood content/flow due to vascular damage. Finally, photobleaching of the photosensitizer, that is, decrease in the optical absorption at the treatment wavelength, changes the spatial distribution of the photosensitizer [4,12,53]. Hence, PDT treatment planning, whether for focal or whole-gland treatment, is complex, requiring information about and optimization of the total drug dose, rate of drug delivery, total light dose, and distribution of optical power ("source strength") per centimeter of diffusing fiber. With most photosensitizers, it is likely that there is a photobiological threshold effect, wherein sufficient light, drug, and $^3O_2$ must be present in a given volume of tissue, that is, there must be a minimum local concentration of the cytotoxic photoproduct, such as $^1O_2$ or other ROS, for clinically significant tissue response such as necrosis to occur [2]. This contrasts with the stochastic (i.e., probabilistic) response of cells and tissues to ionizing radiation and significantly impacts the spatial distribution of PDT damage within the prostate [2,54].

21.1.4 CURRENT PRACTICE OF PDT DOSIMETRY

To quantify the complex photodynamic effect, a dosimetric parameter called "PDT dose" has been introduced, which is defined as the number of photons absorbed by the photosensitizer per gram of tissue. However, this is a generally oversimplistic concept, since accurate determination of PDT dose is confounded by several factors [12,14,53]: (1) the local concentration of the photosensitizer varies from site to site in the tissue and between different patients; (2) the penetration of light into the target depends on the optical properties of that specific tissue; and (3) tissue and blood oxygenation is a central component for PDT and also affects the tissue optical properties. The PDT dose cannot predict the dosimetric consequence if the tissue is intrinsically hypoxic or becomes hypoxic as a result of PDT treatment, since the yield of $^1O_2$ will be reduced. In addition, all of these parameters can change during treatment and each of them can also influence the others [4,12,53,55].

Another dosimetry approach method called "implicit dosimetry" monitors a parameter such as fluorescence photobleaching or tissue blood flow in real time during PDT treatment [4,56,57]. It has been hypothesized, for example, that the photobleaching of the photosensitizer can predict the extent of damage [12]. Measurement of the corresponding fluorescence photobleaching is relatively inexpensive and straightforward to implement, but *in vivo* these measurements must also take into account the effects of light scattering and absorption. In addition, the validity of the relationship between fluorescence photobleaching and $^1O_2$ dose is predicated on the photobleaching being mediated primarily by the $^1O_2$ reaction with the photosensitizer, so that the photobleaching and the tissue PDT response are correlated. However, there is experimental evidence to suggest that other photobleaching mechanisms may be important for some commonly used photosensitizers such as Photofrin [53] and ALA-induced PpIX [58], while the *in vivo* photobleaching of Foscan [59] exhibits features that are not readily interpretable. Hence, care must be exercised in using photobleaching as a metric of PDT dose [12].

The amount of generated ROS is presumed to be predictive of PDT tissue damage. "Explicit dosimetry" then refers to the prediction of ROS dose on the basis of the measurable parameters that underlie the $^1O_2$ generation, namely light distribution, photosensitizer concentration, and tissue oxygenation [55,60–65], each of which must be independently measured *in situ* and used as an input into a photophysical model to calculate the local $^1O_2$ concentration. Alternatively, these steps may be circumvented in the so-called direct dosimetry, where direct measurement of ROS production during PDT is performed, based on either near-infrared (NIR) measurements of the $^1O_2 \rightarrow {}^3O_2$ luminescence decay or indirect assays of ROS detection as a dose metric [55,60]. In the case of $^1O_2$, while its 1270 nm luminescence emission can be measured (singlet oxygen luminescence dosimetry, SOLD), the signal is extremely weak and has a very short lifetime (<1 μs) due to the high reactivity of

$^1O_2$ with the biological environment. Hence, there are currently major practical obstacles for the clinical implementation of SOLD [55,60]. An additional challenge is how to interpret the luminescence signal that arises from the $^1O_2 \rightarrow {}^3O_2$ transition, since this process competes with the reaction of $^1O_2$ with intracellular and extracellular substrates, so that the luminescence can increase under conditions where the substrates for $^1O_2$ are not plentiful although the biological effects may decrease. SOLD is only applicable to type II photosensitizers, for example, it is not viable for type I photosensitizers such as TOOKAD. Nevertheless, SOLD serves as an ultimate "gold standard" for testing and validating other types of PDT dosimetry [12,64].

21.2 SPECTROSCOPIC IMAGING TECHNIQUES FOR CLINICAL PDT OF PROSTATE

For successful PDT, accurate techniques are required for light delivery as well as calculation of photosensitizer concentration and ϕ in the entire prostate volume [4,12]. PDT can cause changes in photosensitizer concentration and oxygenation of blood in tissue, both directly through photochemical $^3O_2$ consumption and indirectly through effects on the vasculature and general immunological/inflammation responses [4,12]. Accurate calculation of the interstitial photosensitizer concentration and ϕ requires accurate characterization of the *in vivo* tissue oxygenation and tissue optical properties at the treatment wavelength: absorption coefficient (μ_a) and reduced scattering coefficient (μ'_s) [4,66]. In this section, we demonstrate the utility of different imaging and spectroscopy techniques for measuring (the spatiotemporal variation of) μ_a and μ'_s, the interstitial drug concentration, ϕ, and blood oxygenation. The current clinical use of these methods in prostate PDT will be also explained.

21.2.1 MEASUREMENT AND MAPPING OF TISSUE OPTICAL PROPERTIES

Several studies on optical properties of primary and locally recurrent prostate cancer have been conducted at different wavelengths, using both continuous-wave (CW) [27,47,56,67–73] and time-resolved [12,20,21] techniques. Figure 21.1 illustrates the spectra of μ_a and μ'_s in human prostates based on published data, indicating the ranges of μ_a and μ'_s as well as their inter- and intra-prostate heterogeneity.

With these overall data and background, we now review the current spectroscopic imaging techniques that have been used clinically to obtain these optical properties.

21.2.1.1 DIFFUSE REFLECTANCE SPECTROSCOPY

CW spatially resolved diffuse reflectance absorption spectroscopy can be obtained from a contact probe used to measure reflected light from a tissue surface. The measured reflectance can be used to determine μ_a and μ'_s by fitting the data with the calculations. If one considers $\mu_t = \mu_a + \mu'_s$ and $z_b = 2AD$, where D is the diffusion constant and A is a constant that depends on the Fresnel reflectance at the surface of the boundary, the reflected flux, R_f, exiting the surface from the tissue is expressed as

$$R_f(\rho) = \frac{1}{4\pi\mu'_t}\left[\left(\mu_{eff} + \frac{1}{r_1}\right)\frac{e^{-\mu_{eff}r_1}}{r_1^2} + \left(\frac{1}{\mu'_t} + 2z_b\right)\left(\mu_{eff} + \frac{1}{r_2}\right)\frac{e^{-\mu_{eff}r_2}}{r_2^2}\right] \tag{21.1}$$

where

r_1 and r_2 are the radial distances from the detector to the two point sources (depth of the measurement $z = 0$ and $z = -2z_b$)

effective attenuation coefficient, μ_{eff}, is given by $\mu_{eff} = \sqrt{3\mu_a\mu'_s}$

A can be determined from the indices of refractions and the numerical aperture of the incident light

Using reflectance measurements, μ_a and μ'_s are obtained within 5%–15%. More detailed description can be found elsewhere [66,74].

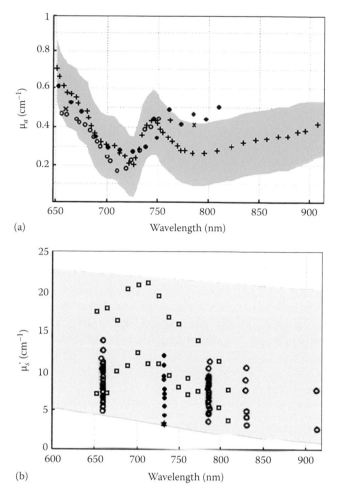

Figure 21.1 (a) Absorption (μ_a) and (b) reduced scattering (μ_s') coefficients of human prostate tissue *versus* wavelength. The grey shaded region is the 95% confidence interval range of μ_a and μ_s'. The different symbols represent results from different published studies [46,47,56,66,70]. (From Sandell, J.L. and Zhu, T., *J. Biophotonics*, 4, 773, 2011. With permission.)

21.2.1.2 TRANSMITTANCE (OR INTERSTITIAL) SPECTROSCOPY

As the spatial distributions of μ_a and μ_s' essentially determine the spatial ϕ distribution [75], one strategy to measure the optical properties without requiring prior knowledge is to perform *in situ* light dosimetry to measure the actual ϕ distribution in the prostate. This can be done pre- and post-PDT. A light source fiber is first placed interstitially within the prostate through a biopsy needle. A detector fiber (preferably with isotropic response) is then placed within the prostate at a known distance from the source fiber. The light fluence rate ϕ at a distance r from a point source with source strength, S, can be expressed by the diffusion approximation [4,66]

$$\phi(r) = \frac{S\mu_{eff}^2}{4\pi r \mu_a}e^{-\mu_{eff}r} = \frac{S3\mu_s'}{4\pi r}e^{-\mu_{eff}r} \tag{21.2}$$

x and h are the parallel and perpendicular distances from the center of the point source and r is given by

$$r = \sqrt{x^2 + h^2} \tag{21.3}$$

For a point source measurement with a given source strength, μ_a and μ'_s can then be determined separately by the slope in ϕ versus r and the magnitude of ϕ near the source. To implement this model clinically, a computer-controlled positioning system capable of moving an isotropic point source and an isotropic detector independently along parallel catheters in the prostate has been developed. ϕ can then be measured at a variety of distances from the point source, and the resulting profile can be fitted to Equation 21.2 to determine the optical properties, applying optimization algorithms [27,66,74]. Then, by moving the source to various positions, the distribution of optical properties throughout the organ can be mapped "point-by-point." If a sufficient number (typically ~800) of such measurements are made, then a modified differential-evolution algorithm can be applied [27] to fit the measured data using Equation 21.2 to generate μ_a and μ'_s. A three-dimensional (3D) map of the optical properties can also be reconstructed with sufficient point-by-point measurements in 3D [4,71].

The spatial variation of fluence rate per unit source intensity (ϕ/S) in human prostate has been reported at 732 nm for different patients [4,27,71]. Comparisons have been made before, during, and after MLu-mediated PDT and differences within and among patients have been studied; the results are summarized in Figure 21.2a. Clearly, there is a significant variability in the optical properties measured at different locations that affected the resulting ϕ distributions. The optical properties, μ_a and μ_{eff}, have also been measured at various sites—right lower quadrant (RLQ), right upper quadrant (RUQ), and left upper quadrant (LUQ)—for several human prostate glands before and after PDT, as shown in Figure 21.2b and c. The effective attenuation coefficients vary by a factor of about 3 over the length of the prostate, indicating significant changes of light penetration depth at different locations. The variation of ϕ at the same site of the same prostate has also been studied before and after MLu-mediated PDT, showing little change in the optical properties during PDT treatment (data not shown).

21.2.1.3 TIME-OF-FLIGHT (TOF) SPECTROSCOPY

Steady-state ϕ measurements are aggravated by the localized bleeding caused by needle insertion, which can prevent proper quantitative derivation of optical and physiological parameters. TOF spectroscopy has been introduced as a tool for interstitial *in vivo* measurements of μ_a and μ'_s by analysis of the temporal dispersion of picosecond laser pulses (~70 ps) [20,21,66]. As pulse shapes, rather than ϕ, are evaluated in TOF, the

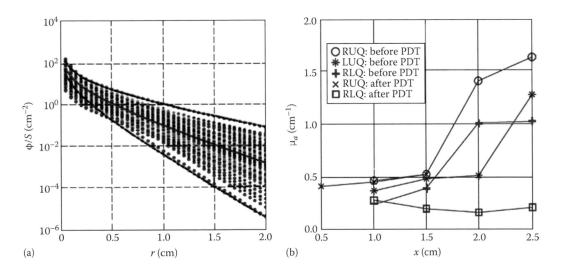

(a)　　　　(b)

Figure 21.2 (a) The spatial variation of light fluence rate per unit source strength (ϕ/S) in human prostate for a point source at 732 nm. The solid line corresponds to the average optical properties: $\mu_a = 0.3$ cm^{-1}, $\mu'_s = 14$ cm^{-1}. The dashed lines correspond to the highest and lowest light penetrations: $\mu_a = 0.04$ cm^{-1}, $\mu'_s = 30$ cm^{-1} and $\mu_a = 1.5$ cm^{-1}, $\mu'_s = 9$ cm^{-1}, respectively. *In vivo* distribution of (b) μ_a and (*Continued*)

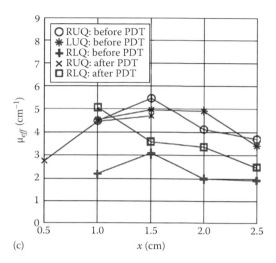

(c)

Figure 21.2 (Continued) (c) μ_{eff} in human prostate at different locations before and after PDT (RUQ, right upper quadrant; LUQ, left upper quadrant; RLQ, right lower quadrant). (Modified from Zhu, T.C. and Finlay, J.C., *Photodiagnosis and Photodyn. Ther.*, 3, 234, 2006; Zhu, T.C. et al., *J. Photochem. Photobiol. B Biol.*, 79, 231, 2005. With permission.)

technique is insensitive to local bleeding at the fiber tips. In TOF, two optical fibers are used to inject and collect the light interstitially. Collected light is sent to a cooled microchannel plate photomultiplier tube (MCP-PMT), which together with a time-correlated single-photon-counting (TCSPC) computer card is used to obtain photon TOF histograms (24.4 ps time resolution).

The recorded photon TOF distributions (at 660, 786, 830, and 916 nm and 1–2 mW average power) have been evaluated in the human prostate by Lund University using time–domain diffusion theory of light propagation and Monte Carlo simulation [20,21]. Although both diffusion theory– and Monte Carlo–based evaluations provide consistent data and good signal-to-noise ratio, Monte Carlo–based TOF evaluation is more reliable because of the additional information provided by the time delay. More detailed description can be found elsewhere [20,21].

21.2.1.4 DIFFUSE OPTICAL TOMOGRAPHY (DOT)

Diffuse optical tomography (DOT) is a spectroscopic imaging modality that generates images of μ_a and μ_s' through a tissue volume [74,76]. Although one can obtain the spatial distribution of optical properties using the point-by-point scanning [74,76], reconstruction methods as used in DOT to solve the inverse diffusion problem can greatly improve the spatial resolution and ensure smoothness of the resulting spatial distribution of optical properties. Based on the data presented in Figure 21.1 and confirmed by TOF measurements [20,21], μ_s' is typically an order higher than the μ_a in prostate tissue, so that DOT techniques are valid.

An interstitial DOT method using multiple cylindrical light-diffusing fibers (CDF-DOT) and isotropic detectors has been developed for characterizing the optical properties of the prostate gland during PDT [73]. In this technique, several parallel catheters containing CDFs and detectors are inserted under ultrasound image guidance. The same fibers can be used as light sources for both DOT and PDT light delivery, simplifying the fiber insertion and reducing the overall operation time, thereby making online dosimetry clinically feasible. For each source position, the isotropic detectors scan and record the ϕ distribution in the direction along the catheter axis [73]. Using a 3D reconstruction model [73,75], volumetric μ_a and μ_s' images of the prostate can be recovered. For each source location, the model utilizes measurements made both above and below the source plane to maximize efficiency. The spatial distribution of ϕ can be described by the steady-state diffusion equation and the calculated ϕ can be matched to the measured data using correct source and detector separation. The tissue optical properties are then reconstructed by solving the inverse problem using a steady-state diffusion model, as described in detail previously [73,75].

A clinical example of *in vivo* point-by-point and CFD-DOT reconstruction of the prostate optical properties is shown in Figure 21.3a and c [73] for one transverse slice through the gland. In the point-by-point methods, the data were taken for each 5×5 mm^2 pixel and assumed homogeneous optical properties within the pixel. The hot spot locations of optical properties reconstructed by CDF-DOT are consistent with those calculated by the point-by-point method.

It has been reported that if the measured ϕ/S at $x = 5$ mm is less than 0.1 cm^{-2}, then bleeding around the source and/or the detector fiber has occurred and this may account for the central hot spots seen in Figure 21.3b [73]. However, it is not clear that the scattering hot spots are also related to bleeding because the current inverse algorithm tends to suffer from cross talk between μ_a and μ_s' in regions with large deviation from the background optical properties ($\mu_a = 0.3$ cm^{-1} and $\mu_s' = 14$ cm^{-1}). The volumetric distributions of μ_a and μ_s' are shown in Figure 21.3b and d, respectively. The hot spots are observed through the central portion of the prostate and heterogeneity in μ_a and μ_s' is present in several planes for the same patient [73]. The two methods were also compared along the x-axis at specific z and y locations and the μ_a profile was consistent for both methods, as shown in Figure 21.3e. The comparison for μ_s' shows a large inconsistency at $x = 1.75$ cm, but

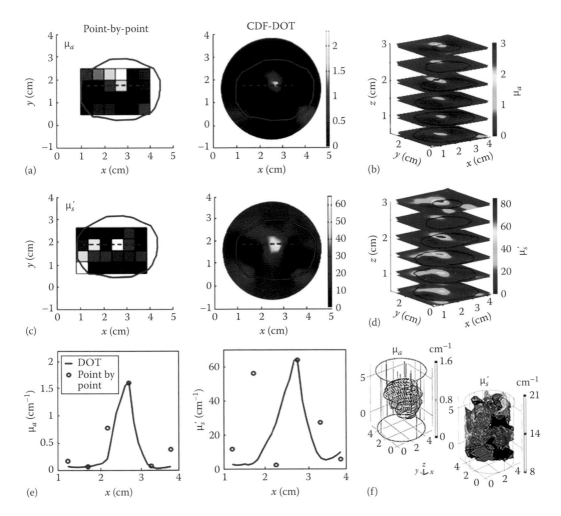

Figure 21.3 (a) *In vivo* mapping of μ_a using point-by-point and CDF-DOT methods for a patient's prostate in one transverse plane ($z = 0.5$ cm). (b) Volumetric distributions of μ_a: the boundary of the prostate is indicated by the red contour lines in each z plane. (c, d) Corresponding plots for μ_s'. (e) Comparison of μ_a and μ_s' between the two methods along the x-axis (blue dashed line in (a) and (c)) at $z = 0.5$ and $y = 1.75$ cm. (f) 3D reconstructed μ_a and μ_s' for the solid prostate phantom. ([a–e]: Modified from Wang, K.K. and Zhu, T.C., *Opt. Express*, 17, 11665, 2009. [f]: Adapted from Liang, X. et al., *Phys. Med. Biol.*, 58, 3461, 2013. With permission.)

the other points appear to be reasonably well matched (Figure 21.3e). A more detailed description of this study has been reported previously [71,73].

To test the feasibility of reconstructing optical properties using interstitial CDF-DOT, simulations and measurements in a solid prostate phantom were used, including anomalies with known heterogeneous optical properties [75]. The prostate boundary in one transverse plane through the center of the prostate was obtained from an ultrasound scan of a patient and was used in the simulation, extending 1 cm axially (along z) [75]. The 3D reconstruction of the spatial distributions of μ_a and μ_s' are shown in Figure 21.3f [75], demonstrating that μ_a is reconstructed in good agreement with the CDF-DOT results. However, the CDF-DOT method is not very sensitive to μ_s'. Detailed description has been published previously [75].

21.2.1.5 TRANSRECTAL ULTRASOUND–COUPLED NEAR-INFRARED OPTICAL TOMOGRAPHY (NIR/TRUS)

The use of endorectal NIR tomography in combination with transrectal ultrasound (TRUS) has been reported as a means to characterize the spatial distribution of optical properties in the intact prostate known to have intra-organ and inter-subject heterogeneities [76–78]. The rationale for this hybrid approach is the inadequacy of conventional TRUS and the limited spatial resolution and long scanning time needed for DOT [75,76]. The combined NIR/TRUS probe and system enable concurrent acquisition of transrectal NIR tomography and TRUS images in the same sagittal plane. Integration with TRUS ensures accurate endorectal positioning of the NIR applicator and the utility of using TRUS spatial *prior* information to guide NIR image reconstruction. A hierarchical reconstruction algorithm has also been developed that implements cascaded initial guesses for nested domains. This image reconstruction method is then applied for evaluating a number of NIR applicator designs for integration with a sagittal TRUS transducer. More detailed description of the technique can be found elsewhere [76–78].

21.2.2 INTERSTITIAL MEASUREMENTS OF INTERSTITIAL PHOTOSENSITIZER CONCENTRATION AND BLOOD OXYGENATION

Direct *in vivo* determination of photosensitizer concentration in the region of treatment is important for assessing PDT efficacy and predicting the treatment outcome. Early PDT clinical protocols specified this quantity only in terms of the mass of photosensitizer administrated per kilogram body weight or per square meter body surface area, which is only indirectly related to the resultant concentration in the target tissue. As indicated earlier, the PDT treatment itself can also cause changes in the photosensitizer concentration and oxygenation of blood in tissue, both directly through photochemical $^3O_2$ consumption and indirectly through effects on the vasculature and general physiological responses [4,12]. Moreover, *in vivo* studies have shown large variation of the tissue photosensitizer concentration for different tumors and normal tissue types and of course the concentration at the time of treatment depends strongly on the drug–light interval used [4,71].

The effect of injected drug dose and drug–light interval on tissue photosensitizer concentration is illustrated in Figure 21.4a for MLu-mediated PDT. Overall, patients who received higher injected MLu doses generally had higher local drug concentrations in the prostate and the concentration tended to decrease with increasing drug–light interval. However, there was also marked intra- and inter-patient variability [4,71] pre- and post-treatment. The total optical absorption in the tissue at the treatment wavelength of 732 nm increased linearly with photosensitizer concentration c, as $\mu_a = 0.658c + 0.227$ [4,71]. This clear dependence on drug concentration is due to the strong absorption peak of MLu at 732 nm and the weak hemoglobin absorption in tissue at this wavelength that results in low intrinsic absorption. This heterogeneity in photosensitizer concentration, which is probably a common phenomenon to a different degree for all photosensitizers, is sufficiently large to motivate the use of *in situ* monitoring of the drug distribution in individual patients. Hence, in the current clinical practice using MLu-PDT, *in situ* fluorescence spectroscopy is used to determine dynamic information related to photosensitizer photobleaching and, at the same time, tissue oxygenation [12]. In this technique, several catheters are placed into the prostate and side-firing optical probes are inserted into each catheter under accurate motor control. The same fiber is used to deliver 460 nm light and measure fluorescence. To measure

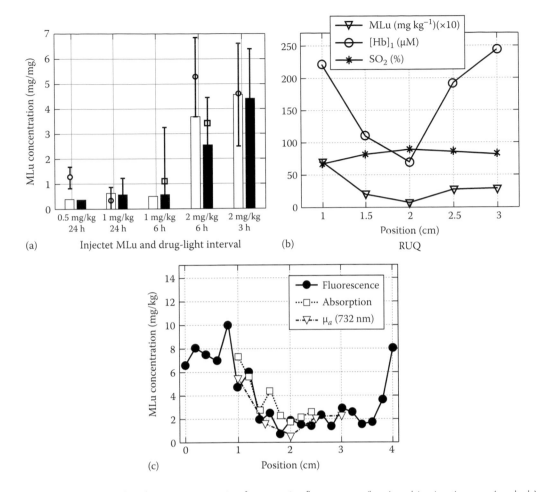

Figure 21.4 (a) Extrapolated MLu concentration from *ex vivo* fluorescence (bars) and *in vivo* tissue μ_a (symbols) measurements as a function of injected MLu concentration: open bars O before and solid bars □ immediately after PDT. Error bars correspond to ±1 standard deviation of the *ex vivo* biopsy and *in vivo* absorption measurements. The large discrepancy between the *in vivo* and *ex vivo* data in the two patients receiving 0.5 mg kg^{-1} is a consequence of uncertainties in the *in vivo* measurements in this early group of patients. In addition, since μ_a for the earlier patients was small (low MLu dose), the relative uncertainty in μ_a is higher. In the group receiving 1 mg kg^{-1} with a 6 h drug–light interval, the large discrepancy between *in vivo* and *ex vivo* measurements is not statistically significant ($n = 1$). (b) Typical *in vivo* distribution of Hb, HbO$_2$, and MLu concentration in human prostate pre-PDT. (c) *In vivo* distributions of MLu determined by absorption spectroscopy (∇), 732 nm absorption measurements (□), and fluorescence spectroscopy (●). Both panels are taken from the right upper quadrant (RUQ). (Modified from Zhu, T.C. and Finlay, J.C., *Photodiagnosis and Photodyn. Ther.*, 3, 234, 2006; Zhu, T.C. et al., *Photochem. Photobiol.*, 81, 96, 2005; Zhu, T.C. et al., *J. Photochem. Photobiol. B Biol.*, 79, 231, 2005. With permission.)

the photosensitizer concentration, the fluorescence signal measured at the tip of the same side-firing fiber is separated from multiply scattered excitation light by a dichroic beam splitter and then corrected for the tissue optical properties using an analytical correction algorithm [55,57,60]. The resultant spectrum is then fitted to determine the contributions of the sensitizer and the tissue autofluorescence. For $^3O_2$ monitoring, broadband illumination and detection are used and the diffuse transmittance spectra are measured, from which the tissue absorption spectrum is derived. The known absorption spectra of oxy- and deoxy-hemoglobin are then fitted to determine the oxygen saturation, $SO_2 = 100 \times [HbO_2]/\{[HbO_2] + [Hb]\}$, the fraction of total Hb that is in its oxygenated state. This can be translated into an estimate of the cellular $^3O_2$ concentration using a model of $^3O_2$ diffusion and consumption [55,60]. This interstitial approach has been investigated in animal models as well as in the human prostate, monitoring the interstitial photosensitizer concentration and tissue oxygenation and correlating the treatment outcome with the changes in these parameters during PDT [79,80].

The spatial distribution of Hb, SO_2, and photosensitizer determined from absorption, scattering, and fluorescence spectroscopy have been reported for MLu-mediated PDT, as illustrated in Figure 21.4b and c. This shows that the photosensitizer concentration can vary up to fourfold at different locations of the same prostate [4,71], which should translate into significantly different tumor response unless both light and oxygen are in excess and the lower photosensitizer concentrations are sufficient to produce an effective local PDT dose that exceeds the tissue necrosis threshold. More detailed description can be found elsewhere [4,71].

21.2.3 REAL-TIME MONITORING OF BLOOD FLOW AND TISSUE OXYGENATION

PDT requires oxygen to cause cellular and vascular damage to tumors. The tissue oxygen concentration, in turn, is influenced by blood flow and blood SO_2 [12,53], so that real-time monitoring of these hemodynamic quantities allows the treatment conditions (e.g., light dose or illumination intensity) to be altered to improve outcome. Different variants of NIR spectroscopy have been used for noninvasive measurement of these quantities deep within tissues [51,53,81–83]. For example, a multi-modality instrument combining diffuse reflectance spectroscopy (DRS) with NIR diffuse correlation spectroscopy (DCS) has been used for continuous measurement of SO_2 and blood flow during interstitial prostate PDT [51,57,79]. This latter technique has been validated against color power Doppler ultrasound in tumors and against laser Doppler in brain. DRS for SO_2 measurements has also been validated in liquid tissue phantoms and different tissues *in vivo*. For clinical application in the prostate, a transparent probe with <1 mm outer diameter has been constructed containing one source fiber (multimode, 200 μm core diameter) and five detector fibers within an 18G catheter, which is inserted into the prostate (Figure 21.5a and b). The source and detector fibers extend to different depths in the tissue, enabling simultaneous measurement in different locations. The source fiber is shared for both DRS and DCS, while three multimode fibers (100 μm) are used for DRS. Two single-mode fibers (7 μm) are employed for DCS. The light is delivered to the tissue surface from amplitude-modulated (70 MHz) lasers at 690, 785, and 830 nm and scattered light is detected in reflectance geometry. These wavelength-dependent data are used to determine the local volume-averaged Hb and HbO_2 concentrations. A narrowband CW laser at 800 nm, four single-photon-counting avalanche photodiodes, and a four-channel autocorrelator are used for blood flow measurements. In order to monitor the hemodynamic changes during illumination and to avoid interference with the optical measurements, optical filters are placed in front of the detectors to attenuate the PDT excitation light. Details of the instrument have been reported elsewhere [51,57,80,84].

21.2.3.1 DRS FOR TISSUE BLOOD OXYGENATION

In DRS the prostate is treated as an infinite homogeneous optically turbid medium and an analytical solution to the photon diffusion equation is used to fit the bulk tissue properties μ_a and μ_s' [12,51,53,85]. The analysis then minimizes

$$\chi^2 = \Sigma \left\| \frac{\phi_m(t)}{\phi_{m\_ref}} - \frac{\phi_c(t)}{\phi_{c\_ref}} \right\|^2 , \qquad (21.4)$$

where

$\phi_m(t)$ and $\phi_c(t)$ are the measured and calculated light fluence rates at time (t), respectively
$\phi_{m\_ref}(t)$ and $\phi_{c\_ref}(t)$ are the corresponding data from a calibration phantom of known optical properties

The summation here is over the large (10 or 15 mm) separation source–detector pairs, ensuring that the same tissue volume is sampled as in the DCS measurements. This method works well in phantoms and *in vivo*, but only μ_{eff} is determined so that independent knowledge of μ_s' is required to extract μ_a. The wavelength-dependent μ_a is then decomposed into HbO_2 and Hb concentrations, which then yield the total hemoglobin concentration (THC = $C_{Hb} + C_{HbO_2}$) and SO_2.

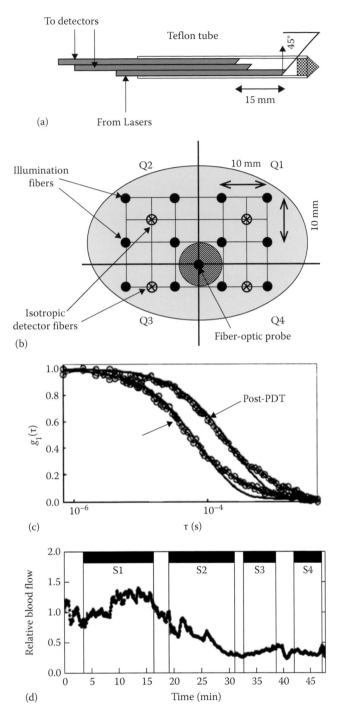

Figure 21.5 (a) The fiber-optic probe used during interstitial prostate PDT. The fiber tips are cleaved and polished at 45° to improve the light coupling (>80%) between the fibers and the tissue. (b) Cross-sectional view of the fiber positions for each quadrant of the prostate. The treatment light is delivered via the cylindrical diffusing fibers inside the catheters (solid circles). The distribution of the treatment light is monitored by an isotropic detector fiber (cross circles) at the center of the source fibers placed prior to treatment. Each quadrant is illuminated sequentially to cover the entire gland. The shaded area indicates the tissue zone monitored by the probe. (c) Typical normalized $g_1(\tau)$ measurements with 10 mm source–detector separation in a prostate cancer patient before and after PDT: the solid lines are fits to a Brownian diffusion model [51,79] and the symbols are measurements. The lower traces show the dynamic changes in (d) relative blood flow [51]. *(Continued)*

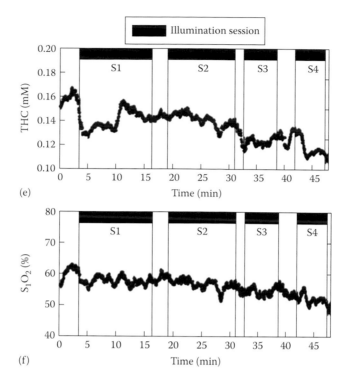

Figure 21.5 (Continued) (e) THC, and (f) SO$_2$ during treatment. (From Yu, G. et al., *Photochem. Photobiol.*, 82, 1279, 2006. With permission.)

21.2.3.2 DCS FOR RELATIVE BLOOD FLOW

Speckle fluctuations of the diffuse light are sensitive to the motion of scattering objects in the tissue such as red blood cells [12,51,53,85]. The temporal autocorrelation function, $G_1(r, \tau)$, of the electric field, $E(r, t)$, or its Fourier transform is explicitly related to this motion and satisfies the correlation diffusion equation in highly scattering media:

$$G_1(r, \tau) = \left\langle E(r, t) E^*(r, t + \tau) \right\rangle, \tag{21.5}$$

where

  τ is the correlation delay time

  the angle brackets denote averages over time

From G_1 value measured by DCS, the normalized electric field temporal autocorrelation function, $g_1(r, \tau)$, is calculated [12,51,53,85] as

$$g_1(r, \tau) = \frac{G_1(r, \tau)}{\left\langle E(r, t) E^*(r, t) \right\rangle} \tag{21.6}$$

The exact form of the correlation diffusion equation depends on the nature and heterogeneity of the particle motion. In the case of diffusive motion, $G_1(r, \tau)$ decays approximately exponentially at early times, τ, at a rate that depends on a parameter α (proportional to the tissue blood volume fraction) and on the mean-square displacement of the blood cells:

$$\left\langle \Delta r^2 (\tau) \right\rangle = 6D_B \tau, \tag{21.7}$$

where D_B is the effective diffusion coefficient of the moving scatterers. Relative changes of αD_B are then correlated with relative changes in tissue blood flow.

Figure 21.5c shows typical DCS $g_1(\tau)$ measurements in a prostate patient before and after PDT. The post-PDT autocorrelation curve decays much slower than that of pre-PDT, indicating a decrease in blood flow. Figure 21.5d through f show the typical time course of changes in hemodynamics that occur during prostate PDT in a patient, demonstrating that both blood flow and total hemoglobin were decreased in each quadrant by the end of treatment, compared with the corresponding pretreatment values. A slight decrease in SO_2 can also be observed. A study in three patients showed ~50% decrease in the average blood flow and ~15% decrease in THC after PDT, while the average SO_2 was essentially unchanged.

21.2.4 MEASUREMENTS OF TISSUE OXYGEN TENSION (pO$_2$)

It is well known that the efficacy of PDT may be affected by the presence of preexisting hypoxic tumor regions, or by oxygen depletion during the PDT light irradiation [7,73]. In a preclinical study on normal dog prostate, the pO_2 was measured prior to PDT using an OxyLite system (Oxford Optronics, Oxford, United Kingdom). The pre-calibrated sensor (operating range up to 100 mmHg) consists of an optical fiber (diameter ~220 μm) that measures pO_2 by determining the oxygen-dependent fluorescence lifetime of a ruthenium chloride coating on the tip. A 22G needle is used to penetrate the capsule and advance the fiber into the prostate. Up to three measurement tracks are obtained for each lobe. Prior to PDT, the inspired oxygen (FIO_2) was adjusted briefly from 95% to 98% to room air breathing (21%) and the pO_2 baseline of each track was recorded 2–3 min thereafter for each pre-irradiated prostate. The FIO_2 was switched back to 95%–98% immediately after pO_2 measurements.

A comparison of the measured pO_2 profiles of prostate glands that had been pre-irradiated (with ionizing radiation) and nonirradiated in dogs before TOOKAD-PDT, which is specifically vascular-targeted, indicated that both nonirradiated and pre-irradiated prostates became hyper-oxygenated [7,73]. However, pre-irradiated prostates were better oxygenated, even under room air breathing conditions; mean pO_2 = 36.8 ± 15.9 and 27.9 ± 14.2 mmHg, respectively (see Figure 21.6). This might be due to reduced cell metabolism and increased noncellular components such as collagen. These findings, if they also hold in patients, indicate that PDT following radical radiation therapy to the prostate should not be limited by treatment-induced hypoxia or, by inference, by inadequate delivery of photosensitizer, at least on a global basis.

21.2.5 REAL-TIME MONITORING OF LIGHT FLUENCE DISTRIBUTION

For successful PDT, the light has to be distributed in a way that the whole tumor volume receives a ϕ above the threshold. This means ensuring that a minimum dose, that is, the dose required to induce direct cell death, is received by all parts of the tumor volume. Optimization of the light dose and distribution for PDT depends upon an accurate light delivery system (with appropriate geometric positions, shape, and power of the light source) and determination of ϕ throughout the prostate volume [4,12,19]. Currently, in the most clinical interstitial PDT protocols, the delivered light dose is based on measurements made with implanted isotropic light detectors, which is a better method than simply relying on the delivered light energy, since it improves the chance of achieving uniform light energy deposition within a given patient cohort at a specific dose level. In some clinical trials, ϕ monitoring with equal weighting for the light delivered from each linear source fiber was employed, which may be inadequate. In addition, the light fluence is monitored at only a few selected points within the treatment volume. It is suggested, therefore, to integrate ultrasound imaging and effective PDT dose calculation into the PDT delivery system, using the measured tissue optical properties and drug uptake in individual patients as input parameters [4,12,19]. This would allow optimization of the light energy delivered from each source fiber, as discussed later in order to improve the uniformity of light fluence throughout the target tissue.

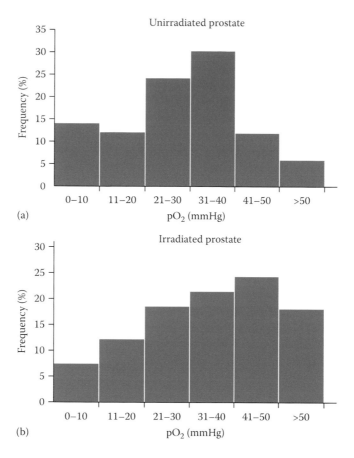

Figure 21.6 Baseline histograms of prostate tissue pO_2 prior to PDT, measured with room air breathing (inspired oxygen FIO_2 = 21%), based on 108 points from two unirradiated prostates and 172 points from four irradiated prostates. The median pO_2 values are 38.0 mmHg for irradiated and 27.3 mmHg for unirradiated prostates and the corresponding means are 36.8 ± 15.9 and 27.9 ± 14.2 mmHg. (From Huang, Z. et al., *Radiat. Res.*, 161, 723, 2004. With permission.)

21.2.5.1 OPTIMIZATION OF THE FIBER POSITIONING AND SOURCE–DETECTOR DISTANCE

Flat-cut optical fibers that serve either as sources or detectors have been adopted by Lund University that allow well-defined positioning and source–detector distance in any measurements conducted with the fibers. Based on the geometry of the tumor and the organs at risk, a dosimetry software has been also developed to calculate the optimum positioning of the fibers. Using this system, predefined values for absorption and scattering can be assigned to different types of tissue and the irradiation times for the individual fibers can be calculated. Based on the treatment-induced changes in the optical properties, the irradiation times can be updated and dosimetry calculations can be performed during treatment. The laser φ through the tumor mass is measured regularly and used to recalculate the optimum light delivery based on the threshold doses set for the treated target tissue and organs at risk in the vicinity of the target tissue. The general procedure and clinical outcome are described elsewhere [19,24].

21.2.5.2 OPTIMIZATION OF SPATIAL LIGHT DISTRIBUTION

A Cimmino algorithm has been developed to optimize the light distribution in PDT of whole prostate by iteratively adjusting the location, length, and intensity of the interstitial light sources [4,66,86–89]. This method is more robust than most optimization algorithms, since it always converges and, if all the constraints are not

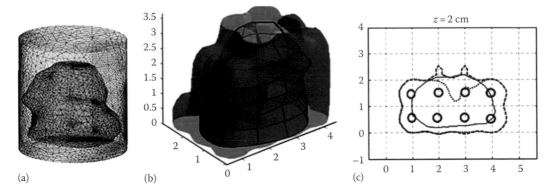

Figure 21.7 (a) Mesh plot of the prostate geometry with a cylindrical outer layer. (b) Isofluence rate surface of 150 mW cm^{-2} for heterogeneous optical properties. (c) Isofluence rate contours in a slice of prostate at $z = 2$ cm: solid line, prostate boundary; dashed line, 150 mW cm^{-2} for homogeneous optical properties; dotted line, 150 mW cm^{-2} for heterogeneous optical properties. The linear source positions are indicated as circles in (c). (Reproduced from Li, J. et al., *Proc. SPIE*, 6139, 61390M, 2006. With permission.)

satisfied, reverts to the best least-squares solution. The algorithm is linear, since the relationship between ϕ and the power of the point (or linear) sources is always linear even though the relationship between ϕ and the distance from the source is nonlinear. Studies to date indicate that it is possible to cover the prostate gland by ensuring delivery of at least a minimum (threshold) light dose while reducing the PDT dose to adjacent critical normal tissues. The algorithm is fast enough (e.g., 300 s on a PC with Intel Pentium 2 GHz CPU) to allow iterative treatment replanning during treatment.

21.2.5.3 MODELING THE LIGHT DISTRIBUTION IN PROSTATE

The finite element–based method (FEM) applied to the P_1 approximation of diffusion theory is currently the main tool for calculating ϕ distributions under conditions of arbitrary geometry and heterogeneous optical properties [4,90]. Figure 21.7 shows an example of linear light sources covering the entire prostate gland with heterogeneous optical properties. The prostate geometry, together with a cylindrical outer layer, is meshed for the calculation, based on 3D transrectal ultrasound images (see Figure 21.7a). The resulting isofluence rate surface is shown in Figure 21.7b and the contour lines are shown in Figure 21.7c, comparing the results for heterogeneous optical properties in an individual patient with those for homogeneous, patient-averaged optical properties ($\mu_a = 0.3$ cm^{-1} and $\mu'_s = 14$ cm^{-1}). The isofluence rate contour for the former misses the top portion of the prostate due to increased absorption in that region, while the latter covers the entire prostate.

21.3 INTERSTITIAL PROSTATE PDT: PRECLINICAL AND CLINICAL RESULTS

Here we will describe several major PDT preclinical and clinical trials done to date using the spectroscopic imaging techniques described earlier. The focus of this section is on the technical aspects of treatment planning, delivery, and monitoring in TOOKAD-, MLu-, and Foscan-mediated PDT.

21.3.1 PRECLINICAL

Most preclinical studies of PDT for prostate cancer have been carried out on transplanted (xenograft) tumors in mice or rats [91,92], either subcutaneously or located in the prostate itself (orthotopic). These models allow assessment of factors such as tumor selectivity. There is no readily available *in vivo* model of prostate cancer in a large animal such as a dog in which one can test light distributions and dosimetry techniques at a size scale that is representative of the clinical situation. Therefore, studies to date have utilized normal (no tumor) adult dog prostate for this purpose, accepting the limitation that there is no target tumor so that the response assessment must be only on normal tissue. The major preclinical study in normal dogs, used to inform the design of subsequent first-in-human clinical trials, was with the vascular-acting photosensitizer TOOKAD [7,44–47,93].

In this study, normal adult male beagle dogs, with or without prior radiation therapy treatment, were prepared following a standard laparotomy procedure [7,44–47,93]. Prostate sizes were determined prior to PDT by computed tomography (CT) scanning. The dogs received antibiotics before and after PDT (IM, Ampicillin, 20 mg kg^{-1}) to prevent possible infection. The animals were variously treated with a single PDT treatment or with two separate procedures. For the latter, the first treatment was carried out at a drug dose of 0.25 or 1 mg kg^{-1} and both lobes received an identical light dose of 50 or 100 J cm^{-1}. The second treatment was carried out 12–13 weeks later at a drug dose of 2 mg kg^{-1} and both lobes received a light dose of 100 or 200 J cm^{-1} [7,12,94]. Pain control consisted of pre- and postoperative injection of morphine, with long-term control provided by Fentanyl patches.

21.3.1.1 LIGHT DELIVERY AND TREATMENT PROCEDURE

The prostate pO$_2$ was measured immediately prior to PDT. The blood clearance of TOOKAD is very fast (see Figure 21.8a) and the intent was to activate the photosensitizer while it was still in the vasculature. Hence, light irradiation was started 4–15 min after the start of sensitizer infusion using a 763 nm diode

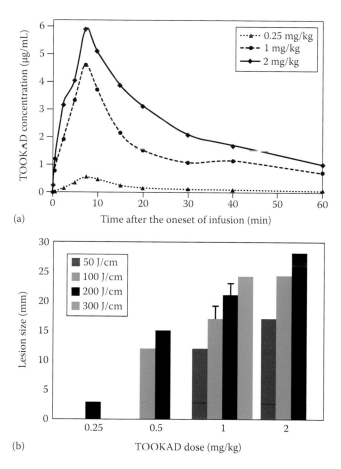

(a)

(b)

Figure 21.8 (a) TOOKAD pharmacokinetics: data points are averages (0.25 mg kg^{-1}, $n = 2$; 1 mg kg^{-1}, $n = 6$; 2 mg kg^{-1}, $n = 2$). (b) Lesion size as a function of TOOKAD and light doses. (Modified from Huang, Z. et al., *Radiat. Res.*, 161, 723, 2004; Huang, Z. et al., *Lasers Surg. Med.*, 36, 390, 2005. With permission.)

laser (CeraLas, Biolitec AG, Germany) with a maximum output of 4 W. A total energy of 50–300 J cm^{-1} of diffusing fiber length was delivered over a period of 5–40 min. The laser output was coupled into a beam splitter that allowed up to four irradiation fields to be treated through separate interstitial fibers simultaneously at identical or varying ϕ. Each interstitial irradiation was delivered through a CDF (1 or 3 cm active length, 1.3 mm outer diameter; CeramOptec GmbH, Bonn, Germany). The CDF tip was placed in the middle section of the right and/or left lobe, either perpendicular (1 cm tip) or parallel (3 cm tip) to the prostatic urethra. An isotropic optical fiber probe (800 μm in diameter) was placed transurethrally into the midpoint of the prostate urethra and coupled to a photometer (Model 88XL, Photodyne, Westlake Village, CA) to monitor the ϕ dynamic changes during PDT; readings of the local ϕ were made every 30 s during PDT. In addition to treating the prostate, direct irradiation of bladder, colon, and abdominal wall surfaces was carried out via an optical fiber fitted with a microlens tip (Medlight S.A., Ecublens, Switzerland) held perpendicular to the serosal surfaces to form a 1 cm diameter irradiation spot.

21.3.1.2 PHOTOSENSITIZER MEASUREMENTS

Blood samples (~3 mL) were taken at timed intervals from the left jugular vein prior to, during, and post-drug infusion to measure the TOOKAD concentration. The samples were immediately transferred to trisodium citrate–pretreated polypropylene tubes in the dark. Plasma extracts were collected after centrifugation and stored at −70°C until high-performance liquid chromatography (HPLC) analysis with ultraviolet (UV) detection was performed. More detailed description of these procedures can be found elsewhere [7,94]. The results for different injected photosensitizer doses, shown in Figure 21.8b, indicate a plasma concentration peak at the end of drug infusion and subsequent rapid clearance. The maximum plasma concentrations for administered TOOKAD doses of 0.25, 1.0, and 2.0 mg kg^{-1} were reported as 0.5, 4.6, and 5.9 μg mL^{-1}, respectively.

21.3.1.3 VASCULAR AND HISTOLOGICAL RESPONSE EVALUATION

In order to evaluate changes in blood flow, blood volume, and permeability inside the treated region, helical contrast-enhanced CT scanning (5 mm slice thickness every 1.8 s for 3 min) using a non-iodinated contrast agent was performed at 48 h and 1 week post-PDT. Marked changes in blood flow, blood volume, and permeability inside the treated region post-PDT were found [53,94]. Following the 1-week scan, the dogs were sacrificed by a barbiturate overdose at 1 week after PDT and the prostate and bladder were removed for histopathology. Typical PDT lesions showed total necrosis of glandular and connective tissues at the center of the irradiated volume, with patchy or diffuse hemorrhage in the case of dogs receiving two PDT treatments and residual fibrosis due to the first treatment [5,7,95].

21.3.1.4 IN VIVO OPTICAL PROPERTIES EVALUATION

Extensive measurements of optical properties were performed in normal canine prostate in Mlu-mediated prostate PDT using 732 nm light [27,47,56,67–73]. The measurements were performed using an interstitial catheter at 0.3–0.7 cm from the central catheter, with a point source. The tissue optical properties can be determined through Equations 21.2 and 21.3, using the same method as described earlier. The basic conclusion is that the light penetration depth in canine prostate is around 0.8 cm. Thus, CDFs spaced 1 cm apart are most suitable to cover the entire prostate for Mlu-mediated PDT at 732 nm. This value in the canine is at least twice as long as those found in prostate for Photofrin-mediated PDT at 630 nm and is considered comparable to the penetration depth for TOOKAD-mediated PDT at 762 nm.

Transrectal NIR optical tomography was conducted concurrently with TRUS on dogs to compare the optical properties of prostate cancer with those of normal intact prostate tissues [96]. In these measurements, the NIR probe was integrated with a 60 mm long sagittal TRUS transducer. The steady-state NIR measurements reconstructed the μ_a and μ'_s images without *a priori* structural information (see Figure 21.9).

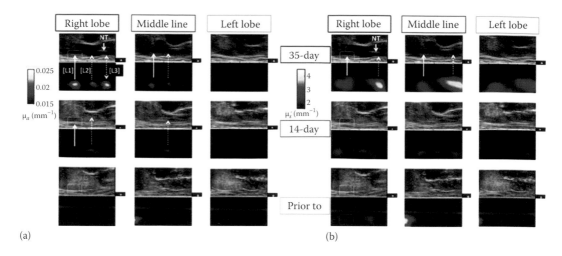

Figure 21.9 *In vivo* transrectal NIR/TRUS in canine pelvic canal. The images were taken before tumor cell injection, 14 days after injection when the ultrasound and rectal examinations showed no evidence of tumor growth, and 35 days after injection when tumor growth was evident both on ultrasound and rectal examinations. (a) NIR/TRUS images of (a) μ_a and (b) μ'_s. (From Jiang, Z. et al., *J. Biomed. Optics*, 14, 030506, 2009. With permission.)

21.3.2 CLINICAL

21.3.2.1 TOOKAD-MEDIATED PDT

In the first human clinical trial for prostate PDT [48,52], for each patient magnetic resonance (MR) images including non-enhanced T2-weighted (T2W), dynamic gadolinium-enhanced T1-weighted (T1W), and delayed contrast-enhanced T1-weighted were acquired 0–36 days before PDT, as well as at 1 week, 4 weeks, and 6 months after treatment. T2W MR images were used by an experienced radiologist to quantify the prostate volume as well as the anatomy and architecture of the prostate gland. The estimation of the necrosis was done using the dynamic contrast-enhanced T1W images. Based on T2W MR images, PDT procedures were planned and the optimized positions and lengths of the fibers were selected. The patients were treated with WST09 or WST11 TOOKAD doses from 2 to 6 mg kg^{-1} of body weight. TOOKAD blood kinetics are very fast and the intent is to activate the photosensitizer while it is still in the vasculature. Thus, light delivery begins 5–15 min after the start of the infusion.

21.3.2.1.1 Treatment procedure and light delivery

Urologists performed the vascular-targeted PDT procedures. Patients were anesthetized and placed in the lithotomy position. By using trocars, surgeons guided the catheters through the perineum to the locations in the prostate that were determined at pretreatment planning. Optical fibers with CDFs for light delivery were inserted within the catheters. WST09 and WST11 TOOKAD were activated using 762 and 753 nm, respectively. In WST11 TOOKAD-mediated PDT, light was delivered through CDFs at the rate of 150 mW cm^{-1} during 1333 s. The diffusing tip of each fiber was positioned according to the security margins from the apex, the base, and the capsule. Insertion was guided by transrectal ultrasound and a perineal template as in brachytherapy. More detailed description can be found elsewhere [48,52].

21.3.2.1.2 Calculation of the PDT-induced necrosis

For each patient, the PDT-induced necrosis was measured. An inflammation of prostatic tissue leading to a swelling of the entire gland occurred due to the catheter insertion and the energy received in the prostate [48,52,97]. The prostate swelling ratio, the ratio between the prostate volumes 7 days after PDT and 0 day before PDT, was evaluated. The induced lesions were quantified by T2W series and T1 gadolinium-enhanced images. The validation protocol consisted in comparing the overlap between the simulated necrosis and the necrosis

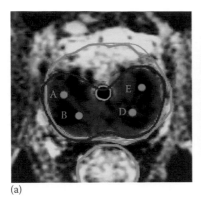
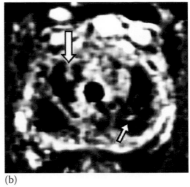

(a)   (b)

Figure 21.10 (a) Color fluence map superimposed on transverse contrast-enhanced T1-weighted MR image. Blue, yellow, and green circles outline the prostate, urethra, and rectum margins, respectively. The fiber locations are shown with blue dots (A, B, D, E). The red region presents the expected necrosis boundary determined by the treatment-planning software, which assumes homogeneous WST09 TOOKAD distribution and tissue sensitivity to PDT. (b) Corresponding T1-weighted MR image obtained 1 week after PDT showing islands of spared enhancing tissue within the expected area of necrosis (small arrow) and irregular treatment boundaries (large arrow). (From Haider, M.A. et al., *Radiology*, 244, 196, 2007. With permission.)

measured by the MR images after swelling correction. Figure 21.10 compares the expected necrosis boundary determined by a treatment-planning software, which assumes homogeneous drug distribution and tissue sensitivity to PDT with necrosis effect observed at contrast-enhanced T1W MR imaging. More detailed description can be found elsewhere [52].

21.3.2.2 MLu-MEDIATED PDT

In this section, the clinical trials carried out at University of Pennsylvania with the photosensitizer MLu will be described in detail. Patients with biopsy-proven, locally recurrent prostate carcinoma following radiation therapy were enrolled for interstitial MLu-mediated PDT after radiation therapy. Each patient had standard history and physical, MRI, radionuclide bone scan, urological evaluation, and laboratory studies including complete blood count, biochemistry profile, lipid panel, and serum prostate-specific antigen (PSA) levels [5]. The biochemical success of prostate treatment is typically measured through the extent of PSA reduction after resolution of the initial therapy-induced spike [2,5] that typically lasts from <1 h to several weeks [5].

Before treatment, the urologist drew the target prostate volume on each slice of transrectal ultrasound images, spaced 0.5 cm apart. A template with 0.5 cm grid spacing projected the locations of light sources relative to the prostate and a treatment plan was then developed for the placement of CDFs and to determine the length of each CDF [56,57].

21.3.2.2.1 Light delivery

A 732 nm diode laser (Model 730, 15-W; Diomed, Ltd., Cambridge, United Kingdom) was used. This wavelength is within the "therapeutic window" [12] in which the photon energy is high enough to excite the photosensitizer, and yet the light has sufficient penetration into the tissue. Interstitial optical fibers connected sequentially to the laser source were placed directly into the prostate at the preplanned locations [66] and the light was delivered at 150 mW cm^{-1} length for a total light delivered fluence from 25 to 150 J cm^{-2} measured at 0.5 cm from the CDFs, depending on tissue optical properties.

21.3.2.2.2 Placement of interstitial CDFs

Before treatment the patients were placed under general anesthesia. Based on the treatment plan, the prostate was divided into four quadrants, as shown in Figure 21.10. Then, four 18G plastic catheters with metal trocars were placed through the template into the prostate (Figure 21.11) for the pre-calibrated isotropic detector fibers, one for each quadrant. For treatment light delivery, four additional catheters were then inserted 0.5 or 0.7 cm distance lateral from the detector catheters; these sources were used during both measurement of the optical

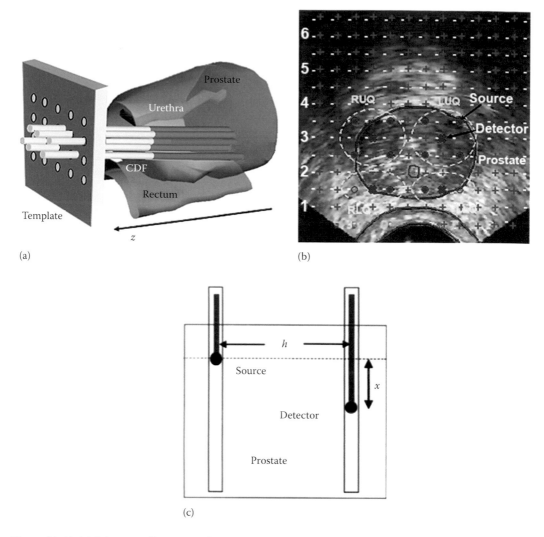

Figure 21.11 (a) Schematic illustration of the prostate and surrounding anatomy as well as its relationship to the template used for placement of the catheters [4]. For simplicity, only six catheters are shown, with their active regions shaded. (b) Transrectal ultrasound image of a human prostate, showing the position of sources (●) and detector (x) fibers. The prostate was divided into four quadrants—right upper quadrant (RUQ), left upper quadrant (LUQ), right lower quadrant (RLQ) and left lower quadrant (LLQ)—as shown with yellow dashed circles. The open circle on the RLQ is for a linear source that passed through the position but was too short to have an active light component in the cross-sectional plane. The grid on the template (+) has 5 mm spacing. (c) Schematic of the measurement geometry, illustrating the coordinates used to determine the source–detector distances [27]. ([a]: Modified from Zhu, T.C. and Finlay, J.C., *Photodiagnosis and Photodyn. Ther.*, 3, 234, 2006; [c]: Zhu, T.C. et al., *Photochem. Photobiol.*, 81, 96, 2005. With permission.)

properties and treatment light delivery. The detector fibers were kept in place during the entire treatment to monitor the light fluence, tissue optical properties, and blood flow. A fifth detector catheter was also placed in the urethra to monitor the light fluence at this location. A transrectal ultrasound unit was used to guide the needle and catheter placement.

21.3.2.2.3 Treatment procedure

After mapping the tissue optical properties over a total time of about 5 min, interstitial PDT was performed with light delivery one quadrant at a time. The 732 nm was delivered at a power of 150 mW cm^{-1} diffusing fiber length and the treatment time for the four fibers was varied to deliver the same cumulative fluence from all four *in situ* detectors lying in a transverse plane at 2 cm from the apex of the prostate. The target fluence ranged from 25 to 150 J cm^{-2} between different patient cohorts. After treatment was completed the optical properties of the prostate in all four quadrants were measured again (over 5 min). The light sources and detectors were then removed and posttreatment biopsies were performed immediately. The tissue specimens were quick-frozen on dry ice, protected from light, and stored at −80°C for subsequent analysis.

The above treatment procedure was performed in a surgical suite with precautions to prevent unplanned photosensitizer activation, including the use of filtered operating room lights and covering of the patient's exposed skin. The total treatment time varied but was always less than 2 h. The details of the dosimetry system and calibration procedures can be found elsewhere [27].

21.3.2.2.4 Prostate optical properties and photosensitizer concentration

In determining the prostate tissue optical properties in these patients, measurements in phantoms with a range of known μ_a and μ_s' values, as well as *ex vivo* measurements of the sensitizer concentration, provided baselines for interpreting interstitial *in vivo* measurements. The liquid phantom comprised a mixture of a scattering medium (liposyn III, 30% Abbott Lab, North Chicago, IL) and a pure absorbing dye (green ink). A second set of phantoms was used to verify that μ_a varies linearly with photosensitizer concentration.

Ex vivo measurements of photosensitizer concentration were made as follows. Biopsies collected pre- and post-PDT from each prostate quadrant were placed in a 2 mL capped polypropylene tube and homogenized in 400 µL of phosphate buffer (24 µM; pH 7.5). The homogenates were then mixed with 400 µL of chloroform, after which 400 µL of methanol was added. After centrifugation (3500 rpm; 15 min), the organic layer was collected and 200 µL was transferred to a cuvette and measured in a spectrofluorometer (FluoroMax-3; JobinYvon, Inc.) with excitation and detection at 474 and 650–850 nm, respectively. The photosensitizer concentration was calculated based on the measured change in fluorescence upon addition of a known amount of photosensitizer after the initial reading. The effect of PDT on tissue photosensitizer was calculated as the ratio of the post- to pre-PDT measurements.

More detailed description of the phantom and *ex vivo* studies for verification of the *in vivo* measurements can be found elsewhere [5,27].

21.3.2.3 FOSCAN-MEDIATED PDT

In this trial at Lund University, interstitial human prostate PDT mediated by Foscan was done 96 h post-drug injection [19–21,23,24]. PDT was performed by using 18 optical fibers that were coupled through a fiber switch to 18 diode lasers (with the wavelength of 652 nm). The optimal positions were found using the random search algorithm explained in Section 21.2.5.1 [19,24], which relies on the knowledge of the 3D anatomy of the prostate and surrounding tissues, retrieved from a transrectal ultrasound scan. Each fiber emits light, while the six neighboring fibers collect the transmitted and fluorescent light of Foscan (broad peak between 710 and 730 nm). Light detection is governed by a set of spectrometers. During treatment the light irradiation was halted, and a sequence of measurements was performed. During a monitoring session, a total of 108 fluorescence recordings were acquired between 54 source–detector pairs.

Optical properties were assessed using spatially resolved measurements as well as TOF spectroscopy as described in Section 21.2.1.3 [19–21,24]. Data acquired during a prostate PDT session was used to reconstruct the 2D and 3D mapping of the photosensitizer distribution in the human prostate. Reconstructions from a patient showing heterogeneous distribution of Foscan photosensitizer in prostate have been shown in Figure 21.12 [23].

21.3.3 COMPARISON OF PROSTATE PDT SYSTEMS

We have described several major clinical trials of whole-prostate PDT done to date, focusing on the technical aspects of treatment planning, delivery, and monitoring, and highlighting the differences in the approach taken. In this section, the differences in light delivery and dosimetry of trials carried out with TOOKAD, MLu, and Foscan photosensitizers will be compared to highlight the advantages and limitations of different methods and technology platforms. The clinical objective of all these trials was to destroy the whole prostate gland, not simply

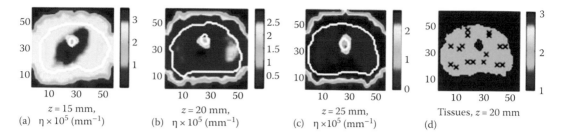

Figure 21.12 (a)–(c) Schematic of the Foscan distribution in cross-sectional slices at $z = 15$, 20, and 25 mm, respectively. The prostate and urethra boundaries are marked with white. (d) One slice of the prostate showing the tissue regions where 1 is normal, 2 is the prostate, and 3 is the urethra; the fiber positions in the xy plane are also shown. These images are reconstructed based on the data obtained from the PDT clinical trial. (From Axelsson, J. et al., *Optics Lett.*, 34, 232, 2009. With permission.)

to target known areas of tumor within it. This poses significant challenges of ensuring complete coverage of the gland, which has a complex 3D shape and varies significantly between patients, and avoiding damage to normal tissues, including the rectal wall, erectile nerves, and urinary sphincter.

Clinical trials of MLu-mediated PDT have been carried out in the United States, at University of Pennsylvania, using a system that includes measurements of the tissue optical properties, interstitial photosensitizer concentration, as well as the real-time monitoring of light fluence distribution, blood flow, and tissue oxygenation. Clinical trials of PDT using the photosensitizer Foscan have been carried out in Sweden using a light delivery and light/photosensitizer/tissue oxygenation dosimetry system developed at University of Lund and commercialized by Spectracure AB, Lund, Sweden [22]. Phase I and II trials using the vascular-targeted photosensitizer TOOKAD have been carried out in Toronto using a customized treatment planning system and separate light dosimetry system.

21.3.3.1 LIGHT DELIVERY COMPARISON

As summarized in Table 21.2, the first significant difference between the Swedish and U.S. trials was the use of interstitial point fiber sources (up to 18) in Lund, rather than cylindrically diffusing fibers (2–4 fibers per quadrant, up to 16 total) that were used in the United States. Further, each point fiber was connected to a separate diode laser and all fibers were activated simultaneously with the output power of each adjusted to 150 mW prior to treatment. The consequence of using many point sources is that, in principle, there is much greater control over the resultant light distribution. In addition, there is the possibility to adjust the output power of each fiber source independently to maintain uniform light delivery throughout the prostate during treatment even if the optical properties and/or photosensitizer concentration are changing. However, placing so many sources accurately is challenging and time-consuming, and determining the optimum placement requires sophisticated pretreatment planning. The Toronto trial was a compromise between these two approaches, in which four to six individual cylindrical fibers were used, powered by two or three diode lasers each having a two-way beam splitter. The light was delivered simultaneously to all the fibers and at the same power. The requirement for simultaneous light delivery from all fibers was due to the fact that TOOKAD is very rapidly cleared from the circulation (within minutes), so that there is a very short time window for light delivery and sequential activation of the fibers is not an option.

21.3.3.2 DOSIMETRY COMPARISON

All three centers developed specific dosimetry systems for whole-prostate PDT and the main characteristics are summarized in Table 21.3.

All three centers had capabilities for *in situ* light dosimetry using isotropic fiber probes placed within the prostate at multiple points. In Toronto, additional probes were placed on the rectal wall and into the space between the prostate and the rectum, and were used to terminate treatment at a certain fluence (4 J cm^{-2}) to avoid overdosing. Probes were also variously used to measure the light dose in the urethra. Various probes

Table 21.2 Comparison of light delivery used in the three major clinical studies of whole-prostate PDT

Trial center	Sources	Beam splitter	Fibers	Fiber placement	Power per fiber	Treatment time per fiber
U. Pennsylvania, USA	15 W diode laser: 4–8 W, 732 nm	Yes	12–18 cylindrical diffusing	As per treatment plan	150 mW cm^{-1}	Variable
U. Lund, Sweden	6–18 diode lasers: 250 mW, 652 nm	No	Up to 18 point	As per treatment plan	150 mW	Fixed
U. Health Network, Canada	2 or 3 diode lasers: 4 W, 763 nm	Yes	4–6 cylindrical diffusers	As per treatment plan	100 mW cm^{-1}	Fixed

More detailed description of the clinical trials at U. Pennsylvania (U. Penn), U. Lund, and U. Health Network Canada can be found in References [4,57,71,88,89,99]; 22; and 44, respectively.

Table 21.3 Comparison of online dosimetry used in the three major clinical studies of whole-prostate PDT

Trial center	Light				Active monitoring/control during treatment	Sensitizer concentration	Tissue oxygenation
	Isotropic probes	Placement	Dynamic feedback	Optical properties			
U. Penn, USA	5 simultaneously scanning along the catheter	One per prostate quadrant urethra	16-channel computerized power control	Multiple clusters of 1 emitting and 4 detector fibers *DOT map*	Manual	*In situ* fluorescence/absorption spectroscopy	Blood flow by NIRS
U. Lund, Sweden	Up to 18, switching from source to detector	As needed based on optimization for uniform light dose		Multiple clusters of 1 emitting and 6 detector fibers	Automatic, based on achieving minimum threshold dose	*In situ* fluorescence spectroscopy *FDOT map*	*In situ* SO$_2$ by NIRS
U. Health Network, Canada	Up to 8 simultaneously	Each prostate lobe urethra rectal wall rectal–prostate space	Rectal wall limited to 4 J cm^{-2}	All source–detector combinations prior to treatment	Manual	Absorption spectroscopy of blood samples *in situ* white-light diffuse transmittance spectroscopy	*In situ* diffuse transmittance NIRS

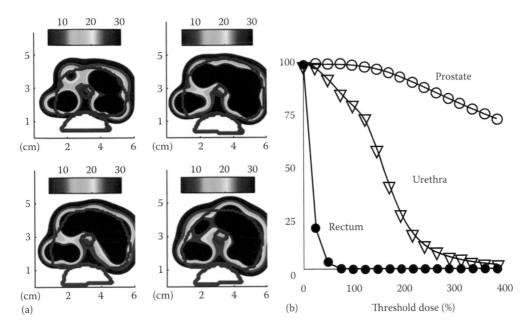

Figure 21.13 Examples of dosimetry results from Lund clinical trial. (a) Light fluence maps (J cm^{-2}) at different craniocaudal positions throughout one patient's prostate, showing the degree of dose uniformity achieved. (b) Example of resulting dose–volume histogram in one patient expressed as a function of the percentage of threshold dose for the target prostate tissue, the urethra, and the rectum. (Modified from Swartling, J. et al., *J. Biomed. Opt.*, 15, 058003, 2010. With permission.)

within the prostate were used to monitor the local light fluence rate during PDT light delivery: for example, in the Lund system, each of the 18 fibers was activated in turn and a cluster of 6 other fibers was switched to detection mode, as shown in the example in Figure 21.13.

The interstitial probes could also be used to map the tissue optical properties, either locally or globally throughout the prostate. The fluence rate or derived optical property measurements can be used to adjust the light delivery to compensate for heterogeneity of the light distribution, and in the integrated dosimetry system developed in Lund this was done automatically using an algorithm to ensure that a minimum PDT dose threshold (5 J cm^{-2}) was achieved throughout the prostate. In the other two trials, the adjustment of the treatment, if any, was carried out manually.

There was also considerable variability between the three trials in their approach to measuring the photosensitizer concentration, and how this information was used. TOOKAD is not fluorescent and is rapidly cleared from the circulation: in fact, light delivery is initiated before completion of the photosensitizer infusion in order to maximize the effective PDT dose. Hence, a simple absorption spectroscopy set up was used in the operating room to measure the photosensitizer concentration in blood samples taken periodically during treatment in order to monitor the pharmacokinetics and, in particular, to monitor the disaggregation of the photosensitizer into the photoactive monomeric state. In addition, *in situ* measurements were made by connecting the urethral fiber to a broadband source and measuring the transmittance spectrum from one of the detector fibers, which allowed the TOOKAD absorption peak around 760 nm to be observed at a few time points during treatment: this was limited by the need to temporarily turn off the treatment laser during measurements so as to avoid saturating the detector. The main value of these measurements was to confirm the optimal interval between the start of drug infusion and the start of light delivery (around 6 min). In the Lund studies the photosensitizer fluorescence was mapped in much the same way as the tissue optical properties, with sequential delivery of blue excitation light to each of the 18 intra-prostatic fibers and using 6 surrounding fibers as fluorescence detectors by switching their output to individual spectrometers. In the Upenn study, the fluorescence for photosensitizer (Mlu) concentration was measured with both absorption and fluorescence spectroscopy. The fluorescence spectroscopy used a single fiber to both emit 460 nm light and detect fluorescent light along a detector catheter connected to a motor to determine photosensitizer concentration versus longitudinal distances for each prostate quadrant.

Finally, for this comparison, some information in individual patients was obtained relating to blood flow or blood oxygenation in the prostate at the time of PDT treatment, based on diffuse transmittance NIR spectroscopy of hemoglobin. However, none of the trials to date has made use of this information to adjust the treatment parameters.

One important feature of the technology platform developed and implemented in clinical trials in Lund was the integration of the light generation, delivery, and multifunctional dosimetry into a single, computer-controlled instrument (see Figure 21.14). A prototype device for 16 channel CDFs via a 1:16 high power beam

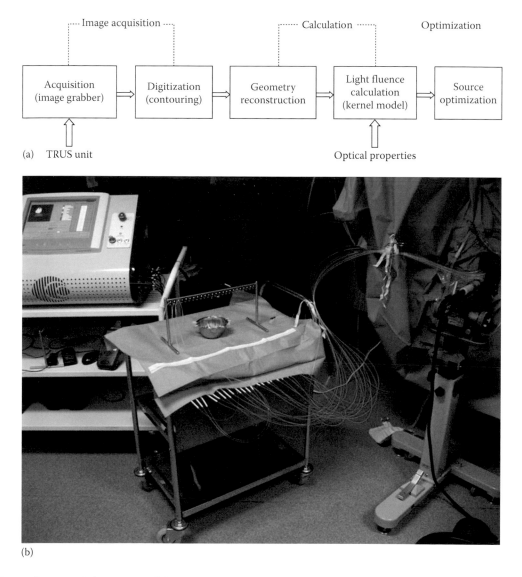

(b)

Figure 21.14 (a) Schematics and (b) integrated light delivery and dosimetry system. ([a]: From Zhu, T.C. and Finlay, J.C., *Photodiagnosis and Photodyn. Ther.*, 3, 234, 2006; Finlay, J.C. et al., *Photochem. Photobiol.*, 82, 1270, 2006; Zhu, T.C. et al., *J. Photochem. Photobiol. B Biol.*, 79, 231, 2005; Zhu, T.C. et al, *Proc. SPIE*, 7551, 75510E, 2011; Li, J. et al., *Proc. SPIE*, 6846, 68450Q, 2008. [b]: Courtesy of Spectracure AB, Lund, Sweden.)

splitter was also developed at Upenn [98]. The latter requires a separate 16-channel detector system to perform light dosimetry, unlike the Lund system, which allows switching between the light source and detector for each point source.

Since the treatment light is coupled into optical fibers for delivery to the prostate and all the light that is utilized for dosimetry is also collected by the same interstitial optical fibers, it is relatively straightforward to use state-of-the-art fiber-optic switching devices to "manage" the light, for example, by switching each fiber from light-delivery mode to light-collection mode, or altering the light for photosensitizer quantification, or tissue oxygenation measurements, all done under computer control.

21.4 SUMMARY AND FUTURE PERSPECTIVES

Treatment options for locally recurrent prostate cancer after radiation therapy are limited. PDT is a minimally invasive treatment option for these patients that has shown efficacy in several clinical trials using different photosensitizers targeting either the vasculature and/or cellular components. The goal for all of them was to achieve complete functional destruction of the prostate, including complete tumor kill. The fact that PDT does not destroy the collagen structure of the tissue means that the prostate is structurally intact and becomes fibrotic following successful treatment. PDT is not generally contradicted by prior radical radiotherapy since the mechanism of action (membrane versus DNA damage) is different, and this has been demonstrated by the successful whole-prostate treatments [1,4,5,18]. The ability to repeat PDT treatments if there is incomplete response [44] has also been demonstrated. The use of PDT for primary focal prostate cancer is also under investigation [99] using WST11, an improved water-soluble version of TOOKAD.

For whole-prostate PDT, different light delivery schemes have been developed to achieve near-complete coverage of the prostate, as summarized in Table 21.2. Analogous to radioactive seeds and wires, interstitial delivery of light has used either point or cylindrically diffusing optical fibers, respectively. The main advantage of the former is that a greater degree of conformity with the irregular shape of the prostate can be achieved. It is not clear how critical this consideration is in practice, given the other uncertainties in PDT dosimetry, and the fact that it is only necessary to exceed a minimum threshold dose throughout the prostate rather than achieve an equal prescribed dose everywhere. This latter point is worth emphasizing. For example, it was demonstrated that sharply demarcated regions of devascularization in the prostate can be accurately mapped using gadolinium contrast-enhanced MRI following TOOKAD-PDT. If one then co-registers these regions with the light distribution based on interstitial fluence rate measurements, it is possible to estimate the threshold dose in individual prostates, which in turn is correlated with the outcome [100].

As we have emphasized, PDT dosimetry is much more complex than dosimetry for radiation therapy, due to two main factors: (1) the much greater degree of heterogeneity in the tissue optical properties and the photosensitizer concentration within the target volume, and (2) the dynamic interdependence of several factors (light, photosensitizer, oxygenation) that contribute to the effective treatment dose [101–103]. On the other hand, unlike radiation therapy, there is the possibility to perform real-time monitoring of these factors and interactively modify the treatment online in order to achieve the optimum therapeutic response, that is, to "personalize" the treatment. This poses significant technical challenges and, as evidenced by the various systems developed to date, there is potential for innovative approaches to fully integrated online treatment dosimetry and delivery.

Since the response of tissue to PDT is also very rapid, there is a further opportunity to integrate different forms of online response monitoring (both imaging and spectroscopic) to provide better feedback and treatment adjustment [101]. The best form of response monitoring will depend on the mechanism of action of the particular photosensitizer, depending on whether the treatment targets the vascular or cellular compartments. As we exploit our growing knowledge of the underlying photochemistry, biology, and physiology of PDT to develop new and better treatments, it will be more important than ever to understand and optimize the key components of treatment over which we have direct control.

LIST OF SYMBOLS

$^1O_2$	singlet oxygen (µM)
$^3O_2$	oxygen (µM)
μ_a	absorption coefficient (cm⁻¹)
μ_s'	reduced scattering coefficient (cm⁻¹)
c	photosensitizer concentration (µM)
μ_{eff}	effective attenuation coefficient (cm⁻¹)
ϕ	fluence rate (mW cm⁻²)
$\phi_m^{(t)}$	measured fluence rate (mW cm⁻²) at time (t)
$\phi_c^{(t)}$	calculated fluence rate (mW cm⁻²) at time (t)
$\phi_{m\_ref}^{(t)}$	measured light fluence rate (mW cm⁻²) from the calibration phantom
$\phi_{c\_ref}^{(t)}$	calculated light fluence rate (mW cm⁻²) from the calibration phantom
S	source strength (mW cm⁻³ sr⁻¹)
r	distance from point source (cm)
x	parallel distance from the center of the point source (cm)
h	perpendicular distance from the center of the point source (cm)
C_{HbO_2}	oxy-hemoglobin concentration (µM)
C_{Hb}	deoxy-hemoglobin concentration (µM)
THC	hemoglobin concentration (µM)
SO_2	blood oxygen saturation
pO_2	tissue oxygen tension (mmHg)
τ	correlation delay time (s)
$E(r,t)$	electric field (V cm⁻¹)
$G_1(r,\tau)$	electric field temporal autocorrelation function (V² cm⁻²)
$g_1(r,\tau)$	normalized electric field temporal autocorrelation function
α	proportional to the tissue blood volume fraction
D_B	effective diffusion coefficient of the moving scatterers (µm² s⁻¹)
αD_B	relative changes in tissue blood flow

ACKNOWLEDGMENTS

This work is supported by grants to T.Z. and R.P. from National Institute of Health (NIH) P01 CA87971 and R01 CA 154562 and to B.W. from the Canadian Cancer Society Research Institute. We are grateful for helpful discussions and insights from Dr. Jarod C. Finlay.

REFERENCES

1. H. Lepor, Vascular targeted photodynamic therapy for localized prostate cancer, *Reviews in Urology*, 10 (2008) 254–261.
2. C.M. Moore, D. Pendse, M. Emberton, Photodynamic therapy for prostate cancer—A review of current status and future promise, *Nature Clinical Practice, Urology*, 6 (2009) 18–30.
3. J. Finkelstein, E. Eckersberger, H. Sadri, S.S. Taneja, H. Lepor, B. Djavan, Open versus laparoscopic versus robot-assisted laparoscopic prostatectomy: The European and US experience, *Reviews in Urology*, 12 (2010) 35–43.
4. T.C. Zhu, J.C. Finlay, Prostate PDT dosimetry, *Photodiagnosis and Photodynamic Therapy*, 3 (2006) 234–246.

5. H. Patel, R. Mick, J. Finlay, T.C. Zhu, E. Rickter, K.A. Cengel, S.B. Malkowicz, S.M. Hahn, T.M. Busch, Motexafin lutetium-photodynamic therapy of prostate cancer: Short- and long-term effects on prostate-specific antigen, *Clinical Cancer Research: An Official Journal of the American Association for Cancer Research*, 14 (2008) 4869–4876.

6. R.L. Siegel, K.D. Miller, A. Jemal, Cancer statistics 2015, *CA: A Cancer Journal for Clinicians*, 65 (2015) 5–29.

7. Z. Huang, Q. Chen, N. Trncic, S.M. LaRue, P.H. Brun, B.C. Wilson, H. Shapiro, F.W. Hetzel, Effects of Pd-bacteriopheophorbide (TOOKAD)-mediated photodynamic therapy on canine prostate pretreated with ionizing radiation, *Radiation Research*, 161 (2004) 723–731.

8. A. Bill-Axelson, L. Holmberg, H. Garmo, J.R. Rider, K. Taari, C. Busch, S. Nordling et al., Radical prostatectomy or watchful waiting in early prostate cancer, *The New England Journal of Medicine*, 370 (2014) 932–942.

9. H. Lepor, A. McCullough, J.D. Engel, Renewing intimacy: Advances in treating erectile dysfunction post-prostatectomy, *Reviews in Urology*, 10 (2008) 245–253.

10. T.M. Beer, A.J. Armstrong, D.E. Rathkopf, Y. Loriot, C.N. Sternberg, C.S. Higano, P. Iversen et al., Enzalutamide in metastatic prostate cancer before chemotherapy, *The New England Journal of Medicine*, 371 (2014) 424–433.

11. R.J. Kumar, A. Barqawi, E.D. Crawford, Adverse events associated with hormonal therapy for prostate cancer, *Reviews in Urology*, 7(Suppl 5) (2005) S37–S43.

12. T.C. Zhu, J.C. Finlay, The role of photodynamic therapy (PDT) physics, *Medical Physics*, 35 (2008) 3127–3136.

13. R. Penjweini, H.-G. Loew, P. Breit, K.W. Kratky, Optimizing the antitumor selectivity of PVP-Hypericin re A549 cancer cells and HLF normal cells through pulsed blue light. *Photodiagnosis and Photodynamic Therapy*, 10 (2013) 591–599.

14. R. Penjweini, B. Liu, M.M. Kim, T.C. Zhu. Explicit dosimetry for 2-(1-hexyloxyethyl)-2-devinyl pyropheophorbide-a-mediated photodynamic therapy: Macroscopic singlet oxygen modeling. *Journal of Biomedical Optics*, 20 (2015) 128003.

15. R. Penjweini, N. Smisdom, S. Deville, M. Ameloot, Transport and accumulation of PVP-Hypericin in cancer and normal cells characterized by image correlation spectroscopy techniques, *Biochimica et Biophysica Acta*, 1843 (2014) 855–865.

16. P. Jichlinski, D. Jacqmin, Photodynamic diagnosis in non-muscle-invasive bladder cancer, *European Urology Supplements*, 7 (2008) 529–535.

17. D. Jocham, H. Stepp, R. Waidelich, Photodynamic diagnosis in urology: State-of-the-art, *European Urology*, 53 (2008) 1138–1150.

18. T. Liu, L.Y. Wu, J.K. Choi, C.E. Berkman, Targeted photodynamic therapy for prostate cancer: Inducing apoptosis via activation of the caspase-8/-3 cascade pathway, *International Journal of Oncology*, 36 (2010) 777–784.

19. K. Svanberg, N. Bendsoe, J. Axelsson, S. Andersson-Engels, S. Svanberg, Photodynamic therapy: Superficial and interstitial illumination, *Journal of Biomedical Optics*, 15 (2010) 041502.

20. T. Svensson, S. Andersson-Engels, M. Einarsdottir, K. Svanberg, In vivo optical characterization of human prostate tissue using near-infrared time-resolved spectroscopy, *Journal of Biomedical Optics*, 12 (2007) 014022.

21. T. Svensson, E. Alerstam, M. Einarsdottir, K. Svanberg, S. Andersson-Engels, Towards accurate in vivo spectroscopy of the human prostate, *Journal of Biophotonics*, 1 (2008) 200–203.

22. J. Swartling, J. Axelsson, G. Ahlgren, K.M. Kalkner, S. Nilsson, S. Svanberg, K. Svanberg, S. Andersson-Engels, System for interstitial photodynamic therapy with online dosimetry: First clinical experiences of prostate cancer, *Journal of Biomedical Optics*, 15 (2010) 058003.

23. J. Axelsson, J. Swartling, S. Andersson-Engels, In vivo photosensitizer tomography inside the human prostate, *Optics Letters*, 34 (2009) 232–234.

24. A. Johansson, J. Axelsson, S. Andersson-Engels, J. Swartling, Realtime light dosimetry software tools for interstitial photodynamic therapy of the human prostate, *Medical Physics*, 34 (2007) 4309–4321.

25. D.E. Dolmans, D. Fukumura, R.K. Jain, Photodynamic therapy for cancer, *Nature Reviews Cancer*, 3 (2003) 380–387.

26. K. Verigos, D.C. Stripp, R. Mick, T.C. Zhu, R. Whittington, D. Smith, A. Dimofte et al., Updated results of a phase I trial of motexafin lutetium-mediated interstitial photodynamic therapy in patients with locally recurrent prostate cancer, *Journal of Environmental Pathology, Toxicology and Oncology: Official Organ of the International Society for Environmental Toxicology and Cancer*, 25 (2006) 373–387.

27. T.C. Zhu, A. Dimofte, J.C. Finlay, D. Stripp, T. Busch, J. Miles, R. Whittington et al., Optical properties of human prostate at 732 nm measured in mediated photodynamic therapy, *Photochemistry and Photobiology*, 81 (2005) 96–105.

28. H.M. Ross, J.A. Smelstoys, G.J. Davis, A.S. Kapatkin, F. Del Piero, E. Reineke, H. Wang et al., Photodynamic therapy with motexafin lutetium for rectal cancer: A preclinical model in the dog, *The Journal of Surgical Research*, 135 (2006) 323–330.

29. D.J. Kereiakes, A.M. Szyniszewski, D. Wahr, H.C. Herrmann, D.I. Simon, C. Rogers, P. Kramer et al., Phase I drug and light dose-escalation trial of motexafin lutetium and far red light activation (phototherapy) in subjects with coronary artery disease undergoing percutaneous coronary intervention and stent deployment: Procedural and long-term results, *Circulation*, 108 (2003) 1310–1315.

30. Z. Huang, A review of progress in clinical photodynamic therapy, *Technology in Cancer Research and Treatment*, 4 (2005) 283–293.

31. J.C. Finlay, A. Darafsheh, Light sources, drugs, and dosimetry, in: *Biomedical Optics in Otorhinolaryngology: Head and Neck Surgery*, B. Wong and J. Ilgner (Eds.), Springer, New York (2016).

32. T. Windahl, S.O. Andersson, L. Lofgren, Photodynamic therapy of localised prostatic cancer, *Lancet*, 336 (1990) 1139.

33. U. Igbaseimokumo, Quantification of in vivo Photofrin uptake by human pituitary adenoma tissue, *Journal of Neurosurgery*, 101 (2004) 272–277.

34. P.V. Marks, P.E. Belchetz, A. Saxena, U. Igbaseimokumo, S. Thomson, M. Nelson, M.R. Stringer, J.A. Holroyd, S.B. Brown, Effect of photodynamic therapy on recurrent pituitary adenomas: Clinical phase I/II trial—An early report, *British Journal of Neurosurgery*, 14 (2000) 317–325.

35. M. Wiedmann, F. Berr, I. Schiefke, H. Witzigmann, K. Kohlhaw, J. Mossner, K. Caca, Photodynamic therapy in patients with non-resectable hilar cholangiocarcinoma: 5-year follow-up of a prospective phase II study, *Gastrointestinal Endoscopy*, 60 (2004) 68–75.

36. M. Wiedmann, K. Caca, F. Berr, I. Schiefke, A. Tannapfel, C. Wittekind, J. Mossner, J. Hauss, H. Witzigmann, Neoadjuvant photodynamic therapy as a new approach to treating hilar cholangiocarcinoma: A phase II pilot study, *Cancer*, 97 (2003) 2783–2790.

37. R.E. Cuenca, R.R. Allison, C. Sibata, G.H. Downie, Breast cancer with chest wall progression: Treatment with photodynamic therapy, *Annals of Surgical Oncology*, 11 (2004) 322–327.

38. T. Momma, M.R. Hamblin, H.C. Wu, T. Hasan, Photodynamic therapy of orthotopic prostate cancer with benzoporphyrin derivative: Local control and distant metastasis, *Cancer Research*, 58 (1998) 5425–5431.

39. B. Chen, B.W. Pogue, X. Zhou, J.A. O'Hara, N. Solban, E. Demidenko, P.J. Hoopes, T. Hasan, Effect of tumor host microenvironment on photodynamic therapy in a rat prostate tumor model, *Clinical Cancer Research: An Official Journal of the American Association for Cancer Research*, 11 (2005) 720–727.

40. N. Solban, P.K. Selbo, A.K. Sinha, S.K. Chang, T. Hasan, Mechanistic investigation and implications of photodynamic therapy induction of vascular endothelial growth factor in prostate cancer, *Cancer Research*, 66 (2006) 5633–5640.

41. Z. Huang, F. Hetzel, K. Dole, J. Beckers, D. Maul, Preliminary study of verteporfin photodynamic therapy in a canine prostate model, *Proceedings of SPIE*, 7380 (2009) 73801Y.

42. K. Svanberg, N. Bendsoe, S. Svanberg, S. Andersson-Engels, Clinical and technical aspects of photodynamic therapy—Superficial and interstitial illumination in skin and prostate cancer, in: *Handbook of Biophotonics*, J. Popp, V.V. Tuchin, A. Chiou, S.H. Heinemann (Eds.), Wiley-VCH Verlag & Co. KgaA, Weinheim, Germany, part 2:3, vol. 18 (2013) pp. 259–287.

43. T.R. Nathan, D.E. Whitelaw, S.C. Chang, W.R. Lees, P.M. Ripley, H. Payne, L. Jones et al., Photodynamic therapy for prostate cancer recurrence after radiotherapy: A phase I study, *The Journal of Urology*, 168 (2002) 1427–1432.

44. J. Trachtenberg, A. Bogaards, R.A. Weersink, M.A. Haider, A. Evans, S.A. McCluskey, A. Scherz et al., Vascular targeted photodynamic therapy with palladium-bacteriopheophorbide photosensitizer for recurrent prostate cancer following definitive radiation therapy: Assessment of safety and treatment response, *The Journal of Urology*, 178 (2007) 1974–1979; discussion 1979.

45. J. Trachtenberg, R.A. Weersink, S.R. Davidson, M.A. Haider, A. Bogaards, M.R. Gertner, A. Evans et al., Vascular-targeted photodynamic therapy (padoporfin, WST09) for recurrent prostate cancer after failure of external beam radiotherapy: A study of escalating light doses, *BJU International*, 102 (2008) 556–562.

46. R.A. Weersink, J. Forbes, S. Bisland, J. Trachtenberg, M. Elhilali, P.H. Brun, B.C. Wilson, Assessment of cutaneous photosensitivity of TOOKAD (WST09) in preclinical animal models and in patients, *Photochemistry and Photobiology*, 81 (2005) 106–113.

47. R.A. Weersink, A. Bogaards, M. Gertner, S.R. Davidson, K. Zhang, G. Netchev, J. Trachtenberg, B.C. Wilson, Techniques for delivery and monitoring of TOOKAD (WST09)-mediated photodynamic therapy of the prostate: Clinical experience and practicalities, *Journal of Photochemistry and Photobiology B: Biology*, 79 (2005) 211–222.

48. N. Betrouni, R. Lopes, P. Puech, P. Colin, S. Mordon, A model to estimate the outcome of prostate cancer photodynamic therapy with TOOKAD soluble WST11, *Physics in Medicine and Biology*, 56 (2011) 4771–4783.

49. K.L. Du, R. Mick, T.M. Busch, T.C. Zhu, J.C. Finlay, G. Yu, A.G. Yodh et al., Preliminary results of interstitial motexafin lutetium-mediated PDT for prostate cancer, *Lasers in Surgery and Medicine*, 38 (2006) 427–434.

50. D. Zaak, R. Sorka, M. Hoopner, Photodynamic therapy by means of 5-ALA induced PPIX in human prostate—Preliminary results, *Medical Laser Application*, 18 (2003) 91–95.

51. G. Yu, T. Durduran, C. Zhou, T.C. Zhu, J.C. Finlay, T.M. Busch, S.B. Malkowicz, S.M. Hahn, A.G. Yodh, Real-time in situ monitoring of human prostate photodynamic therapy with diffuse light, *Photochemistry and Photobiology*, 82 (2006) 1279–1284.

52. M.A. Haider, S.R. Davidson, A.V. Kale, R.A. Weersink, A.J. Evans, A. Toi, M.R. Gertner et al., Prostate gland: MR imaging appearance after vascular targeted photodynamic therapy with palladium-bacteriopheophorbide, *Radiology*, 244 (2007) 196–204.

53. J.C. Finlay, S. Mitra, M.S. Patterson, T.H. Foster, Photobleaching kinetics of Photofrin in vivo and in multicell tumour spheroids indicate two simultaneous bleaching mechanisms, *Physics in Medicine and Biology*, 49 (2004) 4837–4860.

54. K.W. Fornalski, L. Dobrzynski, M.K. Janiak, A stochastic markov model of cellular response to radiation, *Dose-Response: A Publication of International Hormesis Society*, 9 (2011) 477–496.

55. K.K. Wang, J.C. Finlay, T.M. Busch, S.M. Hahn, T.C. Zhu, Explicit dosimetry for photodynamic therapy: Macroscopic singlet oxygen modeling, *Journal of Biophotonics*, 3 (2010) 304–318.

56. T.C. Zhu, S.M. Hahn, A.S. Kapatkin, A. Dimofte, C.E. Rodriguez, T.G. Vulcan, E. Glatstein, R.A. Hsi, In vivo optical properties of normal canine prostate at 732 nm using motexafin lutetium-mediated photodynamic therapy, *Photochemistry and Photobiology*, 77 (2003) 81–88.

57. J.C. Finlay, T.C. Zhu, A. Dimofte, D. Stripp, S.B. Malkowicz, T.M. Busch, S.M. Hahn, Interstitial fluorescence spectroscopy in the human prostate during motexafin lutetium-mediated photodynamic therapy, *Photochemistry and Photobiology*, 82 (2006) 1270–1278.

58. J.S. Dysart, M.S. Patterson, Photobleaching kinetics, photoproduct formation, and dose estimation during ALA induced PpIX PDT of MLL cells under well oxygenated and hypoxic conditions, *Photochemical and Photobiological Sciences: Official Journal of the European Photochemistry Association and the European Society for Photobiology*, 5 (2006) 73–81.

59. J.C. Finlay, S. Mitra, T.H. Foster, In vivo mTHPC photobleaching in normal rat skin exhibits unique irradiance-dependent features, *Photochemistry and Photobiology*, 75 (2002) 282–288.

60. T.C. Zhu, B. Liu, R. Penjweini, Study of tissue oxygen supply rate in a macroscopic photodynamic therapy singlet oxygen model, *Journal of Biomedical Optics*, 20 (2015) 38001.

61. M. Niedre, M.S. Patterson, B.C. Wilson, Direct near-infrared luminescence detection of singlet oxygen generated by photodynamic therapy in cells in vitro and tissues in vivo, *Photochemistry and Photobiology*, 75 (2002) 382–391.

62. M.J. Niedre, A.J. Secord, M.S. Patterson, B.C. Wilson, In vitro tests of the validity of singlet oxygen luminescence measurements as a dose metric in photodynamic therapy, *Cancer Research*, 63 (2003) 7986–7994.

63. M.J. Niedre, C.S. Yu, M.S. Patterson, B.C. Wilson, Singlet oxygen luminescence as an in vivo photodynamic therapy dose metric: Validation in normal mouse skin with topical amino-levulinic acid, *British Journal of Cancer*, 92 (2005) 298–304.

64. M.T. Jarvi, M.J. Niedre, M.S. Patterson, B.C. Wilson, Singlet oxygen luminescence dosimetry (SOLD) for photodynamic therapy: Current status, challenges and future prospects, *Photochemistry and Photobiology*, 82 (2006) 1198–1210.

65. M.T. Jarvi, M.S. Patterson, B.C. Wilson, Insights into photodynamic therapy dosimetry: Simultaneous singlet oxygen luminescence and photosensitizer photobleaching measurements, *Biophysical Journal*, 102 (2012) 661–671.

66. J.L. Sandell, T.C. Zhu, A review of in-vivo optical properties of human tissues and its impact on PDT, *Journal of biophotonics*, 4 (2011) 773–787.

67. M.R. Arnfield, J.D. Chapman, J. Tulip, M.C. Fenning, M.S. McPhee, Optical properties of experimental prostate tumors in vivo, *Photochemistry and Photobiology*, 57 (1993) 306–311.

68. Q. Chen, B.C. Wilson, S.D. Shetty, M.S. Patterson, J.C. Cerny, F.W. Hetzel, Changes in in vivo optical properties and light distributions in normal canine prostate during photodynamic therapy, *Radiation Research*, 147 (1997) 86–91.

69. C. Whitehurst, M.L. Pantelides, J.V. Moore, P.J. Brooman, N.J. Blacklock, In vivo laser light distribution in human prostatic carcinoma, *The Journal of Urology*, 151 (1994) 1411–1415.

70. L.K. Lee, C. Whitehurst, M.L. Pantelides, J.V. Moore, In situ comparison of 665 nm and 633 nm wavelength light penetration in the human prostate gland, *Photochemistry and Photobiology*, 62 (1995) 882–886.

71. T.C. Zhu, J.C. Finlay, S.M. Hahn, Determination of the distribution of light, optical properties, drug concentration, and tissue oxygenation in-vivo in human prostate during motexafin lutetium-mediated photodynamic therapy, *Journal of Photochemistry and Photobiology B: Biology*, 79 (2005) 231–241.

72. J. Li, T.C. Zhu, Determination of in vivo light fluence distribution in a heterogeneous prostate during photodynamic therapy, *Physics in Medicine and Biology*, 53 (2008) 2103–2114.

73. K.K. Wang, T.C. Zhu, Reconstruction of in-vivo optical properties for human prostate using interstitial diffuse optical tomography, *Optics Express*, 17 (2009) 11665–11672.

74. A. Dimofte, J.C. Finlay, T.C. Zhu, A method for determination of the absorption and scattering properties interstitially in turbid media, *Physics in Medicine and Biology*, 50 (2005) 2291–2311.

75. X. Liang, K.K. Wang, T.C. Zhu, Feasibility of interstitial diffuse optical tomography using cylindrical diffusing fibers for prostate PDT, *Physics in Medicine and Biology*, 58 (2013) 3461–3480.

76. D. Piao, K.E. Bartels, Z. Jiang, G.R. Holyoak, J.W. Ritchey, G. Xu, C.F. Bunting, G. Solobodov, Alternative transrectal prostate imaging: A diffuse optical tomography method, *IEEE Journal of Selected Topics in Quantum Electronics*, 16 (2010) 715–729.

77. Z. Jiang, D. Piao, G. Xu, J.W. Ritchey, G.R. Holyoak, K.E. Bartels, C.F. Bunting, G. Slobodov, J.S. Krasinski, Trans-rectal ultrasound-coupled near-infrared optical tomography of the prostate, part II: Experimental demonstration, *Optics Express*, 16 (2008) 17505–17520.

78. G. Xu, D. Piao, C.H. Musgrove, C.F. Bunting, H. Dehghani, Trans-rectal ultrasound-coupled near-infrared optical tomography of the prostate, part I: Simulation, *Optics Express*, 16 (2008) 17484–17504.

79. G. Yu, T. Durduran, C. Zhou, H.W. Wang, M.E. Putt, H.M. Saunders, C.M. Sehgal, E. Glatstein, A.G. Yodh, T.M. Busch, Noninvasive monitoring of murine tumor blood flow during and after photodynamic therapy provides early assessment of therapeutic efficacy, *Clinical Cancer Research: An Official Journal of the American Association for Cancer Research*, 11 (2005) 3543–3552.

80. H.W. Wang, M.E. Putt, M.J. Emanuele, D.B. Shin, E. Glatstein, A.G. Yodh, T.M. Busch, Treatment-induced changes in tumor oxygenation predict photodynamic therapy outcome, *Cancer Research*, 64 (2004) 7553–7561.

81. T. Durduran, R. Choe, J.P. Culver, L. Zubkov, M.J. Holboke, J. Giammarco, B. Chance, A.G. Yodh, Bulk optical properties of healthy female breast tissue, *Physics in Medicine and Biology*, 47 (2002) 2847–2861.

82. T.H. Pham, R. Hornung, M.W. Berns, Y. Tadir, B.J. Tromberg, Monitoring tumor response during photodynamic therapy using near-infrared photon-migration spectroscopy, *Photochemistry and Photobiology*, 73 (2001) 669–677.

83. R. Bays, G. Wagnieres, D. Robert, D. Braichotte, J.F. Savary, P. Monnier, H. van den Bergh, Clinical determination of tissue optical properties by endoscopic spatially resolved reflectometry, *Applied Optics*, 35 (1996) 1756–1766.

84. G. Yu, T. Durduran, D. Furuya, J.H. Greenberg, A.G. Yodh, Frequency-domain multiplexing system for in vivo diffuse light measurements of rapid cerebral hemodynamics, *Applied Optics*, 42 (2003) 2931–2939.

85. D.J. Pine, D.A. Weitz, P.M. Chaikin, E. Herbolzheimer, Diffusing wave spectroscopy, *Physical Review Letters*, 60 (1988) 1134–1137.

86. M.D. Altschuler, T.C. Zhu, J. Li, S.M. Hahn, Optimized interstitial PDT prostate treatment planning with the Cimmino feasibility algorithm, *Medical Physics*, 32 (2005) 3524–3536.

87. J. Li, M.D. Altschuler, S.M. Hahn, T.C. Zhu, Optimization of light source parameters in the photodynamic therapy of heterogeneous prostate, *Physics in Medicine and Biology*, 53 (2008) 3127–3136.

88. T.C. Zhu, M.D. Altschuler, Y. Hu, K. Wang, J.C. Finlay, A. Dimofte, K. Cengel, S.M. Hahn, A heterogeneous optimization algorithm for reacted singlet oxygen for interstitial PDT, *Proceedings of SPIE* 7551 (2011) 75510E.

89. M.D. Altschuler, T.C. Zhu, Y. Hu, J.C. Finlay, A. Dimofte, K. Wang, J. Li, K. Cengel, S.B. Malkowicz, S.M. Hahn, A heterogeneous optimization algorithm for PDT dose optimization for prostate, *Proceedings of SPIE* 7164 (2009) 71640B .

90. J. Li, T.C. Zhu, J.C. Finlay, Study of light fluence rate distribution in photodynamic therapy using finite-element method, *Proceedings of SPIE*, 6139 (2006) 61390M.

91. M.G. Lawrence, R.A. Taylor, R. Toivanen, J. Pedersen, S. Norden, D.W. Pook, M. Frydenberg Australian Prostate Cancer Bioresource et al., A preclinical xenograft model of prostate cancer using human tumors, *Nature Protocols*, 8 (2013) 836–848.

92. T. Lange, S. Ullrich, I. Muller, M.F. Nentwich, K. Stubke, S. Feldhaus, C. Knies et al., Human prostate cancer in a clinically relevant xenograft mouse model: Identification of beta(1,6)-branched oligosaccharides as a marker of tumor progression, *Clinical Cancer Research: An Official Journal of the American Association for Cancer Research*, 18 (2012) 1364–1373.

93. Z. Huang, Q. Chen, K.C. Dole, A.B. Barqawi, Y.K. Chen, D. Blanc, B.C. Wilson, F.W. Hetzel, The effect of Tookad-mediated photodynamic ablation of the prostate gland on adjacent tissues—In vivo study in a canine model, *Photochemical and Photobiological Sciences: Official Journal of the European Photochemistry Association and the European Society for Photobiology*, 6 (2007) 1318–1324.

94. Z. Huang, Q. Chen, D. Luck, J. Beckers, B.C. Wilson, N. Trncic, S.M. Larue, D. Blanc, F.W. Hetzel, Studies of a vascular-acting photosensitizer, Pd-bacteriopheophorbide (Tookad), in normal canine prostate and spontaneous canine prostate cancer, *Lasers in Surgery and Medicine*, 36 (2005) 390–397.

95. Z. Huang, Q. Chen, P.-H. Brun, B.C. Wilson, A. Scherz, Y. Salomon, D. Luck, J. Beckers, F.W. Hetzel, Studies of novel photosensitizer Pd-bacteriopheophorbide (Tookad(R)) for the prostate cancer PDT in canine model, *Proceedings of SPIE*, 5254 (2003) 83–90.

96. Z. Jiang, G.R. Holyoak, K.E. Bartels, J.W. Ritchey, G. Xu, C.F. Bunting, G. Slobodov, D. Piao, In vivo transrectal ultrasound-coupled optical tomography of a transmissible venereal tumor model in the canine pelvic canal, *Journal of Biomedical Optics*, 14 (2009) 030506.

97. O. Tanaka, S. Hayashi, M. Matsuo, M. Nakano, H. Uno, K. Ohtakara, T. Miyoshi, T. Deguchi, H. Hoshi, Effect of edema on postimplant dosimetry in prostate brachytherapy using CT/MRI fusion, *International Journal of Radiation Oncology, Biology, Physics*, 69 (2007) 614–618.

98. J. Li, T.C. Zhu, X. Zhou, A. Dimofte, J.C. Finlay, Integrated light dosimetry system for prostate photodynamic therapy, *Proceedings of SPIE* 6846 (2008) 68450Q .

99. C.M. Moore, A.R. Azzouzi, E. Barret, A. Villers, G.H. Muir, N.J. Barber, S. Bott et al., Determination of optimal drug dose and light dose index to achieve minimally invasive focal ablation of localised prostate cancer using WST11-vascular-targeted photodynamic (VTP) therapy, *BJU International* 116(6) (2015) 888–896. DOI:10.1111/bju.12816.

100. S.R. Davidson, R.A. Weersink, M.A. Haider, M.R. Gertner, A. Bogaards, D. Giewercer, A. Scherz et al., Treatment planning and dose analysis for interstitial photodynamic therapy of prostate cancer, *Physics in Medicine and Biology*, 54 (2009) 2293–2313.

101. B.C. Wilson, M.S. Patterson, The physics, biophysics and technology of photodynamic therapy, *Physics in Medicine and Biology*, 53 (2008) R61–R109.

102. R. Penjweini, H.-G. Loew, M.R. Hamblin, K.W. Kratky, Long-term monitoring of live cell proliferation in presence of PVP-Hypericin: A new strategy using ms pulses of LED and the fluorescent dye CFSE, *Journal of Microscopy*, 245 (2012) 100–108.

103. R. Penjweini, H.-G. Loew, M. Eisenbauer, K.W. Kratky, Modifying excitation light dose of novel photosensitizer PVP-Hypericin for photodynamic diagnosis and therapy. *Journal of Photochemistry and Photobiology B: Biology*, 120 (2013) 120–129.

Fluorescent-guided resection in clinical oncology

RON R. ALLISON

22.1 INTRODUCTION

Surgery is the foundation and bedrock of modern cancer treatment. Through a continuum of innovation surgery retains its preeminence in this field of endeavor. One of the major goals of oncologic surgery is the complete resection of gross and microscopic tumor without undue morbidity to normal tissue and organ function. Achieving this remains both art and science.

Imaging technology has revolutionized the preoperative and also operative management of cancer patients [1]. Radiologic procedures involving x-rays and radioactive pharmaceuticals often allow for a very accurate assessment of tumor extent both locally and systemically for primary lesions and metastasis so long as these lesions approach 1 cm in size or greater. Based on this, it is now routine to obtain a CT scan and PET/CT to evaluate cancer patients for both staging and, if indicated, for surgery. Tumor extent may also be imaged by magnetic resonance imaging (MRI), which may offer a more detailed look [2]. Both x-rays and MRI can also be employed intraoperatively to help the surgeon define the location and extent of disease to improve the accuracy of a biopsy or resection. But neither modality offers real-time feedback and both suffer an inability to reliably and accurately detect volumes much less than 1 cm. That means millions of cancer cells may be left behind as they are too small to be accurately imaged.

This is why optical-based imaging for guiding surgery has gained momentum [3]. Optical imaging during surgery may be able to define lesion extent to the near microscopic level and do this in real time. Currently, during a procedure the surgeon may request "frozen section" evaluation of surgical margins as an aid to determining presence or absence of tumor. As the goal of "curative" surgery is to remove both gross disease and its microscopic fingers, as this reliably improves tumor control and often survival, the frozen section can be critical. But frozen sections may take an hour or more to be determined, which is not a benefit to an anesthetized patient; require extensive and expert staff; and most critical of all may offer false positive or negative results, which is an unfortunate disservice and reality of this procedure [4]. This is a major driver of optical procedures, which offer the possibility of providing evaluation of tumor extent and surgical margins of resection in real time. Further, these optical procedures, in addition to identifying microscopic extent of tumor, can often identify critical normal tissues such as nerves, ducts, and vessels, which may be inadvertently injured during surgery. Therefore, just as importantly optically guided surgery may also minimize the side effects associated with many surgical procedures.

This chapter will review fluorescent-guided clinical resection in surgical oncology. Fluorescent-guided resection is one of several image-guided and optical techniques being explored clinically and preclinically [5]. Unlike other potential image-guided surgery, fluorescent-based procedures have already shown patient benefit, have a number of approved fluorescent probes available, have tools and instruments commercially available to detect fluorescence, and perhaps most importantly appear to be a reliable and relatively simple procedure to undertake during actual surgery [6]. That final point is often what allows widespread introduction of a promising procedure to become an established part of the surgical armamentarium.

22.2 HISTORICAL OVERVIEW

The use of light in medicine dates back to ancient times [7]. Most often topical salves were applied and activated by sunlight to treat cutaneous diseases, including tumors. A modern continuation of an ancient practice is PUVA therapy. Here an applied agent (psoralen) is activated by UV light to successfully ablate cutaneous lesions such as Mycosis Fungoides.

At the turn of the twentieth century, fluorescent phenomena were brought to the forefront of medical science [8]. A medical student, Oscar Raab was studying fluorescence in infusoria via the use of dyes. In conjunction with his professors, Raab additionally discovered Photodynamic Therapy (PDT). Here fluorescent dyes exposed to enough energy from light could cause ablation via the Photodynamic Reaction, which generated toxic singlet oxygen. PDT became a popular treatment for skin cancers and other malignancies. Additional work soon followed showing fluorescence and photodynamic potential of porphyrins. While much work was done, fluorescence and PDT were essentially lost.

It was not until the 1950s and 1960s that fluorescent phenomena (and PDT) were rediscovered. Fluorescent dyes and porphyrins were used to illuminate various organs and vessels. Intentional fluorescence of a breast tumor was reported by Lipson in 1964. Still the intentional use of fluorescence to assist in surgery had to wait for the rebirth of PDT in the late 1970s and 1980s. By fluorescing the photosensitizing agent employed in PDT, surgeons could better identify the target for treatment. Eventually the use of fluorescent agents to guide surgery, rather than as part of PDT, became a field of study in itself [9]. The success of dye-based mapping of sentinel nodes is an example. This also led to early work in bladder and brain. In both, fluorescent agents were better able to detect tumor and define normal tissue leading to promising clinical results, still in progress today.

22.3 PRINCIPLES OF FLUORESCENCE

Fluorescence is an inherent phenomenon of many naturally occurring and synthetic agents [10]. It is related but distinct from phosphorescence, which may occur under anaerobic conditions, whereas fluorescence requires oxygen. Essentially fluorescence occurs when a photon of light energy interacts with a fluorophore. The energy of the light photon is transferred to an electron in the fluorophore that creates an "excited" state. The energized electron will move to a higher (excited) state and then eventually lose this energy and return to its ground state. When the electrons return from its higher state to its previous ground state, visible/detectable emission of light, termed fluorescence, can be observed. This fluorescence may be detectable by the naked eye, but far more commonly by optical detectors.

By definition, some energy will be lost between the absorbed and emitted photon. This energy loss will alter the wavelength of light emitted as fluorescence, as compared to the wavelength of light introduced, and is termed a "Stokes Shift."

In addition to this Stokes Shift, the fluorescent emission photons will also be affected by a complex interaction with tissue, which often includes additional absorption and scattering. Therefore, the clinical measurement and detection of fluorescence is not simple, as will be outlined.

22.4 LIGHT INTERACTIONS WITH TISSUE

The light introduced to activate the fluorescent agent and the light emitted by the fluorescent agent, as well as any light emitted by naturally occurring fluorophores in the body (hemoglobin, melanin, for example), interact with tissue in a number of ways, not all of which are well worked out. To simplify this very complex phenomenon, we will break these interactions down to single pathways, fully realizing that in tissue, all pathways may be active (Figure 22.1).

Absorption: Light photons (energy packets) may be partially or totally absorbed by tissue that they pass through. Since tumor composes only a small portion of tissue, it is likely that most light photons will be absorbed by normal tissues. Blood (hemoglobin) absorbs most visible light (blue 400 nm, green 500 nm light), which allows red light (600 nm) to continue to travel, and gives Caucasian skin a red tint. Water absorbs the more energetic photons, around and above 1000 nm. This essentially means a very limited range of a photon's light wavelength may actually penetrate tissue without being absorbed. Therefore, infrared light is most commonly used for fluorescent surgery as this wavelength range has a chance to penetrate tissue and reach the target.

Scattering: The photon may also be scattered by tissue, which results in a change in direction. Quite often multiple scattering events occur during the photons travels. Essentially, then the fluorescent phenomena may be pointed in a direction far from its origin. Sometimes the photon may never penetrate the outer tissue surface as it is *reflected*. Similarly, the fluorescent emission may never be detected as it too may reflect off the inner surface of the tissue. Another important aspect is *refraction,* which occurs at the interface of different tissues (or air) and also changes the direction of the light photon.

22.5 FLUORESCENCE IMAGING

With all the absorptions, reflections, scattering, and refractions, virtually all the incident photons miss the fluorophore. Even fewer of these fluorescent interactions can be imaged again due to absorption, reflection, scattering, and refractions of this light. Still, even with these significant limitations, fluorescence can be employed clinically to detect tumor, its extent, and even metastasis [11,12]. Because tumor is structurally different than nearby normal tissue, inherent differences in the quality and quantity of naturally

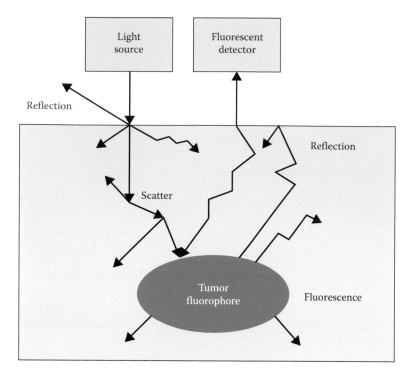

Figure 22.1 An incident photon from the light source may reflect or scatter as it interacts with tissue. Should this photon make contact with the fluorophore, fluorescence may occur. The fluorescent photon will also scatter; some fluorescent photons may then make contact with the detector.

occurring fluorophores (termed autofluorescence) can be exploited to detect tumor location and extent. However, as these structural differences may be subtle, autofluorescence via inherent fluorophores often has a low signal-to-noise ratio. In other words, it is difficult to accurately tell what is tumor and what is not. Clinically, scar tissue autofluoresces similarly to tumor. As often tumor and surrounding normal tissue develop scars particularly after radiation and chemotherapy the use of autofluorescence as a means to detect growing tumor in previously treated cancer is very limited. Clinically this situation occurs in a large oncologic patient population. These individuals would potentially benefit from fluorescent-guided resection to eliminate residual tumor. To enhance the signal-to-noise ratio, a number of innovative strategies have been clinically employed.

22.6 INHERENT FLUOROPHORES DETECTION

As mentioned, a variety of natural and synthetic structures have the ability to fluoresce. Autofluorescence is a technique that exploits the structural and quantitative differences in naturally occurring endogenous fluorophores that are already present in both malignant and normal tissue [13]. As described before, for example, if normal tissue structure is different enough from the structure of tumors, then this difference should potentially provide a different autofluorescent signal for each. By measuring and detecting their differences one may be able to visually detect what is tumor and what is not. As the difference is often subtle, a technique using "*signature emissions*" is often employed. Here the difference in the fluorescent spectrum between the tissues is analyzed (termed "*spectral unmixing*"). Ideally the spectrum is different enough between tumor tissue and normal tissue to be identified. This is not always the case.

Potentially a second method termed "*Fluorescent Lifetime Imaging*" may be of greater clinical utility. In this methodology, the decay rates of fluorescence may be different between tumor and normal tissue.

This decay rate (i.e., fluorescent lifetime) is not dependent on many of the physical characteristics such as fluorophore concentration, light energy, and optics that interfere with the reliability of the previously mentioned spectral unmixing technique. Both lifetime imaging and spectral unmixing require specific imaging equipment, which so far have yielded enticing but still relatively primitive optical imaging.

22.7 APPLIED FLUOROPHORE DETECTION

Currently, a more promising avenue to optically detect the difference between tumor and normal tissue involves application of fluorophores. These may be topically, orally, or intravenously applied to try to enhance the signal-to-noise ratio. Successful agents will essentially concentrate in the tissue/tumor in question. Several applied fluorophores have found clinical utility. They may broadly be categorized as originating from the following concepts.

Nontargeted applied fluorophores: These structures do not appear to seek out or be specific to tumor or tissue [14]. However, they fluoresce at appropriate wavelengths for clinically relevant detection methods and appear to concentrate in highly vascular (angiogenic) and lymphatic pathways. Therefore, in select situations, nonspecific fluorophores may be of clinical benefit. These commonly used agents also have a long track record of safety and importantly are regulatory agency approved (but not necessarily for fluorescent detection and surgery). Moreover, they are commercially available. This category of probes includes Lugol's Iodine, Violet Acetate, Fluorescein, Indocyanine Green (ICG), and Toluidine Blue among others. Again while not originally designed or used for optical surgery, each of these probes has been clinically found to have this ability. As an example ICG has been employed for decades to assess biliary excretion. Recently, ICG was found to also concentrate in liver metastasis, probably due to physical compression by the tumor on biliary excretion [5]. The combination of availability and clinical intuition can allow nonspecific probes to flourish.

Targeted probes: Targeted probes have the added ability of specifically targeting tumor tissue [15]. If successful, these targeted probes should allow for a high chance of differentiating normal from malignant tissue. Currently, the photosynthesizers (and their derivatives) from PDT have the remarkable ability to concentrate in malignant and transforming tissue. As these photosynthesizers also generally fluoresce at clinically useful wavelengths, they have served as a rich source of targeted probes. As many of these photosynthesizers are regulatory approved and commercially available, the expensive and time-consuming hurdle to widespread clinical introduction has already been achieved. Photosensitizers, when intensively illuminated can create the cyto and vasculotoxic photodynamic reaction. When less intensely illuminated these structures reliably fluoresce (Figure 22.2) Conceivably one could both optically detect a tumor and then use PDT as a means of ablation. This will be discussed further in the theranostic section of this chapter. Currently, the photosensitizer ALA (aminolevulinic acid) is a leading targeted agent. It can be applied orally, topically, or intravenously. This Pro-drug, part of the Heme Synthetic Pathway preferentially accumulates in malignant tissue where it is transformed to the active agent protoporphyrin-IX (PpIX). As the drug concentrates to many fold higher levels in tumor compared to surrounding tissue ALA has been an active agent for both PDT and now fluorescent surgery [16]. A hexalated version (HALA) has even greater ability to fluoresce and as will be seen in the clinical section is an excellent probe. Other photosynthesizers such as photofrin, texaphyrin, and verteporfin have also been explored for fluorescent-guided surgery, in addition to PDT.

Targeted and activatable probes: A new generation of probes, some of which have been clinically tested, are currently being explored [17]. These agents may have specific targets they attach to, such as up-regulated proteins or receptors associated with tumors. These include VEGF and folate receptors that are found in high concentrations in tumors.

Other probes may require binding to activate fluorescence. These probes may first bind to cell receptors, peptides, and in particular matrix-metalloproteinases. The binding alters structure to allow for fluorescence.

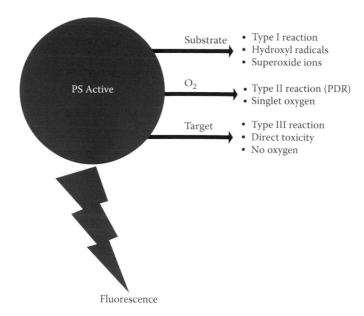

Figure 22.2 The active photosensitizer (fluorophore) may undergo several pathways, one of which is the creation of fluorescence.

The matrix-metalloproteinases now has a family of commercially available probes. Nanoparticles appear to be an important part of these developing probes.

Theranostic probes: Probes that both detect and destroy tumor is a reality [18]. Currently, photosynthesizers as probes can achieve this. While beyond the scope of this chapter, it is easy to imagine theranostic probes that can detect tumor for staging, fluoresce for fluorescent resection, and then when further activated, destroy residual tumor cells. These are likely the probes of the future, but we must get there first.

22.8 QUALITIES OF AN ONCOLOGICALLY SUCCESSFUL FLUORESCENT PROBE

The qualities of a successful probe will vary depending on the criteria and judges. To the surgeon (and the patient) the following qualities of a successful probe are generally required:

1. *High signal-to-noise ratio*: A distinct difference between tumor and normal tissue will allow the surgeon a better chance at resection of malignancy and preservation of normal tissue. This may also be termed high quantum yield to fluorescence.
2. *Specificity*: Ideally, the fluorescent imaging truly shows tumor and its extension, minimizing guesswork.
3. *Versatile agent*: Oral, topical, or intravenous introduction allow for wide clinical application.
4. *Nontoxic*: Direct toxicity of the probe or derivatives will prevent widespread introduction.
5. *Short half-life*: The probe should leave the body rapidly to prevent any potential photosensitivity or long-term morbidity.
6. *Long activation wavelength*: Activation in the infrared (600–1000) allows for deep (1 cm+) tissue penetration and ease of detection.
7. *Amphylicity*: The ability to travel in the blood stream without clumping allows for great versatility in penetration of various tissues.
8. *Available detection devices*: The ability to easily detect fluorescence in the operating room will depend on the widespread availability of these tools.

9. *Commercially available and regulatory agency approved probe*: without these you cannot have fluorescent-guided surgery brought to those who need it.
10. *Seamless procedure*: Ideally, the addition of the fluorescence to the surgical procedure will be easy to accomplish to allow widespread use.

22.8.1 TOOLS OF THE TRADE

Essentially as the majority of fluorophores are in the infrared range, tools are required to detect this fluorescence. Further, the human eye can be injured by the intensity of the light used to generate fluorescence, so eye protection for all involved, including the patient, is mandatory.

A basic requirement is a light source that can be directed to the target to deliver the light energy needed to activate the probe. As each probe may have a preferential wavelength to fluoresce the light source must not only match this wavelength but also be powerful enough to activate the probe. This is why lasers may be preferential as they can be tuned to the wavelength of activation and provide intense light energy. However, lasers are expensive, so light-emitting diodes (LED) may become popular, as they are far less costly to purchase and maintain.

Broad spectrum light sources such as high wattage incandescent bulbs can also be used though appropriate filters are required to optimize the light spectrum.

The next requirement is a light detector to identify the fluorescence emitted. Quite often this is a CCD—camera that has the ability to pick up even faint levels of fluorescence, far beyond the capability of the human eye. The detectors may also be enhanced by computer programs that can enhance the "signal-to-noise" ratio, which may then provide a more accurate level of fluorescent detection.

Ideally these tools would be user friendly and not delay or prolong the surgical procedure. Having fluorescent detection tools that are part of the standard equipment already in use during a particular procedure is what a major goal should be. For example, endoscopes are widely used to examine tissue within the body. Autofluorescent endoscopes are commercially available for the lung and have an excellent clinical track record [19]. Similarly endoscopes able to detect fluorescence from probes applied to the lung and GI tract are also available [20]. Further endoscopes that evaluate the bladder (cystoscopes) can be easily equipped for fluorescent detection [21]. This is likely why pulmonary, GI, and urologic specialists commonly employ fluorescence during evaluation and treatment of malignancy. Not surprisingly, the neurosurgical microscope, which is routinely used in neurosurgical oncology, now has fluorescent detection tools built in [22]. The relative ease of use has made fluorescent-guided neurosurgery an accepted modality. These are the models needed to bring fluorescent surgery to other anatomic sites.

22.9 CLINICAL APPLICATION

Clearly any procedure that can reasonably enhance the outcome of surgery can become an established part of the standard of care. Fluorescent-guided surgery has not yet achieved this status but the clinical outcomes published point in the direction. This section will serve to highlight the peer-reviewed literature in select anatomic sites.

22.9.1 BRAIN AND SPINAL CORD

It is well established that local control of tumor in brain and spinal cord has a direct correlation with outcome and survival. Most tumor recurrence is at or around the primary tumor site. Therefore, highly aggressive measures to achieve local control, which include the combination of surgery, radiation therapy, and chemotherapy are the norm. Still local control, particularly for high-grade tumors such as glioblastoma, is not satisfactory. The neurosurgical operating microscope is ideal for fluorescent detection and resection. This microscope is already commonly used in most neurosurgical procedures during resection. Currently, commercially available fluorescent-enhanced microscopes are widely employed.

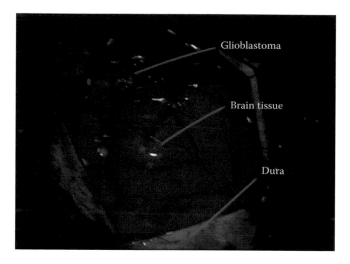

Figure 22.3 Operating room image of fluorescent guided resection: After ALA introduction, the glioblastoma tumor fluoresces red. Normal brain remains blue. This color change allows the surgeon an enhanced resection of tumor and sparing of normal brain. Under the usual white operating room light, tumor and normal brain tissue appear similar in color. (Photo courtesy of professor Sam Eljamel.)

The fluorescent part of the procedure can be turned on or off seamlessly. Therefore, the neurosurgeon can potentially enhance outcomes without significant change in the actual surgical procedure that they are accustomed to (see Figure 22.3).

The majority of reports employ ALA as the fluorophore. The ALA may be brought on board orally or intravenously, several hours to a day prior to the procedure. As ALA is essentially inert, morbidity from ALA is minimal. ALA converts to PpIX, which is a strong fluorescent agent that also is relatively specific to malignancy and its neovascularity. The trained surgeon can easily detect the tumor fluorescence and carefully resect this. Nonfluorescent regions are left alone, meaning less normal tissue damage, which is critical in the brain. A number of clinical papers report improved rates of achieving clear margins with fluorescent-guided neurosurgery compared to the standard of room light-based surgery.

Della-Puppa, using ALA, reported the ability to achieve nearly 100% gross total removal of high-grade gliomas [23]. Summarizing a randomized trial of 243 patients, ALA-based surgery doubled the rate of complete resection and also doubled the rate of progression-free survival. A five mouth overall improvement in survival was reported [24]. In a meta-analysis of ALA-based fluorescent resection, El Jamel reporting on 20 publications showed an overall 75% gross total resection rate with an impressive 6 month survival advantage for glioblastoma [25]. What also has been noted from these studies is that the fluorescent tumor region is usually larger and more irregular than appreciated, even on advanced preoperative imaging such as MRI [26,27]. An innovative approach has used intraoperative MRI and ALA for intraoperative fluorescence. The combination may allow for even higher rates of resection [28]. Similarly the combination of intraoperative ultrasound and fluorescent resection may enhance outcomes [29]. A potential strong application will be in pediatric patients, where preserving normal developing brain tissue is critical [30]. Similarly in spinal cord tumors where surgical resection may result in paralysis, enhanced accuracy has been found for ALA-based guidance. Millesi reporting on 55 spinal cord tumors reported enhanced ability for gross total resection [31]. They also noted that lower grade tumors may not fluoresce. Similarly enhanced ability to resect spinal cord tumors was published by Eiker [32].

It appears important to note that not all CNS tumors fluoresce, but usually high-grade lesions do [33]. And, fluorescent patterns may be different following chemotherapy and radiation [34]. So still much work needs to be done. This can include both fluorescence and photodynamic therapy in a theranostic approach [35]. An exciting possibility is to use the same agent for imaging and for treatment. That would seem to be a near ideal probe [36].

22.9.2 HEAD AND NECK

Here too, local control of tumor correlates with survival. Therefore, tumors of the head and neck are often treated with surgery, chemotherapy, and radiation. Morbidity, even with state-of-the-art tools, is common. A small but growing literature of fluorescent and other types of optical probes show great potential, particularly for minimizing resection of normal tissue [37]. An obstacle is the ability to detect nodal metastasis easily, which is common in tumors of this region.

Fluorescent detection was employed to assess margins of resection in a phase 1 tried by Warram [38]. They found an improved ability to achieve negative margins. Similarly, improved rates of clear resection margins were noted by Atallah [39]. In an attempt to spare normal tissue and reduce morbidity, Yokoyama employed Indocyanine Green to guide para-pharyngeal tumor resection [40]. They concluded this technique improved ease of resection and helped identify critical normal tissue. The same authors found other head and neck tumors amenable to Indocyanine Green-guided resection and the procedure did not add significantly to the length of surgery, an important consideration [41]. An interesting application was to employ fluorescence to examine the sentinel node from oral cavity tumors [42]. A negative node might prevent a highly morbid neck dissection. In an early clinical trial reported by Van der Vorst, this may be possible.

22.9.3 LUNG

A large literature shows that autofluorescence can aid in detection of early endobronchial tumors, which can then be ablated for cure [43]. In particular, the combination of autofluorescence and photosensitizer fluorescence followed by PDT appears to yield superior rates of lesion ablation with higher levels of treatment accuracy [44]. The intentional combination of autofluorescence with photosensitizer fluorescence (Npe6) was reported by Usuda to achieve a virtual 100% detection rate of endobronchial disease, with an over 95% local control rate following 1 or 2 PDT sessions [45]. The use of fluorescent-guided detection for endobronchial evaluation is widespread as the current generation of bronchoscopes have built in autofluorescent and fluorescent detection ability.

The use of fluorescent-guided resection for nonendobronchial lung tumors is to be determined. The ability to improve accuracy of resection margin during removal of a pulmonary tumor is an important potential contribution of fluorescent-guided resection. Many of these patients have limited pulmonary reserve, so preservation of normal functioning lung is also critical. An innovative report by Okusanya employed a folate receptor-based fluorescent agent that was able to accurately image the primary tumor to allow for improved lung resection, but also helped identify unexpected tumor metastasis [46]. The same authors were able to image lung tumors intraoperatively using IV Indocyanine Green [47]. This technique also revealed unexpected metastatic lesions, which were resected.

22.9.4 BREAST/SKIN

Among the earliest uses of fluorescent detection was for sentinel node detection, using blue dyes [48]. The fluorescence of the sentinel node (primary node draining a breast tumor) allowed the breast surgeon both greater accuracy in nodal resection but also the ability to spare uninvolved lymph nodes. A negative sentinel node generally obviates the need for any axillary dissection. This translated into far less arm edema associated with these surgical interventions. The benefit of this was tremendous not only to the patient involved but also as a pathway to more accurate and less morbid therapy [49]. Currently, sentinel node detection is a combination of a dye and radioactive tracer, which has high yield of detection, approaching 95% [50].

Similarly, melanoma patients may undergo sentinel node evaluation, which also can translate into improved survival and a less morbid surgery [51]. The use of fluorescent-guided resection of the primary breast (or melanoma) tumor needs to be further evaluated. This would likely yield a higher chance of clear margins of resection [9]. The use of sentinel node evaluation by fluorescent and radioactive tracer for other cutaneous lesions is an area of active research [52].

22.9.5 GASTROINTESTINAL

Fluorescence and PDT have a long history for endoscopic-based evaluation and treatment of recurrent and advanced esophageal tumors as well as premalignant lesions such as Barrett's Esophagus [53]. As primary and metastatic cancers to the liver are rapidly lethal and as resection is the only proven means to control these lesions, fluorescent resection has been explored for these indications. Aoki reported that ICG allowed for improved anatomic hepatic resection as did Gotoh [54,55]. In these reports ICG delivered IV several days prior to surgery allowed excellent fluorescence of all liver tumors. Fluorescence also revealed a 40% rate of additional lesion detection of tumors not visible or palpable to the surgeon. Additional reports of enhanced liver resection outcomes were summarized by Verbeck [56]. Of interest is the report from Van der Vorst [57]. Again using ICG, 71 liver metastases were resected from 40 patients. In five patients (12.5%), additional metastases were found by the fluorescent techniques that were not detectable by other means. This is clearly a potential benefit for this technique. Fluorescent-guided surgery is commonly used in the biliary tract to define the biliary tree [58]. The use of fluorescent resection in primary tumors of the GI tract including pancreas, intestines, and rectum is yet to be determined.

22.9.6 GENITOURINARY

Currently, one of the fastest growing and particularly beneficial uses of fluorescence surgery is within the GU tract. Bladder cancer is common and a vast majority of patients, even those with in situ tumors, end up with removal of the bladder by cystectomy. Clearly any procedure that can spare bladder and also retain functioning bladder would be welcome.

In that regard, fluorescent-guided resection has found a growing niche in GU oncology. Bladder cancer is felt to start as noninvasive disease of the bladder endothelium and then it progresses, often rapidly to invasive tumor. Invasive tumor is generally treated by radical cystectomy, but due to its very aggressive nature, noninvasive in situ bladder cancer is also often treated by cystectomy. This is due in large part to the lack of successful alternative treatments. Local resection of in situ bladder cancer often fails due to a combination of the tumor being multifocal in origin and also an inability to distinguish the extent of disease, as normal urothelium is visually similar to urothelium containing in situ tumor. Therefore, it is difficult to achieve clear resection margins. If too much bladder is removed, then the remaining organ will hold little urine and functionally this will be troublesome to the patient due to frequent urination needs. This is why cystectomy is so common.

Fluorescent-guided surgery using ALA or its hexalated form HAL has shown an ability to better define the extent of noninvasive bladder cancer allowing surgeons a greater ability to achieve complete resection and preservation of bladder function. This reduction in recurrence rate also translates into cost savings as further surgery is avoided. This is critically important in modern medicine [59]. A randomized trial using HAL showed a nearly 50% residual tumor rate after "complete visual resection." Using HAL fluorescent doubled local control [60].

Similarly HAL-based cystoscopy allowed for far greater detection of in situ bladder tumors, nearly 30% greater than just white light visualization [61]. Based on these and other studies larger population-based trials were initiated. The uroscreen study of over 1600 men at high risk for bladder cancer did not show benefit for screening [62]. However, meta-analysis of fluorescent-guided resection has shown improved local control, improved clean resection margins, and lower local recurrence rates based on randomized trials [63].

Currently, guidelines are moving to greater use of florescent-guided resection of noninvasive bladder cancer, though this is a fluid work in progress [60,64–66].

22.10 FUTURE DIRECTIONS

Fluorescent-guided surgery is promising. The extent of this promise to become a clinically beneficial reality is in progress. To achieve status as a generally accepted part of the oncologic surgeons armamentarium will require excellent clinical trials providing not only improved surgical outcomes (improved tumor control and less morbidity) but also an analysis of cost effectiveness. The tools to enhance this surgery also must include better probes and fluorescent detection systems. All of these are in progress.

Ideally, a simple reliable probe would allow a new level of surgical proficiency to achieve negative margin when combined with a simple to use fluorescent-guided imaging system. Potentially goggles worn by the surgeon to easily detect tumor fluorescence could in addition present enhanced anatomy via virtual reality programs and become a standard of care.

Nanotechnology will provide better probes and ideally these probes will also have theranostic ability to not only detect malignancy but be able to assist in its destruction. With its great promise, fluorescent-guided resection and its father optical-guided resection will likely continue to enhance surgery for the next generation of operators and receivers.

REFERENCES

1. S Hess, BA Blomberg, HJ Zhu, PF Hoilund-Carlsen, A Alavi: The pivotal role of FDG-PET/CT in modern medicine. *Acad. Radiol.* **21**(2), 232–249 (2014).
2. OL Gobbo, F Wetterling, P Vaes et al.: Biodistribution and pharmacokinetic studies of SPION using particle electron paramagnetic resonance, MRI and ICP-MS. *Nanomedicine (Lond.)* **10**(11), 1751–1760 (2015).
3. JV Frangioni: New technologies for human cancer imaging. *J. Clin. Oncol.* **26**(24), 4012–4021 (2008).
4. KJ Chambers, S Kraft, K Emerick: Evaluation of frozen section margins in high-risk cutaneous squamous cell carcinomas of the head and neck. *Laryngoscope* **125**(3), 636–639 (2015).
5. S Keereweer, PB Van Driel, TJ Snoeks et al.: Optical image-guided cancer surgery: Challenges and limitations. *Clin. Cancer Res.* **19**(14), 3745–3754 (2013).
6. E de Boer, NJ Harlaar, A Taruttis et al.: Optical innovations in surgery. *Br. J. Surg.* **102**(2), e56–e72 (2015).
7. RR Allison, HC Mota, CH Sibata: Clinical PD/PDT in North America: An historical review. *Photodiagnosis Photodyn. Ther.* **1**(4), 263–277 (2004).
8. RR Allison, CH Sibata: Photodynamic therapy: Mechanism of action and role in the treatment of skin disease. *G. Ital. Dermatol. Venereol.* **145**(4), 491–507 (2010).
9. RR Allison, CH Sibata, GH Downie, RE Cuenca: A clinical review of PDT for cutaneous malignancies. *Photodiagnosis Photodyn. Ther.* **3**(4), 214–226 (2006).
10. JC Hsiang, AE Jablonski, RM Dickson: Optically modulated fluorescence bioimaging: Visualizing obscured fluorophores in high background. *Acc. Chem. Res.* **47**(5), 1545–1554 (2014).
11. S Luo, E Zhang, Y Su, T Cheng, C Shi: A review of NIR dyes in cancer targeting and imaging. *Biomaterials* **32**(29), 7127–7138 (2011).
12. S Gioux, HS Choi, JV Frangioni: Image-guided surgery using invisible near-infrared light: Fundamentals of clinical translation. *Mol. Imaging* **9**(5), 237–255 (2010).
13. B Zaric, V Stojsic, T Sarcev et al.: Advanced bronchoscopic techniques in diagnosis and staging of lung cancer. *J. Thorac. Dis.* **5**(Suppl 4), S359–S370 (2013).
14. W Polom, M Markuszewski, YS Rho, M Matuszewski: Use of invisible near infrared light fluorescence with indocyanine green and methylene blue in urology. Part 2. *Cent. Eur. J. Urol.* **67**(3), 310–313 (2014).
15. RR Allison, CH Sibata: Oncologic photodynamic therapy photosensitizers: A clinical review. *Photodiagnosis Photodyn. Ther.* **7**(2), 61–75 (2010).
16. H Stepp, T Beck, T Pongratz et al.: ALA and malignant glioma: Fluorescence-guided resection and photodynamic treatment. *J. Environ. Pathol. Toxicol. Oncol.* **26**(2), 157–164 (2007).
17. EA Te Velde, T Veerman, V Subramaniam, T Ruers: The use of fluorescent dyes and probes in surgical oncology. *Eur. J. Surg. Oncol.* **36**(1), 6–15 (2010).
18. J Kuil, AH Velders, FW van Leeuwen: Multimodal tumor-targeting peptides functionalized with both a radio- and a fluorescent label. *Bioconjug. Chem.* **21**(10), 1709–1719 (2010).
19. T Nakajima, K Yasufuku: Early lung cancer: Methods for detection. *Clin. Chest Med.* **34**(3), 373–383 (2013).

20. H Aoki, H Yamashita, T Mori, T Fukuyo, T Chiba: Ultrahigh sensitivity endoscopic camera using a new CMOS image sensor: Providing with clear images under low illumination in addition to fluorescent images. *Surg. Endosc.* **28**(11), 3240–3248 (2014).

21. SP Chen, JC Liao: Confocal laser endomicroscopy of bladder and upper tract urothelial carcinoma: A new era of optical diagnosis? *Curr. Urol. Rep.* **15**(9), 437-014-0437-y (2014).

22. HA Leroy, M Vermandel, JP Lejeune, S Mordon, N Reyns: Fluorescence guided resection and glioblastoma in 2015: A review. *Lasers Surg. Med.* **47**(5), 441–451 (2015).

23. A Della Puppa, P Ciccarino, G Lombardi, G Rolma, D Cecchin, M Rossetto: 5-Aminolevulinic acid fluorescence in high grade glioma surgery: Surgical outcome, intraoperative findings, and fluorescence patterns. *Biomed. Res. Int.* **2014**, 232–561 (2014).

24. MJ Colditz, K Leyen, RL Jeffree: Aminolevulinic acid (ALA)-protoporphyrin IX fluorescence guided tumour resection. Part 2: theoretical, biochemical and practical aspects. *J. Clin. Neurosci.* **19**(12), 1611–1616 (2012).

25. S Eljamel: 5-ALA Fluorescence image guided resection of glioblastoma multiforme: A meta-analysis of the literature. *Int. J. Mol. Sci.* **16**(5), 10443–10456 (2015).

26. P Schucht, S Knittel, J Slotboom et al.: 5-ALA complete resections go beyond MR contrast enhancement: Shift corrected volumetric analysis of the extent of resection in surgery for glioblastoma. *Acta Neurochir. (Wien)* **156**(2), 305–312; discussion 312 (2014).

27. S Eljamel, M Petersen, R Valentine et al.: Comparison of intraoperative fluorescence and MRI image guided neuronavigation in malignant brain tumours, a prospective controlled study. *Photodiagnosis Photodyn. Ther.* **10**(4), 356–361 (2013).

28. S Yamada, Y Muragaki, T Maruyama, T Komori, Y Okada: Role of neurochemical navigation with 5-aminolevulinic acid during intraoperative MRI-guided resection of intracranial malignant gliomas. *Clin. Neurol. Neurosurg.* **130**, 134–139 (2015).

29. A Moiyadi, P Shetty: Navigable intraoperative ultrasound and fluorescence-guided resections are complementary in resection control of malignant gliomas: One size does not fit all. *J. Neurol. Surg. A. Cent. Eur. Neurosurg.* **75**(6), 434–441 (2014).

30. GM Barbagallo, F Certo, K Heiss, V Albanese: 5-ALA fluorescence-assisted surgery in pediatric brain tumors: Report of three cases and review of the literature. *Br. J. Neurosurg.* **28**(6), 750–754 (2014).

31. M Millesi, B Kiesel, A Woehrer et al.: Analysis of 5-aminolevulinic acid-induced fluorescence in 55 different spinal tumors. *Neurosurg. Focus.* **36**(2), E11 (2014).

32. SO Eicker, FW Floeth, M Kamp, HJ Steiger, D Hanggi: The impact of fluorescence guidance on spinal intradural tumour surgery. *Eur. Spine J.* **22**(6), 1394–1401 (2013).

33. S Marbacher, E Klinger, L Schwyzer et al.: Use of fluorescence to guide resection or biopsy of primary brain tumors and brain metastases. *Neurosurg. Focus.* **36**(2), E10 (2014).

34. MA Kamp, J Felsberg, H Sadat et al.: 5-ALA-induced fluorescence behavior of reactive tissue changes following glioblastoma treatment with radiation and chemotherapy. *Acta Neurochir. (Wien)* **157**(2), 207–213, discussion 213–214 (2015).

35. MJ Colditz, RL Jeffree: Aminolevulinic acid (ALA)-protoporphyrin IX fluorescence guided tumour resection. Part 1: Clinical, radiological and pathological studies. *J. Clin. Neurosci.* **19**(11), 1471–1474 (2012).

36. T Hussain, QT Nguyen: Molecular imaging for cancer diagnosis and surgery. *Adv. Drug Deliv. Rev.* **66**, 90–100 (2014).

37. S Keereweer, HJ Sterenborg, JD Kerrebijn, PB Van Driel, RJ Baatenburg de Jong, CW Lowik: Image-guided surgery in head and neck cancer: Current practice and future directions of optical imaging. *Head Neck* **34**(1), 120–126 (2012).

38. JM Warram, E de Boer, LS Moore et al.: A ratiometric threshold for determining presence of cancer during fluorescence-guided surgery, *J. Surg. Oncol.* **112**(1), 2–8 (2015).

39. I Atallah, C Milet, JL Coll, E Reyt, CA Righini, A Hurbin: Role of near-infrared fluorescence imaging in head and neck cancer surgery: From animal models to humans, *Eur. Arch Otorhinolaryngol .* **272**(10), 2593–2600 (2014).

40. J Yokoyama, S Ooba, M Fujimaki et al.: Impact of indocyanine green fluorescent image-guided surgery for parapharyngeal space tumours. *J. Craniomaxillofac. Surg.* **42**(6), 835–838 (2014).

41. J Yokoyama, M Fujimaki, S Ohba et al.: A feasibility study of NIR fluorescent image-guided surgery in head and neck cancer based on the assessment of optimum surgical time as revealed through dynamic imaging. *Onco Targets Ther.* **6**, 325–330 (2013).

42. JR van der Vorst, BE Schaafsma, FP Verbeek et al.: Near-infrared fluorescence sentinel lymph node mapping of the oral cavity in head and neck cancer patients. *Oral Oncol.* **49**(1), 15–19 (2013).

43. M Kitada, Y Ohsaki, Y Matsuda, S Hayashi, K Ishibashi: Photodynamic diagnosis of pleural malignant lesions with a combination of 5-aminolevulinic acid and intrinsic fluorescence observationsystems. *BMC Cancer* **15**, 174-015-1194-0 (2015).

44. Y Ohsaki, K Takeyama, S Nakao et al.: Detection of photofrin fluorescence from malignant and premalignant lesions in the bronchus using a full-color endoscopic fluorescence imaging system. *Diagn. Ther. Endosc.* **7**(3–4), 187–195 (2001).

45. J Usuda, S Ichinose, T Ishizumi et al.: Outcome of photodynamic therapy using NPc6 for bronchogenic carcinomas in central airways >1.0 cm in diameter. *Clin. Cancer Res.* **16**(7), 2198–2204 (2010).

46. OT Okusanya, EM DeJesus, JX Jiang et al.: Intraoperative molecular imaging can identify lung adeno-carcinomas during pulmonary resection. *J. Thorac. Cardiovasc. Surg.* **150**(1), 28-35.e1 (2015).

47. OT Okusanya, D Holt, D Heitjan et al.: Intraoperative near-infrared imaging can identify pulmonary nodules. *Ann. Thorac. Surg.* **98**(4), 1223–1230 (2014).

48. TM Tuttle: Technical advances in sentinel lymph node biopsy for breast cancer. *Am. Surg.* **70**(5), 407–413 (2004).

49. TR Lopez Penha, LM van Roozendaal, ML Smidt et al.: The changing role of axillary treatment in breast cancer: Who will remain at risk for developing arm morbidity in the future? *Breast*, **24**(5), 543–547 (2015).

50. VM Moncayo, JN Aarsvold, NP Alazraki: Lymphoscintigraphy and Sentinel Nodes. *J. Nucl. Med.* **56**(6), 901–907 (2015).

51. MP Doepker, JS Zager: Sentinel lymph node mapping in melanoma in the twenty-first century. *Surg. Oncol. Clin. N. Am.* **24**(2), 249–260 (2015).

52. C Navarrete-Dechent, MJ Veness, N Droppelmann, P Uribe: High-risk cutaneous squamous cell carcinoma and the emerging role of sentinel lymph node biopsy: A literature review. *J. Am. Acad. Dermatol.* **73**(1), 127–137 (2015).

53. RR Allison, C Sheng, R Cuenca, VS Bagnato, C Austerlitz, CH Sibata: Photodynamic therapy for anal cancer. *Photodiagnosis Photodyn. Ther.* **7**(2), 115–119 (2010).

54. T Aoki, D Yasuda, Y Shimizu et al.: Image-guided liver mapping using fluorescence navigation system with indocyanine green for anatomical hepatic resection. *World J. Surg.* **32**(8), 1763–1767 (2008).

55. K Gotoh, T Yamada, O Ishikawa et al.: A novel image-guided surgery of hepatocellular carcinoma by indocyanine green fluorescence imaging navigation. *J. Surg. Oncol.* **100**(1), 75–79 (2009).

56. FP Verbeek, JR van der Vorst, BE Schaafsma et al.: Image-guided hepatopancreatobiliary surgery using near-infrared fluorescent light. *J. Hepatobiliary. Pancreat. Sci.* **19**(6), 626–637 (2012).

57. JR van der Vorst, BE Schaafsma, M Hutteman et al.: Near-infrared fluorescence-guided resection of colorectal liver metastases. *Cancer* **119**(18), 3411–3418 (2013).

58. DL Scroggie, C Jones: Fluorescent imaging of the biliary tract during laparoscopic cholecystectomy. *Ann. Surg. Innov. Res.* **8**, 5-014-0005-7 eCollection 2014 (2014).

59. JA Witjes, J Douglass: The role of hexaminolevulinate fluorescence cystoscopy in bladder cancer. *Nat. Clin. Pract. Urol.* **4**(10), 542–549 (2007).

60. GG Hermann, K Mogensen, S Carlsson, N Marcussen, S Duun: Fluorescence-guided transurethral resection of bladder tumours reduces bladder tumour recurrence due to less residual tumour tissue in Ta/T1 patients: A randomized two-centre study. *BJU Int.* **108**(8 Pt 2), E297–E303 (2011).

61. A Lapini, A Minervini, A Masala et al.: A comparison of hexaminolevulinate (Hexvix((R))) fluores-cence cystoscopy and white-light cystoscopy for detection of bladder cancer: Results of the HeRo obser-vational study. *Surg. Endosc.* **26**(12), 3634–3641 (2012).

62. M Horstmann, S Banek, G Gakis et al.: Prospective evaluation of fluorescence-guided cystoscopy to detect bladder cancer in a high-risk population: Results from the UroScreen-Study. *Springerplus* **3**, 24-1801-3-24, eCollection 2014 (2014).

63. P Shen, J Yang, W Wei et al.: Effects of fluorescent light-guided transurethral resection on non-muscle-invasive bladder cancer: A systematic review and meta-analysis. *BJU Int.* **110**(6 Pt B), E209–E215 (2012).

64. JA Witjes, JP Redorta, D Jacqmin et al.: Hexaminolevulinate-guided fluorescence cystoscopy in the diagnosis and follow-up of patients with non-muscle-invasive bladder cancer: Review of the evidence and recommendations. *Eur. Urol.* **57**(4), 607–614 (2010).

65. M Rink, M Babjuk, JW Catto et al.: Hexyl aminolevulinate-guided fluorescence cystoscopy in the diagnosis and follow-up of patients with non-muscle-invasive bladder cancer: A critical review of the current literature. *Eur. Urol.* **64**(4), 624–638 (2013).

66. H Yuan, J Qiu, L Liu et al.: Therapeutic outcome of fluorescence cystoscopy guided transurethral resection in patients with non-muscle invasive bladder cancer: A meta-analysis of randomized controlled trials. *PLoS One.* **8**(9), e74142 (2012).

Index